Julia Myk ✓ Y0-CAS-204

Basic Neuroscience

ANATOMY AND PHYSIOLOGY

Arthur C. Guyton, M.D.

Professor and Chairman
Department of Physiology and Biophysics
The University of Mississippi Medical Center
Jackson, Mississippi

1987

W.B. SAUNDERS COMPANY

Philadelphia   London   Toronto   Mexico City
Rio de Janeiro   Sydney   Tokyo   Hong Kong

W. B. Saunders Company: West Washington Square
Philadelphia, PA 19105

Library of Congress Cataloging-in-Publication Data

Guyton, Arthur C.

Basic neuroscience.

1. Neurophysiology.   2. Neuroanatomy.   I. Title.
   [DNLM: 1. Nervous System—anatomy.   2. Nervous
   System—physiology. WL 101 G992b]

QP355.2.G89 1987   612'.8   86–3697

ISBN 0–7216–2061–2

Editor: W. B. Saunders Staff
Designer: Bill Donnelly
Production Manager: Bob Butler
Manuscript Editor: Carol Stillman
Illustration Coordinator: Lisa Lambert
Indexer: George Vilk

Basic Neuroscience: Anatomy and Physiology   ISBN 0–7216–2061–2

© 1987 by W. B. Saunders Company.   Copyright under the Uniform Copyright Convention. Simultaneously published in Canada.   All rights reserved.   This book is protected by copyright.   No part of it may be reproduced, stored in a retrieval system, or transmitted in any form or by any means, electronic, mechanical, photocopying, recording, or otherwise, without written permission from the publisher. Made in the United States of America. Library of Congress catalog card number 86-3697.

Last digit is the print number: 9   8   7   6   5   4   3   2   1

Preface

In the past, neuroanatomy and neurophysiology have mostly been taught as separate subjects. However, every course in neuroanatomy almost invariably includes major amounts of neurophysiology as well. And it is literally impossible to teach a course in neurophysiology without teaching neuroanatomy at the same time. Even so, most attempts to present both neuroanatomy and neurophysiology in the same textbook have led to multiauthor books that usually encompass far too much for the student to study in the time that is available to him or her.

Therefore, this text, entitled simply *Basic Neuroscience: Anatomy and Physiology*, is designed to present the basics of both of these subjects as a single integrated discipline. The book is intended for a wide variety of students who have the common desire to know how the nervous system works, whether they be medical or dental students, students of basic neuroanatomy and physiology, students of psychology, students of biology, or others with similar interests.

The text begins with chapters on the gross anatomy of the nervous system, displaying full color pictures of virtually every important neuroanatomical structure. These chapters are intended to give the student a background understanding of the gross organization of the nervous system, along with a beginning concept of its function.

Then, the remainder of the text details the basic functional anatomy and physiology of each part of the nervous system. For instance, all through the text are multiple diagrams of the many nervous tracts that carry information from one neural locus to another. Also, the anatomy of each sensory organ is discussed along with its function—the eyes, the ears, the vestibular apparatus, and the sensory organs of somatic sensation, smell, taste, and so forth. Likewise, the anatomy and function of the neural effector organs—the muscles, heart, and glands—are given. And even the chemical anatomies of the nerve cell membrane, the neuronal cell body, the nerve endings, and the synapses are discussed as a basis for understanding the processing of nerve signals.

The ultimate goal of all this information is to present a total fabric of neural function, so that the student can understand how the nervous system serves as the controller of most bodily activities and yet at the same time as a sensing, feeling, and thinking organ of ideas and behavior.

My own deep interest in the nervous system began when I was still a student. In fact, I put together my first book at that time by photographically enlarging a great many microscopic cross-sectional slides of the nervous system and collecting these together in a large personal atlas of neuroanatomy. Then, later, as a resident in neurosurgery, the study of neuroanatomy once again became of paramount importance in my work. And more recently, my research carried me deeply into various aspects of neural control of the body, especially control of the circulation and to a less extent control of the respiration and endocrine functions. From these varied interests, I have learned to respect the nervous system as a masterpiece of design, with all those magical properties that make life meaningful, thoughtful, and exciting.

Finally, I wish to thank many others who have made this text possible, particularly Mrs. Ivadelle Osberg Heidke and Ms. Gwendolyn Robbins for their excellent secretarial services and to Ms. Tomiko Mita, Ms. Iris Nichols, and Ms. Patricia Johnson for the art work. I am also indebted to the staff of the W.B. Saunders Company for its continued excellence in the publication of this book, especially to Mr. Dana Dreibelbis, Mr. Robert Butler, Mr. William Donnelly, and Ms. Carol Stillman, whose editorial and technical help have been invaluable.

ARTHUR C. GUYTON

Contents

INTRODUCTION

1

Introduction: The Structural and Functional Highlights of the Nervous System

The nervous system is the sensing, thinking, and controlling system of our body. To perform these functions, it collects sensory information from all of the body—from a myriad of special sensory nerve endings in the skin, from the deep tissues, from the eyes, the ears, the equilibrium apparatus, and other sensors—and transmits this information through nerves into the spinal cord and brain. The cord and the brain may react immediately to this sensory information and send signals to the muscles or internal organs of the body to cause some response, called a *motor response*. Or, under other conditions, no immediate reaction might occur at all; instead the sensory information is stored in one of the brain's memory banks. There it is compared with other memories already stored; it is combined with other information; and from the various combinations, new thoughts are achieved. Then, perhaps a few minutes later, a month later, or even several years later, this extensive processing of information might at last lead to some motor response, maybe a very simple one or maybe very complex, such as building a house or piloting a space craft. Also, the nervous activation of the internal organs of the body, such as increasing the heart rate or increasing peristalsis in the intestines, may also be part of a motor response.

Thus, the nervous system is said to subserve three principal functions: (1) *sensory function;* (2) *integrative function,* which includes the memory and thinking processes; and (3) *motor function.*

THE MAJOR DIVISIONS OF THE NERVOUS SYSTEM

Figure 1–1 illustrates the two major divisions of the nervous system: (1) the *central nervous system,* which in turn is comprised of the *brain* and the *spinal cord,* and (2) the *peripheral nervous system.*

The brain is the principal integrative area of the nervous system—the place where memories are stored, thoughts are conceived, emotions are generated, and other functions related to our psyche and to complex control of our body are performed. To perform these complex activities, the brain itself is divided into many separate functional parts, which we shall begin discussing in the following chapter.

The spinal cord serves two functions. First, it serves as a conduit for many nervous pathways to and from the brain. Second, it serves as an integrative area for coordinating many subconscious nervous activities, such as reflex withdrawal of a part of the body from a painful stimulus, reflex stiffening of the legs when a person stands on his feet, and even crude reflex walking movements. Thus, the spinal cord is much more than simply a large peripheral nerve.

The peripheral nervous system is illustrated to the left in Figure 1–1, showing that it is a branching network of nerves that is so extensive that hardly a single cubic millimeter of tissue anywhere in the body is without nerve fibers. These fibers are of two functional types: *afferent fibers* for transmission of sensory information into the spinal cord and brain and *efferent fibers* for transmitting motor signals back from the central nervous system to the periphery, especially to the skeletal muscles (see Chapter 7). Some of the peripheral nerves arise directly from the brain itself and supply mainly the head region of the body. These, called *cranial nerves,* are not illustrated in Figure 1–1, but they will be discussed later. The remainder of the peripheral nerves are *spinal nerves,* one of which leaves each side of the spinal cord through an intervertebral foramen at each vertebral level of the cord.

NERVOUS TISSUE

Nervous tissue, whether it be in the brain, the spinal cord, or the peripheral nerves, contains two basic types of cells:

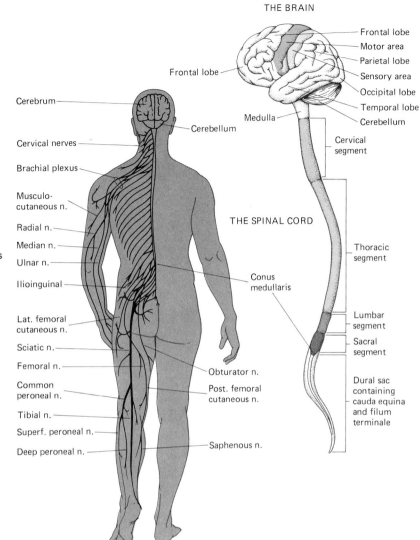

Figure 1–1. The principal anatomical parts of the nervous system.

1. *Neurons* conduct the signals in the nervous system. There are about 100 billion of these in the entire nervous system.

2. *Supporting* and *insulating cells* hold the neurons in place and prevent signals from spreading between the neurons where this is not desired. In the central nervous system these supporting and insulating cells are collectively called the *neuroglia.* In the peripheral nervous system they are the *Schwann cells.*

The Central Nervous System Neuron

Figure 1–2 illustrates a typical neuron of the brain or spinal cord. Its principal parts are the following:

1. *Cell body.* It is from this that other parts of the neuron grow. Also the cell body provides much of the nourishment that is required for maintaining the life of the entire neuron.

2. *Dendrites.* These are multiple branching outgrowths from the cell body. They are the main receptor portions of the neuron. That is, most signals that are to be transmitted by the neuron enter by way of the dendrites, although some enter also through the surface of the cell body. The dendrites of each neuron usually receive signals from literally thousands of contact points with other neurons, points called *synapses,* as we shall discuss later.

3. *Axon.* Each neuron has one axon leaving the cell body. This is the portion of the neuron that is usually called the *nerve fiber.* It may extend only a few millimeters, as is the case for the axons of many small neurons within the brain, or it may be as long as a meter in the case of the axons (nerve fibers) that leave the spinal cord to innervate the feet. The axons carry the nerve signals to the next nerve cell in the brain or spinal cord or to muscles and glands in peripheral parts of the body.

4. *Axon terminals and synapses.* All axons branch near their ends many times, often thousands of times. At the end of each of these branches is a

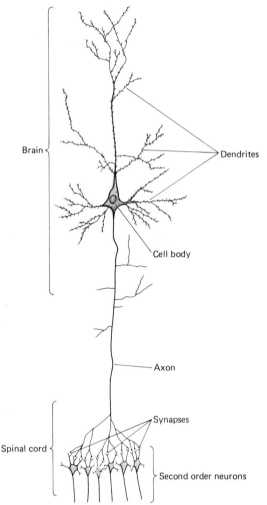

Figure 1–2. Structure of a large neuron of the brain, showing its important functional parts.

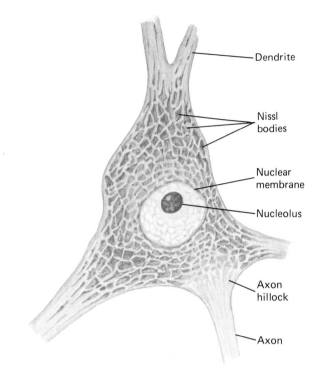

Figure 1–3. The neuronal cell body.

The Neuroglia

Figure 1–4 illustrates a large neuron of the spinal cord surrounded by its supporting tissue, the neuroglia. The cells in the neuroglia are called *glial cells*. Many of them function similarly to the fibroblasts of connective tissue; that is, they form fibers that hold the tissue together. But others serve the same function as the Schwann cells of the peripheral nerves to wrap *myelin sheaths* around the larger nerve fibers, thus providing typical *myelinated nerve fibers* that transmit signals at velocities as great as 100 m a second, the same as in peripheral nerves as will be described in Chapter 6. The very small nerve fibers do not have myelin sheaths and therefore are called *unmyelinated fibers,* but even these are insulated from each other by interposition of glial cells between the fibers, much the same way that Schwann cells insulate the unmyelinated nerve fibers from each other in the peripheral nerves.

specialized axon terminal that, in the central nervous system, is called a *presynaptic terminal, a synaptic knob,* or a *bouton* because of its knoblike appearance. The presynaptic terminal lies on the membrane surface of a dendrite or cell body of another neuron, thus providing a contact point called a *synapse* through which signals can be transmitted from one neuron to the next. When stimulated, the presynaptic terminal releases a minute quantity of a hormone called a *transmitter substance* into the space between the terminal and the membrane of the neuron, and the transmitter substance then stimulates this neuron as well.

Figure 1–3 illustrates more details of the neuronal cell body. It depicts a typical *nucleus* with a very prominent *nucleolus*. Also shown are *Nissl bodies,* which are parts of a specialized endoplasmic reticulum that synthesizes substances required to keep the neuron alive. In fact, these substances are even transported into the axon and dendrites through a system of microtubules called *neurofibrils*. Finally, note in Figure 1–3 that the axon arises from a conical pole of the cell body called the *axon hillock.*

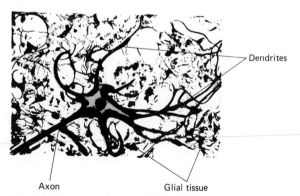

Figure 1–4. A large neuron of the spinal cord surrounded by its supporting tissue called neuroglia.

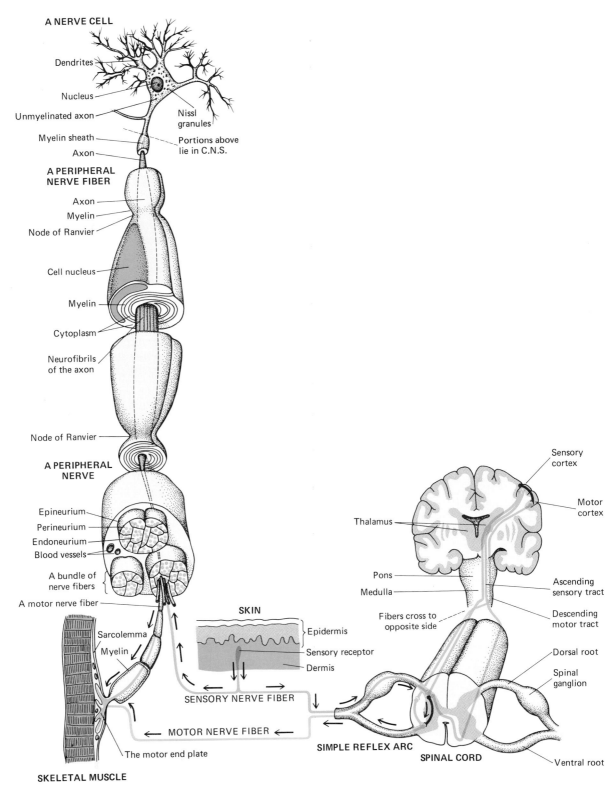

Figure 1-5. The functional components of the nervous system.

RECAPITULATION OF THE FUNCTIONAL STRUCTURE OF THE NERVOUS SYSTEM

Figure 1–5 gives a composite view of the structural highlights of the complete nervous system. To the left is a typical neuron, a motor neuron located in the spinal cord that sends a large myelinated nerve fiber to a muscle through a peripheral nerve. To the right is shown the course of both a sensory and a motor nerve fiber entering and leaving the spinal cord through a peripheral nerve. Also shown is an ascending sensory tract in the cord that carries millions of sensory nerve fibers upward from the cord to the brain and a descending motor tract that carries millions of motor fibers downward.

Note especially the junction points, the synapses, between successive neurons. It is at these synapses that the transmitted signals are controlled and their directions of travel in the nervous system are determined, as will be discussed fully in Chapter 10.

ORGANIZATIONAL PLAN FOR THIS TEXT

The ultimate goal of this text is to explain how the nervous system performs its multiple roles as a sensing, thinking, and controlling system. Obviously, this requires detailed knowledge of the structure of each part of the nervous system as well as an understanding of how each part functions. Therefore, we will begin in Section II (Chapters 2 through 4) with a survey of the *gross anatomy* of the nervous system, principally to provide the basic terminology and interrelationships needed for later discussion. Then, throughout the remainder of the text, the *functional anatomy* of each organ system will be presented, along with its physiology.

In Section III (Chapters 5 through 9), we will present the basic biophysics and physiology of signal transmission in nerves and muscle, as well as the functional role of skeletal, smooth, and heart muscle as the major motor outflow pathway of the nervous system.

The functional anatomy and physiology of the central nervous system will be given in Section IV (Chapters 10 through 21), while Section V (Chapters 22 through 26), will present the special senses.

Finally, Section VI (Chapters 27 through 29) will discuss the many ways in which the nervous system controls most of the functional systems of the non-nervous portions of the body, such as the circulation, respiration, gastrointestinal function, body temperature, most general hormonal secretion, and sexual and reproductive functions.

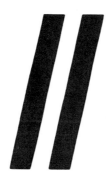

GROSS ANATOMY

2

Gross Anatomy of the Nervous System: I. General Divisions of the Brain; the Cerebrum; the Diencephalon

THE BRAIN AND ITS DIVISIONS

The brain is that portion of the nervous system located in the cranial cavity. Figure 2–1 illustrates a lateral view of the brain, Figure 2–2 an inferior view (its ventral surface), and Figure 2–3 a sagittal view as seen in the median plane of the brain. Unfortunately, several different terminologies are used to describe the different parts of the brain, three of which are listed in Table 2–1. The most widely used terminology in medical circles is given in the right-hand column of the table in which the brain is divided into six separate parts: (1) the *cerebrum*, (2) the *diencephalon*, (3) the *mesencephalon*, (4) the *cerebellum*, (5) the *pons*, and (6) the *medulla oblongata*, usually called simply the "medulla."

It is important to recognize the relationship of this widely used terminology to the classical terminology given in the left-hand column of the table and also to several anglicized classical terms given in the middle column. The cerebrum is the same as the *telencephalon*, and the telencephalon and diencephalon together constitute the *prosencephalon*, or *forebrain*, which is the large massive portion of the brain filling the anterior and superior three fourths of the cranial cavity.

The mesencephalon, also called the *midbrain*, is a minute portion of the brain located at the base of the forebrain, as illustrated in Figures 2–2 and 2–3. Yet, despite its small size, it is the only connecting link between the forebrain and all the lower portions of the brain and spinal cord.

The cerebellum, pons, and medulla all lie in the posterior fossa of the cranial cavity, and together they constitute the *rhombencephalon*, or *hindbrain*.

One can see from the figures that the major mass of the brain is the cerebrum, and it is also clear that the next largest portion of the brain is the cerebellum. This might make one think that the other four parts of the brain—the diencephalon, the mesencephalon, the pons, and the medulla—are of relatively little importance. But, we shall see later that these parts are absolutely crucial to the maintenance of nervous function, indeed, far more so than any equivalent mass of the cerebrum or cerebellum.

THE CEREBRUM

The Cerebral Hemispheres and the Corpus Callosum. For the next few moments let us study the external views of the cerebrum in Figures 2–1, 2–2, and 2–3 and also a horizontal section of the cerebrum shown in Figure 2–4. The first notable feature that one observes about the cerebrum is that it is composed of two large bilateral masses, the *cerebral hemispheres*, illustrated in Figures 2–1, 2–2, and 2–3. These two hemispheres are connected with each other through several bundles of nerve fibers, the two most important of which are discussed here:

1. The *corpus callosum* is illustrated in sagittal section in Figure 2–3 and in horizontal section in Figure 2–4. Note that the corpus callosum is a broad band of fibers extending almost half the length of the cerebral hemisphere. Its importance is made apparent by its extremely large number of fibers, about 20 million.

2. The *anterior commissure* is also shown in Figure 2–3. This is a much smaller bundle, probably no more than a million fibers. It is located several centimeters below the anterior third of the corpus callosum, and it interconnects mainly the anterior and medial portions of the two temporal lobes.

Corresponding points in almost all areas of the two hemispheres interconnect with each other in both directions via the fibers in these two bundles, which allows continuous communication between the two hemispheres. When the corpus callosum and anterior commissure are destroyed, each of the two hemispheres functions as a separate brain, even

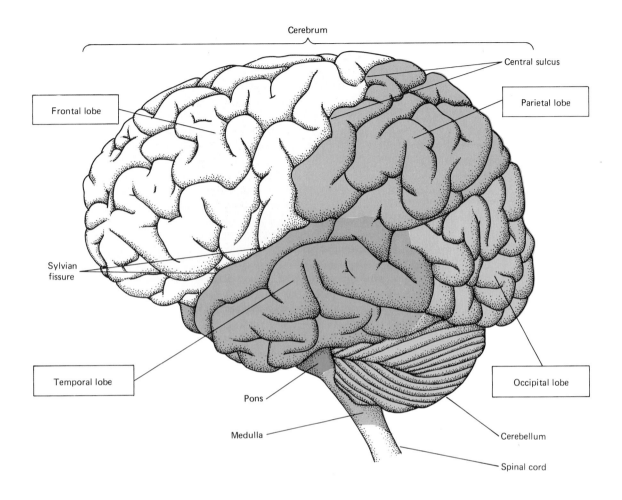

Figure 2–1. Left lateral view of the brain, showing the principal divisions of the brain and the four major lobes of the cerebrum.

Table 2–1. DIVISIONS OF THE BRAIN

Classical terminology	Anglicized terminology	Most widely used terminology
Encephalon	*Brain*	*Brain*
Prosencephalon		
Telencephalon		Cerebrum
Diencephalon		Diencephalon (or thalamus, hypothalamus, and surroundings)
Mesencephalon	Midbrain	Mesencephalon
Rhombencephalon	Hindbrain	
Metencephalon		
Cerebellum		Cerebellum
Pons		Pons
Myelencephalon		
Medulla oblongata		Medulla (or medulla oblongata)

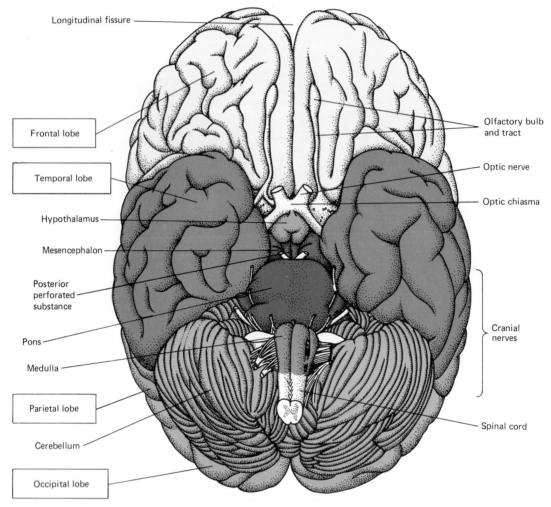

Figure 2–2. Basal view of the brain.

thinking separate thoughts and causing separate reactions in the two sides of the body.

Cerebral Convolutions, Fissures, and Sulci. The next distinctive feature of the cerebrum is the folds in its surface. These are called *cerebral convolutions*, and each convolution is called a *gyrus*. The grooves between the gyri are called either *fissures* or *sulci*, the larger and deeper ones generally being called fissures whereas the great majority, less deep, are the sulci. Four of the principal fissures or sulci are illustrated in Figures 2–1 and 2–2. They are listed here:

1. The *longitudinal fissure* separates the two cerebral hemispheres from each other in the midsagittal plane of the basin.

2. The *central sulcus* extends in an approximate inferosuperior direction on the lateral side of each hemisphere and divides the cerebrum approximately into an anterior half and a posterior half.

3. The *lateral fissure*, also called the *Sylvian fissure*, extends along the lateral aspect of each cerebral hemisphere for about half its length.

4. The *parieto-occipital sulcus* originates from the side of the longitudinal fissure about one quarter

the distance anterior to the posterior pole of the hemisphere and then extends laterally and anteriorly for about 5 cm.

To some extent, these fissures and sulci demarcate separate functional parts of the cerebrum, as we shall discuss.

The Lobes of the Cerebrum. Figures 2–1 through 2–4 illustrate that the cerebrum is divided into four major *lobes* and a fifth minor one. The major lobes are (1) the *frontal lobe*, (2) the *parietal lobe*, (3) the *occipital lobe*, and (4) the *temporal lobe*; the minor lobe is (5) the *insula*.

The central sulcus separates the frontal lobe from the parietal lobe. The lateral fissure demarcates the frontal lobe and the anterior portion of the parietal lobe from the temporal lobe. And the parieto-occipital sulcus separates the superior part of the parietal lobe from the occipital lobe. The separation between the temporal lobe and the occipital lobe is less distinct. We shall see later that the area where the parietal, temporal, and occipital lobes all meet is the major area of the brain where integration of sensory information occurs, with sensory information from the body feeding into this area through

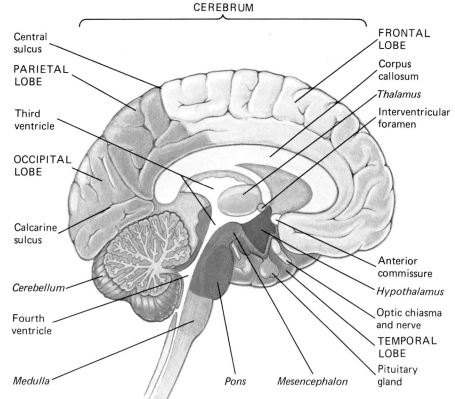

CEREBRUM

Central sulcus

PARIETAL LOBE

Third ventricle

OCCIPITAL LOBE

Calcarine sulcus

Cerebellum

Fourth ventricle

Medulla

Pons

Mesencephalon

FRONTAL LOBE

Corpus callosum

Thalamus

Interventricular foramen

Anterior commissure

Hypothalamus

Optic chiasma and nerve

TEMPORAL LOBE

Pituitary gland

Figure 2–3. Medial view of the left half of the brain, showing especially the relationship of the cerebrum to the brain stem and cerebrum.

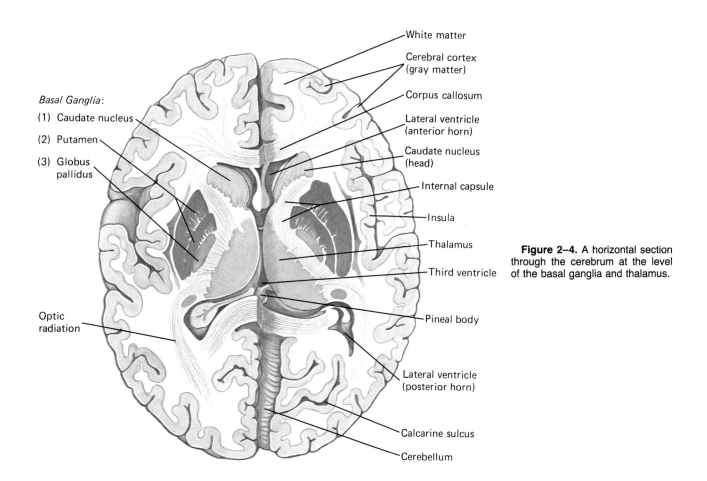

Basal Ganglia:

(1) Caudate nucleus

(2) Putamen

(3) Globus pallidus

Optic radiation

White matter

Cerebral cortex (gray matter)

Corpus callosum

Lateral ventricle (anterior horn)

Caudate nucleus (head)

Internal capsule

Insula

Thalamus

Third ventricle

Pineal body

Lateral ventricle (posterior horn)

Calcarine sulcus

Cerebellum

Figure 2–4. A horizontal section through the cerebrum at the level of the basal ganglia and thalamus.

the parietal lobe, visual information through the occipital lobe, and auditory information through the temporal lobe. In contrast, we shall see that the frontal lobe is concerned primarily with control of muscle movement and also with certain types of thinking processes.

The insula cannot be seen from the surface of the cerebrum. Instead, it lies deep in the lateral fissure. The horizontal section of the brain in Figure 2–4 shows that the lateral sulcus has a broad flat bottom covered by overhanging lips from the frontal, parietal, and temporal lobes. This flat bottom is the *insula*, and the lips are called *opercula* of the other lobes. Unfortunately, we know little about the function of the insula except that it probably acts as part of the limbic system (which will be discussed later) to help control behavior.

Table 2–2 summarizes the structures of the cerebrum and also gives its functional parts, which will be discussed further in the following sections of this chapter.

THE CEREBRAL CORTEX—GRAY MATTER AND WHITE MATTER

Now let us look inside the cerebrum to see how its internal structure is organized. Figure 2–4 shows a horizontal section through the cerebrum. It is composed of areas that appear gray to the naked eye, called *gray matter*, and other areas that appear white, called *white matter*. The gray matter is collections of great numbers of neuronal cell bodies that all together give it its grayish hue. The white matter is comprised of great bundles of nerve fibers leading to or from the nerve cells in the gray matter; its white appearance is caused by the brilliant white color of the myelin sheaths of nerve fibers.

Figure 2–4 shows especially that a thin shell of gray matter covers the entire surface of the cerebrum, including the fissures and sulci. This is the *cerebral cortex*. One of the principal advantages of having the many fissures and sulci is that they triple the total area of the cerebral cortex; the exposed surface area of the brain is only about two thirds of 1 ft² or 600 cm², but the total area of the cerebral cortex is about 2 ft² or 1800 cm².

The cerebral cortex is the portion of the brain most frequently associated with the thinking process, even though it cannot provide thinking without simultaneous action of most deep structures of the brain. Yet, the cerebral cortex is the portion of the brain in which essentially all of our memories are stored, and it is also the area most responsible for our ability to acquire our many muscle skills. We still do not know the basic physiological mechanisms by which the cerebral cortex stores either memories or knowledge of muscle skills, but what we do know about these will be discussed in Chapter 18.

In most areas, the cerebral cortex is about 6 mm thick, and all together it contains an estimated 50

Table 2–2. THE CEREBRUM

	Location and function
The cerebral lobes	
Frontal	Anterior superior
Parietal	Superior midportion
Occipital	Posterior
Temporal	Lateral
Insula	Deep in lateral fissure
Principal fissures and sulci	
Longitudinal fissure	Separates the cerebral hemispheres
Central sulcus	Separates frontal and parietal lobes
Lateral fissure	Separates temporal lobe from frontal lobe and part of the parietal lobe
Parieto-occipital sulcus	Separates superior part of parietal lobe from superior part of occipital lobe
Principal structural parts	
Cerebral cortex (gray matter)	Thin layer on surface comprised mainly of billions of neuronal cell bodies
Deep nuclei (also gray matter)	
Basal ganglia	Most important: (1) caudate nucleus, (2) putamen, (3) globus pallidus
Some of the limbic structures	
White matter	Comprised of billions of nerve fibers, mainly myelinated
Functional areas	
Motor areas:	Located in posterior frontal lobe
Motor cortex	Controls discrete muscle activities
Premotor cortex	Controls patterns of coordinate muscle contractions
Broca's area	Controls speech
Somesthetic cortex	Parietal lobe detects tactile and proprioceptor sensations
Visual area	Occipital lobe detects visual sensations
Auditory area	Superior temporal lobe detects auditory sensations
Wernicke's area	Superior posterior temporal lobe analyzes sensory information from all sources
Short-term memory area	Inferior portions of temporal lobe
Prefrontal area	Anterior half of frontal lobe— "elaboration of thought"

billion or more nerve cell bodies. Also, perhaps a billion nerve fibers lead away from the cortex as well as comparable numbers leading into it, passing to other areas of the cortex, to and from deeper structures of the brain, and some even all the way to the spinal cord.

Functional Areas of the Cerebral Cortex

Until World War I we knew the function of only a few areas of the cerebral cortex. But, at that time soldiers with bullet wounds in discrete parts of the brain were studied systematically for brain functional changes. Also, in more recent years neurosurgeons and neurologists have carefully documented changes in brain function caused by tumors or other specific lesions. Figure 2–5 illustrates the principal functional areas of the cerebral cortex that have been determined by these studies. These are as follows:

The Motor Area: Motor Cortex, Premotor Cortex, and Broca's Area. The motor area lies in front of the central sulcus and occupies the posterior half of the frontal lobe. It, in turn, is divided into three subdivisions, the motor cortex, the premotor cortex, and Broca's area, all of which are concerned with the control of muscle activity.

The *motor cortex*, located in a strip about 2 cm wide immediately anterior to the central sulcus, controls the specific muscles throughout the body, especially the muscles that cause fine movements, such as the finger and thumb motions and the lip and mouth motions for talking and eating, and to a much lesser extent the fine motions of the feet and toes.

The *premotor cortex*, located anterior to the motor cortex, elicits coordinate movements that involve either sequences of individual muscle movements or combined movements of a number of different muscles at the same time. It is in this area that

much of one's knowledge is stored for controlling learned skilled movements such as the special movements required for playing an athletic game.

Broca's area, located anterior to the motor cortex at the lateral margin of the premotor cortex, controls the coordinate movements of the larynx and mouth to produce the words of speech. This area is developed in only one of the two cerebral hemispheres, in the left hemisphere in about 19 out of 20 persons, including all right-handed persons and one half of all left-handed persons.

The Somesthetic Sensory Area. Somesthetic sensations are the sensations from the body such as touch, pressure, temperature, and pain. One can see in Figure 2–5 that the somesthetic sensory area occupies the entire parietal lobe.

Note that this sensory area is divided into a primary area and a secondary area. This is true also of all the other sensory areas. The primary somesthetic sensory area is the portion of the cortex that receives signals directly from the different sensory receptors located throughout the body. In contrast, signals to the secondary somesthetic sensory area are partly processed in deep brain structures or in the primary somesthetic area before being relayed to the secondary area. The primary area can distinguish the specific types of sensation in discrete regions of the body. The secondary area serves mainly to interpret the sensory signals, not to dis-

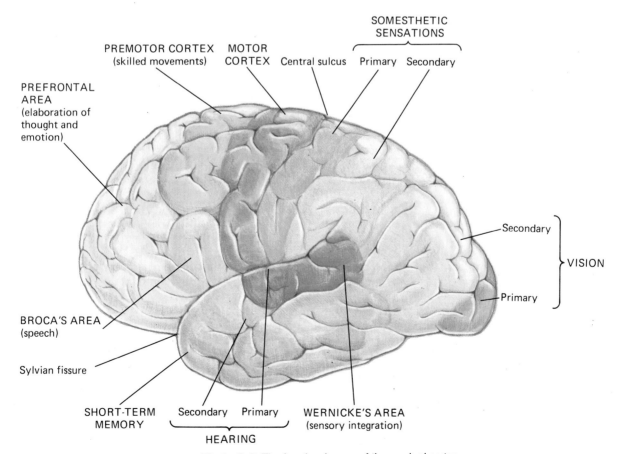

Figure 2–5. The functional areas of the cerebral cortex.

tinguish them, such as interpreting that a hand is feeling a chair, a table, a ball, or so forth.

The Visual Area. Figure 2–5 shows that the visual area occupies the entire occipital lobe. Most of the primary area for vision is located on the medial surface of the cerebral hemisphere along the course of the calcarine sulcus (Figs. 2–3 and 2–4), but a small portion of the primary visual area projects over the outer pole of the occipital lobe as shown in Figure 2–5. This area detects specific light and dark spots as well as orientations of lines and borders in the visual scene. The secondary visual areas occupy the remainder of the occipital lobe, and their function is to interpret the visual information. For instance, it is in these areas that the meanings of written words are interpreted.

The Area for Hearing (the Auditory Area). The hearing area is located in the upper half of the anterior two thirds of the temporal lobe. The primary auditory area is located in the midportion of the superior temporal gyrus. It is here that specific tones, loudness, and other qualities of sound are detected. The secondary areas occupy the other parts of the hearing area. It is in these areas that the meanings of spoken words are interpreted; and portions of these areas are also important for music recognition.

Wernicke's Area for Sensory Integration. Wernicke's area lies in the posterior part of the superior temporal lobe at the point where the parietal and occipital lobes both come in contact with the temporal lobe. It is here that sensory signals from all of the three sensory lobes—the temporal, occipital, and parietal lobes—all come together. This area is exceedingly important for interpreting the ultimate meanings of almost all the different types of sensory information such as the meanings of sentences and thoughts, whether they be heard, read, felt, or even generated within the brain itself. Therefore, destruction of this area of the brain causes extreme loss of thinking ability. This area is well developed only in one of the cerebral hemispheres, usually in the left hemisphere. This unilateral development of Wernicke's area prevents confusion of thought processes between the two halves of the brain.

The Short-Term Memory Area of the Temporal Lobe. The lower half of the temporal lobe seems to be mainly of importance for storing short-term memories, memories that last from a few minutes to several weeks.

The Prefrontal Area. The prefrontal area occupies the anterior half of the frontal lobe. Its function is less well defined than that of any other part of the cerebrum. It has been removed in many psychotic patients to bring them out of depressive states. These persons function quite well without the prefrontal areas. However, they lose their ability to concentrate for long periods of time and also their abilities to plan for the future or to think through deep problems. Therefore, this area is said to be important for elaboration of thought.

We shall discuss in further detail the intellectual function of the cerebral cortex in Chapter 18.

THE BASAL GANGLIA

The horizontal sectional view of the brain in Figure 2–4 shows several areas of gray matter, called *nuclei*, located deep inside the brain. A nucleus is a mass of nerve cell bodies congregated into a cohesive area. Two separate groups of nuclei are shown in the figure: (1) the *basal ganglia*, which are part of the cerebrum, and (2) the *thalamus*, which is composed of multiple small nuclei and is part of the diencephalon, to be described later in this chapter.

Figures 2–6 and 2–7 show still other views of the brain with the basal ganglia high-lighted, Figure 2–6 a coronal view and Figure 2–7 a three-dimensional view to show the locations of the basal ganglia in the cerebral masses and also to show their relationships to the thalamus. The three most important of the basal ganglia are the (1) *caudate nucleus*, (2) *putamen*, and (3) *globus pallidus*. In addition to these three, anatomists also consider the *claustrum* and the *amygdala* to be basal ganglia. However, the function of the claustrum is unknown, and the amygdala functions as part of the limbic system, which we will discuss later in this chapter; it has very little functional relationship to the remainder of the basal ganglia.

On the other hand, the basal ganglia of the cerebrum function in very close association with the *subthalamus* of the diencephalon and the *substantia nigra* and *red nucleus* of the mesencephalon. Therefore, physiologists frequently consider these three bodies also to be part of the basal ganglial system.

The Three-Dimensional Location of the Basal Ganglia in the Cerebrum. Now, let us study in more detail the anatomical locations of the principal basal ganglia. Note in Figure 2–4 in the horizontal section of the brain, that the caudate nucleus, putamen, and globus pallidus lie anterior and lateral to the thalamus. Figure 2–6 shows a coronal section of the brain slightly in front of the anterior end of the thalamus, approximately in the motor region of the cerebrum. In this area the three basal ganglia lie astride one of the major fiber pathways of the cerebrum, called the *internal capsule*. This pathway, which will be described later, is the principal communication link between the cortex and the lower regions of the brain and spinal cord. Many of the fibers in the internal capsule originate in the motor cortex and premotor cortex, and branches of them enter the basal ganglia. Portions of the motor signals are then processed and relayed through these ganglia rather than passing directly from the cerebral cortex to the cord.

Note also in Figure 2–6 the relationship of the basal ganglia to the anterior portions of the two

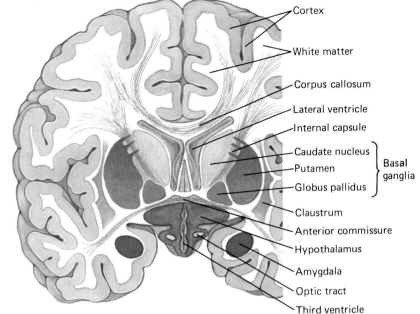

Figure 2–6. A coronal section of the cerebrum in front of the thalamus, showing especially the basal ganglia.

lateral ventricles, which are fluid-filled cavities in the cerebrum. The ventricles lie respectively superior and medial to the caudate nucleus in each of the two cerebral hemispheres.

Finally, the three-dimensional diagram in Figure 2–7 shows especially the relationship of the basal ganglia to the thalamus. One can see the central location of the thalamus in the basal portion of the brain and the location of the basal ganglial system mainly anterior and lateral to the thalamus, but note also the long tail of the caudate nucleus that curls posteriorly through the parietal lobe and thence laterally and inferiorly into the temporal lobe. The amygdala lies at the tip of the caudate nucleus tail in the temporal lobe.

Function of the Basal Ganglia. If the cerebral cortex is removed in a cat but without removing the basal ganglia, the cat can still perform most of its normal motor activities, including walking, fighting, arching its back, spitting, and almost any other movement. On the other hand, in the human being a similar loss of the cerebral cortex, but with the basal ganglia intact, leaves the person with only crude motor activities such as gross trunk movements and movements of the limbs with a stiff-legged, uncontrolled walking.

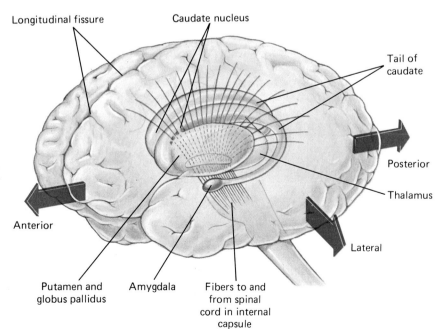

Figure 2–7. Relationship of the basal ganglia to the thalamus, shown in a three-dimensional view.

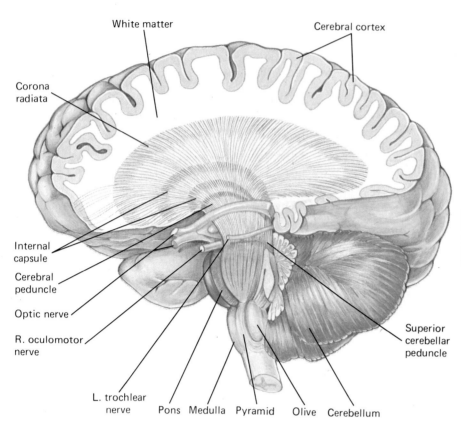

White matter

Cerebral cortex

Corona radiata

Internal capsule

Cerebral peduncle

Optic nerve

R. oculomotor nerve

L. trochlear nerve

Pons   Medulla   Pyramid   Olive   Cerebellum

Superior cerebellar peduncle

Figure 2–8. A deep dissection of the cerebrum showing the radiating nerve fibers, the corona radiata, that conduct signals in both directions between the cerebral cortex and the lower portions of the central nervous system.

Putting this information together, one can deduce that a major function of the basal ganglia in the human being is to control the background gross body movements, whereas the cerebral cortex is necessary for performance of the more precise movements of the arms, hands, fingers, and feet. When the hand is performing some precise activity that requires a background stance of the body, the basal ganglia provide the body movements while the cerebral cortex provides the precise movements.

To achieve the high degree of coordination that is required among the muscles of the body during most motor functions, a very complex circuitry of nerve fibers interconnects (1) the cerebral cortex and basal ganglia in the cerebrum, (2) the thalamus and subthalamus in the diencephalon, (3) the red nucleus and the substantia nigra in the mesencephalon, and (4) the cerebellum in the hindbrain.

THE WHITE MATTER OF THE CEREBRUM

In almost all areas of the cerebrum besides the cerebral cortex and basal ganglia one finds white matter. The white matter is comprised nearly exclusively of nerve fibers, these often organized into specific bundles of fibers called *fiber tracts*. Three of the principal fiber tracts, each containing millions of fibers, are illustrated in Figure 2–4. These are the following:

1. The *corpus callosum*, which was discussed earlier, connects the respective areas of the cerebral cortex in each cerebral hemisphere with corresponding areas in the opposite hemisphere. The corpus callosum is also seen in sagittal section in Figure 2–3 and in coronal section in Figure 2–6.

2. The *optic radiation*, shown in Figure 2–4, passes from the lateral geniculate body of the thalamus back to the calcarine sulcus area of the occipital lobe. This is the final relay pathway for transmission of visual signals from the eyes to the cerebral cortex.

3. The *internal capsule*, shown in Figure 2–4, is found in the areas between the thalamus, the caudate nucleus, and the putamen. It is through this internal capsule that most signals between the cerebral cortex and the lower brain and spinal cord are transmitted.

Figure 2–8 illustrates even more vividly the gray and white matter of the cerebrum. Shown too is the great mass of nerve fibers that extends upward from the internal capsule to the cerebral cortex through an extensive radiation called the *corona radiata*.

THE DIENCEPHALON

The term *diencephalon* means the *between brain*. In primitive animals the diencephalon is a nodular structure, distinct from the remainder of the brain, that links the telencephalon (the cerebrum) with the mesencephalon (the midbrain). In the human being, the diencephalon still provides a similar linkage between the cerebrum and the lower parts of the brain, but anatomically it is so tightly fused with the basal portions of the cerebrum that it is difficult to demarcate its boundaries with the cerebrum. However, the diencephalon is defined as those structures that surround the third ventricle (another fluid-filled cavity in the brain, shown in Figure 2–9 and discussed in the following chapter). Table 2–3 summarizes the important structures and functions of the diencephalon. The most important of the structures are the *thalamus* and *hypothalamus*. Both of these are composed of multiple nuclei that perform many different important nervous functions. In addition to these two, smaller nuclear areas of the diencephalon, located posterior and inferior to the thalamus, are the *epithalamus* and *subthalamus*.

The Thalamus

We have already seen in several figures that the thalamus is located in the very center of the brain, enshrouded on all sides except inferiorly by the cerebrum. Figure 2–9 illustrates another view of the thalamus and its location in a coronal section of the brain. Several specific features of the thalamus are described here:

First, the thalamus is comprised of a number of separate discrete nuclei, as illustrated by the multiple blue-colored areas in the figure.

Second, the thalamus rests directly on top of the mesencephalon (also called the "midbrain"); almost all signals from the midbrain and other lower regons of the brain, as well as from the spinal cord, are relayed through synapses in the thalamus before proceeding to the cerebral cortex.

Third, the thalamus has numerous two-way connections with all parts of the cerebral cortex, carrying a continual traffic of signals from the thalamus to the cortex and also from the cortex to the thalamus.

Fourth, the thalamus lies in close apposition to the basal ganglia. In fact, the thalamus relays many signals from other lower regions of the brain and spinal cord directly to the basal ganglia. And, in turn, the thalamus also functions as a relay station for signals from some of the basal ganglia to the cortex.

In essence, then, the thalamus is a chief traffic relay station for directing sensory and other signals to appropriate points in both the cerebral cortex and the deeper areas of the cerebrum as well. Some examples of the different types of signals that are relayed through the thalamus include:

1. all the *somesthetic sensory signals* from the body (touch, pressure, pain, temperature, and so forth) to the somesthetic cortex of the parietal lobe;

2. *visual signals* to the calcarine sulcus area of the occipital cortex (the part of the thalamus that relays these signals is sometimes classified as the *metathalamus*, which is the posterior end of the thalamus);

3. *auditory signals* to the superior temporal gyrus (also relayed by the metathalamus); and

4. *muscle control signals* from the cerebellum, mesencephalon, and other areas of the lower brain stem to the motor cortex and basal ganglia.

Anatomical Relationship of the Thalamus to the Ventricles. Note especially in Figure 2–9 the relationship of the thalamus to several of the ventricles: (1) the two lateral ventricles lie immediately above the two lateral halves of the thalamus and (2) the third ventricle bisects the thalamus into two halves. Each half of the thalamus functions separately with the cerebral hemisphere on the same side, and there is very little direct communication between the two halves of the thalamus.

The Sensory Interpretive Function of the Thalamus. In lower animals, at about the reptile stage, the cerebral cortex is not developed to a great extent, but the thalamus is an established part of

Table 2–3. THE DIENCEPHALON AND LIMBIC SYSTEM

Structure	Location	Function
Diencephalon		
Thalamus	Central base of brain	Relays sensory signals to cortex, sensory analytic functions
Hypothalamus	Inferior to anterior thalamus	Controls internal body functions, stimulates autonomic nervous system
Subthalamus	Inferior to posterior thalamus	Functions with basal ganglia to control subconscious muscle activity
Epithalamus	Posteroinferior to thalamus	Function unknown; includes pineal gland
Limbic system		
Amygdala	Deep inside anterior end of each temporal lobe	Controls behavior for each social occasion
Hippocampus	Medial border of each cerebral hemisphere	Determines which sensory information will be committed to memory
Mammillary body	Posterior to hypothalamus	Perhaps helps to determine mood and degree of wakefulness
Septum pellucidum	Midline of cerebrum anterior and superior to hypothalamus	Perhaps helps to control temper and autonomic nervous system
Limbic cortex: Cingulate gyrus, cingulum, insula, and parahippocampal gyrus	Ring of cerebral cortex in medial part of cerebrum around deeper limbic structures	Conscious components in the control of behavior

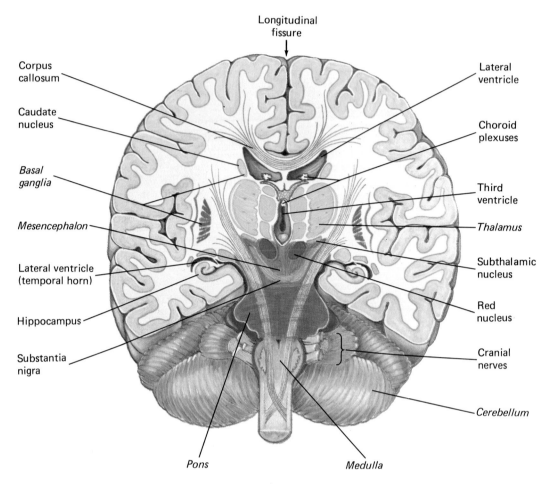

Figure 2–9. A coronal view of the cerebrum looking from anteriorly backward. This section was made immediately anterior to the lower brain stem and through the middle of the thalamus.

the brain. In these animals, the thalamus plays a much greater role in sensory interpretation than it does in man. But, even in man some of its sensory interpretive abilities still persist. This is especially true for pain sensation, for a person can lose most if not all of the somesthetic sensory areas of his cerebral cortex and still retain much if not most of his ability to perceive pain. This is in keeping with the fact that pain is one of the most primitive of our sensations and also that the thalamus is a more primitive portion of the brain than is the cerebrum.

The Thalamocortical Relationship. In addition to the relay pathways through the thalamus to the cerebral cortex, there are also innumerable two-way connections between the thalamus and all areas of the cortex, with nerve fibers going in both directions. Figure 2–10 illustrates by means of a color code the areas of the thalamus that connect with specific areas of the cerebral cortex. For example, the posterior portion of the thalamus (lateral geniculate body and pulvinar) has two-way connections with the occipital lobe of the cortex. The superior medial part of the thalamus (nucleus medialis dorsalis) connects with the prefrontal area of the frontal lobe. And the posterolateral portion of the ventral nucleus (nucleus ventralis posterior lateralis) con-

nects with the primary somesthetic area of the parietal cortex, and so forth.

But what are the purposes of these two-way connections? First, without the thalamus, the cortex is useless. It is the thalamus that drives the cortex to activity, which is another function of the thalamus in addition to relaying signals to the cortex from other areas of the brain and spinal cord. In fact, one can consider most of the cerebral cortex to be mainly an outgrowth of the thalamus; the cortex provides a great memory storehouse to function at the beck and call of the control centers of the thalamus.

The Hypothalamus

Several figures presented earlier in this chapter illustrated a small structure in the middle of the base of the brain called the *hypothalamus*. Study especially Figures 2–2 and 2–3 and locate this structure, but look carefully or otherwise you will miss it. Its small size belies its importance, for it is a major center of the brain for controlling internal body functions.

Figure 2–11 illustrates an enlarged internal view of the hypothalamus, showing in third dimension various nuclei of the hypothalamus. Note that the hypothalamus lies anterior to the red nucleus, which is in the uppermost part of the mesencephalon, and it also lies immediately inferior to the anterior end of the thalamus. There are especially abundant nerve pathways between the hypothalamus and the anterior thalamus and also between the hypothalamus and the mesencephalon.

Some of the Functions of the Nuclei of the Hypothalamus. At many points in this text we shall discuss the importance of one or more of the hypothalamic nuclei for control of some of the internal body functions, and more details of the function of the hypothalamus as a whole will be presented in Chapter 20. However, let us list here some of the important functions of a few of the hypothalamic nuclei.

The *preoptic nucleus,* located anteriorly, is primarily concerned with body temperature control.

The *supraoptic nucleus,* also located anteriorly but inferiorly as well, lying immediately above the optic nerves, controls the secretion of *antidiuretic hormone;* this hormone in turn helps to control the concentration of electrolytes in the body fluids.

The *medial nuclei* of the hypothalamus, when stimulated, gives a person a sense of satiety (that is, he feels satisfied, especially satisfied for food).

Stimulation of the most *lateral regions of the hypothalamus* causes a person to become very hungry, and stimulation anteriorly in the lateral hypothalamus causes a person to become very thirsty.

Stimulation of the *posterior hypothalamus* excites the sympathetic nervous system throughout the body, increasing the overall level of activity of many internal parts of the body, especially increasing heart rate and causing blood vessel constriction.

Finally, stimulation of different areas of the hypothalamus causes its neurons to secrete several hormones called *releasing hormones* that are carried in the venous blood directly to the anterior pituitary

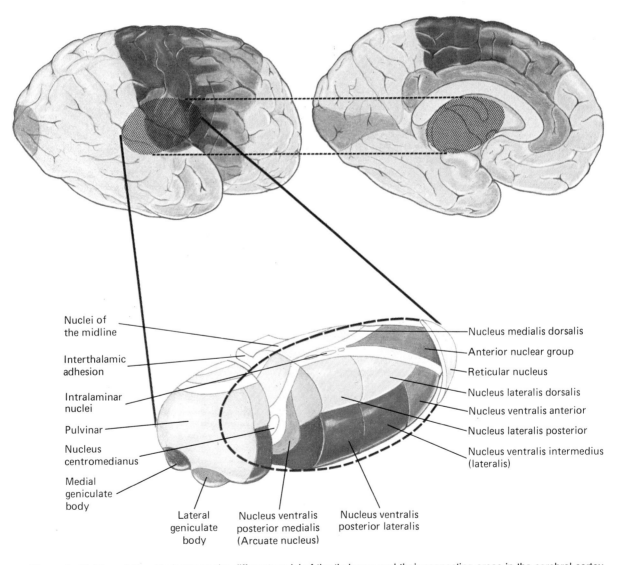

Figure 2–10. The relationship between the different nuclei of the thalamus and their connecting areas in the cerebral cortex. (Reprinted from Warwick and Williams: Gray's Anatomy, 35th British Edition. Philadelphia, W. B. Saunders, 1973.)

gland; here they then cause secretion of the anterior pituitary hormones. The pituitary hormones in turn control such varied activities of the body as the metabolism of carbohydrates, metabolism of proteins, metabolism of fats, functions of the sex glands, and several other functions.

Thus, one cannot help but be impressed by the global importance of this small area of the brain, the hypothalamus, and its multiple roles in the control of our bodies. Therefore, we will be discussing its functions at many points in this text.

THE LIMBIC SYSTEM

The word "limbic" means border; and the *limbic system*, illustrated in Figure 2–12, and summarized in Table 2–3, comprises the border structures of the cerebrum and the diencephalon that mainly surround the hypothalamus. This limbic system func-

tions especially to control our emotional and behavioral activities. Some of the important parts of the limbic system are as follows:

1. The *amygdala* (also called the *amygdaloid body*) is a small nuclear structure located deep inside each anterior temporal lobe and considered by anatomists to be one of the basal ganglia. However, it functions very closely with the hypothalamus, not with the usual basal ganglia. It is believed that the amygdala helps to control the appropriate behavior of the person for each type of social situation.

2. The *hippocampus*, one on each side, is a primitive portion of the cerebral cortex that lies along the medial-most border of the temporal lobe and folds upward and inward to form the inferior surface of the inferior horn of the lateral ventricle. The hippocampus is believed to interpret for the brain the importance of most of our sensory experiences. If the hippocampus determines an experience to be

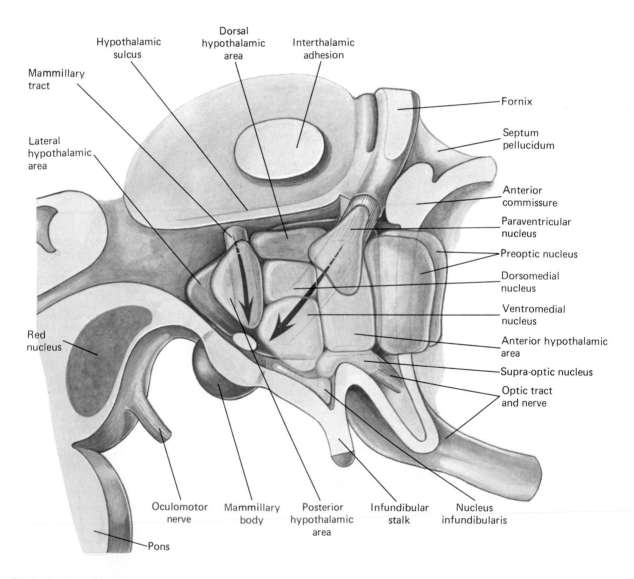

Figure 2–11. A three-dimensional view of one side of the hypothalamus, showing its principal nuclei. (From Nauta and Haymaker: The Hypothalamus. Springfield, Ill., Charles C Thomas, 1969.)

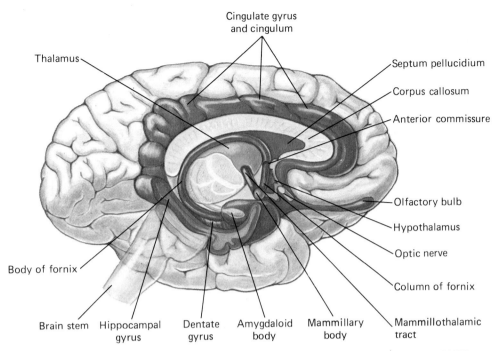

Figure 2–12. The limbic system in the midportion of the cerebrum. (From Warwick and Williams: Gray's Anatomy, 35th British Edition. Philadelphia, W. B. Saunders, 1973.)

important enough, then the experience will be stored as a memory in the cerebral cortex. Without the hippocampus, a person's ability to store memories becomes very deficient.

3. The *mammillary bodies* lie immediately behind the hypothalamus and function in close association with the thalamus, hypothalamus, and brain stem to help control many behavioral functions such as the person's degree of wakefulness and perhaps also his feeling of well-being.

4. The *septum pellucidum* lies anterior to the thalamus, superior to the hypothalamus, and between the basal ganglia in the median plane of the cerebrum. Stimulation in different parts of this septum can cause many different behavioral effects, including the phenomenon of rage.

5. The *cingulate gyrus,* the *cingulum*, the *insula,* and the *parahippocampal gyrus* all together form a ring of cerebral cortex in each cerebral hemisphere around the deeper structures of the limbic system described in the previous few paragraphs. This ring of cortex is believed to allow association between conscious cerebral behavioral functions and subconscious behavioral functions of the deeper limbic system.

Signals from the limbic system leading into the hypothalamus can modify any one or all of the many internal bodily functions controlled by the hypothalamus. And signals feeding from the limbic system into the mesencephalon can control such behavior as wakefulness, sleep, excitement, attentiveness, and even rage or docility. Yet, the precise manner in which the different parts of the limbic system function together to control all these emotional and behavioral functions of the body is still only slightly understood.

References

See References, Chapter 4.

3

Gross Anatomy of the Nervous System: II. Brain Stem; Cerebellum; Spinal Cord; and Cerebrospinal Fluid System

THE BRAIN STEM

The brain stem, illustrated in Figure 3–1, is exactly what its name implies: it is the stem of the brain that connects the forebrain with the spinal cord. Its major divisions are (1) the *mesencephalon*, (2) the *pons*, and (3) the *medulla oblongata*. Some anatomists also consider the *diencephalon*, which was discussed in the previous chapter, to be part of the brain stem because it too is a connecting link.

Several important *fiber tracts* pass both upward and downward through the brain stem, transmitting sensory signals from the spinal cord mainly to the thalamus and motor signals from the cerebral cortex to the cord. In addition, other fiber tracts either originate or terminate in the brain stem, again mainly for the purpose of carrying sensory and motor signals.

However, the brain stem also contains many very important centers that control such physiological variables as respiration, arterial pressure, equilibrium, and others. In fact, centers in the brain stem even determine the level of activity in the cerebrum and also cause the waking-sleeping cycle of the nervous system.

And, finally, the brain stem serves as the connecting link between the cerebellum and the cerebrum superiorly and between the cerebellum and spinal cord inferiorly.

THE MESENCEPHALON

The surface anatomy of the mesencephalon is shown from the left posterolateral side in Figure 3–1, and a horizontal section is illustrated in Figure 3–2. It is divided from anterior to posterior into two major sections: (1) the two *cerebral peduncles*, which constitute the anterior four fifths of the mesencephalon, and (2) the *tectum*, which comprises the posterior surface structures. Passing inferiorly in the posterior part of the tegmentum is the *cerebral aqueduct*, which is a small tubular canal that connects the third ventricle in the diencephalon with the fourth ventricle in the lower brain stem.

The Cerebral Peduncles. The cerebral peduncles veer anteriorly and laterally at the top of the mesencephalon and then project superiorly into the two lateral halves of the diencephalon. Each cerebral peduncle is divided into three separate areas:

1. A thick anterolateral surface layer of *corticospinal* and *corticopontine fibers* conducts motor signals from the cortex to the spinal cord and to the pons.

2. A deeper layer of darkly pigmented nerve cell bodies called the *substantia nigra* lies behind the fiber layer. The neurons of the substantia nigra function as part of the basal ganglial system to control subconscious muscle activities of the body. Destruction of these neurons causes Parkinson's disease, in which the person develops continuous muscle spasm and a shaking tremor in part or all of the body, sometimes so severe that muscle functions become useless.

3. The *tegmentum* is the major mass of the cerebral peduncles medial and posterior to the substantia nigra.

The tegmentum contains several important fiber tracts and nuclei that provide specific functions as follows:

1. The *medial lemniscus* is the major fiber tract for transmitting sensory signals from the body to the thalamus.

2. The *medial longitudinal fasciculus* is a tract that connects many of the nuclei of the brain stem with each other and also with the diencephalon.

3. The *red nucleus*, illustrated in Figure 3–2, occupies a major part of each side of the superior mesencephalic tegmentum. This nucleus functions with the basal ganglia and cerebellum to coordinate muscle movements of the body. It also serves as a

Table 3–1. THE BRAIN STEM AND CEREBELLUM

Structure	Function
Mesencephalon	
Cerebral peduncles	
1. Corticospinal and corticopontine tracts	Motor signals to cord and pons
2. Substantia nigra	Part of basal ganglia motor control system
3. Tegmentum	
a. Red nucleus	Relays signals from cerebellum
b. Reticular formation	Excites whole brain, controls muscular tone
c. Nuclei of cranial nerves III and IV	Control eye movements
d. Medial lemnisci	Sensory signals to thalamus
Tectum	
1. Superior colliculi	Help to control eye movements
2. Inferior colliculi	Cause motor reactions to auditory signals
Pons	
Ventral part	
1. Corticospinal tracts	Pass through ventral pons toward cord
2. Pontine nuclei	Terminis of corticopontine tracts
3. Transverse fibers	Fibers from pontine nuclei to opposite cerebellar hemisphere
Tegmentum	
1. Reticular formation	Same as in mesencephalon, also parts of vasomotor and respiratory centers
2. Nuclei of cranial nerves V, VI, VII, and VIII	Eye and facial movements; facial, auditory, and equilibrium sensations
3. Medial lemnisci	Same as in mesencephalon
Medulla Oblongata	
Pyramids and decussation of pyramids	Downward extensions and crossover of corticospinal tracts
Gracile and cuneate nuclei	Origins of fibers in medial lemnisci
Decussation of medial lemnisci	Crossover of the medial lemnisci
Inferior olivary nuclei	Origin of many input fibers to cerebellum
Nuclei of cranial nerves IX, X, XI, and XII	Motor signals to larynx, pharynx, tongue, some neck muscles; sensory signals from viscera; motor signals to parasympathetic nervous system
Reticular formation	
1. Most of vasomotor center	Controls vascular resistance, arterial pressure, heart activity
2. Most of respiratory center	Controls inspiration and expiration
Cerebellum	
Cerebellar peduncles	
1. Inferior peduncle	Extends from medulla; mainly input signals
2. Middle peduncle	Extends from ventral part of pons; entirely input signals
3. Superior peduncle	Extends to mesencephalon; mainly output signals
Vermis	Midline portion of cerebellum; functions with brain stem and spinal cord
Cerebellar hemispheres	Lateral portions of cerebellum; functions mainly with higher motor centers
Cerebellar cortex	Provides delays in motor signals
Deep nuclei	
1. Dentate nuclei	Output nuclei of cerebellar hemispheres
2. Fastigial, globose, and emboliform nuclei	Output nuclei of vernis

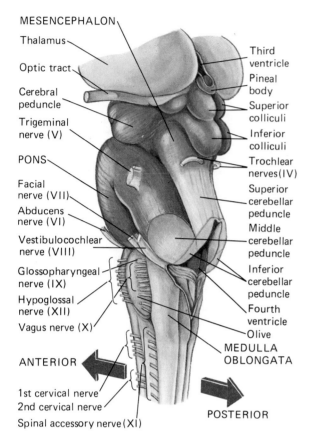

MESENCEPHALON
Thalamus
Optic tract
Cerebral peduncle
Trigeminal nerve (V)
PONS
Facial nerve (VII)
Abducens nerve (VI)
Vestibulocochlear nerve (VIII)
Glossopharyngeal nerve (IX)
Hypoglossal nerve (XII)
Vagus nerve (X)
ANTERIOR
1st cervical nerve
2nd cervical nerve
Spinal accessory nerve (XI)

Third ventricle
Pineal body
Superior colliculi
Inferior colliculi
Trochlear nerves (IV)
Superior cerebellar peduncle
Middle cerebellar peduncle
Inferior cerebellar peduncle
Fourth ventricle
Olive
MEDULLA OBLONGATA
POSTERIOR

Figure 3–1. The brain stem.

relay station for signals transmitted from the cerebellum to the thalamus and cerebrum.

4. The *nuclei of the oculomotor and trochlear nerves* are small collections of nerve cells on each side of the mesencephalon that control most of the muscles for eye movements.

5. The *periaqueductal gray* is a collection of diffuse nuclei around the cerebral aqueduct. This area seems to play a major role in the analysis of the reaction to pain.

6. The *reticular formation* is composed of many widely dispersed nuclei in large portions of the tegmentum. The reticular formation is not only present in the mesencephalon but actually extends all the way from the superior end of the spinal cord to the diencephalon, passing through the medulla oblongata, the pons, the mesencephalon, and even extending into the middle of the thalamus where it is represented by the thalamic intralaminar nuclei. Various collections of nerve cells within the reticular formation control many of the stereotyped body movements, such as *turning motions of the trunk, turning and bending motions of the head,* and *postural motions of the limbs.* But, even more important, the reticular formation is the major center of the entire brain for *controlling the brain's overall level of activity.* Generalized stimulation of the mesencephalic and pontine portions of the reticular formation usually causes a high degree of wakefulness in an animal while increasing the tone of the muscles throughout the body. Therefore, the reticular formation, though dispersed rather broadly in the brain stem, is functionally one of the most important of all the brain structures, as we shall discuss much more fully in later chapters.

The Tectum. The tectum is the posterior fifth of the mesencephalon, and it consists principally of four small nodular bodies, two superior colliculi and two inferior colliculi, that are arranged in a quadrangle on the posterior surface of the mesencephalon, as illustrated in Figure 3–1.

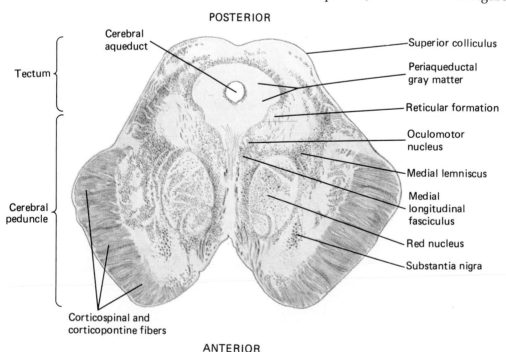

POSTERIOR
Cerebral aqueduct
Tectum
Cerebral peduncle
Corticospinal and corticopontine fibers
ANTERIOR

Superior colliculus
Periaqueductal gray matter
Reticular formation
Oculomotor nucleus
Medial lemniscus
Medial longitudinal fasciculus
Red nucleus
Substantia nigra

Figure 3–2. A horizontal section through the mesencephalon at the level of the superior colliculi.

The two *superior colliculi* are located side by side on the superior portion of the posterior mesencephalon, lying immediately beneath the posterior poles of the thalamus. In lower animals, especially the fish, the superior colliculi are the principal brain terminus for vision. In the human being, the visual functions of these bodies have been lost, but they are still used for *causing eye movements* and even *trunk movements* in response to sudden visual signals such as a flash of light from one side of the field of vision or sudden movement of a person or an animal nearby.

The two *inferior colliculi* are located inferior to the two superior colliculi, also on the posterior surface of the mesencephalon. These serve as way-stations for relaying auditory signals from the ears to the cerebrum. In addition, they play a role in causing a person to turn his or her head or body in response to sounds coming from different directions.

Inferior to the inferior colliculi on the two sides of the mesencephalon are two large bundles of nerve fibers called the *superior cerebellar peduncles* that project inferiorly and posteriorly to connect with the superior portions of the cerebellum. These are one of the major trunk lines between the cerebellum and the remainder of the brain.

THE PONS

The pons, illustrated from the left posterolateral side in Figure 3–1 and in horizontal section in Figure 3–3, has many of the same types of internal structures as the mesencephalon, such as some of the same major fiber pathways that transmit signals both up and down the brain stem and multiple nuclei that perform specific functions. For descriptive purposes, the pons is divided into two parts: the *ventral part* and the *dorsal part,* also called the *tegmentum of the pons,* which is continuous with the tegmentum of the mesencephalon.

The Ventral Part of the Pons. The ventral part of the pons is the large bulbous anterior protrusion illustrated in Figure 3–1 and seen even better in the basal view of the brain in Figure 2–2 of the previous chapter. Its internal structure is illustrated in Figure 3–3.

The same *corticospinal fibers* and *corticopontine fibers* that pass through the cerebral peduncles of the mesencephalon also descend into the ventral part of the pons. The corticospinal fibers then pass through the medulla into the spinal cord. On the other hand, the corticopontine fibers terminate here, synapsing in multiple *pontine nuclei*. From these, transverse fibers cross immediately to the opposite side of the ventral pons and then circle backwards around the two lateral sides of the pons to form the *middle cerebellar peduncles* that extend posteriorly into the two cerebellar hemispheres. In addition, a few fibers also pass directly backward into these peduncles on the same side. Because of the crossing of the transverse fibers and because most of the output fibers leaving the cerebellum to reenter the brain stem also cross to the opposite side, the right half of the cerebellum functions mainly with the left half of the cerebrum, and the left half of the cerebellum functions mainly with the right cerebrum.

The Tegmentum of the Pons. Figure 3–3 shows that the pontine tegmentum contains the following

POSTERIOR

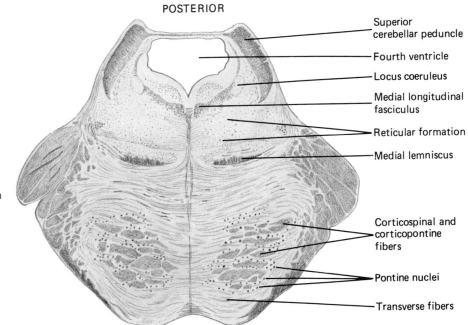

Superior cerebellar peduncle

Fourth ventricle

Locus coeruleus

Medial longitudinal fasciculus

Reticular formation

Medial lemniscus

Corticospinal and corticopontine fibers

Pontine nuclei

Transverse fibers

Figure 3–3. A horizontal section through the pons.

ANTERIOR

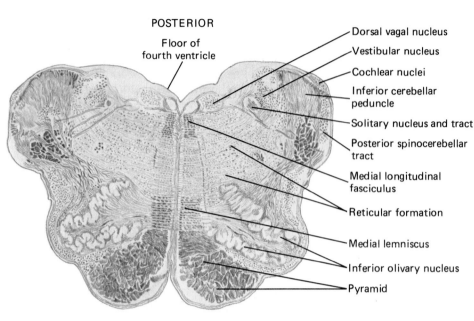

POSTERIOR

Floor of
fourth ventricle

Dorsal vagal nucleus

Vestibular nucleus

Cochlear nuclei

Inferior cerebellar
peduncle

Solitary nucleus and tract

Posterior spinocerebellar
tract

Medial longitudinal
fasciculus

Reticular formation

Medial lemniscus

Inferior olivary nucleus

Pyramid

ANTERIOR

Figure 3–4. A horizontal section through the medulla oblongata.

three structures that are continuous with those in the mesencephalon: the *medial lemniscus,* the *medial longitudinal fasciculus,* and the *reticular formation.* In addition, it contains the nuclei of several cranial nerves: (1) the *abducens nerve,* which helps to control eye movements; (2) the *facial nerve,* which controls the muscles of expression of the face; (3) the *trigeminal nerve,* which controls the muscles of mastication and also transmits sensory signals from the face, mouth, and scalp; and (4) the *vestibulocochlear nerve,* which transmits sensory signals from the ear and from the vestibular apparatus (the equilibrium apparatus of the inner ear).

THE MEDULLA OBLONGATA

The *medulla oblongata,* usually called simply the *medulla,* is illustrated at the lower end of the brain stem in Figure 3–1, and it is seen in cross-section in Figure 3–4. On the surface are two distinguishing characteristics:

1. On the anterior aspect of the medulla are two protruding longitudinal columns called *pyramids* (seen best in Figure 2–2 of the previous chapter but also illustrated in cross-section in Figure 3–4). These carry the same *corticospinal fibers* that pass from the cerebral cortex through the cerebral peduncles of the mesencephalon and through the ventral pons. The fibers in this trunk pass eventually to all levels of the spinal cord, carrying signals that control muscle contraction. In the inferior portion of the medulla, the fibers of the pyramid cross to the opposite side before passing down the spinal cord, which is called the *decussation of the pyramids.* Therefore, the left cerebral cortex controls muscle contraction in the right half of the body while the right cortex controls the left side.

2. An *olive* protrudes from each anterolateral surface of the medulla lateral to the pyramids (Fig. 3–1). Deep to the external projection of the olive is the *inferior olivary nucleus,* which can be seen in cross-section in Figure 3–4. This nucleus functions to relay signals into the cerebellum, functioning similarly to the pontine nuclei. However, it receives its input signals mainly from the basal ganglia and spinal cord and less from the motor cortex. Its outgoing signals go to the contralateral cerebellum through the *inferior cerebellar peduncle* (Fig. 3–1), which is an upward and posteriorly projecting column of nerve fibers extending from the medulla to the cerebellum.

In addition to these specific surface structures, the medulla contains many of the same components as the mesencephalon and pons. Especially prominent are the bilateral *medial lemnisci,* the large fiber tracts through which sensory signals are conducted from the spinal cord to the cerebrum. The fibers in these tracts originate in large bilateral nuclei in the posterior inferior medulla, the *gracile* and *cuneate nuclei,* which themselves receive sensory signals from sensory fibers in the dorsal column of the spinal cord. After leaving these nuclei, the fibers cross to the opposite side of the medulla in the *decussation of the medial lemnisci* to form the medial lemnisci. Because of this crossing, the left side of the brain is excited by sensory stimuli from the right side of the body and the right brain from the left body.

Also present in the medulla are (1) nuclei for *cranial nerves IX, X, XI,* and *XII,* which will be discussed more fully in the following chapter, and (2) the *reticular formation* that makes up a large share of the posterior and lateral medulla.

Some Special Functional Areas of the Reticular Formation in the Medulla and Pons. The reticular formation of the medulla and pons contains two especially important control centers:

1. The *vasomotor center* consists of widely dispersed nerve cells in the formation. This center transmits signals to the heart and blood vessels to increase heart pumping activity and to constrict the vessels. These effects acting together can increase the blood pressure greatly.

2. The *respiratory center* is composed of nerve cells also located widely in the reticular formation. This is an automatic, rhythmically active center that causes the rhythmical respiratory muscle contractions necessary for inspiration and expiration.

In addition to these special centers, the medullary and pontine reticular formation also serves as an important relay station for signals coming from higher brain centers to control many other important internal functions of the body. For instance, signals from the hypothalamus are relayed down the spinal cord to control body temperature, sweating, secretion in the digestive tract, emptying of the urinary bladder, and many other bodily functions. Also, lying in close association with the posterior medullary reticular formation on each side of the midline is the *dorsal motor nucleus of the vagus* (Fig. 3–4). This nucleus relays signals into the vagus nerve to control heart rate, gastric secretion, peristalsis in the gastrointestinal tract, and other internal functions.

THE CEREBELLUM

The *cerebellum* is a large structure of the hindbrain (rhombencephalon) located inferior to the occipital lobe of the cerebrum and posterior to the brain stem. Its location in relation to the remainder of the brain is seen best in Figures 2–6 through 2–8 of the previous chapter, and its specific relationship to the brain stem is illustrated in Figure 3–5.

The cerebellum is an important part of the motor control system. Even though it is located far away from both the motor cortex and the basal ganglia, it interconnects with these through special nerve pathways, and it also interconnects with motor areas in both the reticular formation and the spinal cord. Its primary function is to determine the time sequence of contraction of different muscles during complex movements of parts of the body, especially when these movements occur extremely rapidly.

Surface Anatomy of the Cerebellum. Shown in Figure 3–1 are three different cerebellar peduncles that lead from the posterior surface of each side of the brain stem to the cerebellum; these are: (1) the *superior cerebellar peduncle*, which connects with the mesencephalon, as discussed earlier; (2) the *middle cerebellar peduncle*, which connects with the pons; and (3) the *inferior cerebellar peduncle*, which connects with the medulla. It is through these that signals are transmitted into and away from the cerebellum.

Now, let us study the structure of the cerebellum itself as shown in Figures 3–5 and 3–6. Its major

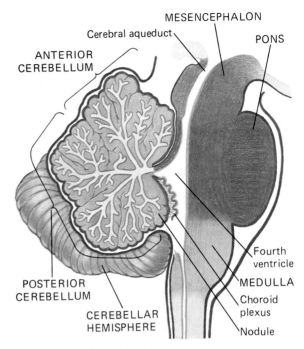

BLUE: arachnoid mater
RED: pia mater
GREEN: ependyma

Figure 3–5. Relationship of the cerebellum to the brain stem.

parts are the *vermis*, which is a midline structure 1 to 2 cm wide extending around the entire cerebellum from anterior to posterior and from superior to inferior, and two *cerebellar hemispheres*, located laterally on the two sides of the cerebellum. Both the vermis and the cerebellar hemispheres can also be divided into the *anterior lobe of the cerebellum*, which is the superior and anterior third of the cerebellum anterior to the primary fissure, and *posterior lobe of the cerebellum*, which is the posterior and inferior two thirds of the cerebellum posterior to the primary fissure.

In the human being, the cerebellar hemispheres make up by far the greater portion of the cerebellar mass. These hemispheres function in concert with the cerebrum to coordinate voluntary movements of the body. The vermis, on the other hand, functions more for coordinating the stereotyped and subconscious body movements, operating mainly in association with the brain stem and spinal cord.

Internal Structure of the Cerebellum. The internal structure of the cerebellum is illustrated in Figure 3–7. Like the cerebrum, it is comprised of three principal structures: (1) the *cerebellar cortex*, (2) the *subcortical white matter* composed almost entirely of nerve fibers, and (3) the *deep nuclei*.

The cerebellar cortex is a 3- to 5-mm thick sheet of nerve cells covering the entire cerebellar surface, containing a total of about 30 billion cells.

The deep nuclei are located in the center of the cerebellar white matter. By far the most prominent of the deep nuclei is the large *dentate nucleus*, which

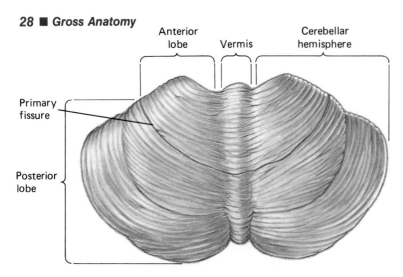

Anterior lobe   Vermis   Cerebellar hemisphere

Primary fissure

Posterior lobe

Figure 3–6. Superior view of the cerebellum.

is located in the center of each cerebellar hemisphere. However, three other smaller deep nuclei are located in each side of the vermis: (1) the *fastigial nucleus,* (2) the *emboliform nucleus,* and (3) the *globose nucleus.*

The deep nuclei give rise to the nerve fibers that transmit signals out of the cerebellum to other parts of the nervous system. The cerebellar cortex is a computing area that receives input information from the cerebral cortex, the basal ganglia, the spinal cord, and the peripheral muscles and integrates all of this to help coordinate the muscle movements.

Note also in Figures 3–5, 3–6 and 3–7 the many folds of the cerebellum, called *folia.* If the cerebellar cortex were stretched out to eliminate these folia, it

would be represented by a flat sheet about 40 cm in length and 8 cm wide. Each area of the cerebellum has almost exactly the same internal neuronal circuitry as all other areas, suggesting that the cerebellum performs almost exactly the same functions in all its separate parts. What it does is to delay signals for short fractions of a second. Thus, when the motor system requires contraction of the biceps to start the arm moving and then contraction of the triceps to stop the movement, the cerebellum determines the appropriate delay before turning off the biceps and simultaneously turning on the triceps. When a person is performing rapid movements, such sequential muscle contractions occur in many separate parts of the body one after the other. Without the appropriate turn-on, turn-off

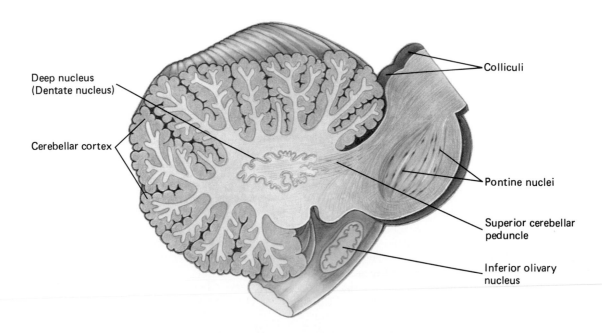

Deep nucleus (Dentate nucleus)

Cerebellar cortex

Colliculi

Pontine nuclei

Superior cerebellar peduncle

Inferior olivary nucleus

Figure 3–7. The internal anatomy of the cerebellar hemisphere and related structures.

sequence of these motor signals, the movements become totally uncoordinated, which is what happens when the cerebellum is destroyed.

THE SPINAL CORD

Figure 3–8 illustrates the *spinal cord* and the *spinal nerves* leaving it to be distributed to all parts of the body, and Table 3–2 summarizes the structural parts of the cord and their functions. Note that a spinal nerve leaves the cord on each side through each *intervertebral* foramen between adjacent vertebrae. Some of these nerves are very large because they innervate large areas of the body, such as the spinal nerves of the lower neck that innervate the arms, forearms, and hands and those of the lumbar and sacral regions that innervate the thighs, legs, and feet. In both of these areas the cord itself is also enlarged because of the great number of nerve cell bodies that are required to relay the signals, giving rise to the *cervical enlargement* of the cord in the lower half of the neck and the *lumbosacral enlargement* at the lower end of the spinal cord.

The spinal cord terminates approximately at the lower end of the second lumbar vertebra. The reason for this is that during growth of the fetus and young child the spinal cord does not continue to lengthen as the vertebral column lengthens, so that the cord becomes located progressively more superiorly in the vertebral canal. Yet the lower lumbar and sacral segments of the spinal cord still exist, and the lumbar and sacral spinal nerves still arise from the cord, but they arise from higher up in the vertebral canal because the levels of the cord segments no longer correspond to the levels of the vertebrae. The nerves then course downward through the lower canal as a large bundle of nerves called the *cauda equina*, and each of them finally emerges through its appropriate lumbar or sacral intervertebral foramen.

The Internal Structure of the Spinal Cord. Like the brain, the spinal cord is composed of areas of *gray matter* and areas of *white matter*, though the white matter is on the surface of the cord, whereas the gray matter is deep. These are illustrated in the cross-sectional view of the cord in Figure 3–9. The *nerve cell bodies* are in the gray matter along with many short nerve fibers as well. But in the white matter, only *fiber tracts* and *glia* exist. Note in Figure 3–9 that the gray matter has the appearance of multiple horns connected by a crossbridge called the *gray commissure* between the two halves of the cord. Many fiber tracts also pass from one side of the cord to the other through *white commissures* that accompany the gray commissure.

The horns of gray matter on each side of the cord are called respectively (1) the *ventral gray horn* (or the *anterior gray horn*), (2) the *dorsal gray horn* (or the *posterior gray horn*), and (3) the *lateral gray horn*.

It is in the ventral horn that the *anterior motor neurons* lie, the nerve cell bodies that send fibers through the spinal nerves to the muscles to cause muscle contraction. In the dorsal gray horn are the nerve cell bodies that receive sensory signals from the spinal nerves. In the lateral gray horn the nerve cells give rise to fibers that lead into the autonomic nervous system, the system that controls many of the internal organs.

Connections of the Spinal Nerves with the Spinal Cord. Note also in Figure 3–9 that each spinal nerve connects with the cord by way of two roots called the *dorsal root* and the *ventral root* (also called *posterior root* and *anterior root*). Each of these roots in turn enters or leaves the cord by way of 7 to 10 small *root filaments*. The dorsal root is also called the *sensory root* because it carries only sensory fibers; and the anterior root is called the *motor root* because it carries only motor fibers leading from the cord to the muscles to cause muscle contraction or to the autonomic nervous system to control the activity of the internal organs. The nerve fibers in the ventral root originate from neurons in the ventral and lateral gray horns and then leave the cord along its anterolateral margin in the ventral root filaments. The dorsal root filaments pierce the cord along its posterolateral border, and its nerve fibers then turn either up or down the cord or enter the dorsal gray horn.

On the dorsal root is an enlargement called the *dorsal root ganglion*. This ganglion contains unipolar nerve cells that have no dendrites but do have the usual single axon. However, immediately after the axon leaves the cell body it divides into two branches, a *peripheral branch* and a *central branch*. The peripheral branch passes through the peripheral portions of the spinal nerve to sensory receptors in the body, and the central branch passes into the spinal cord. About two thirds of the sensory fibers entering the cord terminate in the dorsal gray horn near the point of entry. The other third divides immediately into two branches, one branch terminating in the dorsal horn but the other branch passing all the way up the cord in the white matter and then terminating in the gracile and cuneate nuclei in the lower part of the medulla.

Function of the Spinal Cord Gray Matter. The gray matter of the spinal cord serves two functions. First, its synapses *relay signals between the periphery and the brain* in both directions. It is mainly in the dorsal horns that sensory signals are relayed from the sensory roots of the spinal nerves, then pass superiorly in the white matter of the cord to the various sensory areas of the brain. It is mainly in the ventral and lateral horns that motor signals are relayed from the descending nerve tracts from the brain into the motor roots of the spinal nerves.

Second, the gray matter of the cord functions to *integrate some motor activities*. For instance, when the hand is subjected to a painful stimulus, the sensory signals entering the cord cause an immediate reaction in the gray matter of the cord hand region. Within a fraction of a second this leads to motor signals that cause withdrawal of the hand from the

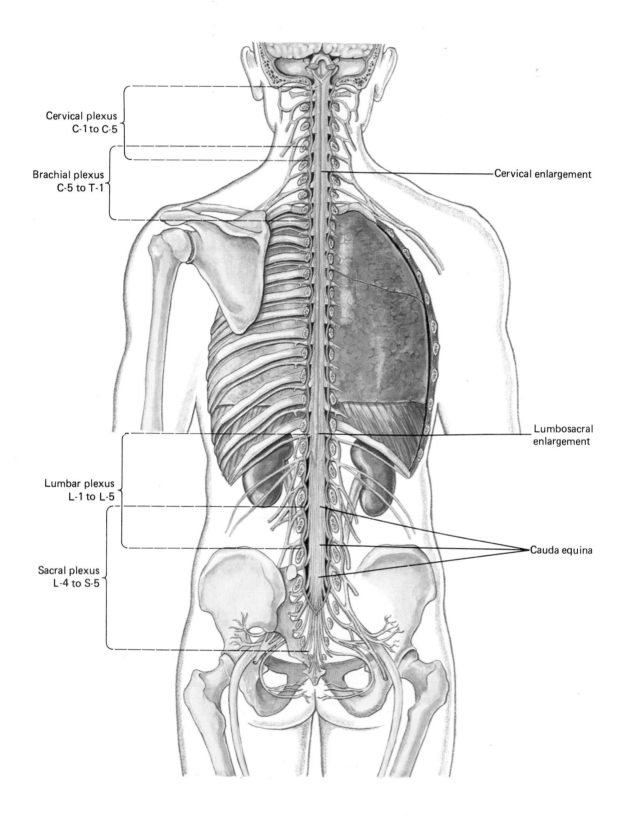

Cervical plexus
C-1 to C-5

Brachial plexus
C-5 to T-1

Cervical enlargement

Lumbosacral
enlargement

Lumbar plexus
L-1 to L-5

Cauda equina

Sacral plexus
L-4 to S-5

Figure 3–8. The spinal cord, its relationship to the peripheral nerves, and the spinal nerve plexuses.

Table 3–2. THE SPINAL CORD

Structure	Function
Gray Matter	
Dorsal horns	Loci of sensory input neurons
Lateral horns	Loci of preganglionic autonomic neurons
Ventral horns	Loci of motor neurons for skeletal muscles
White Matter	
Propriospinal tracts	Signals between cord segments
Long motor tracts	
1. Lateral corticospinal	Motor signals from cortex to spinal cord
2. Ventral corticospinal	Same
3. Rubrospinal	Motor signals from brain stem to spinal cord; most are excitatory,
4. Reticulospinal	a few are inhibitory
5. Olivospinal	
6. Vestibulospinal	
7. Tectospinal	
Long sensory tracts	
1. Fasciculus gracilis and fasciculus cuneatus	Discriminatory sensory signals to gracile and cuneate nuclei, thence to thalamus in medial lemnisci
2. Ventral and lateral spinothalamic	Crude touch, pain, and temperature signals to brain stem and thalamus
3. Ventral and dorsal spinocerebellar	Proprioceptor sensory signals to cerebellum
4. Spino-olivary	Cord signals to inferior olivary nuclei, then relayed to cerebellum
Spinal Nerve Roots	
Dorsal	Sensory input
Ventral	Motor output to muscles and preganglionic output to autonomic nervous system

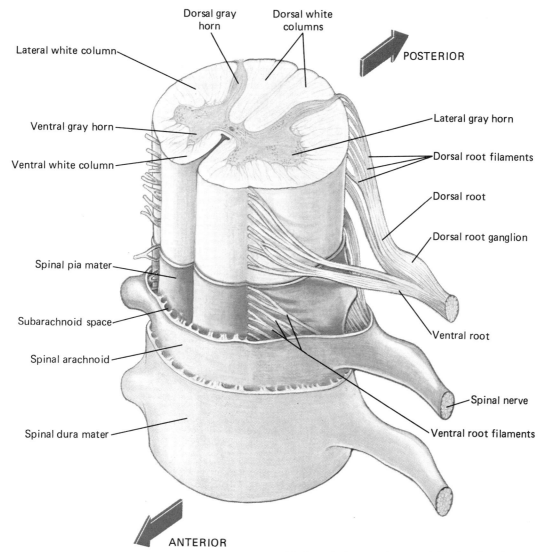

Figure 3–9. Structure of the spinal cord, and its connections with the spinal nerves by way of the dorsal and ventral spinal roots. Note also the coverings of the spinal cord, the meninges.

31

painful stimulus. This is called the *withdrawal reflex* (or flexor reflex or pain reflex). This reaction occurs entirely independently of the higher levels of the nervous system. Some other cord reflexes are (1) reflexes that cause tonic contraction of the extensor muscles of the legs when one stands, thus allowing the legs to support the weight of the body; (2) scratch reflexes in lower animals when they are tickled; (3) stretch reflexes that cause muscles to contract when they are stretched (this is the reflex that causes the knee jerk when the patellar tendon is struck); and (4) even walking reflexes.

The Long Fiber Pathways of the Spinal Cord. Figures 3–9 and 3–10 show that the cord white matter is also divided into columns. These are (1) two *dorsal* (or *posterior*) *white columns* lying between the dorsal gray horns, (2) two *lateral white columns* lying on each side of the cord lateral to the gray matter, and (3) two *ventral* (or *anterior*) *white columns,* lying between and anterior to the ventral gray horns.

All these columns contain fiber tracts that run lengthwise along the cord. Some of these, called *propriospinal tracts,* travel for only a few segments of the cord, connecting separate cord segments of gray matter with one another to help in the performance of the cord reflexes. (A "segment" of the cord is that portion of the cord that corresponds to a single pair of spinal nerves.) The propriospinal tracts lie immediately adjacent to the gray matter, as illustrated in Figure 3–10. The remainder of the white matter contains long fiber tracts that carry sensory information to the brain or motor signals from the brain to the cord. To the left in Figure 3–10 are the motor tracts, and to the right are the sensory tracts. These are described here:

Motor Tracts

1. *Lateral corticospinal tract,* from the motor cortex of the brain.
2. *Ventral corticospinal tract,* also from the motor cortex of the brain.
3. *Rubrospinal tracts,* from the red nucleus of the mesencephalon.
4. *Reticulospinal tracts,* from the reticular substance of the mesencephalon, pons, and medulla.
5. *Olivospinal tract,* from the inferior olive of the medulla.
6. *Vestibulospinal tract,* from the vestibular nuclei of the medulla and pons.
7. *Tectospinal tract,* from the tectum of the mesencephalon.

Sensory Tracts

1. *Fasciculus gracilis* and *fasciculus cuneatus* (the two of which together make up most of the dorsal white columns), carrying signals directly from the spinal sensory roots all the way to the gracile and cuneate nuclei in the lower end of the medulla.
2. *Ventral* and *lateral spinothalamic tracts,* carrying signals relayed in the posterior gray horn, thence through the anterior white commissure, and finally upward on the opposite side of the cord to the brain stem and thalamus.
3. *Ventral* and *dorsal spinocerebellar tracts,* which relay signals from the posterior gray horns upward to the cerebellum.

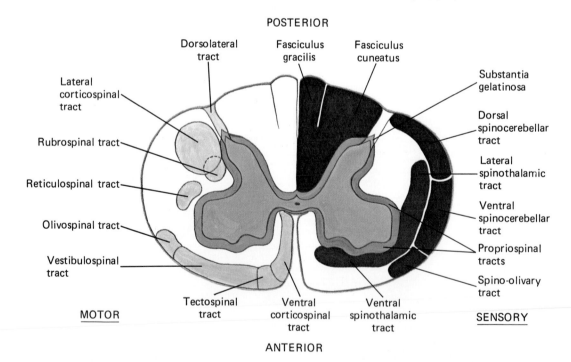

Figure 3–10. A cross-sectional view of the major long nerve fiber pathways of the spinal cord.

4. *Spino-olivary tract*, from the posterior gray horns of the cord to the inferior olive of the medulla.

Stimulation of most motor tracts causes either increased muscle tone or actual muscle contraction, and these tracts are said to be *excitatory tracts;* but stimulation of some tracts can decrease muscle tone, and they are called *inhibitory tracts.*

The sensory signals transmitted in the dorsal column pathways (the fasciculus gracilis and fasciculus cuneatus) are mainly those of fine, discriminatory touch that allow one to recognize the surface locations of sensory stimuli on the skin or the positions of the different parts of the body. The sensory signals transmitted in the spinothalamic tracts are those of crude touch, pain, and temperature. The sensory signals transmitted in the spinocerebellar tracts and also in the spino-olivary tract are mainly signals from the muscles and joints that apprise the cerebellum at all times about the movements and positions of different parts of the body so that the cerebellum can help in coordinating the body's movements.

THE CEREBROSPINAL FLUID SYSTEM—A PROTECTIVE FLUID FLOTATION SYSTEM FOR THE BRAIN AND SPINAL CORD

Even though the brain and spinal cord are crucial to the function of our bodies, nevertheless they are extremely delicate structures. For instance, the brain's tissues are so weak that one can push a finger all the way through it with almost no pressure, and the brain can literally be scooped out of the cranial vault with a spoon. Therefore, the brain requires a special protective system. This protection is achieved by the encasement of both the brain and the spinal cord in a rigid, bony vault comprised of the *cranial cavity* in the skull and the *vertebral canal* in the vertebral column. Within this vault, the brain and spinal cord actually "float" in a bath of fluid called the *cerebrospinal fluid.* This flotation system for the brain is illustrated in Figure 3–11. Now, let us describe this system and the mechanisms for maintaining the fluid in the system.

The Ventricular System in the Brain. In several cross-sectional views of the brain presented in the previous chapter and in the first part of this chapter, large fluid cavities called *ventricles* were shown deep inside the cerebrum, diencephalon, and brain stem. These ventricles, four in number, are illustrated in three-dimensional perspective in Figure 3–12. They are as follows:

1 and 2. The *two lateral ventricles.* Each of these lies near the median plane in each cerebral hemisphere, extending all the way from the center of the frontal lobe anteriorly to the center of the occipital lobe posteriorly. From the parietal region of each of these ventricles an inferior extension turns laterally and anteriorly into the temporal lobe; this is called the *inferior horn of the lateral ventricle.*

3. The *third ventricle.* This lies between the two lateral halves of the thalamus and also extends anteriorly and inferiorly into the midline plane between the two halves of the hypothalamus.

4. The *fourth ventricle.* This lies in the lower brainstem in the space posterior to the pons and medulla but anterior to the cerebellum.

Now, let us study Figure 3–11 to see how the ventricles interconnect with each other. This figure shows the shadow of one of the lateral ventricles deep within a cerebral hemisphere that connects by way of an *interventricular foramen* (also called *foramen of Monro*) with the anterolateral part of the third ventricle. In turn, the third ventricle connects posteriorly and inferiorly with the *cerebral aqueduct* (*aqueduct of Sylvius*), which is a small tube passing downward through the mesencephalon to enter the fourth ventricle lying behind the pontine and medullary regions of the brain stem. Finally, three openings occur in the outer wall of the fourth ventricle through which fluid can flow onto the surface of the brain. One of these is the *medium aperture* (also called the *foremen of Magendie*) in the midline inferior to the cerebellum. The other two, the *lateral apertures* (also called the *foramina of Luschka*), are to the sides of the fourth ventricle.

The Fluid Space Surrounding the Brain and Spinal Cord (Subarachnoid Space), and the Meningeal Coverings of the Brain and Cord. Covering all surfaces of the brain and spinal cord is a thin fluid-filled space several millimeters thick called the *subarachnoid space.* This space is bounded by the coverings of the brain and cord, called the *meninges,* which are illustrated for the spinal cord in Figure 3–9 and shown over a section of the brain in Figure 3–13. There are three layers of meninges:

1. The *dura mater* is a strong fibrous covering that surrounds the entire central nervous system; it is bound tightly to the inner surface of the skull but only loosely to the vertebral canal where there is a loose connective tissue space called the *epidural space.*

2. The *arachnoid* is a delicate structure loosely attached to the inner surface of the dura mater. And beneath the arachnoid is the fluid space that surrounds the brain and cord, the *subarachnoid space.* This space is penetrated by large numbers of small *arachnoidal trabeculae* that are part of the arachnoid.

3. The *pia mater* is a thin fibrous and vascular covering of the brain and cord, attached tightly to their surfaces, even dipping into all fissures and sulci.

The blood vessels that serve the brain have special relations to the meninges. First, note in Figure 3–11 the large *venous sinus,* the superior sagittal sinus, that extends along the midline the entire length of the cerebrum from front to back. This large sinus lies within layers of dura mater, and it has a triangular cross-sectional appearance as shown in

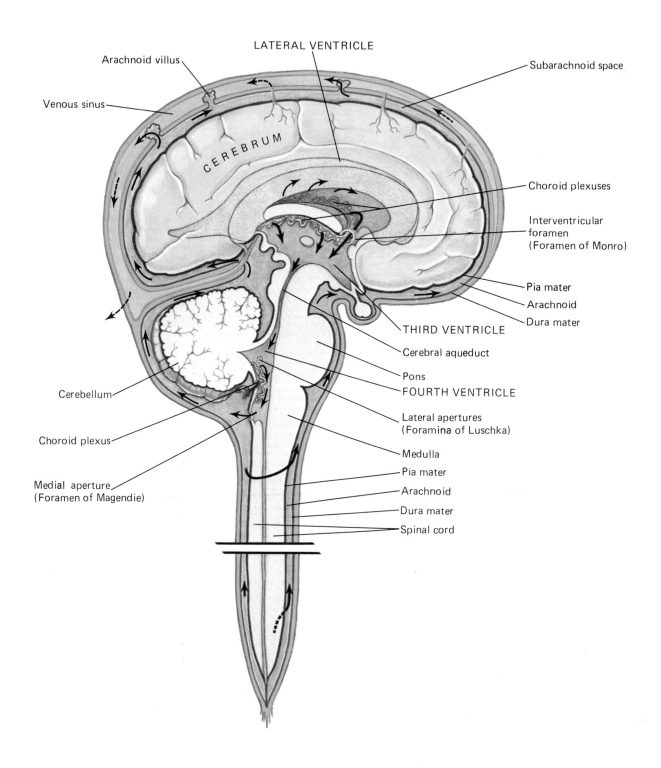

Figure 3–11. The cerebrospinal fluid system and the meningeal coverings of the brain and cord. Note the directions of flow of cerebrospinal fluid indicated by the arrows.

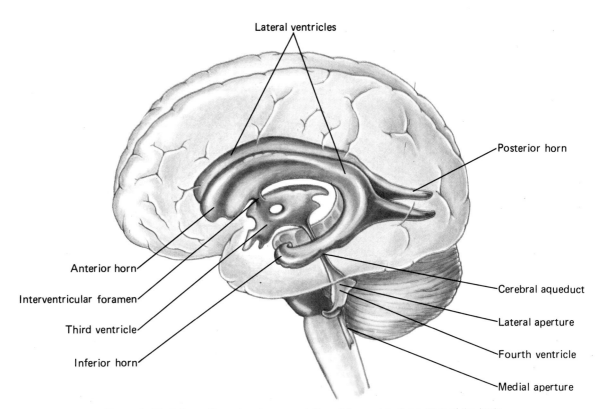

Figure 3–12. A three-dimensional representation of the ventricular system of the brain.

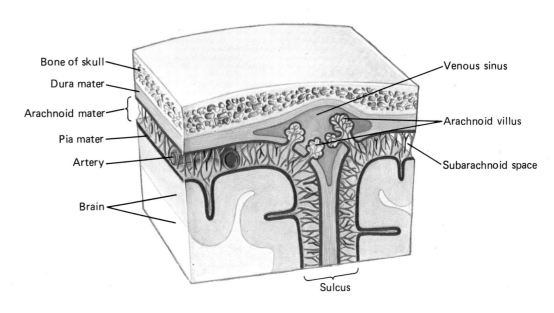

Figure 3–13. An expanded view of the meninges covering a section of the brain. Note also the venous sinus with arachnoid villi protruding into it.

Figure 3–13. Similar venous sinuses lie over other surfaces of the brain and also in the floor of the cranial cavity. All these sinuses interconnect and eventually give rise to the two internal jugular veins.

Next, note in Figures 3–11 and 3–13 the *arachnoid villi* that protrude into the venous sinuses. These are small penetrations of arachnoidal tissue that have made small openings in the walls of the sinuses. Cerebrospinal fluid can flow through these openings from the subarachnoid space into the venous blood. However, the villi function like valves to prevent blood from flowing backward from the venous sinuses into the subarachnoid space.

Finally, observe also in Figure 3–13 the large artery lying on the surface of the brain. Though this artery protrudes into the subarachnoid space, it is actually covered by the pia mater. Such arteries on the surface of the brain and penetrating branches from them provide nutrition to the brain.

Formation of Cerebrospinal Fluid by the Choroid Plexuses, and Fluid Flow Through the System. Most of cerebrospinal fluid is secreted by special secretory structures called *choroid plexuses* that protrude into each of the four ventricles, as shown in Figure 3–11. The most extensive choroid plexuses lie along the inferior surfaces of the lateral ventricles; therefore, most of the cerebrospinal fluid is formed in the lateral ventricles.

A small section of a choroid plexus is illustrated in Figure 3–14. It has a cauliflower-like growth, with large numbers of small capillary blood vessels embedded in loose connective tissue and covered by a thin layer of cuboidal cells that secrete fluid into the ventricle. The secreted cerebrospinal fluid is a clear, watery fluid that contains nearly the same constituents as the plasma portion of the blood except for the plasma proteins.

Once the fluid has been secreted by the choroid plexuses, it flows through the following pathway:

1. From the two lateral ventricles into the third ventricle by way of the two interventricular foramina.

2. From the third ventricle into the fourth ventricle by way of the cerebral aqueduct.

3. From the fourth ventricle into the subarachnoid space surrounding the brain stem through the median aperture and the two lateral apertures.

4. Through the subarachnoid spaces upward around the surfaces of the brain to the arachnoid villi.

5. From the subarachnoid spaces into the venous sinuses through the valvelike structures of the arachnoid villi.

The amount of cerebrospinal fluid formed each day is about 800 ml, and the pressure of this fluid in the cerebrospinal fluid system is about 10 mm Hg, only a very low pressure but enough to support the structures of the brain and spinal cord.

Hydrocephalus. Hydrocephalus is the condition in which there is too much fluid in part or all of the cerebrospinal fluid system of the brain. This can result from any one of several causes: (1) excess formation of fluid by the choroid plexuses, (2) obstruction of its flow at any one of several points in the flow system, or (3) obstruction of its reabsorption through the arachnoid-villi into the venous sinuses.

A common form of hydrocephalus occurs in newborn babies caused by congenital obstruction of the cerbral aqueduct ("congenital" refers to a condition that develops during formation of the fetus). Even normally this aqueduct is a very narrow tubular passage through the mesencephalon. When obstruction occurs, all the fluid formed by the choroid plexuses in the two lateral ventricles and in the third ventricle has no escape route from these inner

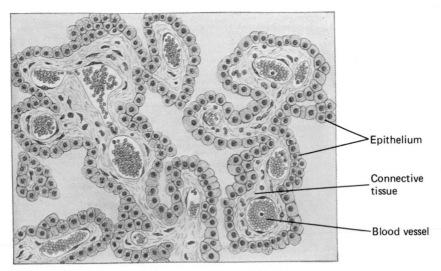

Epithelium

Connective tissue

Blood vessel

Figure 3–14. A microscopic section of a choroid plexus.

recesses of the brain. As a result, the lateral and third ventricles all become extremely enlarged, distending the brain and thinning the layers of the cerebrum. Obviously, this can cause serious mental disturbances if the condition becomes too severe. Also, in the newborn child with this type of hydrocephalus, the flat bones of the skull still have not fused with each other so that, if the condition is not treated, the skull bones are pushed apart and the head becomes tremendous in size—sometimes the size of a watermelon—with commensurate ballooning of the brain as well. Fortunately, though, a surgical procedure can be performed to make an artificial opening from the ventricular system into the subarachnoid space, into one of the veins, or into one of the cavities of the body to allow escape of the fluid. If this is performed early enough in life, the ravages of the process can often be prevented.

REFERENCES

See References, Chapter 4.

4

Gross Anatomy of the Nervous System: III. The Peripheral Nerves

THE CRANIAL NERVES

In several figures of the last two chapters nerves were shown leaving the basal surfaces of the brain. These, called *cranial nerves*, are illustrated in more detail in Figure 4–1, and their connections both in the brain and peripherally are given in Table 4–1.

There are 12 pairs of cranial nerves, numbered in order of their origin on the basal surface of the brain from anterior to posterior, usually using Roman numerals. Each also has its own individual name, which also appears in the figure.

CONNECTIONS OF THE CRANIAL NERVES INSIDE THE BRAIN

Note in Figure 4–1 that the tract to which the olfactory nerves connect arises from the cerebrum, the optic nerve from the diencephalon, and all the remaining ten from the brain stem. Because of their special functional importance for smell and vision, we shall discuss the connections of the olfactory nerves and tract with the brain in Chapter 26 in relation to the sense of smell and of the optic nerve in Chapter 24 in relation to vision. The connecting areas of the other cranial nerves in the brain stem are illustrated in Figure 4–2.

Some of the cranial nerves are entirely *sensory nerves*, some entirely *motor* (that is, they only innervate muscles to cause contraction), and some are combined nerves that have both sensory and motor components. To the left in Figure 4–2 are illustrated the *motor nuclei* to which the different motor and combined motor-sensory nerves connect. To the right are the *sensory nuclei*.

The Motor Nuclei of the Brain Stem. Beginning from the top in Figure 4–2, the important motor nuclei for the cranial nerves are as follows:

The *oculomotor, trochlear,* and *abducens nuclei* (nerves III, IV, and VI) send nerve fibers to the different muscles of the orbit for causing movement of the eye. The upper portion of the oculomotor nucleus is called the *Edinger-Westphal nucleus*. It controls the muscles inside the eye for focusing and for pupillary constriction.

The *trigeminal motor nucleus* (nerve V) controls the muscles of mastication (the muscles for chewing).

The *facial nucleus* (nerve VII) controls the many muscles of expression of the face.

The *dorsal vagal nucleus* (nerve X) is the important nucleus of the parasympathetic nervous system. It controls motor activity in many of the viscera, especially the heart (slowing of the heart), and of the upper digestive tract (increased peristalsis of the stomach and intestines and increased secretion).

The *nucleus ambiguus* sends signals through three different nerves, the glossopharyngeal, the vagus, and the accessory nerves (nerves IX, X, and XI). This nucleus controls such muscles as those for swallowing and the speech muscles of the larynx. The lower end of the nucleus ambiguus is continuous with the anterior horn of the spinal cord from which signals are transmitted through the spinal roots of the accessory nerve to control portions of the trapezius and sternocleidomastoid muscles.

The *hypoglossal nucleus* (nerve XII) controls primarily the movements of the tongue.

THE SENSORY NUCLEI OF THE BRAIN STEM

To the right in Figure 4–2 are the sensory nuclei of the brain stem. From above downward these are the following:

The *trigeminal nuclei* (nerve V) extends all the way from the mesencephalon downward into the upper part of the spinal cord. It has three major divisions: the *main sensory nucleus*, which subserves principally the function of tactile sensation for the face, mouth, and scalp; the *mesencephalic nucleus*, which receives signals mainly from muscles and other deep structures of the head; and the *spinal nucleus*, which is the principal nucleus for receipt of pain signals from the face, mouth, and scalp.

The *cochlear nucleus* (part of nerve VIII) is the receptor area for sound signals from the ear.

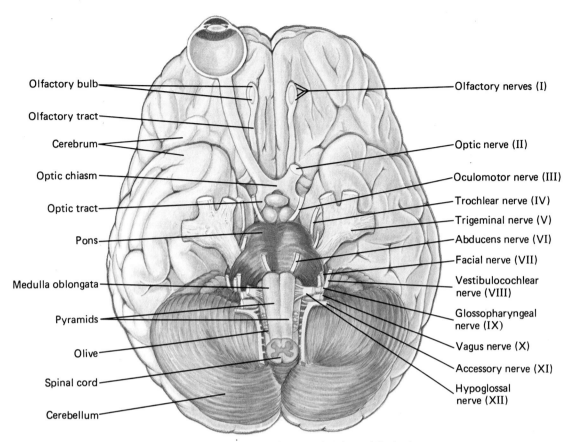

Figure 4–1. Origin of the cranial nerves from the ventral surface of the brain.

Table 4–1. THE CRANIAL NERVES

Nerve	Connection with Brain	Function
I. Olfactory nerves and tract	Anterior ventral cerebrum	Sensory: from olfactory epithelium of superior nasal cavity
II. Optic nerve	Lateral geniculate body of the thalamus	Sensory: from retinae of eyes
III. Oculomotor nerve	Mesencephalon	Motor: to four eye-movement muscles and levator palpebrae Parasympathetic: smooth muscle in eyeball
IV. Trochlear nerve	Mesencephalon	Motor: to one eye-movement muscle, the superior oblique
V. Trigeminal nerve		
Ophthalmic branch	Pons	Sensory: from forehead, eye, superior nasal cavity
Maxillary branch	Pons	Sensory: from inferior nasal cavity, face, upper teeth, mucosa of superior mouth
Mandibular branch	Pons	Sensory: from surfaces of jaw, lower teeth, mucosa of lower mouth, and anterior tongue Motor: to muscles of mastication
VI. Abducens	Pons	Motor: to one eye-movement muscle, the lateral rectus
VII. Facial	Junction pons and medulla	Motor: to facial muscles of expression and cheek muscle, the buccinator
VIII. Vestibulocochlear		
Vestibular branch	Junction pons and medulla	Sensory: from equilibrium sensory organ, the vestibular apparatus
Cochlear branch	Junction pons and medulla	Sensory: from auditory sensory organ, the cochlea
IX. Glossopharyngeal	Medulla	Sensory: from pharynx and posterior tongue, including taste Motor: superior pharyngeal muscles
X. Vagus	Medulla	Sensory: much of viscera of thorax and abdomen Motor: larynx and middle and inferior pharyngeal muscles Parasympathetic: heart, lungs, most of digestive system
XI. Accessory	Medulla and superior spinal segments	Motor: to several neck muscles, sternocleidomastoid and trapezius
XII. Hypoglossal	Medulla	Motor: to intrinsic and extrinsic muscles of tongue

MOTOR   SENSORY

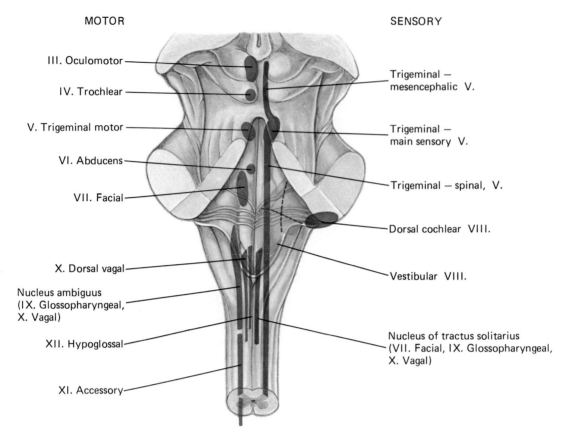

Figure 4–2. The motor and sensory nuclei of the cranial nerves in the brain stem (as seen posteriorly). The motor nuclei are illustrated to the left and the sensory to the right.

The *vestibular nucleus* (the other part of nerve VIII) receives signals from the vestibular apparatus, the sensory organ for equilibrium.

The *nucleus of the tractus solitarius* is the principal nucleus for receipt of visceral sensory signals from such organs as the heart, stomach, special blood pressure receptors (the baroreceptors), and taste buds of the mouth. This nucleus receives signals through the facial, glossopharyngeal, and vagus nerves (nerves VII, IX, and X).

THE EXTERNAL DISTRIBUTIONS OF THE CRANIAL NERVES

The Olfactory Nerves and Olfactory Tract (I). The olfactory nerves and olfactory tract are the sensory pathway for smell. The olfactory nerves are about 20 small nerves, each 1 to 2 cm in length, that arise from the olfactory epithelium, the sensory organ for smell located in the superiormost portion of the nasal cavity on the surfaces of the septum and superior concha. These 20 small olfactory nerves pass through an equal number of foramina in the cribriform plate of the ethmoid bone that forms the superior boundary of the nasal cavity and separates this cavity from the anterior fossa of the cranial cavity. Lying on the superior surface of the cribriform plate and inferior surface of the frontal

lobe of the cerebrum is the *olfactory bulb*, and leading posteriorly from this is the *olfactory tract* that terminates in the *olfactory areas of the cerebrum* located in and between the inferior medial portions of the two temporal lobes. After the olfactory nerves pass through the cribriform plate, some of their fibers terminate at synapses in the olfactory bulb, whereas others continue posteriorly in the olfactory tract, terminating in the cerebral olfactory areas, which will be discussed in Chapter 26.

Optic Nerve (II). Also illustrated in Figure 4–1 is the entire extent of the optic nerve. After leaving the eye, this nerve passes through the posterior recesses of the orbit, then through the optic foramen of the sphenoid bone, finally reaching the basal surface of the brain at the posteromedial limit of the frontal lobes. At this point the lateral half of the optic nerve continues posteriorly along the lateral surface of the hypothalamus, while the medial half abruptly bends medially and crosses to the opposite side through the *optic chiasm* lying anterior to the inferior hypothalamus. The crossed medial fibers then combine with the uncrossed lateral fibers on the opposite sides to form the two *optic tracts*, which course posteriorly along the lateral surfaces of the hypothalamus and terminate in the *lateral geniculate bodies* in the posterior thalamus.

Oculomotor Nerve (III), Trochlear Nerve (IV), and Abducens Nerve (VI). These are the nerves that control the eye movements. Note in Figure 4–1 that the oculomotor nerve leaves the brain stem near the midline of the anterior surface of the mesencephalon. The trochlear nerve arises from the lower posterolateral surface of the mesencephalon and then wraps around its side to its anterior aspect. The abducens nerve arises from the pons at its medullary junction. All these nerves then course through the *superior orbital fissure* into the orbit and innervate the extraocular and intraocular muscles as illustrated in Figure 4–3. The extraocular muscles attach to the eyes to cause the eye movements, and the intraocular muscles control focusing of the eyes and constriction of the pupil.

Trigeminal Nerve (V). As illustrated in Figure 4–1, the trigeminal nerve arises from the anterolateral surface of the midpons. It immediately enlarges for a distance of 1 cm to a diameter about two times its original diameter. This portion of the nerve is called the *trigeminal ganglion*; it contains the cell bodies of the nerve's sensory fibers and therefore is analogous to the dorsal root ganglia of the spinal nerves. Arising from the trigeminal ganglion are three major branches of the nerve illustrated in Figure 4–4: (1) the *ophthalmic division*, (2) the *maxillary division*, and (3) the *mandibular division*.

The ophthalmic and maxillary divisions are both entirely sensory. The ophthalmic nerve passes through the upper reaches of the orbit and branches onto the surface of the nose and superiorly over the forehead, supplying sensory nerves to these areas of the face and scalp and to the eye itself. It also sends branches to the nasal cavity and to the air sinuses.

The maxillary nerve leaves the cranial cavity through the *foramen rotundum*; then it passes through the inferior orbit and eventually through a bony canal underneath the eye to distribute over the anterior and lateral sides of the face to provide sensation. This nerve also supplies sensation to the upper teeth, the upper portions of the oral mucosa, and the mucosa of the nasal cavity and nasopharynx.

The mandibular nerve has both a sensory division and a motor division. This nerve passes through the foramen ovale into the space anterior and inferior to the temporal bone and medial to the ramus of the mandible, a space called the *infratemporal fossa*. The sensory division provides sensation to the most lateral portions of the face, the outer surfaces of the lower jaw and chin, the lower teeth, and the lower portions of the oral mucosa, including the anterior two thirds of the tongue. The motor division of the mandibular nerve innervates the muscles of mastication: the *temporalis*, the *masseter*, and the *medial* and *lateral pterygoid muscles*.

Facial Nerve (VII). The facial nerve arises from the brain stem at the posterolateral junction of the pons and the medulla (Fig. 4–1). It immediately passes through the internal auditory meatus and enters the facial canal in the temporal bone (shown in Fig 4–4) and enters the posterior facial region anterior and inferior to the ear, as illustrated in Figure 4–5. It then spreads through the superficial layers of the entire lateral and anterior facial regions to innervate all the muscles of facial expression as well as the buccinator muscle of the cheek. In its early course anterior to the ear it passes through or

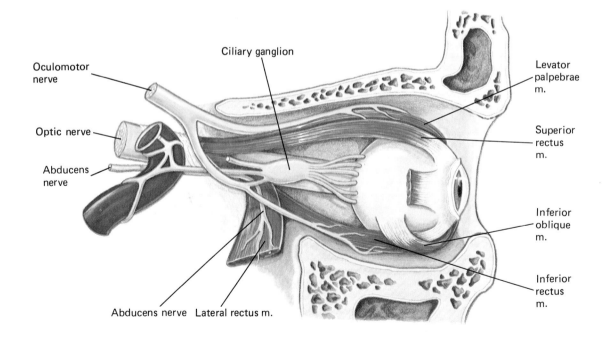

Figure 4–3. The oculomotor nerve (III), trochlear nerve (IV) and abducens nerve (VI) innervating the eye muscles and also the internal structures of the eyeball through the ciliary ganglion.

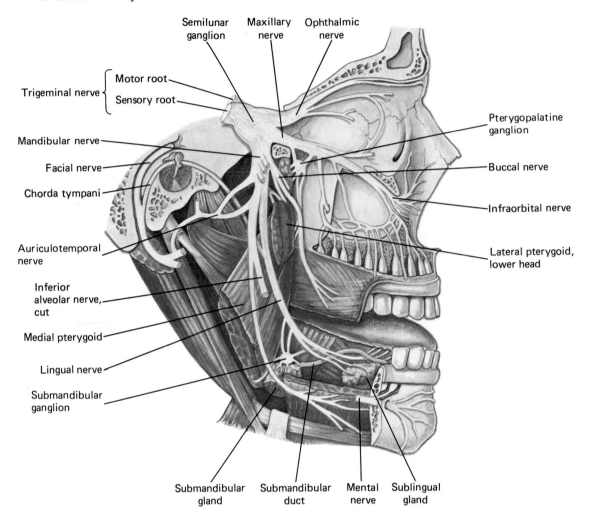

Figure 4–4. The trigeminal nerve (V) and its branches. Note also the chorda tympani that connects the lingual nerve (a branch of the trigeminal) to the facial nerve.

adjacent to the parotid gland, one of the glands for secretion of saliva. This gland on occasion becomes cancerous, in which case the facial nerve is often destroyed by the cancer or by the surgery required to remove the cancer. The person then loses all capability of emotional expression on that side of the face. He also becomes unable to close his eye completely and cannot keep his lips closed adequately on that side, and his cheek bulges outward with food everytime he eats. This combination is an extremely depressing and even debilitating condition for the patient.

Note also in Figure 4–4 a branch of the facial nerve called the *chorda tympani* that passes through the middle ear and eventually combines with the *lingual nerve,* one of the branches of the mandibular nerve. The fibers from the chorda tympani finally terminate (1) in the *submandibular ganglion,* from which nerves then extend to the submandibular and sublingual glands to control salivary secretion, and (2) in the anterior two thirds of the tongue to provide taste sensation. The sensory ganglion of the facial nerve is called the *geniculate ganglion,* and it is located in the facial canal.

Vestibulocochlear Nerve (VIII). The vestibulocochlear nerve arises from the pons-medullary junction just lateral to the facial nerve (Fig. 4–1). It is a short nerve that immediately enters the *internal auditory meatus* to innervate both the *vestibular apparatus* (the organ of equilibrium) and the *cochlea* (the organ of hearing). Both of these organs are contained within the petrous portion of the temporal bone itself.

Glossopharyngeal Nerve (IX). The glossopharyngeal nerve arises from the upper lateral border of the medulla (Fig. 4–1) and passes immediately from the cranial vault via the jugular foramen into the posterior pharyngeal region. Figure 4–6 illustrates this nerve leaving the cranial vault along with the vagus and accessory nerves. The glossopharyngeal nerve provides sensory innervation for the mucous membrane of the pharynx as well as for the posterior third of the tongue, including both general sensory and taste sensation from this area.

A motor branch of the glossopharyngeal also innervates the superior pharyngeal muscles that are important for swallowing.

Vagus Nerve (X). The vagus nerve arises from the lateral border of the medulla (Fig. 4–1) inferior to the glossopharyngeal nerve. Its entry into the cervical region via the jugular foramen, along with the glossopharyngeal and accessory nerves, is illustrated in Figure 4–6. It then courses inferiorly into the thorax alongside the common carotid artery and internal jugular vein. Branches from the vagus nerves in the neck and upper thorax supply the muscles of the larynx for control of speech. At the superior border of the heart, parasympathetic nerve branches from the vagi, together with sympathetic branches from the thoracic sympathetic chains, form the *cardiac plexus* from which nerves then innervate the heart. The distal portions of the vagus nerves continue inferiorly through the thorax alongside the esophagus and pass through the diaphragm to form *anterior* and *posterior gastric nerves.*

These give parasympathetic innervation to the stomach, the entire small intestine, the proximal colon, and other viscera of the abdominal cavity. Thus, the vagus nerve carries the majority of the parasympathetic nerve fibers that help to control the internal organs of the body, such as those controlling heart rate, stomach secretion, intestinal peristalsis, and so forth. The distal colon and pelvic organs receive parasympathetic innervation via sacral spinal nerves, as we shall discuss later.

The vagus nerve also conducts sensory nerve fibers to the medulla from all the same visceral areas that receive vagal sympathetic fibers.

The Accessory Nerve (XI). The accessory nerve arises from the lateral border of the inferior medulla as well as from the anterolateral surface of the upper five segments of the spinal cord (Fig. 4–7). It leaves the cranial vault via the jugular foramen along with the glossopharyngeal and vagus nerves, as illustrated in Figure 4–7. Some of its fibers then join the vagus nerve and innervate the muscles of

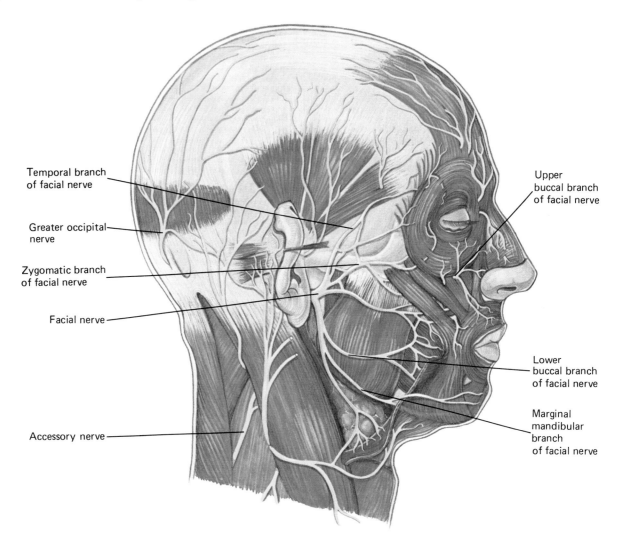

Temporal branch of facial nerve

Greater occipital nerve

Zygomatic branch of facial nerve

Facial nerve

Accessory nerve

Upper buccal branch of facial nerve

Lower buccal branch of facial nerve

Marginal mandibular branch of facial nerve

Figure 4–5. The facial nerve (VII) and the upper cervical portion of the accessory nerve (XI). Note the many branches of the facial nerve to the muscles of facial expression.

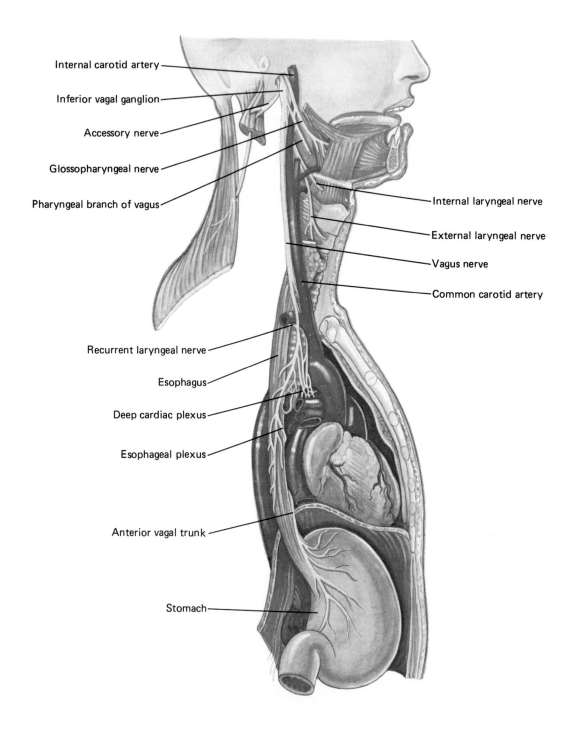

Internal carotid artery

Inferior vagal ganglion

Accessory nerve

Glossopharyngeal nerve

Pharyngeal branch of vagus

Internal laryngeal nerve

External laryngeal nerve

Vagus nerve

Common carotid artery

Recurrent laryngeal nerve

Esophagus

Deep cardiac plexus

Esophageal plexus

Anterior vagal trunk

Stomach

Figure 4–6. The glossopharyngeal nerve (IX), the vagus nerve (X), and the accessory nerve (XI).

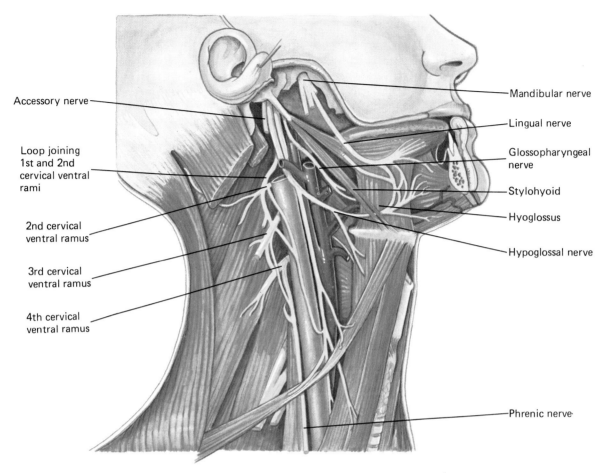

Figure 4–7. The lingual portion of the trigeminal nerve (V), the glossopharyngeal nerve (IX), the hypoglossal nerve (XII), and branches of the cervical plexus.

the larynx and the pharynx, but all of the fibers from the spinal roots of the accessory nerve course downward along the posterolateral portion of the neck to innervate portions of the sternocleidomastoid and trapezius muscles, as illustrated in Figure 4–6. These muscles also receive fibers from the cervical plexus in the neck region.

The Hypoglossal Nerve (XII). The hypoglossal nerve arises from the lateral border of the lower medulla (Fig. 4–1) anterior to the origins of the vagus and accessory nerves. It leaves the skull via the hypoglossal foramen. Figure 4–7 illustrates the entry of the hypoglossal nerve into the inframandibular region of the neck and its distribution to all the muscles of the tongue, including the hypoglossus, genioglossus, styloglossus, and intrinsic tongue muscles.

THE SPINAL NERVES

The anatomy of the spinal cord was discussed in the previous chapter, as was also the origin of the spinal nerves from the cord. To recapitulate, there is one pair of spinal nerves for each vertebral segment of the cord, and these nerves leave the

sides of the vertebral canal through the two *intervertebral foramina* between each two successive vertebrae. The purpose of the remainder of this chapter will be to describe the distributions of the peripheral extensions of the spinal nerves.

Referring again to Figure 3–8 in the previous chapter, showing an overview of the entire spinal cord and its spinal nerves, one can count *eight* pairs of cervical spinal nerves, specified as nerves C-1 through C-8; *twelve* pairs of thoracic spinal nerves, T-1 through T-12; *five* pairs of lumbar spinal nerves, L-1 through L-5; *five* pairs of sacral spinal nerves, S-1 through S-5; and *one* pair of extremely small coccygeal spinal nerves, Co.

The thoracic spinal nerves (those of the chest region) are relatively small. However, branches from these control the deep back muscles as well as the very large latissimus dorsi, the "climbing" muscle of the arm. Also, the thoracic spinal nerves give rise to the *intercostal nerves* that course around the body inferior to the ribs to supply the intercostal muscles and also to provide cutaneous innervation for the chest and abdomen. Extensions of the lower intercostal nerves also supply most of the muscles of the anterior abdominal wall.

By contrast the spinal nerves of the cervical,

lumbar, and sacral regions are very large; it is these nerves that provide motor control and sensation for the neck region, the back of the head, the shoulders and upper extremities, the lower trunk, and the lower extremities. Note also that all of these nerves, shortly after leaving the vertebral canal, interconnect among themselves to form four major plexuses:

1. The *cervical plexus,* formed by spinal nerves C-1 through C-5, supplies the neck, the back of the head, portions of the shoulder, and the diaphragm.

2. The *brachial plexus,* formed by C-5 through T-1, supplies most of the shoulder region, the arm, the forearm, and the hand.

3. The *lumbar plexus,* from L-1 through L-4, supplies some muscles of the lower back, the lower abdomen, and the anterior and medial thigh.

4. The *sacral plexus,* from L-4 through S-5, supplies the gluteal region, the posterior and lateral thigh, the leg, and the foot.

Now, let us look at these plexuses individually to see some of the details of their organizations and distributions.

THE CERVICAL PLEXUS

Figure 4–8 illustrates the cervical plexus that originates mainly between C-1 and C-4 but also receives a small nerve bundle from C-5. Two upper branches of the cervical plexus, the *lesser occipital* and the *greater auricular nerves,* supply sensation to the back of the scalp and the region around the ear. Branching from the lower border of the plexus, several *supraclavicular nerves* supply sensation to the lower neck, and branching anteriorly is the *transverse cutaneous nerve* that provides sensation for the anterior neck. The muscles supplied by the cervical plexus are most of the deep neck muscles, the superficial anterior neck muscles, the levator scapulae, and portions of the trapezius and sternocleidomastoid.

The Phrenic Nerve. Note especially the origin of the *phrenic nerve* from the cervical plexus between C-3 and C-5. This is the principal nerve that controls respiration. The phrenic nerves on the two sides course downward through the neck, then through the thorax on each side of the heart, and finally terminate in the diaphragm to control the breathing movements of this important respiratory muscle. Fractures of the cervical vertebrae, which occur especially in diving accidents, often crush the spinal cord. If the fracture occurs at the fifth through seventh cervical vertebra, as frequently is the case, the connections to the phrenic nerve will remain intact and the person can still breathe. However, all the other spinal nerves below this level will not

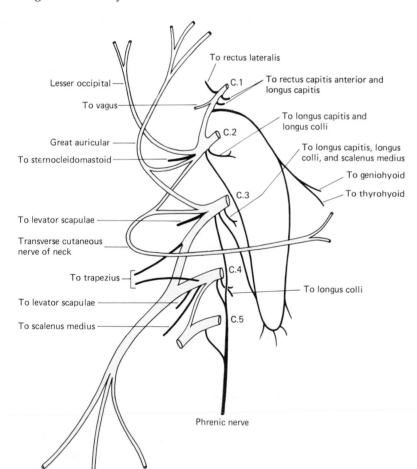

Lesser occipital

To vagus

Great auricular

To sternocleidomastoid

To levator scapulae

Transverse cutaneous nerve of neck

To trapezius

To levator scapulae

To scalenus medius

To rectus lateralis

C.1

To rectus capitis anterior and longus capitis

To longus capitis and longus colli

C.2

To longus capitis, longus colli, and scalenus medius

To geniohyoid

To thyrohyoid

C.3

C.4

To longus colli

C.5

Phrenic nerve

Supraclavicular

Figure 4–8. The cervical plexus and its branches.

receive appropriate signals from higher centers, and the entire body except for the neck muscles and this major breathing muscle, the diaphragm, will be paralyzed. This is the condition called *quadriplegia*.

THE BRACHIAL PLEXUS

Figure 4–9 illustrates the brachial plexus, arising from C-5 through T-1. These five spinal nerves are all very large. They unite to form *upper*, *middle*, and *lower trunks*, each of which splits into an *anterior* and a *posterior division*. All the divisions pass under the clavicle and over the first rib into the axilla (the armpit) where they again fuse into three large bundles called the (1) *lateral cord*, (2) *posterior cord*, and (3) *medial cord*. All along the course of this plexus multiple nerves are given off to provide both motor and sensory innervation to the shoulder, the superior portion of the anterior and lateral thorax, the arm, the forearm, and the hand. Table 4–2 gives the principal nerve branches of this plexus and the muscles that they innervate. In addition, multiple cutaneous branches conduct sensory signals from skin areas that roughly overlie these muscles.

In the cervical region, several medium-sized nerves are given off from the brachial plexus to cause contraction of the shoulder and anterior thoracic muscles. These nerves are the (1) *dorsal scapular*, (2) *long thoracic*, (3) *suprascapular*, (4) *subscapular*, and (5) *anterior thoracic*. The muscles that they innervate are given in Table 4–2.

At the termination of the brachial plexus in the axilla, the cords align themselves around the axillary artery and give rise to multiple branch nerves that extend into the upper extremity, the most important of which are (1) the *musculocutaneous nerve*, (2) the *radial nerve*, (3) the *median nerve*, and (4) the *ulnar nerve*.

Courses of the Major Nerves in the Upper Extremity. Figure 4–10 illustrates the courses of the four major nerves in the upper extremity. These supply both sensation to the skin and motor signals to the muscles along their courses.

The *musculocutaneous nerve*, upon leaving the plexus, curves laterally through the deep portions of the anterior arm and then continues superficially down the lateral surface of the forearm to provide sensory innervation. As it passes through the arm it innervates the anterior arm muscles listed in Table 4–2, the most important of which is the *biceps brachii*, which causes flexion of the forearm.

The *radial nerve*, after leaving the brachial plexus, curves posteriorly and laterally behind the humerus and enters the forearm over the lateral epicondyle of the humerus. Thereafter it follows mainly the lateral border of the radius and finally continues into the posterior portions of the thumb and first three fingers. Along its course in the arm, forearm, and dorsum of the hand the radial nerve gives off branches to muscles and to the skin to provide cutaneous sensation. The list in Table 4–2 of muscles innervated by this nerve demonstrates its importance in controlling movements of the upper extremity. Careful study will show that they are the muscles in the posterior arm and dorsal and lateral aspects of the forearm and hand. The principal movements that they cause are (1) extension of the elbow, (2) supination of the forearm and hand, (3)

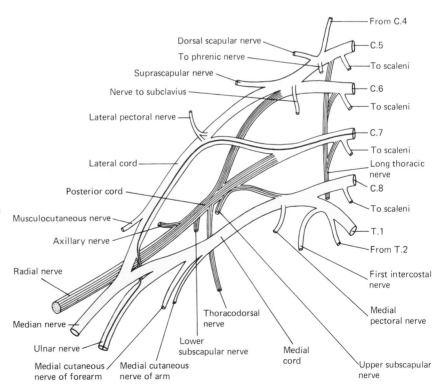

Figure 4–9. The brachial plexus and its branches.

Table 4-2. MAJOR NERVES FROM THE BRACHIAL PLEXUS, AND THE MUSCLES INNERVATED

Nerve	Spinal Cord Segment	Muscle
Dorsal scapular	C-5	Rhomboideus major
Long thoracic	C-5,6,7	Serratus anterior
Suprascapular	C-5,6	Supraspinatus Infraspinatus
Subscapular	C-5,6	Teres major Subscapularis
Anterior thoracic	C-5 through T-1	Pectoralis minor Pectoralis major
Musculo-cutaneous	C-5,6,7	Biceps brachii Coracobrachialis Brachialis
Radial	C-5 through T-1	Triceps brachii Brachialis Brachioradialis Supinator Extensor carpi radialis longus and brevis Extensor carpi ulnaris Extensor digitorum Extensor pollicis longus Extensor pollicis brevis Extensor indicis Abductor pollicis longus
Median	C-6 through T-1	Pronator teres Pronator quadratus Palmaris longus Flexor carpi radialis Flexor digitorum superficialis Flexor digitorum profundus (radial half) Flexor pollicis longus Flexor pollicis brevis (shared with ulnar nerve) Abductor pollicis brevis Opponens pollicis Lumbricals (on radial side of hand)
Ulnar	C-8, T-1	Flexor carpi ulnaris Flexor digitorum profundus (ulnar half) Flexor pollicis brevis (shaped with median nerve) Flexor digiti minimi brevis Abductor digiti minimi Adductor pollicis Opponens digiti minimi Lumbricals (on ulnar side of hand) Interossei

NOTE: The above nerves are listed in the approximate order that they leave the brachial plexus.

extension of the wrist, fingers, and thumb, and (4) abduction of the thumb.

The *median nerve*, after leaving the brachial plexus, passes down the anteromedial portion of the arm, then distally in the anterolateral portions of the forearm, passing next into the hand's lateral palm and into the anterior compartments of the thumb and first two fingers and lateral half of the third

finger. Again, along the course of this nerve, cutaneous branches give sensation to the skin. Table 4-2 shows that the median nerve also innervates approximately the lateral two thirds of the muscles in the anterior compartment of the forearm and lateral third of the anterior muscles of the hand. The major movements that these muscles cause are (1) pronation of the forearm and hand, (2) flexion of the wrist, fingers, and thumb, (3) abduction of the wrist, (4) abduction of the thumb, and (5) opponens motion of the thumb.

The *ulnar nerve* passes down the posteromedial portion of the arm, then behind the medial epicondyle of the humerus at the elbow joint, and finally alongside the ulna to enter the medial border of the hand, supplying both the anterior and posterior surfaces of the little finger and the medial half of the third finger. Along the course of this nerve, cutaneous branches provide sensation for the anteromedial surface of the forearm and the surface of the hand medial to the midline of the third finger. Also, Table 4-2 shows that the ulnar nerve innervates approximately the medial third of the muscles in the anterior forearm and the medial two thirds of the muscles in the anterior hand. These muscles cause mainly (1) flexion of the wrist and fingers (shared functions with the median nerve), (2) abduction of the fingers, (3) adduction of the fingers and thumb, and (4) opponens motion of the little finger.

Though it is not important at this point to memorize the exact distributions of all these nerves, surgeons find it essential to know these distributions precisely. When a nerve injury occurs, the surgeon can determine which nerve is damaged as well as where it is damaged by studying the areas of sensory loss on the skin and the specific muscles that are paralyzed. One of the most common points for severe damage is in the brachial plexus itself. For instance, if the arm is pulled upward with tearing force, the medial cord of the brachial plexus is especially likely to be damaged. From Figures 4-9 and 4-10 one will see that this can completely sever the fibers to the ulnar nerve and can destroy many of the fibers to the median nerve as well, mainly paralyzing the muscles along the medial side of the anterior forearm and hand and also causing sensory loss along these surface areas.

THE LUMBAR PLEXUS AND THE FEMORAL NERVE

The lumbar spinal nerves between L-1 and L-4 and a small branch from T-12 form the lumbar plexus, illustrated in Figure 4-11. This plexus lies on the posterior wall of the lumbar region of the abdominal cavity, then sends branches inferiorly along the lateral wall of the pelvis. Near its origin, branches from the plexus innervate a few muscles in the abdominal and back regions, including the low back muscles, the psoas major, the quadratus

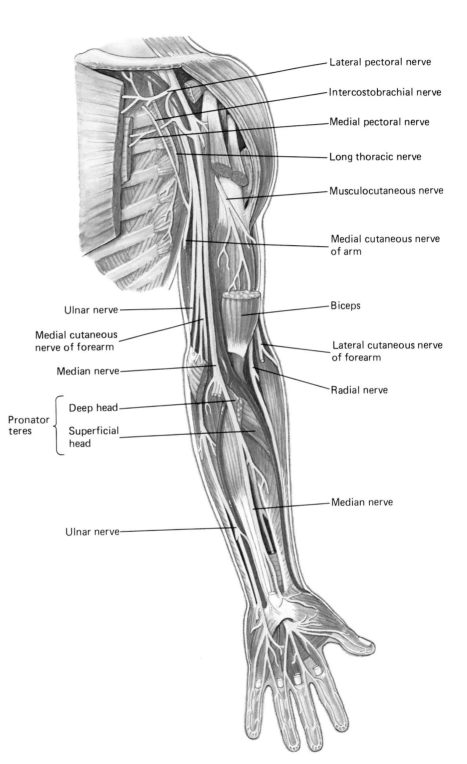

Lateral pectoral nerve

Intercostobrachial nerve

Medial pectoral nerve

Long thoracic nerve

Musculocutaneous nerve

Medial cutaneous nerve of arm

Biceps

Ulnar nerve

Medial cutaneous nerve of forearm

Lateral cutaneous nerve of forearm

Median nerve

Radial nerve

Deep head

Pronator teres

Superficial head

Median nerve

Ulnar nerve

Figure 4–10. The courses of the musculocutaneous, radial, median, and ulnar nerves down the arm, forearm, and hand.

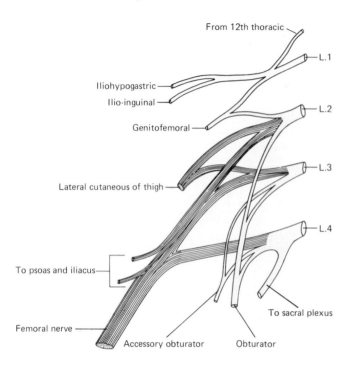

From 12th thoracic

L.1

Iliohypogastric

Ilio-inguinal

Genitofemoral

L.2

Lateral cutaneous of thigh

L.3

L.4

To psoas and iliacus

To sacral plexus

Femoral nerve

Accessory obturator   Obturator

Figure 4–11. The lumbar plexus and its branches, especially the femoral nerve.

lumborum, and the most inferior portions of the abdominal muscles. However, this plexus mainly sends nerves into the thigh, the three most important of which are as follows:

1. The *lateral femoral cutaneous nerve* (illustrated in Fig. 4–12A) enters the anterolateral thigh from underneath the inguinal ligament. This then passes downward along the lateral side of the thigh to provide sensory innervation to the skin.

2. The *obturator nerve* (Figs. 4–11 and 4–12A) originates from the lower portion of the lumbar plexus and enters the medial side of the thigh. This is mainly a motor nerve, controlling the large array of adductor muscles of the thigh that are listed in Table 4–3.

3. The *femoral nerve* (Figs. 4–11 and 4–12A) is by far the largest of the nerves from the lumbar plexus. Figure 4–12A shows that this nerve runs for a short distance parallel to the femoral artery in the upper thigh but divides into multiple large branches about 10 cm below the inguinal ligament. Some of these are muscular branches and some cutaneous. As shown in Figure 4–12A, and also in Table 4–3, the *muscular branches* innervate all the muscles of the anterior thigh, the most important of which are all the four heads of the very large quadriceps femoris muscle and also the sartorius muscle. These are both the principal flexors of the thigh and the single massive extensor muscle for the leg. In addition to these muscular branches, there are two principal cutaneous branches: the *anterior femoral cutaneous* nerve that innervates the skin of the anteromedial thigh all the way to the knee and the *saphenous nerve* that innervates the medial surfaces of the leg from the knee all the way to the foot.

THE SACRAL PLEXUS AND THE SCIATIC NERVE

The sacral plexus derives mainly from spinal nerves L-5 through S-3, but also from small branches of L-4 and S-4 to Co, as illustrated in Figure 4–13. This plexus lies along the posterior wall of the pelvis. Its principal branches are the following:

1. The *superior* and *inferior gluteal nerves* exit laterally from the pelvis to control mainly the gluteal muscles of the buttock and lateral hip, which cause both extension and abduction at the hip joint.

2. The *posterior femoral cutaneous nerve* passes down the back of the thigh and upper portion of the leg.

3. The *pudendal nerve* passes to the perineum and to the external genital organs, including the penis and scrotum in the male and the vagina in the female, to subserve sexual functions and sensations.

4. *Pelvic parasympathetic nerve branches* derived from sacral spinal nerves S-2 through S-4 pass to the pelvic organs to initiate such functions as defecation (emptying the rectum) and micturition (emptying the bladder), as well as playing roles in the involuntary acts of erection, orgasm, and ejaculation during sexual intercourse.

5. Several small nerves derived from spinal nerves S-3 and S-4 control the voluntary muscle sphincters around the anus and around the external urethra. These allow the person to prevent defecation or micturition when these are inconvenient.

6. The very large *sciatic nerve* is so important that it deserves special consideration as follows.

The Sciatic Nerve. The sciatic nerve, illustrated

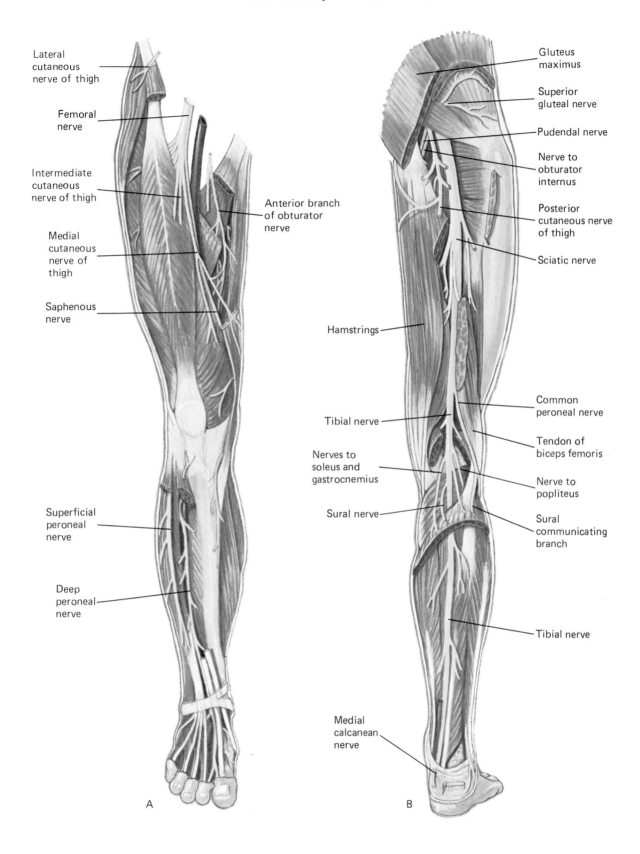

Figure 4–12. The principal nerves of the lower limbs shown in anterior (A) and posterior (B) views.

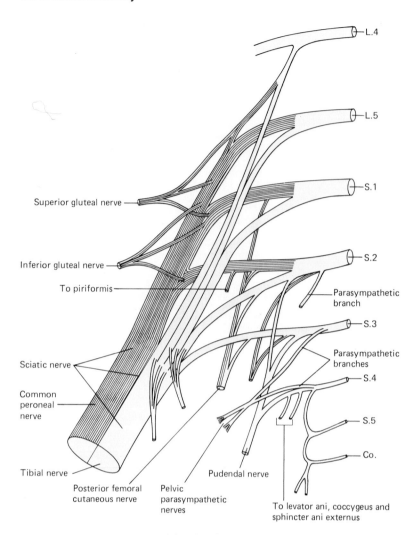

L.4

L.5

S.1

S.2

S.3

S.4

S.5

Co.

Superior gluteal nerve

Inferior gluteal nerve

To piriformis

Parasympathetic branch

Parasympathetic branches

Sciatic nerve

Common peroneal nerve

Tibial nerve

Posterior femoral cutaneous nerve

Pelvic parasympathetic nerves

Pudendal nerve

To levator ani, coccygeus and sphincter ani externus

Figure 4–13. The sacral plexus and its branches, especially the sciatic nerve.

in Figures 4–12B and 4–13, is by far the largest nerve of the body. It originates in the sacral plexus mainly from spinal segments L-5 to S-2, then leaves the posterior pelvis medial to the ischial tuberosity and courses distally in the posterior compartment of the thigh embedded between the hamstring muscles. Along this course, it supplies muscular branches to all the deep muscles posterior to the hip joint, listed in Table 4–3, and also the hamstring muscles. These muscles all cause extension of the thigh, and the hamstrings are also strong flexors of the leg.

At the lower end of the thigh, immediately above the knee joint, the sciatic nerve divides into two major branches, the *tibial nerve* and the *common peroneal nerve.* The tibial nerve continues distally in the posterior compartment of the leg, lying in the interval between the tibia and the fibula. It finally enters the medial side of the foot behind the medial malleolus. In this course it supplies sensory branches to the skin as well as branches to all the muscles of the back of the leg, especially to the soleus, the gastrocnemius, the tibialis posterior, and the flexors of the toes. The principal functions of

these muscles are to plantar flex the foot and toes and also to invert the foot.

The common peroneal nerve wraps around the lateral side of the fibula, where it divides into the *superficial* and *deep peroneal nerves.* The superficial peroneal nerve descends in the lateral leg to provide motor innervation to the peroneus muscles and cutaneous innervation to the dorsum of the foot. These muscles are the everters of the foot. The deep peroneal nerve descends in the anterior compartment of the leg in relation to the anterolateral muscles (the tibialis anterior and the extensor muscles of the toes) and controls them. Their principal function is dorsiflexion of the foot.

THE DERMATOMES

Each spinal nerve provides sensory innervation to a "segmental field" of the skin called a dermatome. This is true even though most of the spinal nerves appear to become mixed up with other spinal nerves as they pass through the plexuses. The different dermatomes for the separate spinal nerves

Table 4–3. MAJOR NERVES FROM THE LUMBAR AND SACRAL PLEXUSES, AND THE MUSCLES INNERVATED

Nerve	Spinal Cord Segment	Muscle
Lumbar Plexus		
Obturator	L-2,3,4	Pectineus (shared with femoral nerve)
		Adductor longus
		Adductor magnus (shared with sciatic)
		Adductor brevis
		Gracilis
Femoral	L-2,3,4	Sartorius
		Iliacus
		Pectineus (shared with obturator nerve)
		Quadriceps femoris
		1. Rectus femoris
		2. Vastus medialis
		3. Vastus lateralis
		4. Vastus intermedius
Other muscular branches	L-2,3	Psoas major
		Quadratus lumborum
Sacral Plexus		
Superior gluteal	L-4,5,S-1	Gluteus medius
		Gluteus minimus
		Tensor fasciae latae
Inferior gluteal	L-5,S-1,2	Gluteus maximus
Sciatic	L-4 through S-3	Adductor magnus (shared with obturator nerve)
		Obturator internus
		Superior gemellus
		Inferior gemellus
		Quadratus femoris
Tibial portion of the sciatic	L-4 through S-3	Biceps femoris (shared with peroneal nerve)
		Semitendinosus
		Semimembranosus
		Gastrocnemius
		Soleus
		Popliteus
		Tibialis posterior
		Flexor digitorum longus
		Flexor hallucis longus
		Plantar and medial foot muscles
Peroneal portion of the sciatic	L-4 through S-2	Biceps femoris (shared with tibial nerve)
		Tibialis anterior
		Peroneus longus
		Peroneus brevis
		Extensor digitorum longus
		Extensor hallucis longus
		Dorsal and lateral foot muscles
Pudendal	S-2,3,4	Muscles of urogenital triangle
Other muscular branches	S-3,4	Levator ani
		Coccygeus
		External anal sphincter

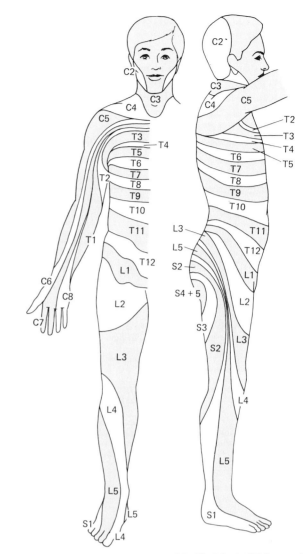

Figure 4–14. The dermatomes. (Modified from Grinker and Sahs: Neurology. Springfield, Ill., Charles C Thomas, 1966.)

are illustrated in Figure 4–14. However, in this figure, the dermatomes are shown as if there were distinct borders between the adjacent dermatomes. This is only partly true because the distal branches of the nerves invade one another's territory. For this reason, an entire single spinal nerve can often be destroyed without significant loss of sensation in the skin, but when several adjacent spinal nerves are destroyed, one can easily establish the extent of sensory loss and from this determine the segmental level of the nerve injury.

Figure 4–14 shows that the anal region of the body lies in the dermatome of the most distal cord segments, S-4 and S-5. In the embryo, this is the tail region and the most distal portion of the body. The lower limbs develop from the lumbar and upper sacral levels of the embryo rather than from the distal sacral segments, which is also evident from the dermatomal map, for the dermatomes of this limb are L-2 through S-2.

Note also in Figure 4–14 that the face and anterior half of the head are not designated by spinal nerve dermatomes. But remember that sensation in these areas is served by the three branches of the fifth cranial nerve (the trigeminal nerve).

THE AUTONOMIC NERVOUS SYSTEM

The autonomic nervous system is the collection of nerves that control most of the automatic subconscious functions of the body. It is so important to the function of almost every physiological system of the body that it will be discussed in detail in Chapter 21. However, at this point let us merely note that branches from all of the thoracic spinal nerves, the first three lumbar nerves, sacral nerves S-2 through S-5, and several cranial nerves—especially the vagus nerve—form the autonomic nervous system. It will become evident in Chapter 21 that this system has special properties that are uniquely different from those of all other portions of the peripheral nervous system.

REFERENCES

Anderson, J. E.: The cranial nerves. *In* Grant's Atlas of Anatomy. Baltimore, Williams & Wilkins, 1978, pp. 8–1 to 8–12.

Anderson, J. E.: The head. *In* Grant's Atlas of Anatomy. Baltimore, Williams & Wilkins, 1978, pp. 7–1 to 7–168.

Bloom, W., and Fawcett, D. W.: The nervous tissue. *In* A Textbook of Histology, 10th Ed. Philadelphia, W. B. Saunders, 1975, pp. 333–385.

Carpenter, M. D.: Human Neuroanatomy, 18th Ed. Baltimore, Williams & Wilkins, 1983.

Copenhaver, W. M., Kelly, D. E., and Wood, R. L.: Nervous system. *In* Bailey's Textbook of Histology, 17th Ed. Baltimore, Williams & Wilkins, 1978, pp. 290–357.

Figge, F. H. J.: The central nervous system. *In* Sobotta/Figge Atlas of Human Anatomy. Vol. III. Baltimore, Urban & Schwarzenberg, 1977, pp. 1–131.

Fujita, T., Tanaka, K., and Tokunaga, J.: Muscles, nerves, and brain. *In* SEM Atlas of Cells and Tissues. New York, Igaku-Shoin, 1981, pp. 312–328.

Goss, C. M.: The nervous system. *In* Gray's Anatomy of the Human Body, 29th Ed. Philadelphia, Lea & Febiger, 1973, pp. 777–1089.

Ham, A. W., and Cromack, D. H.: Nervous tissue. *In* Histology, 8th Ed. Philadelphia, J. B. Lippincott, 1979, pp. 483–539.

Hammersen, F.: Nervous system. *In* Sobotta/Hammersen Histology. Baltimore, Urban & Schwarzenberg, 1980, pp. 203–216.

Hammersen, F.: Nervous tissue and neuroglia. *In* Sobotta/Hammersen Histology. Baltimore, Urban & Schwarzenberg, 1980, pp. 80–93.

Langman, J., and Woerdeman, M. W.: Head and neck. *In* Atlas of Medical Anatomy. Philadelphia, W. B. Saunders, 1978, pp. 351–472.

Leeson, T. S., and Leeson, C. R.: Nervous tissue. *In* A Brief Atlas of Histology. Philadelphia, W. B. Saunders, 1979, pp. 89–104.

Leeson, T. S., and Leeson, C. R.: Nervous tissue. *In* Histology, 4th Ed. Philadelphia, W. B. Saunders, 1981, pp. 216–256.

Netter, F. H.: Nervous system. *In* The CIBA Collection of Medical Illustrations. Vol. 1, Summit, N.J., CIBA Medical Education Division, 1972.

Pernkopf, E.: Brain and meninges. *In* Atlas of Topographical and Applied Human Anatomy. Vol. I. Philadelphia, W. B. Saunders, 1980, pp. 29–135.

Snell, R. S.: Clinical Neuroanatomy. Boston, Little, Brown, 1980.

Williams, P. L., and Warwick, R.: The nervous system. *In* Gray's Anatomy, 36th British Edition. Philadelphia, W. B. Saunders, 1980, pp. 802–1215.

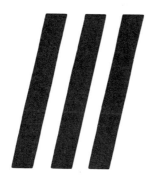

MEMBRANE BIOPHYSICS, NERVE, AND MUSCLE

5

Transport of Ions Through the Cell Membrane

The transmission of nerve signals is the basis of function in the nervous system. However, to understand nerve transmission, one must first be familiar with the biophysics of the nerve cell membrane, especially with the transport of ions through this membrane and the development of electrical potentials across it. It is the purpose of this chapter to discuss the basic principles of these phenomena; the following chapter will utilize these basic principles to explain nerve transmission itself.

Concentrations of Ions and Other Substances on the Outside and Inside of the Cell Membrane

Figure 5–1 gives the approximate compositions of both the extracellular and intracellular fluids. Note that the extracellular fluid contains large quantities of *sodium ions* but only small quantities of *potassium ions*. Exactly the opposite is true of the intracellular fluid, with very large quantities of potassium ions

	Extracellular fluid	Intracellular fluid
Na⁺	142 mEq/L	10 mEq/L
K⁺	4 mEq/L	140 mEq/L
Ca⁺⁺	5 mEq/L	< 1 mEq/L
Mg⁺⁺	3 mEq/L	58 mEq/L
Cl⁻	103 mEq/L	4 mEq/L
HCO₃⁻	28 mEq/L	10 mEq/L
Phosphates	4 mEq/L	75 mEq/L
SO₄⁻⁻	1 mEq/L	2 mEq/L
Glucose	90 mg %	0 to 20 mg %
Amino acids	30 mg %	200 mg % ?
Cholesterol Phospholipids Neutral fat	0.5 g %	2 to 95 g %
Po₂	35 mm Hg	20 mm Hg ?
Pco₂	46 mm Hg	50 mm Hg ?
pH	7.4	7.0
Proteins	2 g % (5 mEq/L)	16 g % (40 mEq/L)

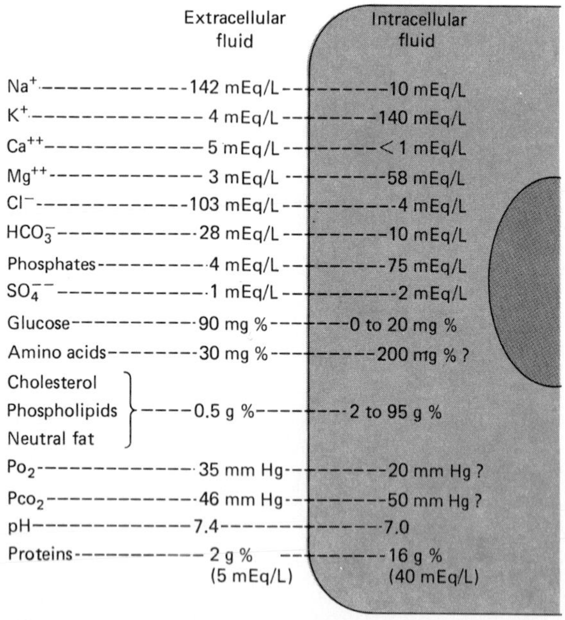

Figure 5–1. Chemical compositions of extracellular and intracellular fluids.

inside the cell but relatively small quantities of sodium ions. Also, inside the cell are high concentrations of phosphates and proteins, both of which are negatively charged. These ionic differences between the inside and the outside of the cell membrane are especially important in causing the negative electrical potential normally present inside all cells of the body, including the nerve fibers. Let us examine how these differences in ionic concentrations are brought about by the transport mechanisms of the cell membrane.

Structure of the Cell Membrane. The cell membrane consists of a *lipid bilayer* with large numbers of protein molecules floating in the lipid, many if not most of them penetrating all the way through, as illustrated in Figure 5–2.

The lipid bilayer is not miscible with either the extracellular or the intracellular fluid. Therefore, it constitutes a barrier for the movement of most water-soluble substances between the extracellular and intracellular fluid compartments. However, as illustrated by the left-hand arrow of Figure 5–2, a few substances can penetrate this bilayer and can either enter the cell or leave it, passing directly through the lipid substance itself.

The protein molecules, on the other hand, have entirely different transport properties. Their molecular structures interrupt the continuity of the lipid bilayer and therefore constitute an alternate pathway through the cell membrane. Most of these proteins, therefore, are *transport proteins*. Different proteins function differently. Some have watery spaces all the way through the molecule and allow free movement of certain ions or molecules; these are called *channel proteins*. Others, called *carrier proteins*, bind with substances that are to be transported, and conformational changes in the protein molecules then move the substances through the interstices of the molecules to the other side of the membrane. Both the channel proteins and the carrier proteins are highly selective in the type or types of molecules or ions that are allowed to cross the membrane.

Diffusion Versus Active Transport. Transport through the cell membrane, either directly through the lipid bilayer or through the proteins, occurs by one of two basic processes, *diffusion* (which is also

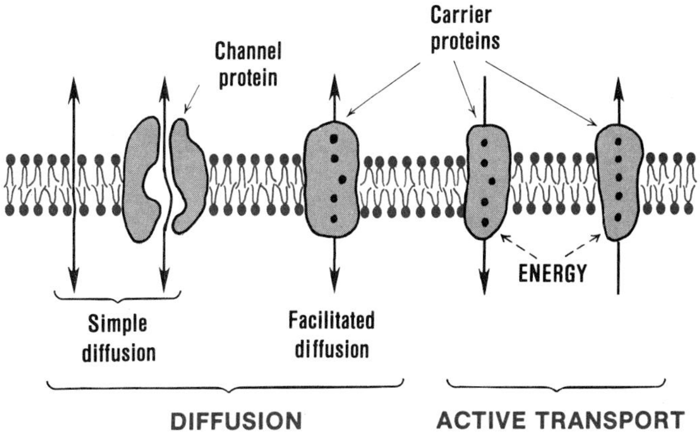

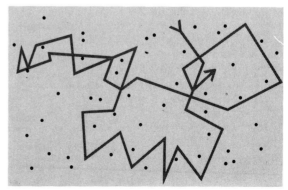

Figure 5–2. Transport pathways through the cell membrane and the basic mechanisms of transport.

called "passive transport") or *active transport.* Though there are many different variations of these two basic mechanisms, as we shall see later in this chapter, diffusion means random molecular movement of substances either through openings in the membrane or in combination with a carrier protein caused by the normal kinetic motion of matter. By contrast, active transport means movement of ions or other substances across the membrane in combination with a carrier protein but additionally *against an energy gradient*, such as from a low concentration state to a high concentration state, a process that requires chemical energy to cause the movement. Let us examine in more detail the basic physics and physical chemistry of these two separate processes.

DIFFUSION

All molecules and ions in the body fluids, including both water molecules and dissolved substances, are in constant motion, each particle moving its own separate way. Motion of these particles is what physicists call heat—the greater the motion, the higher the temperature—and motion never ceases under any conditions except at absolute zero temperature. When a moving molecule, A, approaches a stationary molecule, B, the electrostatic and internuclear forces of molecule A repel molecule B, adding some of the energy of motion to molecule B. Consequently, molecule B gains kinetic energy of motion while molecule A slows down, losing some of its kinetic energy. Thus, as shown in Figure 5–3, a single molecule in solution bounces among the other molecules first in one direction, then another, then another, and so forth, bouncing randomly billions of times each second.

This continual movement of molecules among each other in liquids, or in gases, is called *diffusion.* Ions diffuse in exactly the same manner as whole molecules, and even suspended colloid particles diffuse in a similar manner, except that they diffuse far less rapidly than molecular substances because of their very large sizes.

DIFFUSION THROUGH THE CELL MEMBRANE

Simple Diffusion

Diffusion through the cell membrane is divided into two separate subprocesses called *simple diffusion* and *facilitated diffusion.* Simple diffusion means the molecular kinetic movement of molecules or ions through a membrane opening without the necessity of binding with carrier proteins in the membrane. The rate of diffusion is determined by the amount of substance available, by the velocity of kinetic motion, and by the number of openings in the cell membrane through which the molecules or ions can move. On the other hand, facilitated diffusion requires the interaction of the molecules or ions with a carrier protein that aids its passage through the membrane, probably by binding chemically with it and shuttling it through the membrane in this form.

Simple diffusion can occur through the cell membrane by two pathways: through the interstices of the lipid bilayer and through watery channels in some of the transport proteins, as illustrated to the left in Figure 5–2.

Diffusion Through the Lipid Bilayer

Diffusion of Lipid-Soluble Substances. In experimental studies, the lipids of cells have been sepa-

Figure 5–3. Diffusion of a fluid molecular during a billionth of a second.

rated from the proteins and then reconstituted as artificial membranes consisting of a lipid bilayer but without any transport proteins. Using such an artificial membrane, the transport properties of the lipid bilayer by itself have been determined.

One of the most important factors that determines how rapidly a substance will move through the lipid bilayer is the lipid solubility of the substance. For instance, the lipid solubilities of oxygen, nitrogen, and alcohols are very high, so that all these can dissolve directly in the lipid bilayer and diffuse through the cell membrane in exactly the same manner that diffusion occurs in a watery solution. For obvious reasons, the rate of diffusion of these substances through the membrane is directly proportional to their lipid solubility.

Transport of Water and Other Lipid-Insoluble Molecules. Even though water is highly insoluble in the membrane lipids, nevertheless it penetrates the cell membrane very readily, most of it passing directly though the lipid bilayer and still more passing through protein channels as well. The rapidity with which water molecules can penetrate the cell membrane is astounding. As an example, the total amount of water that diffuses in each direction through the red cell membrane during each second is approximately 100 times as great as the volume of the red cell itself.

The reason for the extreme diffusion of water through the lipid bilayer is still not certain, but it is believed that the water molecules are small enough and their kinetic energy great enough that they can simply penetrate like bullets though the lipid portion of the membrane before the "hydrophobic" character of the lipids can stop them.

Other lipid-insoluble molecules also can pass through the lipid bilayer in the same way as water molecules if they are small enough. However, as they become larger, their penetration falls off extremely rapidly. For instance, the diameter of the urea molecule is only 20 per cent greater than that of water. Yet its penetration of the cell membrane is about a thousand times less than that of water. Even so, remembering the astonishing rate of water penetration, this amount of penetration still allows rapid transport of urea through the cell membrane. The glucose molecule, which has a diameter of less than three times that of the water molecule, penetrates the lipid bilayer 100,000 times less rapidly than water, thus illustrating that the only lipid-insoluble molecules that can penetrate the lipid bilayer are the very small ones.

Failure of Ions to Diffuse Through the Lipid Bilayer. Even though water and other very small uncharged molecules diffuse easily through the lipid bilayer, ions—even small ones such as hydrogen ions, sodium ions, potassium ions, and so forth—penetrate the lipid bilayer about one million times less rapidly than does water. Therefore, any significant transport of these through the cell membrane must occur through channels in the proteins, as we shall discuss shortly.

The reason for the impenetrability of the lipid bilayer to ions is the electrical charge of the ions; this impedes ionic movement in two separate ways: (1) The electrical charge of these ions causes multiple molecules of water to become bonded to the ions, forming so-called *hydrated ions.* This greatly increases the sizes of ions, which alone impedes penetration of the lipid bilayer. (2) Even more important, the electrical charge of the ion also interacts with the charges of the lipid bilayer in the following way. It will be recalled that each half of the bilayer is composed of "polar" lipids that have an excess of negative charge facing toward the surfaces of the membrane and an excess of positive charge in the central portion of the membrane. Therefore, when a charged ion tries to penetrate either the negative or the positive electrical barrier, it is instantaneously repulsed.

Diffusion Through Protein Channels and "Gating" of These Channels

The protein channels are believed to be watery pathways through the interstices of the protein molecules. Therefore, substances can diffuse directly through these channels from one side of the membrane to the other. However, the protein channels are distinguished by two important characteristics: (1) They are often selectively permeable to certain substances. (2) Many of the channels can be opened or closed by *gates.*

Selective Permeability of Different Protein Channels. Most, but not all, protein channels are highly selective for the transport of one or more specific ions or molecules. This results from the characteristics of the channel itself, such as its diameter, its shape, and the nature of the electrical charges along its surfaces. To give an example, one of the most important of the protein channels, the so-called *sodium channels,* are only 0.3 by 0.5 nm in size, but more importantly the inner surfaces of these channels are *strongly negatively charged,* as illustrated by the negative signs in the top panel of Figure 5–4. These strong negative charges pull the sodium ions more than they pull other physiologically important ions into the channels, because the ratio of pulling force to ionic diameter is far greater for sodium than for the others. Once in the channel, the sodium ion then diffuses in either direction according to the usual laws of diffusion. Thus, the sodium channel is specifically selective for the passage of sodium ions.

On the other hand, another set of protein channels is selective for potassium transport, illustrated in the lower panel of Figure 5–4. These channels are slightly smaller than the sodium channels, only 0.3 by 0.3 nm, but *they are not negatively charged.* Therefore, no strong attractive force is pulling ions into the channels. On the other hand, the hydrated form of the potassium ion is considerably smaller than the hydrated form of sodium because the sodium ion has one whole orbital set of electrons

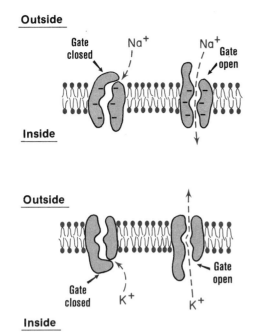

Figure 5–4. Transport of sodium and potassium ions through protein channels. Also shown are conformational changes of the channel protein molecules that open or close the "gates" guarding the channels.

less than the potassium ion, which allows the sodium nucleus to attract far more water molecules than can the potassium. Therefore, the smaller hydrated potassium ions can pass easily through this channel whereas sodium ions are mainly rejected, thus once again providing selective permeability for a specific ion.

Gating of Protein Channels. Gating of protein channels provides a means for controlling the permeability of the channels. This is illustrated in the upper and lower panels of Figure 5–4 for both the sodium and the potassium ion. It is believed that the gates are actual gate-like extensions of the transport protein molecule, which can close over the opening of the channel or can be lifted away from the opening by a conformational change in the shape of the protein molecule itself. In the case of the sodium channels, this gate opens and closes on the outer surface of the cell membrane, whereas for the potassium channels it opens and closes on the inner surface.

The opening and closing of gates are controlled in at least two principal ways:

1. *Voltage gating.* In this instance, the molecular conformation of the gate responds to the electrical potential across the cell membrane. For instance, when there is a strong negative charge on the inside of the cell membrane, the sodium gates remain tightly closed; yet when the inside of the membrane loses its negative charge these gates open suddenly and allow tremendous quantities of sodium to pass inward through the sodium pores (until still another set of gates at the cytoplasmic ends of the channels closes them, as explained in Chapter 6). This is the basic cause of action potentials in nerves that are responsible for nerve signals. The potassium gates also open when the cell membrane becomes positively charged inside the cell. However, this response is different from that of the sodium gates for they open much more slowly; the resulting outflow of potassium ions from the cell helps in the recovery of the nerve fiber membrane at the end of the action potential. These events will be discussed in the following chapter.

2. *Ligand gating.* Some protein channel gates are opened by the binding of another molecule with the protein, thus causing a conformational change in the protein molecule that opens or closes the gate. This is called *ligand gating,* and the substance that binds is the *ligand.* One of the most important instances of ligand gating is the effect of acetylcholine on the so-called *acetylcholine channel.* This opens the gate of this channel, providing a pore about 0.65 nm in diameter that allows all molecules and positive ions smaller than this diameter to pass through. This gate is exceedingly important in the transmission of signals from one nerve cell to another (Chapter 10) and from nerve cells to muscle cells (Chapter 8).

Figure 5–5 illustrates an especially interesting characteristic of voltage-gated channels. This figure shows two recordings of electrical current flowing through a sodium channel when there was an approximate 25 millivolt potential gradient across the pore. Note that the pore conducts current either all or none. That is, the gate of the pore snaps open and then snaps closed, each snapping event occurring within a few millionths of a second. This illustrates the rapidity with which the conformational changes can occur in the shape of the protein molecular gates. The figure also shows in the lower recording another important characteristic: at one voltage potential the pore may remain closed all the time or almost all the time, whereas at another

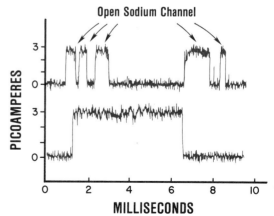

Figure 5–5. Record of current flow through a single voltage-gated sodium pore, demonstrating the all-or-none principle for opening the pore. (This type of record is obtained using a "patch-clamp," which is a minute pipette the tip of which abuts tightly against a small area of the cell membrane and allows current flow to be measured through individual pores.)

voltage level it may remain open either all or most of the time. However, at in-between voltages, the pores tend to snap open and closed as illustrated in the upper recording, giving an average current flow somewhere between the minimum and the maximum.

NET DIFFUSION THROUGH THE PROTEIN CHANNELS OF THE CELL MEMBRANE AND FACTORS THAT AFFECT IT

By now it is evident that many different substances can diffuse either through the lipid bilayer of the cell membrane or through protein channels. However, please understand clearly that substances that diffuse in one direction can also diffuse in the opposite direction. Usually, what is important to the cell is not the total substance diffusing in both directions but the difference between these two, which is the *net rate of diffusion* in one direction. The factors that affect this are (1) the permeability of the membrane, (2) the difference in concentration of the diffusing substance between the two sides of the membrane, (3) the pressure difference across the membrane, and (4) in the case of ions, the electrical potential difference between the two sides of the membrane.

The Permeability of the Membrane. The permeability of a membrane is defined as the rate of transport through a unit area of membrane for a given concentration difference. Among the factors that affect the total permeability of the membrane protein channels are: (1) the *number* of channels through which the substance can diffuse, (2) the *length* of the channels, (3) the degree of impediment to movement through each channel—that is, the *resistance* of the channel, (4) the *molecular weight* of the diffusing substance, and (5) the *temperature*. The effect of each of these on the permeability is obvious, with the possible exception of temperature and molecular weight.

A higher temperature increases the permeability because the thermal motion of all the molecules and ions in a solution increases directly with the temperature, thus causing more diffusion through the channels.

The molecular weight affects diffusion of molecules and ions mainly because the velocity of kinetic motion in a solution is inversely proportional to the square root of the molecular weight. Therefore, in general, the permeability of the membrane is also approximately inversely proportional to the square root of the molecular weight.

The following formula gives the approximate effect of all the above factors together on the permeability of the membrane for diffusion of any given substance:

$$\text{Permeability} = \frac{\text{Number of channels per unit area} \times \text{temperature}}{\text{Resistance of channels per unit length} \times \text{length of channel} \times \text{square root of molecular weight}}$$

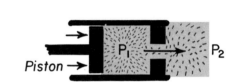

A.

OUTSIDE *Membrane* INSIDE

$C_o \longrightarrow C_i$

B.

C.

Piston → P_1 P_2

Figure 5–6. Effect of (*A*) concentration difference, (*B*) electrical difference, and (*C*) pressure difference on net diffusion of molecules and ions through a cell membrane.

Effect of a Concentration Difference. Figure 5–6*A* illustrates a membrane with a substance in high concentration on the outside and low concentration on the inside. The rate at which the substance diffuses *inward* is proportional to the concentration of molecules on the outside, for this concentration determines how many of the molecules strike the outside of the channel each second. On the other hand, the rate at which the molecules diffuse *outward* is proportional to their concentration *inside* the membrane. Obviously, therefore, the rate of net diffusion into the cell is proportional to the concentration on the outside *minus* the concentration on the inside or

$$\text{Net diffusion} \propto P (C_o - C_i)$$

in which C_o is the concentration on the outside, C_i is the concentration on the inside, and P is the permeability of the membrane for the substance.

Effect of an Electrical Potential Difference. If an electrical potential is applied across the membrane as shown in Figure 5–6*B*, because of their electrical charges ions will move through the membrane even though no concentration difference exists to cause their movement. Thus, to the left in the figure, the concentrations of negative ions are exactly the same on both sides of the membrane, but a positive charge has been applied to the right side of the membrane and a negative charge to the left, creating an electrical gradient across the membrane. The positive charge attracts the negative ions while the negative charge repels them. Therefore, net diffusion occurs from left to right. After much time large quantities of negative ions will have moved to the right (if we neglect, for the time being, the disturbing effects of the positive ions of the solution), creating the condition illustrated on the right in Figure 5–6B, in which a concentration difference of the same ions has developed in the direction opposite to the electrical potential difference. Obviously, the concentration difference is now tending to move the ions to the left, while the electrical difference is tending to move them to the right. When the concentration difference rises high enough, the two effects will exactly balance each other. At normal body temperature (38°C), the electrical difference that will exactly balance a given concentration difference of *univalent* ions, such as Na^+, K^+, or Cl^-, can be determined from the following formula called the *Nernst equation:*

$$\text{EMF (in millivolts)} = \pm 61 \log \frac{C_1}{C_2}$$

in which EMF is the electromotive force (voltage) between side 1 and side 2 of the membrane, C_1 is the concentration on side 1, and C_2 is the concentration on side 2. The polarity of the voltage on side 1 in the above equation is $+$ for negative ions and $-$ for positive ions. This relationship is extremely important in understanding the transmission of nerve impulses, for which reason it is discussed in even greater detail in Chapter 6.

Effect of a Pressure Difference. At times considerable pressure difference develops between the two sides of a membrane. This occurs, for instance, at the capillary membrane, which has a pressure approximately 23 mm Hg greater inside the capillary than outside. Pressure actually means the sum of all the forces of the different molecules striking a unit surface area at a given instant. Therefore, when the pressure is higher on one side of a membrane than the other, this means that the sum of all the forces of the molecules striking the channels on that side of the membrane is greater than on the other side. This can result either from greater numbers of molecules striking the membrane per second or from greater kinetic energy of the average molecule striking the membrane. In either event, increased amounts of energy are available to cause net movement of molecules from the high pressure side toward the low pressure side. This effect is illustrated in Figure 5–6C, which shows a piston developing high pressure on one side of a cell membrane, thereby causing net diffusion through the membrane to the other side.

For the usual red cell membrane, 1 mm Hg pressure difference causes approximately 10^{-4} cubic micron of net diffusion of water through each square micron of membrane each second. This ap-

pears to be only a very minute rate of fluid movement through the membrane, but in relation to the normal cell size and the very large diffusion pressure that can develop at the cell membrane because of osmotic forces, as discussed later in the chapter, this rate can represent tremendous transport of fluid in only a few seconds.

ACTIVE TRANSPORT

Often only a minute concentration of an ion is present in the extracellular fluid, and yet a large concentration of the ion is required in the intracellular fluid. For instance, this is true of potassium ions. Conversely, other ions frequently enter cells and must be removed even though their concentrations inside are far less than outside. This is true of sodium ions.

From the discussion thus far it is evident that *no ions can diffuse against an "electrochemical gradient,"* which is the sum of all the diffusion forces acting at the membrane—the forces caused by concentration difference, electrical difference, and pressure difference. That is, it is often said that ions cannot diffuse "uphill." To cause movement of an ion uphill, energy must be imparted to the ion. This is analogous to the compression of air by a pump. Compression causes the concentration of the air molecules to increase, but to create this greater concentration, energy must be imparted to the air molecules by the piston of the pump as they are compressed. Likewise, as ions are transported through a cell membrane from a dilute solution to a concentrated solution, energy must be imparted to the ions to concentrate them. When a cell membrane moves ions uphill against a concentration gradient (or uphill against an electrical or pressure gradient) the process is called *active transport.*

Among the different ions that are actively transported through cell membranes are sodium ions, potassium ions, calcium ions, iron ions, hydrogen ions, chloride ions, iodide ions, urate ions, and the amino acids.

BASIC MECHANISM OF ACTIVE TRANSPORT

Active transport depends on transport of substances by *carrier proteins* that penetrate through the membrane, the same as is true for facilitated diffusion. However, in active transport, the carrier functions differently from the carrier in facilitated diffusion, because the carrier protein must now impart energy to the substance that is being transported to move it against an electrochemical gradient. The energy for this purpose is derived from ATP. Furthermore, the active transport carrier proteins have ATPase activity, which means that they can cleave ATP to form ADP or AMP with release of the energy from the high energy phosphate bonds. Unfortunately, though, the manner in which this energy is coupled to cause transport of the substance against the electrochemical gradient is not yet clear.

The Sodium-Potassium "Pump"

The most ubiquitous active transport mechanism in the body is the one that transports sodium ions out of cells to the exterior and at the same time pumps potassium ions from the outside to the inside; it is called the *sodium-potassium pump*. This pump is present in all cells of the body, and it is responsible for maintaining the sodium and potassium concentration differences across the cell membrane as well as for establishing a negative electrical potential inside the cells. Indeed, we shall see in the next chapter that this pump is the basis of nerve function to transmit signals throughout the nervous system.

Figure 5–7 illustrates the basic components of the Na^+-K^+ pump. The *carrier protein* is a complex of two separate globular proteins, a larger one with a molecular weight of about 100,000 and a smaller one with a molecular weight of 45,000. Though the function of the smaller protein is not known, the larger protein has three specific features that are important for function of the pump:

(1) It has three *receptor sites for binding sodium ions* on the portion of the protein that protrudes to the interior of the cell.

(2) It has two *receptor sites for potassium ions* on the outside.

(3) The inside portion of this protein adjacent to or near to the sodium-binding sites has ATPase activity.

Now to put the pump into perspective: When three sodium ions bind on the inside of the carrier protein and two potassium ions on the outside, the ATPase function of the protein becomes activated. This then cleaves 1 molecule of ATP, splitting it to ADP and liberating a high energy phosphate bond

of energy. This energy is then believed to cause a conformational change in the protein carrier molecule, extruding the sodium ions to the outside and the potassium ions to the inside.

Note also in Figure 5–7 that the concentration of sodium on the inside, as designated by the small size of the Na^+ symbol, is very slight, whereas the concentration of the sodium on the outside is very great. Conversely, the potassium ion concentration on the outside is very slight whereas its concentration on the inside is very great. Thus, both these ions are transported against very large energy gradients.

The Electrogenic Nature of the Na^+-K^+ Pump. The fact that the Na^+-K^+ pump moves three sodium ions to the exterior for every two potassium ions to the interior means that a net of one positive charge is moved from the interior of the cell to the exterior for each revolution of the pump. This obviously creates positivity outside the cell but leaves a deficit of positive ions inside the cell; that is, it causes negativity on the inside. Therefore, the sodium-potassium pump is said to be *electrogenic*, because it creates an electrical potential across the cell membrane as it pumps.

The Calcium Pump

Another very important pump is the calcium pump. Calcium ions are normally maintained at extremely low concentration in the intracellular fluid, at a concentration about 10,000 times less than that in the extracellular fluid. This is achieved by two calcium pumps: One is in the cell membrane and pumps calcium to the outside of the cell. The other pumps calcium ions into one or more of the internal vesicular organelles of the cell, such as into the sarcoplasmic reticulum of muscle cells and into the mitochondria in all cells. In both instances, the carrier protein responsible for pumping the calcium ions is an ATPase having the same capability to cleave ATP as the ATPase sodium carrier protein. The difference is that this protein has a binding site for calcium instead of sodium.

Saturation of Active Transport

When the concentration of the substance to be transported is small, the rate of transport increases approximately in proportion to the increase in concentration. However, at large concentrations, active transport approaches a maximum, which is also called the V_{max}. This saturation is caused by limitation of the rates at which the chemical reactions of binding, release, and carrier conformational changes can occur.

Energetics of Active Transport

The amount of energy required to transport a substance actively through a membrane (aside from energy lost as heat in the chemical reactions) is determined by the degree that the substance is

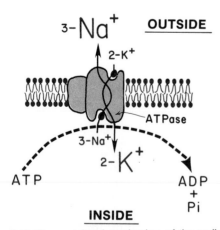

Figure 5–7. The postulated mechanism of the sodium-potassium pump.

concentrated during transport. Compared to the energy required to concentrate a substance tenfold, to concentrate it 100-fold requires twice as much energy, and to concentrate it 1000-fold requires three times as much. In other words, the energy required is proportional to the logarithm of the degree that the substance is concentrated, as expressed by the following formula:

$$\text{Energy (in calories per osmole)} = 1400 \log \frac{C_1}{C_2}$$

That is, in terms of calories, the amount of energy required to concentrate 1 osmole of substance tenfold is about 1400 calories. One can see that the energy expenditure for concentrating substances in cells or for removing substances from cells against a concentration gradient can be tremendous. Some cells, such as those lining the renal tubules as well as many glandular cells, perhaps expend as much as 90 per cent of their energy for this purpose alone.

REFERENCES

Agnew, W. S.: Voltage-regulated sodium channel molecules. *Annu. Rev. Physiol.,* 46:517, 1984.

Almers, W., and Stirling, C.: Distribution of transport proteins over animal cell membranes. *J. Membr. Biol.,* 77:169, 1984.

Armstrong, C. M.: Sodium channels and gating currents. *Physiol. Rev.,* 61:644, 1981.

Auerbach, A., and Sachs, F.: Patch clamp studies of single ionic channels. *Annu. Rev. Biophys. Bioeng.,* 13:269, 1984.

Blaustein, M. P., and Hamlyn, J. M.: Sodium transport inhibition, cell calcium, and hypertension. The natriuretic hormone/Na^+–Ca^{2+} exchange/hypertension hypothesis. *Am. J. Med.,* 77:45, 1984.

Chase, H. S., Jr.: Does calcium couple the apical and basolateral membrane permeabilities in epithelia? *Am. J. Physiol.,* 247:F869, 1984.

Dawson, K. G.: Endocrine physiology of electrolyte metabolism. *Drugs,* 28(Suppl. 1):98, 1984.

DiPolo, R., and Beauge, L.: The calcium pump and sodium-calcium exchange in squid axons. *Annu. Rev. Physiol.,* 45:313, 1983.

Ellis, D.: Na-Ca exchange in cardiac tissues. *Adv. Myocardiol.,* 5:295, 1985.

Flatman, P. W.: Magnesium transport across cell membranes. *J. Membr. Biol.,* 80:1, 1984.

Gadsby, D. C.: The Na/K pump of cardiac cells. *Annu. Rev. Biophys. Bioeng.,* 13:373, 1984.

Guyton, A. C., et al.: Dynamics and Control of the Body Fluids. Philadelphia, W. B. Saunders Co., 1975.

Hess, G. P., et al.: Acetylcholine receptor-controlled ion translocation: Chemical kinetic investigations of the mechanism. *Annu. Rev. Biophys. Bioeng.,* 12:443, 1983.

Hobbs, A. S., and Albers, R. W.: The structure of proteins involved in active membrane transport. *Annu. Rev. Biophys. Bioeng.,* 9:259, 1980.

Katz, A. M.: Basic cellular mechanisms of action of the calcium-channel blockers. *Am. J. Cardiol.,* 55:2B, 1985.

Keynes, R. D.: Ion channels in the nerve-cell membrane. *Sci. Am.,* 240(3):126, 1979.

Kregenow, F. M.: Osmoregulatory salt transporting mechanisms: Control of cell volume in anisotonic media. *Annu. Rev. Physiol.,* 43:493, 1981.

Latorre, R., and Alvarez, O.: Voltage-dependent channels in planar lipid bilayer membranes. *Physiol. Rev.,* 61:77, 1981.

Lindermann, B.: Fluctuation analysis of sodium channels in epithelia. *Annu. Rev. Physiol.,* 46:497, 1984.

Lodish, H. F., and Rothman, J. E.: The assembly of cell membranes. *Sci. Am.,* 240(1):48, 1979.

Malhotra, S. K.: The Plasma Membrane. New York, John Wiley & Sons, 1983.

Miller, C.: Integral membrane channels: Studies in model membranes. *Physiol. Rev.,* 63:1209, 1983.

Miller, C.: Ion channels in liposomes. *Annu. Rev. Physiol.,* 46:549, 1984.

Reuter, H.: Ion channels in cardiac cell membranes. *Annu. Rev. Physiol.,* 46:473, 1984.

Sakmann, B., and Neher, E.: Patch clamp techniques for studying ionic channels in excitable membranes. *Annu. Rev. Physiol.,* 46:455, 1984.

Schatzmann, H. J.: The red cell calcium pump. *Annu. Rev. Physiol.,* 45:303, 1983.

Schultz, S. G.: A cellular model for active sodium absorption by mammalian colon. *Annu. Rev. Physiol.,* 46:435, 1984.

Sjodin, R. A.: Ion transport in skeletal muscle. New York, John Wiley & Sons, 1982.

Smith, P. L., and McCabe, R. D.: Mechanism and regulation of transcellular potassium transport by the colon. *Am. J. Physiol.,* 247:G445, 1984.

Wright, E. M.: Electrophysiology of plasma membrane vesicles. *Am. J. Physiol.,* 246:F363, 1984.

6

Membrane Potentials and Action Potentials

Electrical potentials exist across the membranes of essentially all cells of the body, and some cells, such as nerve and muscle cells, are "excitable"—that is, capable of self-generation of electrochemical impulses at their membranes and, in some instances, employment of these impulses to transmit signals along the membranes. In still other types of cells, such as glandular cells, macrophages, and ciliated cells, changes in membrane potentials probably play significant roles in controlling many of the cell's functions. However, the present discussion is concerned with membrane potentials generated both at rest and during action by nerve and muscle cells.

BASIC PHYSICS OF MEMBRANE POTENTIALS

Before beginning this discussion, let us first recall that the fluids both inside and outside the cells are electrolytic solutions containing 150 to 160 mEq per liter of positive ions and the same concentration of negative ions. Generally, a very minute excess of negative ions (anions) accumulates immediately inside the cell membrane along its inner surface, as illustrated in Figures 6–1A and 6–2, and an equal

number of positive ions (cations) accumulates immediately outside the membrane. The effect of this is the establishment of a *membrane potential* between the inside and outside of the cell.

The two basic means by which membrane potentials can develop are (1) diffusion of ions through the membrane as a result of ion concentration differences between the two sides of the membrane, thus creating an imbalance of negative and positive charges on the two sides of the membrane, and (2) active transport of ions through the membrane, thus also creating an imbalance of charges.

MEMBRANE POTENTIALS CAUSED BY DIFFUSION

Figures 6–1A and B illustrate a nerve fiber when there is no active transport of either sodium or potassium. In Figure 6–1A the potassium concentration is very great inside the membrane while that outside is very low. Furthermore, the membrane is very permeable to the potassium ions but not to any other ions. Because of the large potassium concentration gradient from the inside toward the outside, there is a strong tendency for potassium ions to diffuse outward. As they do so, they carry positive charges to the outside, thus creating a state of electropositivity outside the membrane, and electronegativity on the inside because of the negative

DIFFUSION POTENTIALS

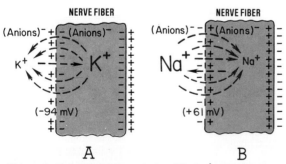

Figure 6–1. *A*, Establishment of a diffusion potential across a cell membrane, caused by potassium ions diffusing from inside the cell to the outside through a membrane that is selectively permeable only to potassium. *B*, Establishment of a diffusion potential when the membrane is permeable only to sodium ions. Note that the internal membrane potential is negative when potassium ions diffuse and positive when sodium ions diffuse because of opposite concentration gradients of these two ions.

ELECTROGENIC POTENTIAL

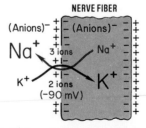

Figure 6–2. Establishment of a membrane potential as a result of sodium and potassium being pumped through the nerve membrane by the $Na^+ - K^+$ electrogenic pump, with three sodium ions passing outward through the membrane for each two potassium ions passing inward.

anions that remain behind, which do not diffuse outward along with the potassium. This potential difference across the membrane tends to repel the potassium ions in a backward direction from outside toward the inside. And within a millisecond or so the potential becomes great enough to block further diffusion of potassium ions to the exterior. The potential at this point is the *Nernst potential for the potassium ions,* as we shall discuss.

Figure 6–1B illustrates the same effect as that in Figure 6–1A but with a high concentration of sodium ions outside the membrane and a low sodium concentration inside. These ions are also positively charged. However, this time the membrane is highly permeable to the sodium ions and impermeable to all other ions. Diffusion of the sodium ions to the inside creates a membrane potential now of opposite polarity, with negativity outside and positivity inside, and, again, the membrane potential rises high enough within milliseconds to block further net diffusion of the sodium ions to the inside, but this time the potential is called the *Nernst potential for the sodium ions.*

Thus, in both parts of Figure 6–1 we see that a concentration difference of ions across a semipermeable membrane can, under appropriate conditions, cause the creation of a membrane potential. In later sections of this chapter, we shall also see that many of the membrane potential changes observed during the course of nerve and muscle impulse transmission result from the occurrence of rapidly changing diffusion membrane potentials of this nature.

Relationship of the Diffusion Potential to the Concentration Difference—The Nernst Equation. When a concentration difference of a single type of ion across a membrane causes diffusion of ions through the membrane, thus creating a membrane potential, the magnitude of the potential *inside* the membrane versus the *outside* is determined by the ratio of the tendency for the ions to diffuse in one direction or the other direction, which is determined for positive ions by the following formula (*at body temperature, 37° C):*

$$\text{EMF (millivolts)} = -61 \log \frac{\text{Conc. inside}}{\text{Conc. outside}}$$

Thus, when the concentration of positive ions on the inside of a membrane is ten times that on the outside, the log of 10 is 1, and the potential difference calculates to be −61 millivolts. This equation is called the *Nernst equation,* and the developed potential is the *Nernst potential.*

However, two conditions are necessary for this Nernst potential to develop as a result of diffusion: (1) The membrane must be selectively permeable, allowing a single type of ion to diffuse through the channels while all other ions do not diffuse. (2) The concentration of the diffusible ions must be greater on one side of the membrane than on the other side.

Using the Nernst equation, let us now calculate the Nernst potential across the nerve membrane, first, when the membrane is permeable only to sodium ions and, second, when the membrane is permeable only to potassium ions:

The normal concentration of sodium ions inside the nerve membrane is approximately 14 mEq per liter and outside approximately 142 mEq per liter. Thus, the ratio of these two is 0.10, and the logarithm of 0.10 is −1.00. Multiplying this by −61 millivolts gives a Nernst potential for sodium of +61 millivolts inside the nerve fiber membrane.

The normal concentration of potassium ions inside the nerve fiber is approximately 140 mEq per liter and 4 mEq per liter on the outside. The ratio of these two is 35. The logarithm of 35 is 1.54; this times −61 millivolts equals a Nernst potential for potassium of −94 millivolts inside the membrane.

Therefore, if there were no pumping of ions through the nerve membrane and if the membrane were permeable only to sodium but not at all to other ions, the potential inside the nerve fiber would be +61 millivolts. Conversely, if the membrane were permeable to potassium but not permeable to any other ions, the membrane potential would be −94 millivolts. We shall see later in this discussion that under resting conditions the membrane potential averages about −90 millivolts, which is very near the −94 millivolts potassium Nernst potential. This is true because in the resting state the membrane is very permeable to potassium and only slightly permeable to sodium. On the other hand, when a nerve impulse is transmitted, the membrane, for a minute fraction of a second, becomes much more permeable to sodium than to potassium. Therefore, during this split second, the membrane potential rises to approximately +45 millivolts, which is much nearer the sodium Nernst potential than the potassium Nernst potential.

Calculation of the Diffusion Potential When the Membrane Is Permeable to Several Different Ions

When a membrane is permeable to several different ions, the diffusion potential that will develop depends on three factors: (1) the polarity of the electrical charge of each ion, (2) the permeability of the membrane (*P*) to each ion, and (3) the concentration (*C*) of the respective ions on the inside (*i*) and outside (*o*) of the membrane. Thus, the following formula, called the *constant field equation,* the *Goldman equation,* or the *Goldman-Hodgkin-Katz equation,* gives the calculated membrane potential on the *inside* of the membrane when two univalent positive ions, sodium (Na^+) and potassium (K^+), and one univalent negative ion, chloride ion (Cl^-), are involved.

$$\text{EMF (millivolts)} =$$
$$-61 \cdot \log \frac{C_{Na^+_i} P_{Na^+} + C_{K^+_i} P_{K^+} + C_{Cl^-_o} P_{Cl^-}}{C_{Na^+_o} P_{Na^+} + C_{K^+_o} P_{K^+} + C_{Cl^-_i} P_{Cl^-}}$$

Now, let us study the importance and the meaning of this equation. First, sodium, potassium, and chloride ions are the ions most importantly involved in the development of membrane potentials in nerve and muscle fibers, as well as in the neuronal cells in the central nervous system. The concentration gradient of each of these ions across the membrane helps determine the voltage of the membrane potential.

Second, the degree of importance of each of the ions in determining the voltage is proportional to the membrane permeability for that particular ion. Thus, if the membrane is impermeable to both potassium and chloride ions, then the membrane potential becomes entirely determined by the concentration gradient of sodium ions alone, and the resulting potential will be exactly equal to the Nernst potential for sodium. The same principle holds for each of the other two ions if the membrane should become selectively permeable for either one of them alone.

Third, a positive ion concentration gradient from *inside* the membrane *to the outside* causes electronegativity inside the membrane. The reason for this is that positive ions diffuse to the outside when their concentration is higher inside than outside. This carries positive charges to the outside but leaves the negative anions on the inside. Exactly the opposite effect occurs when there is a negative ion gradient. That is, a chloride ion gradient from the *outside to the inside* causes negativity inside the cell, because negatively charged chloride ions then diffuse to the inside while leaving the positive ions on the outside.

Fourth, we shall see later that the permeabilities of the sodium and potassium channels undergo very rapid changes during conduction of the nerve impulse, whereas the permeability of the chloride channels does not change greatly during this process. Therefore, the changes in the sodium and potassium permeabilities are primarily responsible for signal transmission in the nerves, which is the subject of most of the remainder of this chapter.

MEMBRANE POTENTIALS CAUSED BY ACTIVE TRANSPORT—THE SODIUM-POTASSIUM "ELECTROGENIC PUMP"

Figure 6–2 illustrates another method by which a membrane potential can develop—by active transport. It will be recalled from the discussions in the last chapter that the sodium-potassium pump pumps three sodium ions out of the cell for every two potassium ions pumped in. Thus, for each cycle of the pump the inside of the nerve fiber loses one positive charge. Because the membrane is not permeable to most of the negatively charged ions (anions) inside the cell, continuation of this process will lead to an excess of positive charges on the outside and an excess of negative charges inside, as illustrated in Figure 6–2. Thus, once again,

the nerve membrane becomes negatively charged on the inside. And, because of the ability of the Na^+-K^+ pump to create such a membrane potential, it is called an *electrogenic pump.*

It was also clear from the discussions of the previous chapter that the Na^+-K^+ pump is responsible for establishing the normal sodium and potassium gradients across the cell membrane. That is, the continual pumping of sodium to the exterior leads to the normally greatly reduced sodium concentration inside the nerve fiber, whereas the pumping of the potassium ions to the interior helps establish the high concentration of potassium on the inside. We shall see later in the chapter that after many nerve impulses have been transmitted, the concentration gradients across the cell membrane of both sodium and potassium decrease because of diffusion of these ions through the membrane during the action potentials. But the Na^+-K^+ pump will soon re-establish the appropriate concentration gradients.

MEASURING THE MEMBRANE POTENTIAL

The method for measuring the membrane potential is simple in theory but often very difficult in practice because of the small sizes of many of the fibers. Figure 6–3 illustrates a small pipette filled with a very strong electrolyte solution (KCl) that is impaled through the cell membrane to the interior of the fiber. Then another electrode, called the "indifferent electrode," is placed in the interstitial fluids, and the potential difference between the inside and outside of the fiber is measured using an appropriate voltmeter. This is a highly sophisticated electronic apparatus that is capable of measuring very small voltages despite extremely high resistance to electrical flow through the tip of the micropipette, which has a diameter usually less than 1 micron and a resistance often as great as a billion ohms. For recording rapid *changes* in the membrane potential during the transmission of nerve impulses, the microelectrode is connected to an oscilloscope, as will be explained later in the chapter.

THE CELL MEMBRANE AS AN ELECTRICAL CAPACITOR

In each of the figures shown thus far, the negative and positive ionic charges that cause the membrane potential

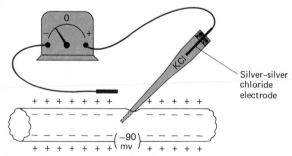

Figure 6–3. Measurement of the membrane potential of the nerve fiber using a microelectrode.

have been shown to be lined up against the membrane, and we have not spoken of the arrangement of the charges elsewhere in the fluids, either inside the nerve fiber or on the outside in the interstitial fluid. However, Figure 6–4 illustrates this, showing that everywhere except adjacent to the surfaces of the cell membrane itself, the negative and positive charges are exactly equal. This is called the principle of *electrical neutrality*; that is, for every positive ion there is a negative ion nearby to neutralize it, or otherwise electrical potentials of billions of volts would appear within the fluids.

When positive charges are pumped to the outside of the membrane, these positive charges line up along the outside of the membrane, and on the inside the anions line up that have been left behind. This creates a *dipole layer* of positive and negative charges between the outside and inside of the membrane, but it still leaves equal numbers of negative and positive charges everywhere else within the fluids. This is the same effect that occurs when the plates of an electrical capacitor becomes electrically charged—that is, lining up of negative and positive charges on the opposite sides of the dielectric membrane between the plates. Therefore, the lipid bilayer of the cell membrane actually functions as a *dielectric* of a cell membrane capacitor, much as mica, paper, and Mylar function as dielectrics in electrical capacitors.

Because of the extreme thinness of the cell membrane (only 7 to 10 nanometers), its capacitance is tremendous for its area—about *1 microfarad per square centimeter.*

The lower part of Figure 6–4 illustrates the electrical potential that will be recorded at each point in or near the nerve fiber membrane, beginning at the left side of the figure and passing to the right. As long as the electrode is outside the nerve membrane, the potential that is recorded is zero, which is the potential of the extracellular fluid. Then, as the recording electrode passes through the electrical dipole layer at the cell membrane, the potential decreases immediately to −90 millivolts. Again, the electrical potential remains at a steady level as the electrode passes across the interior of the fiber but reverses back to zero the instant it passes through the opposite side of the membrane.

The fact that the nerve membrane functions as a ca-

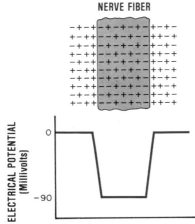

NERVE FIBER

Figure 6–4. Distribution of positively and negatively charged ions in the interstitial fluid surrounding a nerve fiber and in the fluid inside the fiber; note the dipolar alignment of negative charges along the inside surface of the membrane and positive charges along the outside surface. In the lower panel are illustrated the abrupt changes in membrane potential that occur at the membranes on the two sides of the fiber.

pacitor has one especially important point of significance: to create a negative potential inside the membrane, only enough positive ions must be transported outward to develop the electrical dipole layer at the membrane itself. All the remaining ions inside the nerve fiber can still be both positive and negative ions. Therefore, an incredibly small number of ions needs to be transferred through the membrane to establish the normal potential of −90 millivolts inside the nerve fiber—only about 1/500,000 of the total positive charges inside the fiber need be so transferred. Also, an equally small number of positive ions moving to the inside of the fiber can reverse the potential from −90 millivolts to as much as +35 millivolts within as little as 1/10,000 of a second. This rapid shifting of ions in this manner causes the nerve signals that we will discuss in the subsequent sections of this chapter.

THE RESTING MEMBRANE POTENTIAL OF NERVES

The membrane potential of large nerve fibers when they are not transmitting nerve signals—that is, when they are in the so-called "resting" state—is about −90 millivolts (mv). That is, the potential *inside the fiber* is 90 mv more negative than the potential in the interstitial fluid on the outside of the fiber. In the next few paragraphs we will explain how this potential comes about, but before doing so we must describe the transport properties of the resting nerve membrane for sodium and potassium.

Active Transport of Sodium and Potassium Ions Through the Membrane—The Sodium-Potassium Pump. First, let us recall from the discussions of the previous chapter that all cell membranes of the body have a powerful sodium-potassium pump and that this continually pumps sodium to the outside of the fiber and potassium to the inside. Further, let us remember that this is an *electrogenic pump*, because more positive charges are pumped to the outside than to the inside, leaving a net deficit of positive ions on the inside; this is the same as causing a negative charge inside the cell membrane.

This sodium-potassium pump causes the tremendous concentration gradients for sodium and potassium across the resting nerve membrane. These gradients are the following:

Na$^+$ (outside):	142 mEq/L
Na$^+$ (inside):	14 mEq/L
K$^+$ (outside):	4 mEq/L
K$^+$ (inside):	140 mEq/L

And the ratios of these two respective ions from the inside to the outside are

$$Na^+_{inside}/Na^+_{outside} = 0.1$$
$$K^+_{inside}/K^+_{outside} = 35.0$$

Leakage of Potassium and Sodium Through the Nerve Membrane. To the right in Figure 6–5 is illustrated a channel type of transport protein in

OUTSIDE

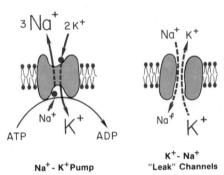

Figure 6–5. The functional characteristics of the Na⁺−K⁺ pump and also of the potassium-sodium "leak" channels.

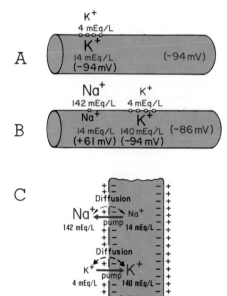

Figure 6–6. Establishment of resting membrane potentials in nerve fibers under three separate conditions: *A*, when the membrane potential is caused entirely by potassium diffusion alone; *B*, when the membrane potential is caused by diffusion of both sodium and potassium ions; and *C*, when the membrane potential is caused by diffusion of both sodium and potassium ions plus pumping of both these ions by the Na⁺−K⁺ pump.

the cell membrane through which potassium and sodium ions can leak. The channels through these proteins are called *potassium-sodium "leak" channels.* The emphasis is on the potassium because these channels are far more permeable to potassium than to sodium, normally about 100 times as permeable. We shall see later that this differential in permeability is exceedingly important in the establishment of the normal resting membrane potential.

ORIGIN OF THE NORMAL RESTING MEMBRANE POTENTIAL

Figure 6–6 illustrates the important factors in the establishment of the normal resting membrane potential of −90 mv. These are

Contribution of the Potassium Diffusion Potential. In Figure 6–6A, we make the assumption that the only movement of ions through the membrane is the diffusion of potassium ions, as illustrated by the open channel between the potassium inside the membrane and the outside. Because of the high ratio of potassium ions inside to the potassium ions outside, 35 to 1, the Nernst potential corresponding to this ratio is −94 mv. That is, the *diffusion potential* caused by the potassium would be −94 mv, as illustrated to the right inside the nerve fiber, if this were the only factor causing the resting nerve potential.

Contribution of Sodium Diffusion Through the Nerve Membrane. Figure 6–6B illustrates the addition of very slight permeability of the nerve membrane to sodium ions, caused by the minute diffusion of the sodium ions through the K⁺-Na⁺ leak channels. The ratio of sodium ions from inside to outside the membrane is 0.1, and this gives a calculated Nernst potential for the inside of the membrane of +61 mv. But also shown in Figure 6–6B is the Nernst potential for potassium diffusion of −94 mv. How do these interact with each other, and what will be the summated potential? This can be answered by using the Goldman equation described earlier. However, intuitively, one can see

that if the membrane is highly permeable to potassium but only very slightly permeable to sodium, it is logical that the diffusion of potassium will contribute far more to the membrane potential than will the diffusion of sodium. In the normal nerve fiber, the permeability of the membrane to potassium is about 100 times as great as to sodium. Using this value in the Goldman equation gives an internal membrane potential of −86 mv, as shown to the right in Figure 6–6B.

Contribution of the Na⁺-K⁺ Pump. Finally, in Figure 6–6C the additional contribution of the sodium-potassium pump is illustrated. In this figure, there is very slight diffusion of sodium ions, much greater diffusion of potassium ions, and continuous pumping of sodium ions to the outside and simultaneous pumping of potassium ions to the inside of the membrane, but with a ratio of sodium to potassium pumping of three to two, as discussed earlier. The fact that more sodium ions are being pumped to the outside than potassium to the inside causes a continual loss of positive charges from inside the membrane, and this creates an additional degree of negativity on the inside beyond that which can be accounted for by diffusion alone. Therefore, as illustrated in Figure 6–6C, the net membrane potential with all these factors operative at the same time is −90 mv.

In summary, the diffusion potentials alone caused by potassium and sodium diffusion would give a membrane potential of approximately −86 mv, almost all of this being determined by the potassium diffusion. Then, an additional −4 mv is contributed to the membrane potential by the electrogenic Na⁺-K⁺ pump, giving a net resting membrane potential of −90 mv.

The resting membrane potential in large skeletal muscle fibers is approximately the same as that in large nerve fibers, also −90 mv. However, in both small nerve fibers and small muscle fibers—smooth muscle, for instance—as well as in many of the neurons of the central nervous system, the membrane potential is often as little as −40 to −60 mv instead of −90 mv.

THE NERVE ACTION POTENTIAL

Nerve signals are transmitted by *action potentials*, which are rapid changes in the membrane potential. Each action potential begins with a sudden change from the normal resting negative potential to a positive membrane potential and then ends with an almost equally rapid change back again to the negative potential. To conduct a nerve signal, the action potential moves along the nerve fiber until it comes to the fiber's end. The upper panel of Figure 6–7 shows the disturbances that occur at the membrane during the action potential, with transfer of positive charges to the interior of the fiber at its onset and return of positive charges to the exterior at its end. The lower panel illustrates graphically the successive changes in the membrane potential over a period of a few 10,000ths of a second, illustrating the explosive onset of the action potential and the almost equally as rapid recovery.

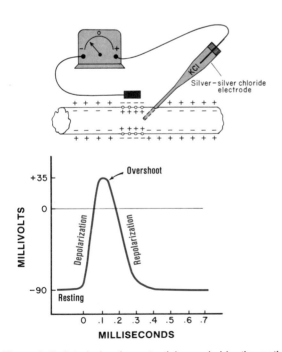

Figure 6–7. A typical action potential recorded by the method illustrated in the upper panel of the figure.

The successive stages of the action potential are described by the following terms:

Resting Stage. This is the resting membrane potential before the action potential occurs. The membrane is said to be "polarized" during this stage because of the very large negative membrane potential that is present.

Depolarization Stage. At this time, the membrane suddenly becomes very permeable to sodium ions, allowing tremendous numbers of sodium ions to flow to the interior of the axon. The normal "polarized" state of −90 mv is lost, with the potential rising rapidly in the positive direction. This is called *depolarization*. In large nerve fibers, the membrane potential actually "overshoots" beyond the zero level and becomes slightly positive, but in some smaller fibers as well as many central nervous system neurons, the potential merely approaches the zero level and does not overshoot to the positive state.

Repolarization Stage. Within a few 10,000ths of a second after the membrane becomes highly permeable to sodium ions, the sodium channels close almost as rapidly as they had opened. Then, rapid diffusion of potassium ions to the exterior re-establishes the normal negative resting membrane potential. This is called *repolarization* of the membrane.

To explain more fully the factors that cause both the depolarization and repolarization processes, we need now to describe the special characteristics of yet two other types of transport channels through the nerve membrane: the voltage-gated sodium and potassium channels.

THE VOLTAGE-GATED SODIUM AND POTASSIUM CHANNELS

The principal actor in causing both depolarization and repolarization of the nerve membrane during the action potential is the *voltage-gated sodium channel*. However, the *voltage-gated potassium channel* also plays an important role in some nerve fibers for the rapid repolarization of the membrane. *These two voltage-gated channels are in addition to the Na⁺-K⁺ pump and also in addition to the Na⁺-K⁺ leak channels.*

The Voltage-Gated Sodium Channel— "Activation" and "Inactivation" of the Channel

The upper panel of Figure 6–8 illustrates the voltage-gated sodium channel in three separate states. This channel has two separate gates, one near the outside of a channel called the *activation gate* and another near the inside called the *inactivation gate*. To the left is shown the state of these two gates in the normal resting membrane when the membrane potential is −90 mv. In this state the activation gate is closed, which prevents any entry of sodium ions to the interior of the fiber through

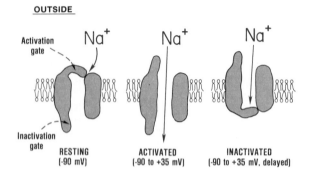

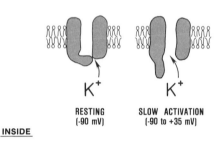

Figure 6–8. Characteristics of the voltage-gated sodium and potassium channels, showing both activation and inactivation of the sodium channels but activation of the potassium channels only when the membrane potential is changed from the normal resting negative value to a positive value.

these sodium channels. On the other hand, the inactivation gate is open and does not at this time constitute any barrier to the movement of sodium ions.

Activation of the Sodium Channel. When the membrane potential becomes less negative than during the resting state, rising from −90 mv toward zero, it finally reaches a voltage, usually somewhere between −70 and −50 mv, that causes a sudden conformational change in the activation gate, flipping it to the open position. This is called the *activated state*, and during this state sodium ions can literally pour inward through the channel, increasing the sodium permeability of the membrane as much as 500- to 5000-fold.

Inactivation of the Sodium Channel. To the far right in the upper panel of Figure 6–8 is illustrated a final state of the sodium channel. The same increase in voltage that opens the activation gate also closes the inactivation gate. However, closure of the inactivation gate occurs a few 10,000ths of a second after the activation gate opens. That is, the conformational change that flips the inactivation gate to the closed state is a slower process, while the conformational change that opens the activation gate is a very rapid process. Therefore, after the sodium channel has remained open for a few 10,000ths of a second, it suddenly closes, and sodium ions can no longer pour to the inside of the membrane. At this point the membrane potential begins to recover back toward the resting membrane state, which is the repolarization process.

A very important characteristic of the sodium channel inactivation process is that *the inactivation gate will not reopen again until the membrane potential returns either to or nearly to the original resting membrane potential level.* Therefore, it is not possible for the sodium channels to open again without the nerve fiber first repolarizing.

The Voltage-Gated Potassium Channels and Their Activation

The lower panel of Figure 6–8 illustrates the voltage-gated potassium channel in two separate states: during the resting membrane state and during the action potential. During the resting state, the gate of the potassium channel is closed, as illustrated to the left in the figure, and potassium ions are prevented from passing to the exterior. When the membrane potential rises from −90 mv toward zero, this voltage change causes a slow conformational opening of the gate and allows increased potassium diffusion outward through the membrane. However, because of the slowness of opening of these potassium channels, they open at the same time that the sodium channels are becoming inactivated and therefore are closing. Thus, the decrease in sodium entry to the cell and simultaneous increase in potassium exit from the cell greatly speeds the repolarization process, leading within a few 10,000ths of a second to full recovery of the resting membrane potential.

The Research Method for Measuring the Effect of Voltage on Opening and Closing of the Voltage-Gated Channels—The Voltage Clamp. The original research that led to our quantitative understanding of the sodium and potassium channels was so ingenious that it led to Nobel prizes for the scientists responsible, Hodgkin and Huxley. The essence of these studies is illustrated in Figures 6–9 and 6–10.

Figure 6–9 illustrates the experimental apparatus called the *voltage clamp*, which is used to measure the flow of ions through the different channels. Let us explain the

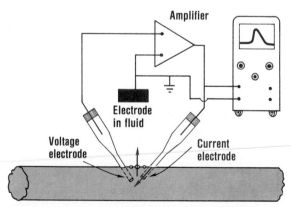

Figure 6–9. The "voltage clamp" method for studying flow of ions through specific channels.

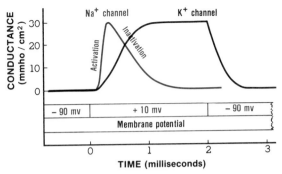

Figure 6–10. Changes in conductance of sodium and potassium ion channels when the membrane potential is suddenly increased from the normal resting value of −90 mv to a positive value of +10 mv for 2 milliseconds. This figure illustrates that the sodium channels open (activate) and then close (inactivate) before the end of the 2 milliseconds whereas the potassium channels only open (activate).

voltage clamp. Two electrodes are inserted into the nerve fiber. One of these is for the purpose of measuring the voltage of the membrane potential. The other is to conduct electrical current either into or out of the nerve fiber. This apparatus is used in the following way: The investigator decides what voltage he or she wishes to establish inside the nerve fiber. He then adjusts the electronic portion of the apparatus to the desired voltage, and this automatically injects either positive or negative electricity through the current electrode at whatever rate is required to hold the voltage, as measured by the voltage electrode, at the level set by the operator. For instance, when the membrane potential is suddenly increased by this voltage clamp from −90 mv to zero, the voltage-gated sodium and potassium channels open, and sodium and potassium ions begin to pour through the channels. Furthermore, electrical current is injected through the current electrode of the voltage clamp to maintain the intracellular voltage at the zero level. To achieve this, the current injected through the current electrode must be exactly equal to but of opposite polarity to the net current flow through the membrane channels. To measure how much current flow is occurring at each instant, the current electrode is connected to an oscilloscope that records the flow, as illustrated on the screen of the oscilloscope in the figure. Finally, the investigator adjusts the concentrations of the ions to desired levels both inside and outside the nerve fiber and repeats the study. This can be done very easily when using very large nerve fibers removed from some crustaceans, especially the giant squid axon that is sometimes as large as 1 mm in diameter. When sodium is the only permeant ion in the solutions inside and outside the squid axon, then the voltage clamp will measure current flow only through the sodium channels. When potassium is the only permeant ion, then current flow only through the potassium channels will be measured.

Another means for studying the flow of ions through individual channels is to block one type of channel at a time. For instance, the sodium channels can be blocked by a toxin called *tetrodotoxin* when this is applied to the outside of the cell membrane where the sodium activation gates are located. Conversely, *tetraethylammonium ion* will block the potassium pores when it is applied to the interior of the nerve fiber.

Figure 6–10 illustrates the changes in conductance of the voltage-gated sodium and potassium channels when the membrane potential is suddenly changed by use of the voltage clamp from −90 mv to +10 mv and 2 milliseconds later back again to −90 mv. Note the sudden opening of the sodium channels (the activation stage) within a very small fraction of a millisecond after the membrane potential was increased to the positive value. However, during approximately the next millisecond, the sodium channels automatically closed (the inactivation stage) and were fully closed within about 1.5 milliseconds after the onset of the positive membrane potential. Thus, long before the membrane potential returned to its original resting value, the sodium channels had already completely closed, or "inactivated."

Now, note the difference in the opening (activation) of the potassium channels. These opened slowly, reaching the full open state only after the sodium channels had already become almost completely closed. Furthermore, once the potassium channels opened, they remained open for the entire duration of the positive membrane potential and did not close again until after the membrane potential was decreased back to −90 mv.

Finally, let us recall that the voltage-gated channels normally flip to the open state or the closed state very suddenly, which was illustrated in Figure 5–5 in the previous chapter. Therefore, how is it that the curves in Figure 6–10 are so smooth? The answer is that these curves represent the flow of sodium and potassium ions through literally thousands of channels at the same time. Some open at one voltage level, others at another voltage, and so forth. Likewise, some become inactivated at different points in the cycle from the others. Thus, the illustrated curves represent summated current flows through the many channels.

SUMMARY OF THE EVENTS THAT CAUSE THE ACTION POTENTIAL

Figure 6–11 illustrates in summary form the sequential events that occur during and shortly after the action potential. These are:

At the bottom of the figure are shown the changes in membrane conductances for sodium and potassium ions. During the resting state, before the action potential begins, the conductance for potassium ions is shown to be already 50 to 100 times as great as the conductance for sodium ions. This is caused by much greater leakage of potassium ions through the leak channels than the leakage of sodium ions. However, at the onset of the action potential, the sodium channels instantaneously become activated and allow an up to 5000-fold increase in sodium conductance. Then the inactivation process almost as rapidly closes the sodium channels within another few fractions of a millisecond. The onset of the action potential also causes voltage gating of the potassium channels, causing them to begin opening a fraction of a millisecond after the sodium channels open. And at the end of the action potential, the return of the membrane potential to the negative state causes the potassium channels to

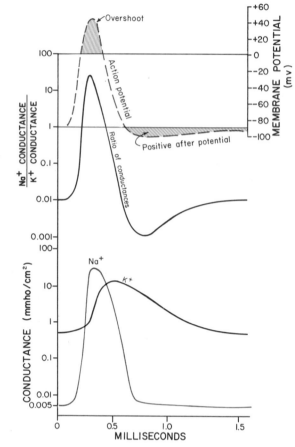

Figure 6–11. Changes in sodium and potassium conductances during the course of the action potential. Note that sodium conductance increases several thousandfold during the early stages of the action potential, whereas potassium conductance increases only about 30-fold during the latter stages of the action potential and for a short period thereafter. (Curves constructed from data in Hodgkin and Huxley papers but transposed from squid axon to apply to the membrane potentials of large mammalian nerve fibers.)

close back to their original status, but again only after a short delay.

In the middle portion of Figure 6–11 is shown the ratio of sodium conductance to potassium conductance at each instant during the action potential, and above this is shown the action potential itself. During the early portion of the action potential, this ratio increases more than a thousand-fold. Therefore, far more sodium ions now flow to the interior of the fiber than do potassium ions to the exterior. This is what causes the membrane potential to become positive. At this time the sodium channels become inactivated but at the same time the potassium channels open, and the ratio of conductance now shifts far in favor of high potassium conductance but low sodium conductance. This allows extremely rapid loss of potassium ions to the exterior while essentially no sodium ions flow to the interior. Consequently, the action potential quickly returns to its baseline level.

The Positive After-Potential

Note also in Figure 6–11 that the membrane potential becomes even more negative than the original resting membrane potential for a few milliseconds after the action potential is over. This is called the *positive after-potential,* which is really a misnomer because the positive after-potential is actually somewhat more negative than the resting potential. However, the reason for calling it "positive" is that, historically, the first potential measurements were made on the outside of the nerve fiber membrane rather than inside, and when measured on the outside this potential caused a positive record on the meter rather than a negative one.

The cause of the positive after-potential is mainly that many potassium channels remain open for several milliseconds after the repolarization process of the membrane is complete. This allows excess potassium ions to diffuse out of the nerve fiber, leaving an extra deficit of positive ions on the inside, which means more negativity.

ROLES OF OTHER IONS DURING THE ACTION POTENTIAL

Thus far, we have considered only the roles of sodium and potassium ions in the generation of the action potential. However, at least three other types of ions must be considered. These are:

The Impermeant, Negatively Charged Ions (Anions) Inside the Axon. Inside the axon are many negatively charged ions that cannot go through the membrane channels. These include protein molecules, many organic phosphate compounds, sulfate compounds, and so forth. Since these cannot leave the interior of the axon, any deficit of positive ions inside the membrane leaves an excess of the impermeant negative ions. Therefore, these impermeant negative ions are responsible for the negative charge inside the fiber.

Calcium Ions. The cell membranes of almost all, if not all, cells of the body have a calcium pump similar to the sodium pump. And, like the sodium pump, this pump pumps calcium ions from the interior to the exterior of the cell membrane, creating a calcium ion gradient of about 10,000-fold, leaving an internal concentration of calcium ions of about 10^{-7} molar in contrast to an external concentration of about 10^{-3} molar.

In addition, there are also voltage-gated calcium channels. These channels are slightly permeable to sodium ions as well as to calcium ions; when they open both calcium and sodium ions flow to the interior of the fiber. Therefore, these channels are frequently called *Ca^{++}-Na$^+$ channels.* The Ca^{++}-Na$^+$ channels are very slow to become activated, requiring 10 to 20 times as long for activation as the normal sodium channels. Therefore, they are also frequently called *slow channels,* in contrast to the normal sodium channels that are called *fast channels.*

The Ca^{++}-Na$^+$ channels are very numerous in both cardiac muscle and smooth muscle. In fact, in some types of smooth muscle, the fast sodium channels are hardly present at all, so the action potentials then are caused almost entirely by activation of the slow Ca^{++}-Na$^+$ channels.

Increased Permeability of the Sodium Channels When There Is a Deficit of Calcium Ions. The concentration of calcium ions in the interstitial fluid also has a profound effect on the voltage level at which the sodium channels become activated. When there is a deficit of calcium ions, the sodium channels can be activated by very little increase of the membrane potential above the normal resting level. Therefore, the nerve fiber becomes highly excitable, sometimes discharging repetitively without any provocation rather than remaining in the resting state. In fact, the calcium ion concentration needs to fall only 30 to 50 per cent below normal before spontaneous discharge occurs in many peripheral nerves, often causing muscle "tetany" that can actually be lethal because of tetanic contraction of the respiratory muscles. On the other hand, an increase in calcium ion concentration above normal decreases the excitability of the nerve fiber for opposite reasons.

The probable way in which calcium ions affect the sodium channels is the following: These ions appear to bind to the exterior surfaces of the sodium channel protein molecule. The positive charges of these calcium ions, in turn, alter the electrical state of the channel protein itself, in this way increasing the voltage level required to open the gate.

Chloride Ions. Chloride ions leak through the resting membrane in the same way that small quantities of potassium and sodium ions leak through. In the usual nerve fiber, the rate of chloride diffusion through the membrane is about one half as great as the diffusion of potassium ions. Therefore, the question must be asked: why have we not considered the chloride ions in our explanation of the action potential? The answer is that the chloride ions function passively in this process. The permeability of the chloride leak channels does not change significantly during the action potential.

In the normal resting state of the nerve fiber, the -90 mv inside the fiber repels most of the chloride ions from the fiber. Therefore, the concentration of chloride ions inside the fiber is only 3 to 4 mEq per liter, whereas the concentration outside the fiber is about 103 mEq per liter. The Nernst potential for this ratio of chloride ions is exactly equal to the -90 mv membrane potential, which is what one would expect for an ion that is not actively pumped.

During the action potential, small quantities of chloride ions do diffuse into the nerve fiber because of the temporary loss of the internal negativity. This movement of the chloride ions serves to alter slightly the timing of the successive voltage changes during the action potential, but it does not alter the fundamental process.

INITIATION OF THE ACTION POTENTIAL

Up to this point, we have explained the changing sodium and potassium permeabilities of the membrane as well as the development of the action potential itself, but we have not explained what initiates the action potential. The answer to this is really quite simple:

First, as long as the membrane of the nerve fiber remains totally undisturbed, no action potential will occur in the normal nerve. However, if any event at all causes enough initial rise in the membrane potential from -90 mv up toward the zero level, the rising voltage itself will directly affect the voltage-gated sodium channels, causing them to be-

come activated (opened). This allows rapid inflow of sodium ions, which causes still further rise of the membrane potential, thus opening still more voltage-gated sodium channels and more streaming of sodium ions to the interior of the fiber, with the process continuing in a positive-feedback circle until all the voltage-gated sodium channels have become totally activated. But then within another fraction of a millisecond the rising membrane potential causes inactivation of the sodium channels, and the action potential soon terminates.

Threshold for Initiation of the Action Potential. An action potential will not occur until the initial rise in membrane potential is great enough to create the circle described in the last paragraph. Usually, a sudden rise in membrane potential of 15 to 30 mv is required. Therefore, a sudden increase in the membrane potential in a large nerve fiber of from -90 mv up to about -65 mv will usually cause the explosive development of the action potential. This level of -65 mv is said to be the *threshold* for stimulation.

Accommodation of the Membrane—Failure to Fire Despite Rising Voltage. If the membrane potential rises very slowly—over many milliseconds instead of a fraction of a millisecond—the slow, inactivating gates of the sodium channels will then have time to close at the same time that the activating gates are opening. Consequently, the opening of the activating gates will not be as effective in increasing the flow of sodium ions as normally because many of the inactivating gates will already be closed. Therefore, a slow increase in the internal potential of a nerve fiber either will require a higher threshold voltage than normal to cause firing or will prevent firing entirely at times, even with a voltage rise all the way to zero or even to positive voltage. This phenomenon is called *accommodation* of the membrane to the stimulus.

PROPAGATION OF THE ACTION POTENTIAL

In the preceding paragraphs we have discussed the action potential as it occurs at one spot on the membrane. However, an action potential elicited at any one point on an excitable membrane usually excites adjacent portions of the membrane, resulting in propagation of the action potential. The mechanism of this is illustrated in Figure 6–12. Figure 6–12A shows a normal resting nerve fiber, and Figure 6–12B shows a nerve fiber that has been excited in its midportion—that is, the midportion has suddenly developed increased permeability to sodium. The arrows illustrate a "local circuit" of current flow between the depolarized areas of the membrane and the adjacent resting membrane areas; positive electrical charges flow inward through the depolarized membrane and then for several millimeters along the core of the axon. These positive charges increase the voltage for a distance of 1 to 3 mm inside large fibers to above the threshold voltage value for initiating an action po-

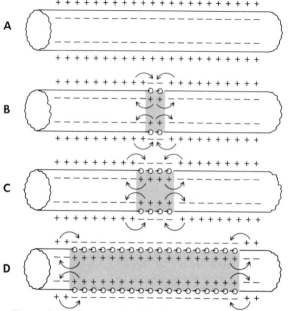

Figure 6–12. Propagation of action potentials in both directions along a conductive fiber.

tential. Therefore, the sodium channels in these new areas immediately activate, and, as illustrated in Figure 6–12C and D, the explosive action potential spreads. And these newly depolarized areas cause local circuits of current flow still further along the membrane, causing progressively more and more depolarization. Thus, the depolarization process travels in both directions along the entire extent of the fiber. The transmission of the depolarization process along a nerve or muscle fiber is called a *nerve* or *muscle impulse.*

Direction of Propagation. It is now obvious that an excitable membrane has no single direction of propagation, but that the action potential can travel in both directions away from the stimulus—and even along all branches of a nerve fiber—until the entire membrane has become depolarized.

The All-or-Nothing Principle. It is equally obvious that, once an action potential has been elicited at any point on the membrane of a normal fiber, the depolarization process will travel over the entire membrane. This is called the *all-or-nothing principle,* and it applies to all normal excitable tissues. Occasionally, though, when the fiber is in an abnormal state, the action potential will reach a point on the membrane at which it does not generate sufficient voltage to stimulate the adjacent area of the membrane. When this occurs, the spread of depolarization will stop. Therefore, for normal propagation of an impulse to occur, the ratio of action potential to threshold for excitation, called the *safety factor,* must at all times be greater than 1.

Propagation of Repolarization. The action potential normally lasts almost the same length of time at each point along a fiber. Therefore, repolarization normally occurs first at the point of original stimulus

and then spreads progressively along the membrane, moving in the same direction that depolarization had previously spread. Figure 6–13 illustrates the same nerve fiber as that in Figure 6–12, showing that the repolarization process is propagated in the same direction as the depolarization process but a few 10,000ths of a second later.

"RECHARGING" THE FIBER MEMBRANE AFTER ACTION POTENTIALS—IMPORTANCE OF ENERGY METABOLISM

Transmission of each impulse along the nerve fiber reduces the concentration differences of sodium and potassium between the inside and outside of the membrane because of diffusion of sodium ions to the inside during depolarization and diffusion of potassium ions to the outside during repolarization. For a single action potential, this effect is so minute that it cannot even be measured. Indeed, 100,000 to 500,000 impulses can be transmitted by nerve fibers before the concentration differences have run down to the point that action potential conduction ceases. Yet, even so, with time it becomes necessary to re-establish the sodium and potassium membrane concentration differences. This is achieved by the action of the Na^+-K^+ pump in exactly the same way as that described earlier in the chapter for establishment of the original resting potential. That is, the sodium ions that, during the action potentials, have diffused to the interior of the cell and the potassium ions that have diffused to the exterior are returned to their original state by the sodium and potassium pump. Since this pump requires energy for operation, this process of "recharging" the nerve fiber is an active metabolic one, utilizing energy derived from the adenosine triphosphate energy "currency" system of the cell.

A special feature of the sodium-potassium ATPase membrane pumping system is that its degree of activity is very strongly stimulated by excess sodium ions inside the cell membrane. In fact, the pumping activity increases approximately in proportion to the third power of the sodium concentration. That is, if the internal sodium concentration rises from 10 to 20 mEq per liter, the activity of the pump does not merely double but instead increases approximately eightfold. Therefore, it can easily be

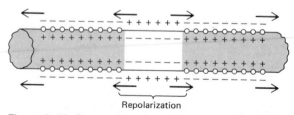

Figure 6–13. Propagation of repolarization in both directions along a conductive fiber.

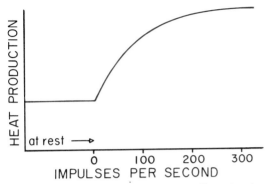

Figure 6–14. Heat production in a nerve fiber at rest and at progressively increasing rates of stimulation.

understood how the recharging process of the nerve fiber can rapidly be set into motion whenever the concentration differences of sodium and potassium across the membrane begin to "run down."

Heat Production by the Nerve Fiber. Figure 6–14 illustrates the relationship of heat production in a nerve fiber to the number of impulses transmitted by the fiber each second. The rate of heat production is a measure of the rate of metabolism in the nerve, because heat is always liberated as a product of the chemical reactions of energy metabolism. Note that the heat production increases markedly as the number of impulses per second increases. It is this increased use of energy that causes the "recharging" process.

THE SPIKE POTENTIAL
AND THE AFTER-POTENTIALS

Figure 6-15 illustrates an action potential recorded with a much slower time scale than that illustrated in Figure 6–7; many milliseconds of recording are shown in comparison with only the first millisecond of the action potential in Figure 6–7.

The Spike Potential. The initial very large change in membrane potential shown in Figure 6–15 is called the spike potential. In large, type A myelinated nerve fibers

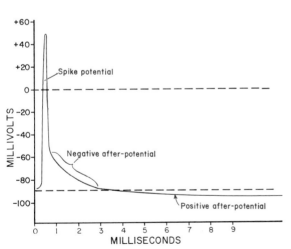

Figure 6–15. An idealized action potential, showing the initial spike followed by a negative after-potential and a positive after-potential.

it lasts for about 0.4 millisecond. The spike potential is the same as the action potential that has been discussed in the preceding paragraphs and is also called the *nerve impulse*.

The Negative After-Potential. At the termination of the spike potential, the membrane potential sometimes fails to return all the way to its resting level for another few milliseconds, as shown in Figure 6–15. This is particularly likely to occur after a series of rapidly repeated action potentials. This is called the *negative after-potential*. It is believed to result at least partly from a buildup of potassium ions immediately outside the membrane; this causes the concentration ratio of potassium across the membrane to be temporarily less than normal and therefore prevents full return of the normal resting membrane potential for a few additional milliseconds.

The Positive After-Potential. Once the membrane potential has returned to its resting value, it then becomes a little more negative than its normal resting value; this is the *positive after-potential* that was discussed earlier. It is a fraction of a millivolt to a few millivolts more negative than the normal resting membrane potential, but it can last from 50 milliseconds to as long as many seconds.

The first part of this positive after-potential is caused by the excess permeability of the nerve membrane to potassium ions at the end of the spike potential, as discussed earlier. However, the prolonged continuance of this potential is caused principally by the electrogenic pumping of excess sodium outward through the nerve fiber membrane, which is the recharging process that was discussed previously. If the active transport processes are poisoned, this part of the positive after-potential is lost.

PLATEAU IN SOME ACTION
POTENTIALS

In some instances the excitable membrane does not repolarize immediately after depolarization, but, instead, the potential remains on a plateau near the peak of the spike sometimes for many milliseconds before repolarization begins. Such a plateau is illustrated in Figure 6–16, from which one can readily see that the plateau greatly prolongs the period of depolarization. This type of action potential occurs in the heart, where the plateau lasts for as long as three- to four-tenths second and causes contraction of the heart muscle during this entire period of time.

The cause of the action potential plateau is a combination of several different factors. First, in heart muscle, two separate types of channels enter into the depolarization process: (1) the usual voltage-activated sodium channels, called the *fast channels*, and (2) the voltage-activated calcium-sodium channels, which are slow to be activated and therefore are called *slow channels*—these channels allow diffusion mainly of calcium ions but also of some sodium ions as well. Activation of the fast channels causes the spike portion of the action potential, whereas the slow but prolonged activation of the slow channels is mainly responsible for the plateau portion of this type of action potential.

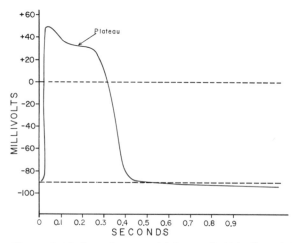

Figure 6–16. An action potential from a Purkinje fiber of the heart, showing a "plateau."

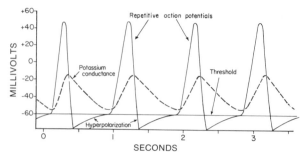

Figure 6–17. Rhythmic action potentials, and their relationship to potassium conductance and to the state of hyperpolarization.

A second factor partly responsible for the plateau is that the voltage-gated potassium channels are slow to be activated in some excitable tissues, often not opening until the very end of the plateau. This delays the return of the membrane potential toward the resting value. But, then, this opening of the potassium channels at the same time that the slow channels begin to close at the end of the plateau causes rapid return of the action potential from its plateau level back to the negative resting level.

RHYTHMICITY OF CERTAIN EXCITABLE TISSUES— REPETITIVE DISCHARGE

All excitable tissues can discharge repetitively if the threshold for stimulation is reduced low enough. For instance, even nerve fibers and skeletal muscle fibers, which normally are highly stable, discharge repetitively when they are placed in a solution containing the drug veratrine or when the calcium ion concentration falls below a critical value. Repetitive discharges, or rhythmicity, occur normally in the heart, in most smooth muscle, and also in many of the neurons of the central nervous system. It is these rhythmical discharges that cause the heart beat, that cause peristalsis, and that cause such neuronal events as the rhythmical control of breathing.

The Re-Excitation Process Necessary for Rhythmicity. For rhythmicity to occur, the membrane, even in its natural state, must already be permeable enough to sodium ions (or to calcium and sodium ions through the Ca^{++}-Na^+ slow channels) to allow automatic membrane depolarization. Thus, Figure 6–17 shows that the "resting" membrane potential is only -60 to -70 millivolts. This is not enough negative voltage to keep the sodium and calcium-sodium channels closed. That is, (1) sodium and calcium ions flow inward; (2) this further increases the membrane permeability; (3) still more ions flow inward; (4) the permeability increases more, and so forth, thus eliciting the regenerative process of sodium and calcium-sodium channel openings until an action potential is generated. Then, at the end of the action potential the membrane repolarizes. But shortly thereafter, the depolarization process begins again and a new action potential occurs spontaneously—this cycle continuing again and again and causing self-induced rhythmical excitation of the excitable tissue.

Yet, why does the membrane not depolarize immediately after it has become repolarized rather than delaying for nearly a second before the onset of the next action potential? The answer to this can be found by referring back to Figure 6–11, which shows that toward the end of all action potentials, and continuing for a short period thereafter, the membrane becomes excessively permeable to potassium. The excessive outflow of potassium ions carries tremendous numbers of positive charges to the outside of the membrane, creating inside the fiber considerably more negativity than would otherwise occur for a short period after the preceding action potential is over, thus drawing the membrane potential nearer to the potassium Nernst potential. This is a state called *hyperpolarization*, which is illustrated in Figure 6–17. As long as this state exists, re-excitation will not occur; but gradually the excess potassium conductance (and the state of hyperpolarization) disappears, thereby allowing the membrane potential to increase until it reaches the *threshold* for excitation; then suddenly a new action potential results, the process occurring again and again.

SPECIAL ASPECTS OF SIGNAL TRANSMISSION IN NERVE TRUNKS

Myelinated and Unmyelinated Nerve Fibers. Figure 6–18 illustrates a cross-section of a typical small nerve trunk, showing a few very large nerve fibers that compose most of the cross-sectional area and many more small fibers lying between the large ones. The large fibers are *myelinated* and the small ones are *unmyelinated*. The average nerve trunk contains about twice as many unmyelinated fibers as myelinated fibers.

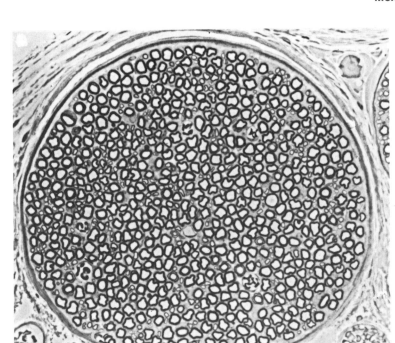

Figure 6–18. Cross-section of a small nerve trunk containing myelinated and unmyelinated fibers.

Figure 6–19 illustrates a typical myelinated fiber. The central core of the fiber is the *axon*, and the membrane of the axon is the actual *conductive membrane*. The axon is filled in its center with *axoplasm*, which is a viscid intra-cellular fluid. Surrounding the axon is a *myelin sheath* that is often thicker than the axon itself, and about once every millimeter along the extent of the axon the myelin sheath is interrupted by a *node of Ranvier*.

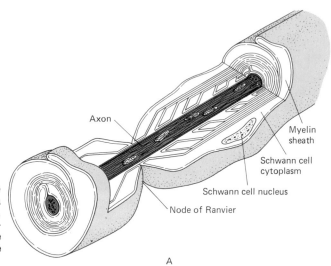

Figure 6–19. Function of the Schwann cell to insulate nerve fibers. *A,* The wrapping of a Schwann cell membrane around a large axon to form the myelin sheath of the myelinated nerve fiber. (Modified from Leeson and Leeson: Atlas of Histology. Philadelphia, W. B. Saunders Company, 1979.) *B,* Evagination of the membrane and cytoplasm of a Schwann cell around multiple umyelinated nerve fibers.

Axon

Myelin sheath

Schwann cell cytoplasm

Schwann cell nucleus

Node of Ranvier

A

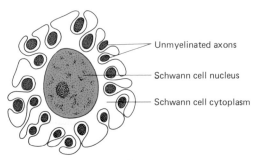

Unmyelinated axons

Schwann cell nucleus

Schwann cell cytoplasm

B

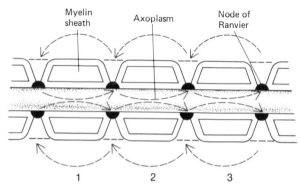

Figure 6–20. Saltatory conduction along a myelinated axon.

The myelin sheath is deposited around the axon by Schwann cells in the following manner: The membrane of a Schwann cell first envelops the axon. Then the cell rotates around the axon many times, laying down multiple layers of cellular membrane containing the lipid substance *sphingomyelin*. This substance is an excellent insulator that prevents almost all flow of ions. In fact, it increases the resistance to ion flow through the membrane approximately 5000-fold and also decreases the membrane capacitance as much as 50-fold. However, at the juncture between each two successive Schwann cells along the axon, a small uninsulated area remains where ions can still flow with ease between the extracellular fluid and the axon. This area is the node of Ranvier.

"Saltatory" Conduction in Myelinated Fibers from Node to Node. Even though ions cannot flow significantly through the thick myelin sheaths of myelinated nerves, they can flow with considerable ease through the nodes of Ranvier. Therefore, action potentials can occur only at the nodes. Yet, the action potentials are conducted from node to node, as illustrated in Figure 6–20; this is called *saltatory conduction*. That is, electrical current flows through the surrounding extracellular fluids and also through the axoplasm from node to node, exciting successive nodes one after another. Thus, the nerve impulse jumps down the fiber, which is the origin of the term "saltatory."

Saltatory conduction is of value for two reasons: First, by causing the depolarization process to jump long intervals along the axis of the nerve fiber, this mechanism increases the velocity of nerve transmission in myelinated fibers an average of five- to sevenfold. Second, saltatory conduction conserves energy for the axon, for only the nodes depolarize, allowing perhaps a hundred times smaller loss of ions than would otherwise be necessary and therefore requiring little extra metabolism for reestablishing the sodium and potassium concentration differences across the membrane after a series of nerve impulses.

Still another feature of saltatory conduction in large myelinated fibers is the following: The excellent insulation afforded by the myelin membrane and the 50-fold decrease in membrane capacitance allows the repolarization process to occur with very little transfer of ions. Therefore, at the end of the action potential when the sodium channels close, repolarization occurs so rapidly that the potassium channels usually have not yet begun to open significantly. Therefore, conduction of the nerve impulse in the myelinated nerve fiber is accomplished almost entirely by the sequential changes in the voltage-gated sodium channels, with very little contribution by the potassium channels.

VELOCITY OF CONDUCTION IN NERVE FIBERS

The velocity of conduction in nerve fibers varies from as little as 0.5 meter per second in very small unmyelinated fibers to as high as 100 meters per second (the length of a football field) in very large myelinated fibers. The velocity increases approximately with the fiber diameter in myelinated nerve fibers and approximately with the square root of fiber diameter in unmyelinated fibers.

EXCITATION—THE PROCESS OF ELICITING THE ACTION POTENTIAL

Chemical Stimulation. Basically, any factor that causes sodium ions to begin to diffuse inward through the membrane in sufficient numbers will set off the automatic regenerative opening of the sodium channels, as noted earlier in the chapter, that eventuates in the action potential. Thus, certain chemicals can stimulate a nerve fiber by increasing the membrane permeability. Such chemicals include acids, bases, almost any salt solution of very strong concentration, and, most importantly, the substance *acetylcholine*. Many nerve fibers, when stimulated, secrete acetylcholine at their endings where they synapse with other neurons or where they end on muscle fibers. The acetylcholine in turn stimulates the successive neuron or muscle fiber by opening pores in the membrane with diameters of 0.6 to 0.7 nanometer, large enough for sodium (as well as other ions) to go through with ease. This is discussed in much greater detail in Chapter 8, and it is one of the most important means by which nerve and muscle fibers are stimulated. Likewise, *norepinephrine* secreted by sympathetic nerve endings can stimulate cardiac muscle fibers and some smooth muscle fibers, and still other hormonal *transmitter substances* can stimulate successive neurons in the central nervous system.

Mechanical Stimulation. Crushing, pinching, or pricking a nerve fiber can cause a sudden surge of sodium influx and, for obvious reasons, can elicit an action potential. Even slight pressure on some specialized nerve endings can stimulate these; this will be discussed in Chapter 12 in relation to sensory perception.

Electrical Stimulation. An electrical current artificially induced through a nerve causes excess flow of ions through the axonal membrane; this too can initiate an action potential. However, not all methods of applying electrical stimuli result in excitation, and, since this is the usual means by which nerve fibers are excited when they are studied in the laboratory, the process of electrical excitation deserves more comment.

Cathodal Versus Anodal Currents. If two electrodes are placed on a nerve bundle and direct electrical current is made to flow through the electrodes with one electrode positive and the other negative, the nerve fibers are stimulated at the negative electrode, called the "cathode." On the other hand, at the positive electrode, called the "anode," the nerve fibers actually become more resistant to excitation than normal. Therefore, it is said that a *cathodal current* excites a nerve fiber while an *anodal current* inhibits it.

The cause of these effects is the following: remember that the action potential is initiated by the opening of voltage-gated sodium channels. Furthermore, these chan-

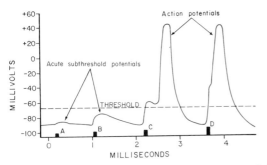

Figure 6–21. Effect of stimuli on the potential of the excitable membrane, showing the development of "acute subthreshold potentials" when the stimuli are below the threshold value required for eliciting an action potential.

nels are opened by a decrease in the electrical voltage across the membrane. The negative current from the cathode reduces the voltage immediately outside the membrane, drawing this voltage nearer to the voltage of the negative resting membrane potential inside the fiber. This decreases the electrical voltage across the membrane and allows activation of the sodium channels, thus resulting in an action potential. Conversely, at the anode, the injection of positive charges on the outside of the nerve membrane heightens the voltage difference across the membrane rather than lessening it. And this causes a state of "hyperpolarization," which decreases the excitability of the fiber.

Threshold for Excitation and "Acute Subthreshold Potential." A very weak electrical, mechanical, or chemical stimulus may not be able to excite a fiber. But, when this stimulus is progressively increased, there comes a point at which excitation takes place. Figure 6–21 illustrates the effects of successively applied stimuli of progressing strength. A very weak stimulus at point *A* causes the membrane potential to change from −90 to −85 millivolts, but this is not sufficient change for the automatic regenerative processes of the action potential to develop. At point *B* the stimulus is greater, but, here again, the intensity still is not enough to set off the automatic action potential. Nevertheless, the membrane voltage is disturbed for as long as a millisecond or more after both of the weak stimuli; the potential changes during these short intervals of time are called *acute subthreshold potentials,* as illustrated in the figure.

At point *C* in Figure 6–21 the stimulus elicits an acute membrane potential that is not subthreshold but slightly more than the threshold value, and, after a short "latent period," it initiates an action potential. At point *D* the stimulus is still stronger, and the acute membrane potential initiates the action potential even sooner. Thus, this figure shows that even a very weak stimulus always causes a local potential change at the membrane, but that the intensity of the *local potential* must rise to a *threshold value* before the automatic action potential will be set off.

Excitability Curve of Nerve Fibers. A so-called "excitability curve" of a nerve fiber is shown in Figure 6–22. To obtain this curve a high voltage electrical stimulus (4 volts, in this instance) is applied to the fiber, and the minimum duration of stimulus required to excite the fiber is found. The voltage and duration are plotted as point *A.* Then a stimulus voltage of 3 volts is applied, and the duration required is again determined; the results are plotted as point *B.* The same is repeated at 2 volts, 1 volt,

0.5 volt, and so forth, until the least voltage possible at which the membrane is stimulated has been reached. On connection of these points, the excitability curve is generated.

The excitability curve of Figure 6–22 is that of a large myelinated nerve fiber. The least possible voltage at which it will fire is called the *rheobase,* and the time required for this least voltage to stimulate the fiber is called the *utilization time.* Then, if the voltage is increased to twice the rheobase voltage, the time required to stimulate the fiber is called the *chronaxie.* The chronaxie is often used as a means of expressing relative excitabilities of different excitable tissues. For instance, the chronaxie of a large type A fiber is about 0.0001 to 0.0002 second; of smaller myelinated nerve fibers, approximately 0.0003 second; of unmyelinated fibers, 0.0005 second; of skeletal muscle fibers, 0.00025 to 0.001 second; and of heart muscle, 0.001 to 0.003 second.

The Refractory Period. A second action potential cannot occur in an excitable fiber as long as the membrane is still depolarized from the preceding action potential. The reason for this is that shortly after the action potential is initiated, the sodium channels become inactivated, and any amount of excitatory signal applied to these channels at this point will not open the inactivation gates. The only condition that will reopen them is for the membrane potential to return either to or almost to the original resting membrane potential level. Then, within another small fraction of a second, the inactivation gates of the sodium channels open, and a new action potential can then be initiated.

The period of time during which a second action potential cannot be elicited, even with a very strong stimulus, is called the *absolute refractory period.* This period for large myelinated nerve fibers is about 1/2500 second. Therefore, one can readily calculate that such a fiber can carry a maximum of about 2500 impulses per second.

Following the absolute refractory period is a *relative refractory period* lasting about one quarter to one half as long. During this time, stronger than normal stimuli can excite the fiber. The cause of this relative refractoriness is twofold: (1) during this time some of the sodium channels still have not been reversed from their inactivation state, and (2) the potassium channels are usually wide open at this time, causing a state of hyperpolarization that makes it more difficult to stimulate the fiber.

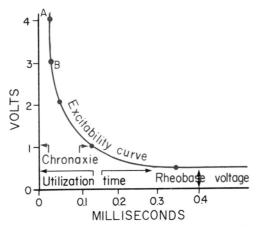

Figure 6–22. Excitability of a large myelinated nerve fiber.

INHIBITION OF EXCITABILITY—"STABILIZERS" AND LOCAL ANESTHETICS

Contrary to the factors that increase nerve excitability, still others, called *membrane-stabilizing factors*, can decrease excitability. For instance, a *high extracellular fluid calcium ion concentration* decreases the membrane permeability and simultaneously reduces its excitability, as was explained earlier. Therefore, calcium ions are said to be a "stabilizer." Also, *low potassium ion concentration* in the extracellular fluids, because it has the direct effect of decreasing the permeability of the potassium channels, likewise acts as a stabilizer and reduces membrane excitability. Indeed, in a hereditary disease known as *familial periodic paralysis*, the extracellular potassium ion concentration is often so greatly reduced that the person actually becomes paralyzed but reverts to normal instantly after intravenous administration of potassium.

Local Anesthetics. Among the most important stabilizers are the many substances used clinically as local anesthetics, including *cocaine, procaine, tetracaine,* and many other drugs. These act directly on the activation gates of the sodium channels, making it much more difficult for these gates to open and thereby reducing the membrane excitability. When the excitability has been reduced so low that the ratio of *action potential strength to excitability threshold* (called the "safety factor") is reduced below 1.0, a nerve impulse fails to pass through the anesthetized area.

RECORDING MEMBRANE POTENTIALS AND ACTION POTENTIALS

The Cathode Ray Oscilloscope. Earlier in this chapter we noted that the membrane potential changes occur very rapidly throughout the course of an action potential. Indeed, most of the action potential complex of large nerve fibers takes place in less than $\frac{1}{1000}$ second. In some figures of this chapter an electrical meter has been shown recording these potential changes. However, it must be understood that any meter capable of recording them must be capable of responding extremely rapidly. For practical purposes the only type of meter that is capable of responding accurately to the very rapid membrane potential changes of most excitable fibers is the cathode ray oscilloscope.

Figure 6–23 illustrates the basic components of a cathode ray oscilloscope. The cathode ray tube itself is composed basically of an *electron gun* and a *fluorescent surface* against which electrons are fired. Where the electrons hit the surface, the fluorescent material glows. If the electron beam is moved across the surface, the spot of glowing light also moves and draws a fluorescent line on the screen.

In addition to the electron gun and fluorescent surface, the cathode ray tube is provided with two sets of plates: one set, called the *horizontal deflection plates,* is positioned on either side of the electron beam, and the other set, called the *vertical deflection plates,* is positioned above and below the beam. If a negative charge is applied to the left-hand plate and a positive charge to the right-hand plate, the electron beam will be repelled away from the left plate and attracted toward the right plate, thus

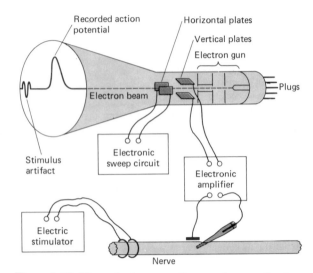

Figure 6–23. The cathode ray oscilloscope for recording transient action potentials.

bending the beam toward the right, and this will cause the spot of light on the fluorescent surface of the cathode ray screen to move to the right. Likewise, positive and negative charges can be applied to the vertical deflection plates to move the beam up or down.

Since electrons travel at extremely rapid velocity and since the plates of the cathode ray tube can be alternately charged positively or negatively within less than a millionth of a second, it is obvious that the spot of light on the face of the tube can also be moved to almost any position in less than a millionth of a second. For this reason, the cathode ray tube oscilloscope can be considered to be an inertialess meter capable of recording with extreme fidelity almost any change in membrane potential.

To use the cathode ray tube for recording action potentials, two electrical circuits must be employed. These are (1) an *electronic sweep circuit* that controls the voltages on the horizontal deflection plates and (2) an *electronic amplifier* that controls the voltages on the vertical deflection plates. The sweep circuit automatically causes the spot of light to begin at the left-hand side and move slowly toward the right. When the spot reaches the right side, it jumps back immediately to the left-hand side and starts a new trace.

The electronic amplifier amplifies signals that come from the nerve. If a change in membrane potential occurs while the spot of light is moving across the screen, this change in potential will be amplified and will cause the spot to rise above or fall below the mean level of the trace, as illustrated in the figure. In other words, the sweep circuit provides the lateral movement of the electron beam while the amplifier provides the vertical movement in direct proportion to the changes in membrane potentials picked up by appropriate electrodes.

Figure 6–23 also shows that an electric stimulator is used to stimulate the nerve. When the nerve is stimulated, a small *stimulus artifact* usually appears on the oscilloscope screen prior to the action potential.

Recording the Monophasic Action Potential. Throughout this chapter "monophasic" action potentials have been shown in the different diagrams. To record these, an electrode such as that illustrated earlier in the chapter

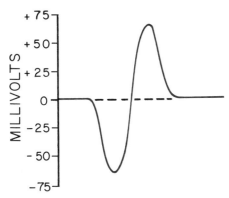

Figure 6–24. Recording of a biphasic action potential.

recorded as illustrated earlier in the chapter in Figures 6–7, 6–11, and 6–15.

Recording a Biphasic Action Potential. When one wishes to record impulses from a whole nerve trunk, it is not feasible to place electrodes inside the nerve fibers. Therefore, the usual method of recording is to place two electrodes on the outside of fibers. However, the record that is obtained is then biphasic for the following reasons: When an action potential moving down the nerve fiber reaches the first electrode, it becomes charged negatively while the second electrode is still unaffected. This causes the oscilloscope to record in the negative direction. Then as the action potential proceeds still farther down the nerve, there comes a point when the membrane beneath the first electrode becomes repolarized while the second electrode is negative, and the oscilloscope records in the opposite direction. When these changes are recorded by the oscilloscope, a graphic record such as that illustrated in Figure 6–24 is recorded, showing a potential change first in one direction and then in the opposite direction.

in Figure 6–3 must be inserted into the interior of the fiber. Then, as the action potential spreads down the fiber, the changes in the potential inside the fiber are

---

REFERENCES

Adams, D. J., *et al.:* Ionic currents in molluscan soma. *Annu. Rev. Neurosci.,* 3:141, 1980.

Adrian, R. H.: Charge movement in the membrane of striated muscle. *Annu. Rev. Biophys. Bioeng.,* 7:85, 1978.

Agnew, W. S.: Voltage-regulated sodium channel molecules. *Annu. Rev. Physiol.,* 45:517, 1984.

Aguayo, A. J., and Karpati, G. (eds.): Current Topics in Nerve and Muscle Research. New York, Elsevier/North-Holland, 1979.

Armstrong, C. M.: Sodium channels and gating currents. *Physiol. Rev.,* 61:644, 1981.

Asbury, A. K., and Johnson, P. C.: Pathology of Peripheral Nerve. Philadelphia, W. B. Saunders Co., 1978.

Auerbach, A., and Sachs, F.: Patch clamp studies of single ionic channels. *Annu. Rev. Biophys. Bioeng.,* 13:269, 1984.

Baker, P. F., *et al.:* Replacement of the axoplasm of giant nerve fibers with artificial solutions. *J. Physiol. (Lond.),* 164:330, 1962.

Baker, P. F., *et al.:* The effects of changes in internal ionic concentrations on the electrical properties of perfused giant axons. *J. Physiol. (Lond.),* 164:355, 1962.

Brinley, F. J., Jr.: Calcium buffering in squid axons. *Annu. Rev. Biophys. Bioeng.,* 7:363, 1978.

Carmeliet, E., and Vereecke, J.: Electrogenesis of the action potential and automaticity. *In* Berne, R. M., *et al.* (eds.): Handbook of Physiology. Sec. 2, Vol. 1. Baltimore, Williams & Wilkins, 1979, p. 269.

Catterall, W. A.: Neurotoxins that act on voltage-sensitive sodium channels in excitable membranes. *Annu. Rev. Pharmacol. Toxicol.,* 20:15, 1980.

Ceccarelli, B., and Clementi, F. (eds.): Neurotoxins, Tools in Neurobiology. New York, Raven Press, 1979.

Cole, K. S.: Electrodiffusion models for the membrane of squid giant axon. *Physiol. Rev.,* 45:340, 1965.

Cooper, S. A.: New peripherally-acting oral analgesic agents. *Annu. Rev. Pharmacol. Toxicol.,* 23:617, 1983.

Cuénod, M., *et al.* (eds.): Development and Chemical Specificity of Neurons. New York, Elsevier/North-Holland, 1979.

DiFrancesco, D., and Noble, D.: A model of cardiac electrical activity incorporating ionic pumps and concentration changes. *Phil. Trans. R. Soc. Lond. (Biol.),* 307:353, 1985.

DiPolo, R., and Beauge, L.: The calcium pump and sodium-calcium exchange in squid axons. *Annu. Rev. Physiol.,* 45:313, 1983.

Fozzard, H. A.: Conduction of the action potential. *In* Berne, R. M., *et al.* (eds.): Handbook of Physiology. Sec. 2, Vol. I. Baltimore, Williams & Wilkins, 1979, p. 335.

French, R. J., and Horn, R.: Sodium channel gating: Models, mimics, and modifiers. *Annu. Rev. Biophys. Bioeng.,* 12:319, 1983.

Goldin, S. M., *et al.:* Isolation and reconstitution of neuronal ion transport proteins. *Annu. Rev. Neurosci.,* 6:419, 1983.

Gospodarowicz, D.: Epidermal and nerve growth factors in mammalian development. *Annu. Rev. Physiol.,* 43:251, 1981.

Greene, L. A., and Shooter, E. M.: The nerve growth factor: Biochemistry, synthesis, and mechanism of action. *Annu. Rev. Neurosci.,* 3:353, 1980.

Guroff, G.: Molecular Neurobiology. New York, Marcel Dekker, 1979.

Harris, W. A.: Neural activity and development. *Annu. Rev. Physiol.,* 43:689, 1981.

Hille, B.: Gating in sodium channels of nerve. *Annu. Rev. Physiol.,* 38:139, 1976.

Hodgkin, A. L.: The Conduction of the Nervous Impulse. Springfield, Ill., Charles C Thomas, 1963.

Hodgkin, A. L., and Horowicz, P.: The effect of sudden changes in ionic concentrations on the membrane potential of single muscle fibers. *J. Physiol. (Lond.),* 153:370, 1960.

Hodgkin, A. L., and Huxley, A. F.: Movement of sodium and potassium ions during nervous activity. *Cold Spr. Harb. Symp. Quant. Biol.,* 17:43, 1952.

Hodgkin, A. L., and Huxley, A. F.: Quantitative description of membrane current and its application to conduction and excitation in nerve. *J. Physiol. (Lond.),* 117:500, 1952.

Jonsson, G.: Chemical neurotoxins as denervation tools in neurobiology. *Annu. Rev. Neurosci.,* 3:169, 1980.

Katz, B.: Nerve, Muscle, and Synapse. New York, McGraw-Hill, 1968.

Keynes, R. D.: Ion channels in the nerve-cell membrane. *Sci. Am.* 240(3):126, 1979.

Kostyuk, P. G.: Intracellular perfusion of nerve cells and its effects on membrane currents. *Physiol. Rev.,* 64:435, 1984.

Latorre, R., and Alvarez, O.: Voltage-dependent channels in lipid bilayer membranes. *Physiol. Rev.,* 61:77, 1981.

Latorre, R., *et al.:* K^+ channels gated by voltage and ions. *Annu. Rev. Physiol.,* 46:485, 1984.

Malhotra, S. K.: The Plasma Membrane. New York, John Wiley & Sons, 1983.

Menaker, M., *et al.:* The physiology of circadian pacemakers. *Annu. Rev. Physiol.,* 40:501, 1978.

Moody, W., Jr.: Effects of intracellular H^+ on the electrical properties of excitable cells. *Annu. Rev. Neurosci.,* 7:257, 1984.

Naftalin, R. J.: The thermostatics and thermodynamics of cotransport. *Biochem. Biophys. Acta,* 778:155, 1984.

Noble, D.: Applications of Hodgkin-Huxley equations to excitable tissues. *Physiol. Rev.,* 46:1, 1966.

Patrick, J., *et al.:* Biology of cultured nerve and muscle. *Annu. Rev. Neurosci.,* 1:417, 1978.

Pfenninger, K. H.: Organization of neuronal membrane. *Annu. Rev. Neurosci.,* 1:445, 1978.

Rall, W.: Core conductor theory and cable properties of neurons. *In* Brookhart, J. M., and Mountcastle, V. B. (eds.): Handbook of Physiology. Sec. 1, Vol. 1. Baltimore, Williams & Wilkins, 1977, p. 39.

Requena, J.: Calcium transport and regulation in nerve fibers. *Annu. Rev. Biophys. Bioeng.,* 12:237, 1983.

Rogart, R.: Sodium channels in nerve and muscle membrane. *Annu. Rev. Physiol.*, 43:711, 1981.

Sakmann, B., and Neher, E.: Patch clamp techniques for studying ionic channels in excitable membranes. *Annu. Rev. Physiol.*, 46:455, 1984.

Schubert, D.: Developmental Biology of Cultured Nerve, Muscle and Glia. New York, John Wiley & Sons, 1984.

Schwartz, J. H. Axonal transport: Components, mechanisms, and specificity. *Annu. Rev. Neurosci.*, 2:476, 1979.

Schwartz, W., and Passow, H.: Ca^{2+}-activated K^+ channels in erythrocytes and excitable cells. *Annu. Rev. Physiol.*, 45:359, 1983.

Shanes, A. M.: Electrochemical aspects of physiological and pharmacological action in excitable cells. *Pharmacol. Rev.*, 10:59, 165, 1958.

Sjodin, R. A.: Ion Transport in Skeletal Muscle. New York, John Wiley & Sons, 1982.

Snell, R. M. (ed.): Transcellular Membrane Potentials and Ionic Fluxes. New York, Gordon Press Pubs., 1984.

Sperelakis, N.: Hormonal and neurotransmitter regulation of Ca^{++} influx through voltage-dependent slow channels in cardiac muscle membrane. *Membr. Biochem.*, 5:131, 1984.

Stefani, E., and Chiarandini, D. J.: Ionic channels in skeletal muscle. *Annu. Rev. Physiol.*, 44:357, 1982.

Stevens, C. F.: The neuron. *Sci. Am.*, 241(3):54, 1979.

Swadlow, H. A., *et al.*: Modulation of impulse conduction along the axonal tree. *Annu. Rev. Biophys. Bioeng.*, 9:143, 1980.

Tsien, R. W.: Calcium channels in excitable cell membranes. *Annu. Rev. Physiol.*, 45:341, 1983.

Ulbricht, W.: Kinetics of drug action and equilibrium results at the node of Ranvier. *Physiol. Rev.*, 61:785, 1981.

Vinores, S., and Guroff, G.: Nerve growth factor: Mechanism of action. *Annu. Rev. Biophys. Bioeng.*, 9:223, 1980.

Walker, J. L., and Brown, H. M.: Intracellular ionic activity measurements in nerve and muscle. *Physiol. Rev.*, 57:729, 1977.

Wallick, E. T., *et al.*: Biochemical mechanism of the sodium pump. *Annu. Rev. Physiol.*, 41:397, 1979.

Waxman, S. G. (ed.): Physiology and Pathobiology of Axons. New York, Raven Press, 1978.

Weiss, D. C. (ed.): Axioplasmic Transport in Physiology and Pathology. New York, Springer-Verlag, 1982.

Windhager, E. E., and Taylor, A.: Regulatory role of intracellular calcium ions in epithelial Na transport. *Annu. Rev. Physiol.*, 45:519, 1983.

Wright, E. M.: Electrophysiology of plasma membrane vesicles. *Am. J. Physiol.*, 246:F363, 1984.

Zigmond, R. E., and Bowers, C. W.: Influence of nerve activity on the macromolecular content of neurons and their effector organs. *Annu. Rev. Physiol.*, 43:673, 1981.

7
Contraction of Skeletal Muscle

Approximately 40 per cent of the body is skeletal muscle and almost another 10 per cent is smooth and cardiac muscle. Many of the same principles of contraction apply to all these different types of muscle, but in the present chapter the function of skeletal muscle is considered mainly; the specialized functions of smooth muscle will be discussed in the following chapter and those of cardiac muscle in Chapter 9.

PHYSIOLOGICAL ANATOMY OF SKELETAL MUSCLE

THE SKELETAL MUSCLE FIBER

Figure 7–1 illustrates the organization of skeletal muscle, showing that all skeletal muscles are made of numerous fibers ranging between 10 and 80 microns in diameter. Each of these fibers in turn is made up of successively smaller subunits, also illustrated in Figure 7–1, that will be described in subsequent paragraphs.

In most muscles the fibers extend the entire length of the muscle, and, except for about 2 per cent of the fibers, each is innervated by only one nerve ending, located near the middle of the fiber.

The Sarcolemma. The sarcolemma is the cell membrane of the muscle fiber. However, the sarcolemma consists of a true cell membrane, called the *plasma membrane,* and an outer coat consisting of a thin layer of polysaccharide material containing numerous thin collagen fibrillae. At the end of the muscle fiber, this surface layer of the sarcolemma fuses with a tendon fiber, and the tendon fibers in turn collect into bundles to form the muscle tendons and thence insert into the bones.

Myofibrils; Actin and Myosin Filaments. Each muscle fiber contains several hundred to several thousand *myofibrils,* which are illustrated by the many small open dots in the cross-sectional view of Figure 7–1C. Each myofibril (Figure 7–1D) in turn has, lying side-by-side, about 1500 *myosin filaments* and 3000 *actin filaments,* which are large polymerized protein molecules that are responsible for muscle contraction. These can be seen in longitudinal view

in the electron micrograph of Figure 7–2 and are represented diagrammatically in Figure 7–1E. The thick filaments are *myosin* and the thin filaments are *actin.* Note that the myosin and actin filaments partially interdigitate and thus cause the myofibrils to have alternate light and dark bands. The light bands, which contain only actin filaments, are called *I bands* because they are mainly *isotropic* to polarized light. The dark bands, which contain the myosin filaments as well as the end of the actin filaments where they overlap the myosin, are called *A bands* because they are *anisotropic* to polarized light. Note also the small projections from the sides of the myosin filaments. These are called *cross-bridges.* They protrude from the surfaces of the myosin filaments along the entire extent of the filament, except in the very center. It is interaction between these cross-bridges and the actin filaments that causes contraction.

Figure 7–1E also shows that the actin filaments are attached to the so-called *Z disc,* and the filaments extend on either side of the Z disc to interdigitate with the myosin filaments. The Z disc, which itself is composed of several filamentous proteins different from the actin and myosin filaments, also passes from myofibril to myofibril, attaching the myofibrils to each other all the way across the muscle fiber. Therefore, the entire muscle fiber has light and dark bands, as is also true of the individual myofibrils. These bands give skeletal and cardiac muscle their striated appearance.

The portion of a myofibril (or of the whole muscle fiber) that lies between two successive Z discs is called a *sarcomere.* When the muscle fiber is at its normal fully stretched resting length, the length of the sarcomere is about 2.0 microns. At this length the actin filaments completely overlap the myosin filaments and are just beginning to overlap each other. We shall see later that at this length the sarcomere also is capable of generating its greatest force of contraction.

When a muscle fiber is stretched beyond its resting length, as it is in Figure 7–1, the ends of the actin filaments pull apart, leaving a light area in the center of the A band. This light area, called the *H zone,* is illustrated in Figure 7–2. Such an H zone rarely occurs in the normally functioning muscle

Skeletal muscle

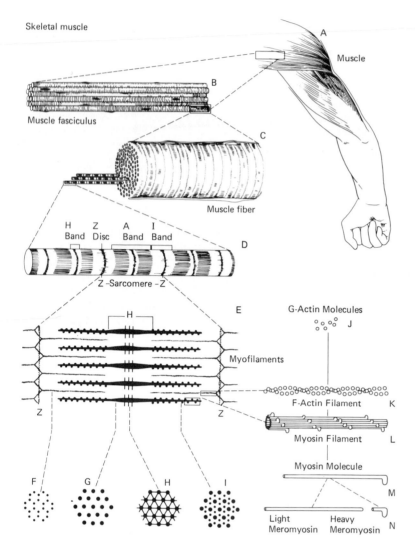

Figure 7–1. Organization of skeletal muscle, from the gross to the molecular level. *F, G, H,* and *I* are cross-sections at the levels indicated. (Drawing by Sylvia Colard Keene. From Bloom and Fawcett: A Textbook of Histology. Philadelphia, W. B. Saunders Company, 1975.)

because normal sarcomere contraction occurs when the length of the sarcomere is between 2.0 microns and 1.6 microns. In this range the ends of the actin filaments not only overlap the myosin filaments but also overlap each other.

The Sarcoplasm. The myofibrils are suspended inside the muscle fiber in a matrix called *sarcoplasm,* which is composed of usual intracellular constituents. The fluid of the sarcoplasm contains large quantities of potassium, magnesium, phosphate, and protein enzymes. Also present are tremendous numbers of *mitochondria* that lie between and parallel to the myofibrils, a condition which is indicative of the great need of the contracting myofibrils for large amounts of ATP formed by the mitochondria.

The Sarcoplasmic Reticulum. Also in the sarcoplasm is an extensive endoplasmic reticulum, which in the muscle fiber is called the *sarcoplasmic reticulum.* This reticulum has a special organization that is extremely important in the control of muscle contraction, which will be discussed later in the chapter. The electron micrograph of Figure 7–3 illustrates the arrangement of this sarcoplasmic reticulum and shows how extensive it can be. The more rapidly contracting types of muscle have especially extensive sarcoplasmic reticula, indicating that this structure is important in causing rapid muscle contraction, as will also be discussed later.

MOLECULAR MECHANISM OF MUSCLE CONTRACTION

Sliding Mechanism of Contraction. Figure 7–4 illustrates the basic mechanism of muscle contraction. It shows the relaxed state of a sarcomere (above) and the contracted state (below). In the relaxed state, the ends of the actin filaments derived from two successive Z discs barely overlap each other while at the same time completely overlapping the myosin filaments. On the other hand, in the contracted state these actin filaments have been pulled inward among the myosin filaments so that they now overlap each other to a major extent. Also, the Z discs have been pulled by the actin

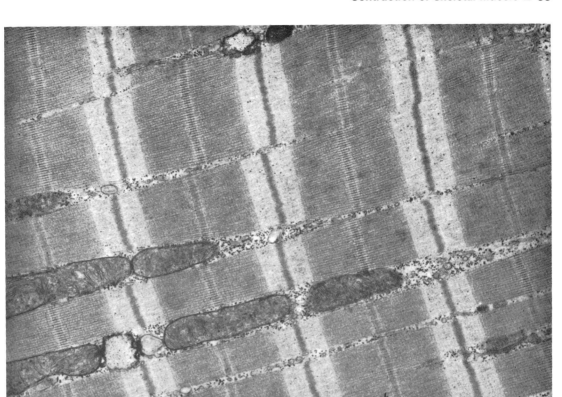

Figure 7–2. Electron micrograph of muscle myofibrils, showing the detailed organization of actin and myosin filaments. Note the mitochondria lying between the myofibrils. (From Fawcett: The Cell. Philadelphia, W. B. Saunders Company, 1981.)

filaments up to the ends of the myosin filaments. Indeed, the actin filaments can be pulled together so tightly that the ends of the myosin filaments actually buckle during very intense contraction. Thus, muscle contraction occurs by a *sliding filament mechanism*.

But what causes the actin filaments to slide inward among the myosin filaments? Almost certainly, this is caused by mechanical, chemical, or electrostatic forces generated by the interaction of the cross-bridges of the myosin filaments with the actin filaments, as we shall discuss in the following sections.

Under resting conditions, the sliding forces between the actin and myosin filaments are inhibited, but when an action potential travels over the muscle fiber membrane, this causes the release of large quantities of calcium ions into the sarcoplasm sur-

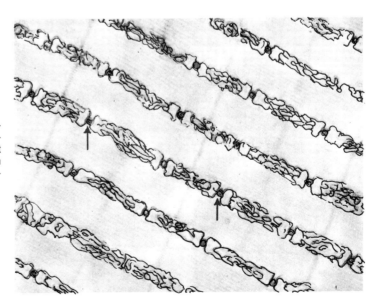

Figure 7–3. Sarcoplasmic reticulum surrounding the myofibril, showing the longitudinal system paralleling the myofibrils. Also shown in cross-section are the T tubules that lead to the exterior of the fiber membrane and that contain extracellular fluid (arrows). (From Fawcett: The Cell. Philadelphia, W. B. Saunders Company, 1981.)

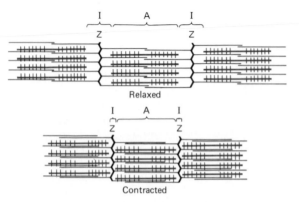

Figure 7–4. The relaxed and contracted states of a myofibril, showing sliding of the actin filaments (black) into the channels between the myosin filaments (red).

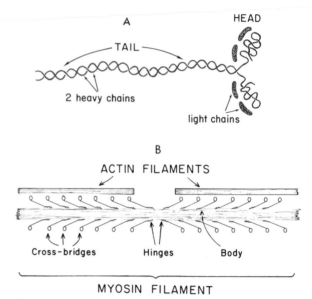

Figure 7–5. *A*, The myosin molecule. *B*, Combination of many myosin molecules to form a myosin filament. Also shown are the cross-bridges and the interaction between the heads of the cross-bridges and adjacent actin filaments.

rounding the myofibrils. These calcium ions activate the forces between the filaments and contraction begins. But energy is also needed for the contractile process to proceed. This energy is derived from the high energy bonds of adenosine triphosphate (ATP), which is degraded to adenosine diphosphate (ADP) to give the energy required.

In the next few sections we will describe what is known about the details of the molecular processes of contraction. To begin this discussion, however, we must first characterize in detail the myosin and actin filaments.

MOLECULAR CHARACTERISTICS OF THE CONTRACTILE FILAMENTS

The Myosin Filament. The myosin filament is composed of multiple myosin molecules, each having a molecular weight of about 480,000. Figure 7–5A illustrates an individual molecule; section B illustrates the organization of the molecules to form a myosin filament, as well as its interaction with the ends of two actin filaments.

The *myosin molecule* is comprised of six polypeptide chains, two *heavy chains* each with a molecular weight of about 200,000, and four *light chains* with molecular weights of about 20,000 each. The two heavy chains coil around each other to form a double helix. However, one end of each of these chains is folded into a globular protein mass called the myosin *head*. Thus, there are two free heads lying side by side at one end of the double helix myosin molecule; the other end of the coiled helix is called the *tail*. The four light chains are also parts of the myosin heads, two to each head. These light chains help control the function of the head during the process of muscle contraction.

The *myosin filament* is made up of about 200 individual myosin molecules. The central portion of one of these filaments is illustrated in Figure 7–5B, showing the tails of the myosin molecules bundled together to form the *body* of the filament, while many heads of the molecules hang outward to the sides of the body. Also, part of the helix portion of each myosin molecule extends to the side along with the head, thus providing an *arm* that extends the head outward from the body as shown in the figure. The protruding arms and heads together are called *cross-bridges*, and each of these is believed to be flexible at two points called *hinges*, one where the arm leaves the body of the myosin filament and the other where the two heads attach to the arm. The hinged arms allow the heads to be extended either far outward from the body of the myosin filament or to be brought close to the body. The hinged heads are believed to participate in the actual contraction process, as we shall discuss in the following sections.

The total length of the myosin filament is 1.6 microns. However, note that there are no cross-bridge heads in the very center of the myosin filament for a distance of about 0.2 micron because the hinged arms extend toward both ends of the myosin filament away from the center; therefore, in the center there are only tails of the myosin molecules and no heads.

Now, to complete the picture, the myosin filament itself is twisted so that each successive set of cross-bridges is axially displaced from the previous set by 120 degrees. This insures that the cross-bridges extend in all directions around the filament.

ATPase Activity of the Myosin Head. Another feature of the myosin head that is essential for muscle contraction is that it can function as an ATPase enzyme. As we shall see later, this property allows the head to cleave ATP and to use the energy derived from the ATP's high energy phosphate bond to energize the contraction process.

The Actin Filament. The actin filament is also complex. It is composed of three different components: *actin, tropomyosin,* and *troponin.*

The backbone of the actin filament is a double-stranded F-actin protein molecule, illustrated in Figure 7–6. The two strands are wound in a helix in the same manner as the myosin molecule, but with a complete revolution every 70 nanometers.

Each strand of the double F-actin helix is composed of polymerized G-actin molecules, each having a molecular weight of 42,000. There are approximately 13 of these molecules in each revolution of each strand of helix. Attached to each one of the G-actin molecules is one molecule of ADP. It is believed that these ADP molecules are the active sites on the actin filaments with which the cross-bridges of the myosin filaments interact to cause muscle contraction. The active sites on the two F-actin strands of the double helix are staggered, giving one active site on the overall actin filament approximately every 2.7 nanometers.

Each actin filament is approximately 1 micron long. The bases of the actin filaments are inserted strongly into the Z discs, while their other ends protrude in both directions into the adjacent sarcomeres to lie in the spaces between the myosin molecules, as illustrated in Figure 7–4.

The Tropomyosin Strands. The actin filament also contains two additional protein strands that are polymers of *tropomyosin* molecules, each molecule having a molecular weight of 70,000 and extending a length of 40 nanometers. It is believed that each tropomyosin strand is loosely attached to an F-actin strand and that in the resting state it physically covers the active sites of the actin strands so that interaction cannot occur between the actin and myosin to cause contraction.

Troponin and Its Role in Muscle Contraction. Attached approximately two thirds the distance along each tropomyosin molecule is a complex of three globular protein molecules called *troponin.* One of the globular proteins (troponin I) has a strong affinity for actin, another (troponin T) for tropomyosin, and a third (troponin C) for calcium ions. This complex is believed to attach the tropomyosin to the actin. The strong affinity of the troponin for calcium ions is believed to initiate the contraction process, as will be explained in the following section.

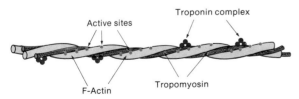

Figure 7–6. The actin filament, composed of two helical strands of F-actin and two tropomyosin strands that lie in the grooves between the actin strands. Attaching the tropomyosin to the actin are several troponin complexes.

Interaction of Myosin and Actin Filaments to Cause Contraction

Inhibition of the Actin Filament by the Troponin-Tropomyosin Complex; Activation by Calcium Ions. A pure actin filament without the presence of the troponin-tropomyosin complex binds strongly with myosin molecules in the presence of magnesium ions and ATP, both of which are normally abundant in the myofibril. But, if the troponin-tropomyosin complex is added to the actin filament, this binding does not take place. Therefore, it is believed that the active sites on the normal actin filament of the relaxed muscle are inhibited (or perhaps physically covered) by the troponin-tropomyosin complex. Consequently, they cannot interact with the myosin filaments to cause contraction. Before contraction can take place, the inhibitory effect of the troponin-tropomyosin complex must itself be inhibited.

Now, let us discuss the role of the calcium ions. In the presence of large amounts of calcium ions, the inhibitory effect of the troponin-tropomyosin on the actin filaments is itself inhibited. The mechanism of this is not known, but one suggestion is the following: When calcium ions combine with troponin C, each molecule of which can bind strongly with up to four calcium ions even when they are present in minute quantities, the troponin complex supposedly undergoes a conformational change that in some way tugs on the tropomyosin protein strand and supposedly moves the tropomyosin strand deeper into the groove between the two actin strands. This "uncovers" the active sites of the actin, thus allowing contraction to proceed. Though this is a hypothetical mechanism, nevertheless it does emphasize that the normal relationship between the tropomyosin-troponin complex and actin is altered by calcium ions—a condition that leads to contraction.

Interaction Between the "Activated" Actin Filament and the Myosin Cross-Bridges—The "Walk-Along" Theory of Contraction. As soon as the actin filament becomes activated by the calcium ions, it is believed that the heads of the cross-bridges from the myosin filaments immediately become attracted to the active sites of the actin filament, and this in some way causes contraction to occur. Though the precise manner by which this interaction between the cross-bridges and the actin causes contraction is still unknown, a suggested hypothesis for which considerable evidence exists is the *"walk-along" theory of contraction.*

Figure 7–7 illustrates the postulated walk-along mechanism for contraction. This figure shows the heads of two cross-bridges attaching to and disengaging from the active sites of an actin filament. It is postulated that when the head attaches to an active site this attachment simultaneously causes profound changes in the intramolecular forces in the head and arm of the cross-bridge. The new alignment of forces causes the head to tilt toward

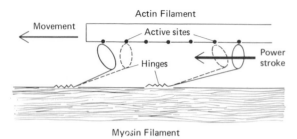

Figure 7-7. The "walk along" mechanism for contraction of the muscle.

the arm and to drag the actin filament along with it. This tilt of the head of the cross-bridge is called the *power stroke*. Then, immediately after tilting, the head automatically breaks away from the active site and returns to its normal perpendicular direction. In this position it combines with an active site farther down along the actin filament; then, a similar tilt takes place again to cause a new power stroke, and the actin filament moves another step. Thus, the heads of the cross-bridges bend back and forth and walk step by step along the actin filament, pulling the action toward the center of the myosin filament.

Each one of the cross-bridges is believed to operate independently of all others, each attaching and pulling in a continuous but random cycle. Therefore, the greater the number of cross-bridges in contact with the actin filament at any given time, the greater, theoretically, is the force of contraction.

ATP as the Source of Energy for Contraction—Chemical Events in the Motion of the Myosin Heads. When a muscle contracts against a load, work is performed and energy is required. It is found that large amounts of ATP are cleaved to form ADP during the contraction process. Furthermore, the greater the amount of work performed by the muscle, the greater the amount of ATP that is cleaved, which is called the *Fenn effect*. Though it is still not known exactly how ATP is used to provide the energy for contraction, the following is a sequence of events that has been suggested as the means by which this occurs:

1. Before contraction begins, the heads of the cross-bridges bind with ATP. The ATPase activity of the myosin head immediately cleaves the ATP but leaves the cleavage products, ADP plus Pi, bound to the head. In this state, the conformation of the head is such that it extends perpendicularly toward the actin filament but is not yet attached to the actin.

2. Next, when the inhibitory effect of the troponin-tropomyosin complex is itself inhibited by calcium ions, active sites on the actin filament are uncovered and the myosin heads do then bind with these, as illustrated in Figure 7-7.

3. The bond between the head of the cross-bridge and the active site of the actin filament causes a conformational change in the head, causing the

head to tilt backward toward the arm of the cross-bridge. This provides the *power stroke* for pulling the actin filament. The energy that activates the power stroke is the energy already stored in the head at the time of cleavage of the ATP.

4. Once the head of the cross-bridge is tilted, this allows release of the ADP and Pi and exposes a site on the head where new ATP can bind. Therefore, a new molecule of ATP binds, and this binding in turn causes detachment of the head from the actin.

5. After the head has split away from the actin, the new molecule of ATP is also cleaved, and the energy again "cocks" the head back to its perpendicular condition ready to begin a new power stroke cycle.

6. Then, when the cocked head, with its stored energy derived from the cleaved ATP, binds with a new active site on the actin filament, it becomes uncocked and once again provides the power stroke.

7. Thus, the process proceeds again and again until the actin filament pulls the Z membrane up against the ends of the myosin filaments or until the load on the muscle becomes too great for further pulling to occur.

DEGREE OF ACTIN AND MYOSIN FILAMENT OVERLAP—EFFECT ON TENSION DEVELOPED BY THE CONTRACTING MUSCLE

Figure 7-8 illustrates the effect of sarcomere length on the tension developed by a single, contracting, *isolated* muscle fiber. To the right are illustrated different degrees of overlap of the myosin and actin filaments at different sarcomere lengths. At point D on the diagram, the actin filament has pulled all the way out to the end of the myosin filament with no overlap at all. At this point, the

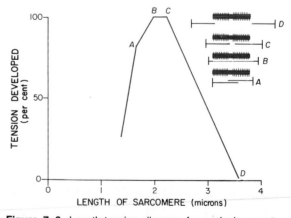

Figure 7-8. Length-tension diagram for a single sarcomere, illustrating maximum strength of contraction when the sarcomere is 2.0 to 2.2 microns in length. At the upper right are shown the relative positions of the actin and myosin filaments at different sarcomere lengths from point A to point D. (Modified from Gordon, Huxley, and Julian: *J. Physiol., 171:*28P, 1964.)

tension developed by the activated muscle is zero. Then, as the sarcomere shortens and the actin filament overlaps the myosin filament progressively more and more, the tension increases progressively until the sarcomere length decreases to about 2.2 microns. At this point the actin filament has already overlapped all the cross-bridges of the myosin filament but has not yet reached the center of the myosin filament. Upon further shortening, the sarcomere maintains full tension until point *B* at a sarcomere length of approximately 2.0 microns. At this point the ends of the two actin filaments begin to overlap. As the sarcomere length falls from 2 microns down to about 1.65 microns at point *A*, the strength of contraction decreases. It is at this point that the two Z discs of the sarcomere abut the ends of the myosin filaments. Then, as contraction proceeds to still shorter sarcomere lengths, the ends of the myosin filaments are actually crumpled, and, as illustrated in Figure 7–8, the strength of contraction also decreases precipitously.

This diagram illustrates that maximum contraction occurs when there is maximum overlap between the actin filaments and the cross-bridges of the myosin filaments, and it supports the idea that the greater the number of cross-bridges pulling the actin filaments, the greater the strength of contraction.

Relation of Force of Contraction of the Intact Muscle to Muscle Length. The upper curve of Figure 7–9 is similar to that in Figure 7–8, but this illustrates the intact whole muscle rather than the isolated muscle fiber. The whole muscle has a large amount of connective tissue in it; also, the sarcomeres in different parts of the muscle do not necessarily contract exactly in unison. Therefore, the curve has somewhat different dimensions from those illustrated for the individual muscle fiber, but it nevertheless exhibits the same form.

Note in Figure 7–9 that when the muscle is at its normal resting length and is then activated, it contracts with maximum force of contraction. If the muscle is stretched to much greater than normal length prior to contraction, a large amount of *resting*

tension develops in the muscle even before contraction takes place; this tension results from the elastic forces of the connective tissue, of the sarcolemma, the blood vessels, the nerves, and so forth. However, the *increase* in tension during contraction, called *active tension*, decreases as the muscle is stretched beyond its normal length. This is demonstrated by the decrease in the arrow length in the figure.

RELATION OF VELOCITY OF CONTRACTION TO LOAD

A muscle contracts extremely rapidly when it contracts against no load—to a state of full contraction in approximately 0.1 second for the average muscle. However, when loads are applied, the velocity of contraction becomes progressively less as the load increases, as illustrated in Figure 7–10. When the load increases to equal the maximum force that the muscle can exert, then the velocity of contraction becomes zero and no contraction at all results, despite activation of the muscle fiber.

This decreasing velocity with load is caused by the fact that a load on a contracting muscle is a reverse force that opposes the contractile force caused by muscle contraction. Therefore, the net force that is available to cause velocity of shortening is correspondingly reduced.

INITIATION OF MUSCLE CONTRACTION: EXCITATION-CONTRACTION COUPLING

Initiation of contraction in skeletal muscle begins with action potentials in the muscle fibers. These elicit electrical currents that spread to the interior of the fiber where they cause release of calcium ions from the sarcoplasmic reticulum. It is the calcium ions that in turn initiate the chemical events of the contractile process. This overall process for controlling muscle contraction is called *excitation-contraction coupling.*

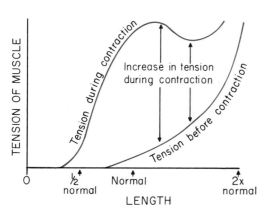

Figure 7–9. Relation of muscle length to force of contraction.

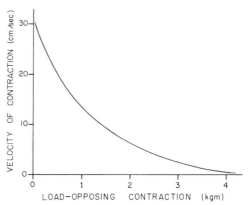

Figure 7–10. Relation of load to velocity of contraction in a skeletal muscle 8 centimeters long.

THE MUSCLE ACTION POTENTIAL

Almost everything discussed in Chapter 6 regarding initiation and conduction of action potentials in nerve fibers applies equally well to skeletal muscle fibers, except for quantitative differences. Some of the quantitative aspects of muscle potentials are the following:

1. Resting membrane potential: approximately −90 millivolts in skeletal fibers—the same as in large myelinated nerve fibers.

2. Duration of action potential: 1 to 5 milliseconds in skeletal muscle—about five times as long as large myelinated nerves.

3. Velocity of conduction: 3 to 5 meters per second—about $\frac{1}{18}$ the velocity of conduction in the large myelinated nerve fibers that excite skeletal muscle.

Excitation of Skeletal Muscle Fibers by Nerves. In normal function of the body, skeletal muscle fibers are excited by large myelinated nerve fibers. These attach to the skeletal muscle fibers at the neuromuscular junction, which will be discussed in detail in the following chapter. Except for 2 per cent of the muscle fibers, there is only one neuromuscular junction to each muscle fiber; this junction is located near the middle of the fiber. Therefore, the action potential spreads from the middle of the fiber toward its two ends. This dual direction of spreading from the center is important because it allows nearly coincident contraction of all sarcomeres of the muscles so that they can all contract together rather than separately.

Spread of the Action Potential to the Interior of the Muscle Fiber by Way of the Transverse Tubule System

The skeletal muscle fiber is so large that action potentials spreading along its surface membrane cause almost no current flow deep within the fiber. Yet, to cause contraction, these electrical currents must penetrate to the vicinity of all the separate myofibrils. This is achieved by transmission of the action potentials along *transverse tubules* (T tubules) that penetrate all the way through the muscle fiber from one side to the other. The T tubule action potentials in turn cause the sarcoplasmic reticulum to release calcium ions in the immediate vicinity of all the myofibrils, and it is these calcium ions that in turn cause contraction. Now, let us describe this system in much greater detail.

The Transverse Tubule–Sarcoplasmic Reticulum System. Figure 7–11 illustrates a group of myofibrils surrounded by the transverse tubule–sarcoplasmic reticulum system. The transverse tubules penetrate all the way from one side of the muscle fiber to the opposite side. Not shown in the figure is the fact that these tubules branch among themselves so that they form entire *planes* of T tubules interlacing among all the separate myofibrils. Also, it should

be noted that where the T tubules originate from the cell membrane they are open to the exterior. Therefore, they communicate with the fluid surrounding the muscle fiber and contain extracellular fluid in their lumens. In other words, the T tubules are internal extensions of the cell membrane. Therefore, when an action potential spreads over a muscle fiber membrane, it spreads along the T tubules to the deep interior of the muscle fiber as well. The action potential currents surrounding these transverse tubules then elicit the muscle contraction.

Figure 7–11 shows the extensiveness of the *sarcoplasmic reticulum* as well. This is composed of two major parts: (1) long *longitudinal tubules* that terminate in (2) large chambers called *terminal cisternae* that abut the transverse tubules. When the muscle fiber is sectioned longitudinally and electron micrographs are made, one sees this abutting of the cisternae against the transverse tubule, which gives the appearance of a *triad* with a small central tubule and a large cisterna on either side. This is illustrated in Figure 7–11 and is also seen in the electron micrograph of Figure 7–3.

In the muscle of lower animals such as the frog, there is a single T tubule network for each sarcomere, located at the level of the Z disc as illustrated in Figure 7–11. Cardiac muscle also has this type of T tubule system. However, in mammalian skeletal muscle there are two T tubule networks for each sarcomere located near the two ends of the myosin filaments, which are the points where the actual mechanical forces of muscle contraction are created. Thus, mammalian skeletal muscle is optimally organized for rapid excitation of muscle contraction.

RELEASE OF CALCIUM IONS BY THE SARCOPLASMIC RETICULUM

One of the special features of the sarcoplasmic reticulum is that it contains calcium ions in very high concentration, and many of these ions are released when the adjacent T tubule is excited.

Figure 7–12 shows that the action potential of the T tubule causes current flow through the cisternae where they abut the T tubule. The cisternae project *junctional feet* that surround the T tubule, presumably facilitating passage of electrical current from the T tubule into the cisternae. This current flow causes rapid release of calcium ions from the cisternae and perhaps from the longitudinal tubules as well. Presumably this results from the opening of calcium channels similar to the opening of sodium channels at the onset of the action potential, though the actual mechanism is still unknown.

The calcium ions that are thus released from the sarcoplasmic reticulum diffuse to the adjacent myofibrils where they bind strongly with troponin C, as discussed in an earlier section, and this in turn elicits the muscle contraction, as has also been discussed. However, the calcium ions also bind less

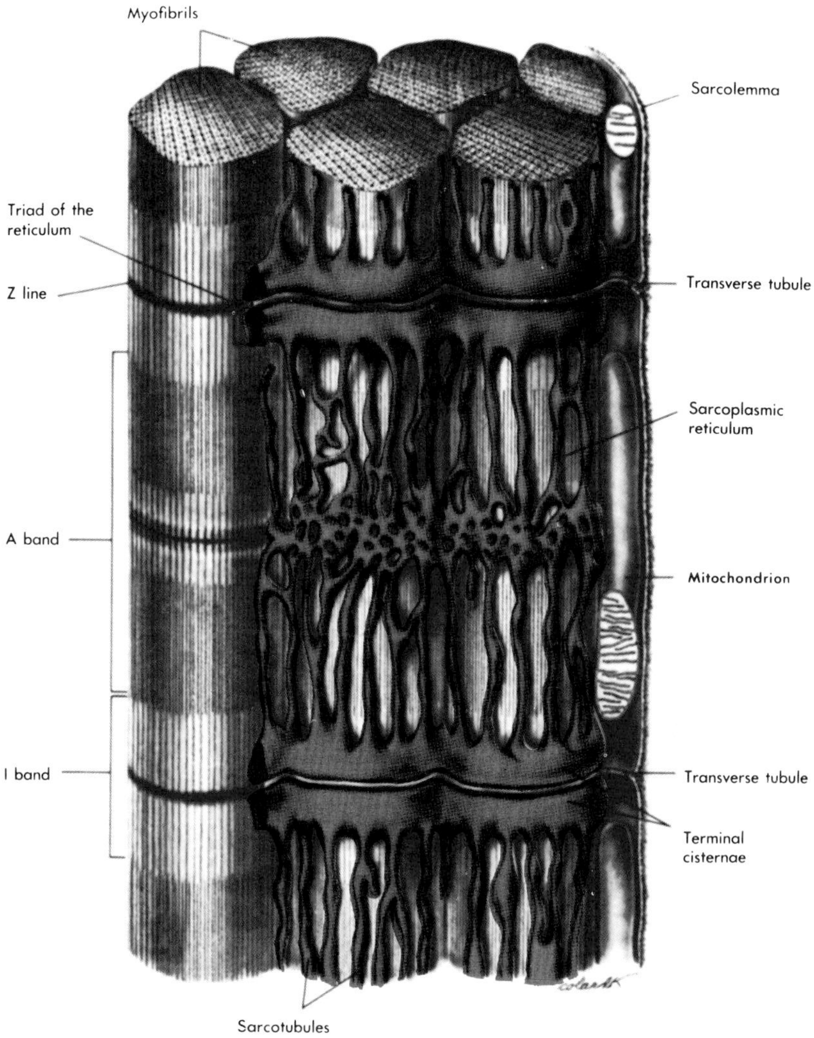

Myofibrils

Sarcolemma

Triad of the
reticulum

Z line

Transverse tubule

Figure 7–11. The transverse tubule-sarco-
plasmic reticulum system. Note the *longitudinal
tubules* that terminate in large *cisternae*. The
cisternae in turn abut the transverse tubules.
Note also that the transverse tubules communicate with the outside of the cell membrane.
This illustration was drawn from frog muscle,
which has one transverse tubule per sarcomere,
located at the Z line. A similar arrangement is
found in mammalian heart muscle, but mammalian skeletal muscle has two transverse tubules per sarcomere, located at the A-I junctions. (From Bloom and Fawcett: A Textbook of
Histology. Philadelphia, W. B. Saunders Company, 1975. Modified after Peachey: *J. Cell Biol.
25*:209, 1965. Drawn by Sylvia Colard Keene.)

Sarcoplasmic
reticulum

A band

Mitochondrion

I band

Transverse tubule

Terminal
cisternae

Sarcotubules

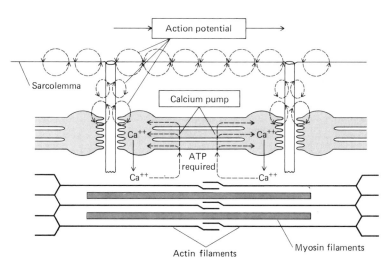

Figure 7–12. Excitation-contraction coupling in the
muscle, showing an action potential that causes release of calcium ions from the sarcoplasmic reticulum
and then reuptake of the calcium ions by a calcium
pump.

strongly with the myosin filaments, which theoretically could be another factor in initiating contraction.

The Calcium Pump for Removing Calcium Ions from the Sarcoplasmic Fluid. Once the calcium ions have been released from the cisternae and have diffused to the myofibrils, muscle contraction will then continue as long as the calcium ions remain in high concentration in the sarcoplasmic fluid. However, a continually active calcium pump located in the walls of the sarcoplasmic reticulum pumps calcium ions out of the sarcoplasmic fluid back into the vesicular cavities of the reticulum. This pump can concentrate the calcium ions about 10,000-fold inside the sarcoplasmic reticulum. In addition, inside the reticulum is a protein called *calsequestrin* that can bind 40 times as much calcium as that in the ionic state, thus providing another 40-fold increase in the storage of calcium. Thus, this massive transfer of calcium in the sarcoplasmic reticulum causes total depletion of calcium ions in the fluid of the myofibrils. Therefore, except immediately after an action potential, the calcium ion concentration in the myofibrils is kept at an extremely low level.

The Excitatory "Pulse" of Calcium Ions. The normal concentration (less than 10^{-7} molar of calcium ions in the cytosol) that bathes the myofibrils is too little to elicit contraction. Therefore, in the resting state, the troponin-tropomyosin complex keeps the actin filaments inhibited and maintains a relaxed state of the muscle.

On the other hand, full excitation of the T tubule–sarcoplasmic reticulum system causes enough release of calcium ions to increase the concentration in the myofibrillar fluid to as high as 2×10^{-4} molar concentration, which is several times the level required to cause maximum muscle contraction (about 2×10^{-5} molar). Immediately thereafter, the calcium pump depletes the calcium ions again. The total duration of this calcium "pulse" in the usual skeletal muscle fiber lasts about $\frac{1}{30}$ of a second, though it may last several times as long as this in some skeletal muscle fibers and be several times shorter in others (in heart muscle the pulse lasts for as long as 0.3 second because of the long duration of the cardiac action potential). It is during this calcium pulse that muscle contraction occurs. If the contraction is to continue without interruption for longer intervals, a series of such pulses must be initiated by a continuous series of repetitive action potentials, as will be discussed in more detail later in the chapter.

THE SOURCE OF ENERGY
FOR MUSCLE CONTRACTION

We have already seen that muscle contraction depends upon energy supplied by ATP. Most of this energy is required to actuate the "walk-along" mechanism by which the cross-bridges pull the actin filaments, but small amounts are required for (1) pumping calcium from the sarcoplasm into the sarcoplasmic reticulum, and (2) pumping sodium and potassium ions through the muscle fiber membrane to maintain an appropriate ionic environment for the propagation of action potentials.

However, the concentration of ATP present in the muscle fiber, about 4 mM, is sufficient to maintain full contraction for only a few seconds at most. Fortunately, after the ATP is broken into ADP, the ADP is rephosphorylated to form new ATP within a fraction of a second. There are several sources of the energy for this rephosphorylation:

The first source of energy that is used to reconstitute the ATP is the substance *phosphocreatine,* which carries a high energy phosphate bond similar to that of ATP. The high energy phosphate bond of the phosphocreatine has a slightly higher amount of free energy than that of the ATP bond. Therefore, it is instantly cleaved and the released energy causes bonding of a new phosphate ion to ADP to reconstitute the ATP. However, the total amount of phosphocreatine is also very little—only about five times as great as the ATP. Therefore, the combined energy of both the stored ATP and the phosphocreatine in the muscle is still capable of causing maximal muscle contraction for no longer than a few more seconds.

The next source of energy used to reconstitute both the phosphocreatine and the ATP is energy released from foodstuffs—from carbohydrates, fats, and proteins. A small amount of this energy is released during the initial breakdown of glucose and glycogen in the cells, which is the process of *glycolysis.* However, about 95 per cent of the energy is released during final oxidation of the foodstuffs, which occurs almost entirely in the mitochondria. Both these processes utilize the energy released from the foodstuffs to form new ATP. The importance of glycolysis is that energy can be released to form new ATP about 2.5 times as rapidly by this mechanism as by the oxidative mechanism. However, the glycolytic mechanism also rapidly builds up glycolytic end-products in the muscle cells so that glycolysis can usually sustain maximum muscle contraction for only about one minute. On the other hand, oxidative release of energy is exceedingly efficient and can also use other food substrates such as fats and proteins in addition to glucose and glycogen, thus allowing continued muscle activity for many hours, though at a level of energy release only about one fourth that which can be achieved during the first few seconds of exercise.

Efficiency of Muscle Contraction. The "efficiency" of an engine or a motor is calculated as the percentage of energy input that is converted into work instead of heat. The percentage of the input energy to a muscle (the chemical energy in the nutrients) that can be converted into work is less than 20 to 25 per cent, the remainder becoming heat. The reason for this low efficiency is that about half of the energy in the foodstuffs is lost during the formation of ATP, and even then only 40 to 45 per cent of the energy in the ATP itself can later be converted into work. Maximum efficiency can be realized only when the muscle contracts at a moderate velocity. If the muscle contracts very slowly or without any movement at all, large amounts of *maintenance heat* are released during the process of contraction even though little or no work is being performed, thereby decreasing the efficiency. On the other hand, if contraction is too rapid, large proportions of the energy are used to overcome the viscous friction within the muscle itself, and this, too, reduces the efficiency of contraction. Ordinarily, maximum efficiency is developed when the velocity of contraction is about 30 per cent of maximum.

CHARACTERISTICS OF A SINGLE MUSCLE TWITCH

Many features of muscle contraction can be especially well demonstrated by eliciting single *muscle twitches*. This can be accomplished by instantaneously exciting the nerve to a muscle or by passing a short electrical stimulus through the muscle itself, giving rise to a single, sudden contraction lasting for a fraction of a second.

Isometric Versus Isotonic Contraction. Muscle contraction is said to be *isometric* when the muscle does not shorten during contraction and *isotonic* when it shortens with the tension on the muscle remaining constant. Systems for recording the two types of muscle contraction are illustrated in Figure 7–13.

To the right is the isometric system in which the muscle is suspended between a solid rod and a lever of an electronic force transducer. This transducer records force with almost zero movement of the lever; therefore, in effect, the muscle is bound between fixed points so that it cannot contract significantly. To the left is shown an isotonic recording system: the muscle simply lifts a pan of weights so that the force against which the muscle contracts remains constant, though the length of the muscle changes considerably.

There are several basic differences between isometric and isotonic contractions. First, isometric contraction does not require much sliding of myofibrils among each other. Second, in isotonic contraction a load is moved, which involves the phenomenon of inertia. That is, the weight or other type of object being moved must first be accelerated, and once a velocity has been attained the load has momentum that causes it to continue moving even after the contraction is over. Therefore an isotonic con-

traction is likely to last considerably longer than an isometric contraction of the same muscle. Third, isotonic contraction entails the performance of external work. Therefore, in accordance with the Fenn effect discussed previously, a greater amount of energy is used by the muscle.

In comparing the rapidity of contraction of different types of muscle, isometric recordings such as those illustrated in Figure 7–14 are usually used instead of isotonic recordings because the duration of an isotonic recording is almost as dependent on the inertia of the recording system as on the contraction itself, and this makes it difficult to compare time relationships of contractions from one muscle to another.

Muscles can contract both isometrically and isotonically in the body, but most contractions are actually a mixture of the two. When standing, a person tenses the quadriceps muscles to tighten the knee joints and to keep the legs stiff. This is isometric contraction. On the other hand, when a person lifts a weight using the biceps, this is mainly an isotonic contraction. Finally, contractions of leg muscles during running are a mixture of isometric and isotonic contractions—isometric mainly to keep the limbs stiff when the legs hit the ground and isotonic mainly to move the limbs.

The Series Elastic Component of Muscle Contraction. When muscle fibers contract against a load, those portions of the muscle that do not contract—the tendons, the sarcolemmal ends of the muscle fibers where they attach to the tendons, and perhaps even the hinged arms of the cross-bridges—will stretch slightly as the tension increases. Consequently, the muscle must shorten an extra 3 to 5 per cent to make up for the stretch of these elements. The elements of the muscle that stretch during contraction are called the *series elastic component* of the muscle.

Characteristics of Isometric Twitches Recorded from Different Muscles. The body has many different sizes of skeletal muscles—from the very small stapedius muscle of only a few millimeters length and a millimeter or so in diameter up to the very large quadriceps muscle. Furthermore, the fibers may be as small as 10 microns in diameter or as large as 80 microns. And, finally, the energetics of muscle contraction vary considerably from one muscle to another. These different physical and chemical characteristics often manifest themselves in the form of different characteristics of contraction—some muscles contract rapidly while others contract slowly.

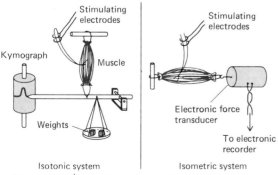

Figure 7–13. Isotonic and isometric recording systems.

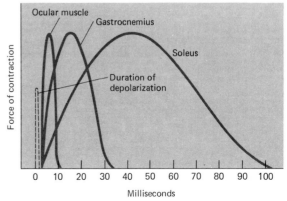

Figure 7–14. Duration of isometric contractions of different types of mammalian muscles, showing also a latent period between the action potential and muscle contraction.

Figure 7–14 illustrates isometric contractions of three different types of skeletal muscles: an ocular muscle, which has a duration of contraction of less than $1/100$ second; the gastrocnemius muscle, which has a duration of contraction of about $1/30$ second; and the soleus muscle, which has a duration of contraction of about $1/10$ second. It is interesting that these durations of contractions are adapted to the function of each of the respective muscles, for ocular movements must be extremely rapid to maintain fixation of the eyes upon specific objects, the gastrocnemius muscle must contract moderately rapidly to provide sufficient velocity of limb movement for running and jumping, while the soleus muscle is concerned principally with slow reactions for continual support of the body against gravity.

Fast Versus Slow Muscle Fibers. Every muscle of the body is composed of a mixture of so-called *fast* and *slow* muscle fibers, with still other fibers graduated between these two extremes. The muscles that react very rapidly are composed mainly of the fast fibers with only small numbers of the slow variety. And, conversely, the muscles that respond slowly but with a prolonged period of contraction are composed mainly of the slow type of fibers. The differences between these two types of fibers are the following:

Fast fibers: (1) Much larger fibers for great strength of contraction. (2) Extensive sarcoplasmic reticulum for rapid release of calcium ions to initiate contraction. (3) Large amounts of glycolytic enzymes for rapid release of energy by the glycolytic process. (4) Less extensive blood supply because oxidative metabolism is of secondary importance. (5) Fewer mitochondria, also because oxidative metabolism is secondary.

Slow fibers: (1) Smaller fibers. (2) Also innervated by smaller nerve fibers. (3) More extensive blood vessel system to supply extra amounts of oxygen. (4) Greatly increased numbers of mitochondria, also to support high levels of oxidative metabolism. (5) Fibers contain large amounts of myoglobin, an iron-containing protein similar to hemoglobin in red blood cells. Myoglobin combines with oxygen and holds this inside the muscle cell until it is needed by the mitochrondria.

From these descriptions, one can see that the fast fibers are adapted for very rapid and very powerful muscle contractions, such as for jumping or for short-distance powerful running. On the other hand, the slow fibers are adapted for prolonged, continued muscle activity, such as support of the body against gravity and long-continuing athletic events like marathon races.

The slow muscle is frequently also called *red muscle* because the excess myoglobin in the slow fibers gives them a slightly reddish tint. On the other hand, the relative deficiency of myoglobin in the fast fibers gives them a whitish appearance, so that this muscle is frequently called *white muscle*.

MECHANICS OF SKELETAL MUSCLE CONTRACTION

THE MOTOR UNIT

Each motor neuron that leaves the spinal cord usually innervates many different muscle fibers, the number depending on the type of muscle. All the muscle fibers innervated by a single motor nerve fiber are called a *motor unit*. In general, small muscles that react rapidly and whose control is exact have few muscle fibers (as few as two to three in some of the laryngeal muscles) in each motor unit and have a large number of nerve fibers going to each muscle. On the other hand, the large muscles that do not require a very fine degree of control, such as the gastrocnemius muscle, may have several hundred muscle fibers in a motor unit. An average figure for all the muscles of the body can be considered to be about 150 muscle fibers to the motor unit.

Usually muscle fibers of adjacent motor units overlap, with small bundles of 10 to 15 fibers from one motor unit lying among similar bundles of the second motor unit. This interdigitation allows the separate motor units to contract in support of each other rather than entirely as individual segments.

Macromotor Units. Loss of some of the nerve fibers to a muscle causes the remaining nerve fibers to sprout forth and innervate many of the paralyzed muscle fibers. When this occurs, such as following poliomyelitis, one occasionally develops *macromotor units*, which can contain as many as five times the normal number of muscle fibers. This obviously decreases the degree of control that one has over the muscles but, nevertheless, allows the muscles to regain function.

SUMMATION OF MUSCLE CONTRACTION

Summation means the adding together of individual muscle twitches to make strong and concerted muscle movements. In general, summation occurs in two different ways: (1) by increasing the number of motor units contracting simultaneously, and (2) by increasing the rapidity of contraction of individual motor units. These are called, respectively, *multiple motor unit summation* and *wave summation* (or spatial summation and temporal summation).

Multiple Motor Unit Summation. Even within a single muscle, the numbers of muscle fibers and their sizes in the different motor units vary tremendously, so that one motor unit may be as much as 50 times as strong as another. The smaller motor units are far more easily excited than are the larger ones because they are innervated by smaller nerve fibers whose cell bodies in the spinal cord have a naturally high level of excitability. This effect causes the gradations of muscle strength during weak muscle contraction to occur in very small steps, while the steps become progressively greater as the intensity of contraction increases because the larger motor units then begin to contract.

Wave Summation. Figure 7–15 illustrates the principles of wave summation, showing in the lower left-hand corner several single muscle twitches followed by successive muscle twitches at increasing frequencies. When the frequency of twitches rises above ten per second, the first muscle twitch is not completely over by the time the second one begins. Therefore, since the muscle is already in a partially contracted state when the second twitch begins, the degree of muscle shortening this time is slightly greater than that which occurs with the single muscle twitch. At more rapid rates of contraction, the degree of summation of successive contractions becomes greater and greater, because the successive contractions appear at earlier times following the preceding contraction.

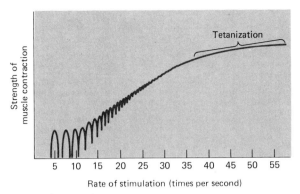

Figure 7-15. Wave summation and tetanization.

Tetanization. When a muscle is stimulated at progressively greater frequencies, a frequency is finally reached at which the successive contractions fuse together and cannot be distinguised one from the other. This state is called *tetanization*, and the lowest frequency at which it occurs is called the *critical frequency*.

Tetanization results partly from the viscous properties of the muscle and partly from the nature of the contractile process itself. The muscle fibers are filled with sarcoplasm, which is a viscous fluid, and the fibers are encased in fasciae and muscle sheaths that have a viscous resistance to change in length. Therefore, these viscous factors play a role in causing the successive contractions to fuse with each other.

But in addition to the viscous property of muscle, the activation process itself lasts for a definite period of time, and successive pulsatile states of activation of the muscle fiber can occur so rapidly that they fuse into a long continual state of activation; that is, the level of free calcium ions in the myofibrils remains continuously above the level required for full activation of the contractile process, providing an uninterrupted stimulus for maintenance of contraction. Once the critical frequency for tetanization is reached, further increase in rate of stimulation increases the force of contraction only a few more per cent, as shown in Figure 7-15.

Asynchronous Summation of Motor Units. Actually it is rare for either multiple motor unit summation or wave summation to occur separately from each other in normal muscle function. Instead, special neurogenic mechanisms in the spinal cord normally increase both the impulse rate and the number of motor units firing at the same time. If a motor unit fires at all, it usually fires at least five times per second, but this can increase to as high as 50 per second for most muscles or much more than this for the very fast muscles—to frequencies sufficient to cause complete tetanization.

Yet, even when tetanization of individual motor units of a muscle is not occurring, the tension exerted by the whole muscle is still continous and nonjerky because *the different motor units fire asynchronously;* that is, while one is contracting another is relaxing; then another fires, followed by still another, and so forth. Consequently, even when motor units fire as infrequently as five times per second, the muscle contraction, though weak, is nevertheless very smooth.

Maximum Strength of Contraction. The maximum strength of tetanic contraction of a muscle operating at a normal muscle length is about 3.5 kilograms per square centimeter of muscle, or 50 pounds per square inch. Since a quadriceps muscle can at times· have as much as 16 square inches of muscle belly, as much as 800 pounds of tension may at times be applied to the patellar tendon. One can readily understand, therefore, how it is possible for muscles sometimes to pull their tendons out of the insertions in bones. This often occurs where the patellar tendon inserts in the tibia, and it occurs even more frequently where the Achilles tendon of the gastrocnemius muscle inserts at the heel.

Changes in Muscle Strength at the Onset of Contraction—The Staircase Effect (Treppe). When a muscle begins to contract after a long period of rest, its initial strength of contraction may be as little as one half its strength 30 to 50 muscle twitches later. That is, the strength of contraction increases to a plateau, a phenomenon called the *staircase effect* or *treppe.*

Though all the possible causes of the staircase effect are not yet known, it is believed to be caused primarily by electrolyte changes that occur when a series of contractions begins. For instance, there is a net increase in calcium ions inside the muscle fiber because of movement of calcium ions inward through the membrane with each action potential. There is probably also further increase of calcium ions in the cytosol because of release of these ions from the sarcoplasmic reticulum and failure to recapture the ions immediately. In addition, there is decreased potassium inside the cell as well as increased sodium; it has been suggested that the changes in these two ions increase the rate of liberation of calcium ions from the sarcoplasmic reticulum. Recalling the earlier discussion of the relationship of calcium ions to the contractile process, one can readily understand that progressive increase in calcium ion concentration in the sarcoplasm, caused either directly or as a consequence of sodium and potassium movement, could progressively increase the strength of muscle contraction, giving rise to the staircase effect.

SKELETAL MUSCLE TONE

Even when muscles are at rest, a certain amount of tautness usually remains. This residual degree of contraction in skeletal muscle is called *muscle tone.* Since skeletal muscle fibers do not contract without an actual action potential to stimulate the fibers except in certain pathological conditions, it is believed that skeletal muscle tone results entirely from nerve impulses coming from the spinal cord. These in turn are controlled partly by impulses transmitted from the brain to the appropriate anterior motor neurons and partly by impulses that originate in *muscle spindles* located in the muscle itself.

Muscle spindles are sensory receptors that exist throughout essentially all skeletal muscles to detect the degree of muscle contraction. These will be discussed in detail in Chapter 15, but, briefly, they transmit impulses almost continually through the posterior roots into the spinal cord, where they excite the anterior motor neurons, which in turn provide nerve stimuli for muscle tone. Simply cutting the posterior roots, thereby blocking the muscle spindle impulses, usually reduces muscle tone to such a low level that the muscle becomes almost completely flaccid.

Many other neurogenic factors, originating especially in the brain, enter into the control of muscle tone. These will be discussed in relation to muscle spindle and spinal cord function in Chapter 15.

MUSCLE FATIGUE

Prolonged and strong contraction of a muscle leads to the well-known state of muscle fatigue. Studies in athletes have shown that muscle fatigue increases in almost direct proportion to the rate of depletion of muscle glycogen. Therefore, most fatigue probably results simply from inability of the contractile and metabolic processes of the muscle fibers to continue supplying the same work output. However, experiments have also shown that transmission of the nerve signal through the neuromuscular junction can occasionally diminish following prolonged muscle activity, thus further diminishing muscle contraction.

Interruption of blood flow through a contracting muscle leads to almost complete muscle fatigue in a minute or more because of the obvious loss of nutrient supply—especially loss of oxygen.

THE LEVER SYSTEMS OF THE BODY

Muscles obviously operate by applying tension to their points of insertion into bones, and the bones in turn form various types of lever systems. Figure 7–16 illustrates the lever system activated by the biceps muscle to lift the forearm. If we assume that a large biceps muscle has a cross-sectional area of 6 square inches, then the maximum force of contraction would be about 300 pounds. When the forearm is exactly at right angles with the upper arm, the tendon attachment of the biceps is about 2 inches anterior to the fulcrum at the elbow, and the total length of the forearm lever is about 14 inches. Therefore, the amount of lifting power that the biceps would have at the hand would be only one seventh of the 300 pounds force, or about 43 pounds. When the arm is in the fully extended position, the attachment of the biceps is much less than 2 inches anterior to the fulcrum, and the force with which the forearm can be brought forward is much less than 43 pounds.

In short, an analysis of the lever systems of the body depends on (1) a discrete knowledge of the point of muscle insertion and (2) its distance from the lever's fulcrum, as well as (3) the length of the lever arm and (4) the position of the lever. Obviously, many different types of movement are required in the body, some of which need great strength and others large distances of move-

ment. For this reason there are all·varieties of muscles; some are long and contract a long distance and some are short but have large cross-sectional areas and therefore can provide extreme strengths of contraction over short distances. The study of different types of muscles, lever systems, and their movements is called *kinesiology* and is a very important phase of human physioanatomy.

Accommodation of Muscle Length to the Length of the Lever System. If a bone is broken and then heals in a shortened state, the force of contraction of the muscles lying along this broken bone would obviously become decreased because of the shortened lengths of muscles. However, muscles shortened in this manner undergo *physical shortening* during the next few weeks. This results from actual loss of sarcomeres at the ends of the muscle fibers. In this way the new muscle length becomes approximately equal to that required for optimal force of contraction. Conversely, if muscles are overstretched for weeks at a time, new sarcomeres develop at the ends of the fibers, again re-establishing optimal force of contraction.

The same shortening process also occurs in muscles of limbs immobilized for several weeks in casts if the muscles during this time are in a shortened position. When the cast is removed, the muscles must often be restretched over a period of weeks before full mobility is restored.

SPECIAL FEATURES AND ABNORMALITIES OF SKELETAL MUSCLE FUNCTION

MUSCLE HYPERTROPHY

Forceful muscular activity causes the muscle size to increase, a phenomenon called *hypertrophy*. Most of the hypertrophy results from increase in the diameters of the fibers already present in the muscle, but the numbers of fibers probably also can increase to a slight extent by splitting of fibers already present; this is called *hyperplasia*. As the diameters of the muscle fibers increase, the sarcoplasm increases, and the fibers gain in various nutrient and intermediary metabolic substances, such as adenosine triphosphate, phosphocreatine, glycogen, intracellular lipids, and even many additional mitochondria. It is likely that the myofibrils also increase in size and perhaps in numbers as well, but this has not been proved. Briefly, muscular hypertrophy increases both the motive power of the muscle and the nutrient mechanisms for maintaining increased motive power.

Weak muscular activity, even when sustained over long periods of time, does not result in significant hypertrophy. Instead, hypertrophy results mainly from *very* forceful muscle activity, though the activity might occur for only a few minutes each day. For this reason, strength can be developed in muscles much more rapidly when "resistive" or "isometric" exercise is used rather than simply prolonged mild exercise. Indeed, essentially no enlargement of the muscle fibers occurs unless the muscle contracts to at least 75 per cent of its maximum tension.

On the other hand, prolonged muscle activity does increase muscle endurance, causing increases in the oxidative enzymes, myoglobin, and even blood capillaries—all of which are essential to increased muscle metabolism.

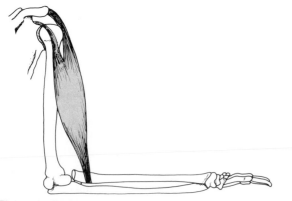

Figure 7–16. The lever system activated by the biceps muscle.

MUSCLE ATROPHY

Muscle atrophy is the reverse of muscle hypertrophy; it results any time a muscle is not used or even when a muscle is used only for very weak contractions. Atrophy is particularly likely to occur when limbs are placed in casts, thereby preventing muscular contraction. As little as one month of disuse can sometimes decrease the muscle size to one-half normal.

Atrophy Caused by Muscle Denervation. When a muscle is denervated, it immediately begins to atrophy, and the muscle continues to decrease in size for several years. If the muscle becomes reinnervated during the first three to four months, full function of the muscle usually returns, but after four months of denervation some of the muscle fibers usually will have degenerated. Reinnervation after two years rarely results in return of any function at all. Pathological studies show that the muscle fibers have by that time been replaced by fat and fibrous tissue.

PREVENTION OF MUSCLE ATROPHY BY ELECTRICAL STIMULATION

Strong electrical stimulation of denervated muscles, particularly when the resulting contractions occur against loads, will delay and in some instances prevent muscle atrophy despite denervation. This procedure is used to keep muscles alive until reinnervation can take place.

PHYSICAL CONTRACTURE OF MUSCLE FOLLOWING DENERVATION

When a muscle is denervated, its fibers tend to shorten if the muscle is kept in a shortened position, and even the associated nerves and fasciae shorten. That is, unless continual movement keeps stretching the muscle and other structures, they will creep toward a shortened length. This is one of the most difficult problems in the treatment of patients with denervated muscles, such as occur in poliomyelitis or nerve trauma. Unless passive stretching is applied daily to the muscles, they may become so shortened that even when reinnervated they will be of little value. But, more important, the shortening can often result in extremely contorted positions of different parts of the body.

RIGOR MORTIS

Several hours after death all the muscles of the body go into a state of *contracture* called rigor mortis; that is, the muscle contracts and becomes rigid even without action potentials. This rigidity is caused by loss of all the ATP, which is required to cause separation of the cross-bridges from the actin filaments during the relaxation process. The muscles remain in rigor until the muscle proteins are destroyed, which usually results from autolysis caused by enzymes released from the lysosomes some 15 to 25 hours later.

FAMILIAL PERIODIC PARALYSIS

Occasionally, a hereditary disease called *familial periodic paralysis* occurs. In persons so afflicted, the extracellular fluid potassium concentration periodically falls to very low levels, causing various degrees of paralysis. The paralysis is caused in the following manner: the initial decrease in extracellular fluid potassium causes an increase in the gradient of potassium from the inside of the muscle fiber to the outside, and this in turn increases the muscle fiber membrane potential to a value greater than normal, an effect called *hyperpolarization*. For a long time it was believed that this hyperpolarization made the muscle fiber membranes less excitable than usual and caused the paralysis. However, with modern methods of study, it has been learned that this initial hyperpolarization is not the culprit. Instead, when the extracellular fluid potassium concentration falls even lower (below about 3 mEq/liter), this low potassium level has the direct effect of decreasing the permeability of the potassium channels. Therefore, potassium now contributes much less to the membrane potential than normally, so that the intracellular membrane potential *decreases* below normal, often decreasing low enough that many or most of the sodium channels become inactivated. It will be recalled from the previous chapter that inactivation of the sodium channels prevents the transmission of action potentials; therefore, this can lead to paralysis.

THE ELECTROMYOGRAM

Each time an action potential passes along a muscle fiber, a small portion of the electrical current spreads away from the muscle as far as the skin. If many muscle fibers contract simultaneously, the summated electrical potentials at the skin may be very great. By placing two electrodes on the skin or inserting needle electrodes into the muscle, an electrical recording called the *electromyogram* can be made when the muscle is stimulated. Figure 7–17 illustrates a typical electromyographic recording from the gastrocnemius muscle during a moderate contraction. Electromyograms are frequently used clinically to discern abnormalities of muscle excitation. Two such abnormalities are muscle *fasciculation* and *fibrillation*.

Muscle Fasciculation. When an abnormal impulse occurs in a motor nerve fiber, its whole motor unit contracts. This often causes sufficient contraction in the muscle that one can see a slight ripple in the skin over the muscle. This process is called fasciculation.

Fasciculation occurs especially following destruction of anterior motor neurons in poliomyelitis or following traumatic interruption of a nerve. As the peripheral nerve

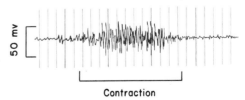

Figure 7–17. Electromyogram recorded during contraction of the gastrocnemius muscle.

fibers die, spontaneous impulses are generated during the first few days, and fasciculatory muscle movements result in the muscle. Typical electromyographic records of weak periodic potentials can be obtained from the skin overlying the muscle.

Muscle Fibrillation. After all nerves to a muscle have been destroyed and the nerve fibers themselves have become nonfunctional, which requires three to five days, spontaneous impulses begin to appear in the denervated muscle fibers. At first, these occur at a rate of once every few seconds, but, after a few more days or a few weeks, the impulses become as rapid as three to ten times per second. Thus skeletal muscle fibers, several days after loss of their innervation, develop an intrinsic rhythmicity. This is associated with, and probably caused by, the spread of large numbers of acetylcholine receptor proteins over the surfaces of the muscle fibers, which is believed to increase the permeability of the fiber membranes. After several more weeks the muscle fibers atrophy to such an extent that the fibrillatory impulses finally cease. To record an electromyogram of fibrillation, minute bipolar needle electrodes must be inserted into the muscle belly itself because adjacent muscle fibers do not fire simultaneously and, therefore, do not summate. As a result, the potentials are not strong enough to record from the surface of the skin.

REFERENCES

Aguayo, A. J., and Karpati, G. (eds.): Current Topics in Nerve and Muscle Research. New York, Elsevier/North-Holland, 1979.

Alexander, R. M.: Mechanics of skeleton and tendons. *In* Brooks, V. B. (ed.): Handbook of Physiology. Sec. 1, Vol. II. Bethesda, American Physiological Society, 1981, p. 17.

American Physiological Society: Skeletal Muscle. Baltimore, Waverly Press, 1983.

Armstrong, R. B.: Mechanisms of exercise-induced delayed onset muscular soreness: A brief review. *Med. Sci. Sports Exerc.*, 16:529, 1984.

Barany, M., and Barany, K.: Phosphorylation of the myofibrillar proteins. *Annu. Rev. Physiol.*, 42:275, 1980.

Buchthal, F., and Schmalbruch, H.: Motor unit of mammalian muscle. *Physiol. Rev.*, 60:90, 1980.

Burke, R. E.: Motor units: Anatomy, physiology, and functional organization. *In* Brooks, V. B. (ed.): Handbook of Physiology. Sec. 1, Vol. 11. Bethesda, American Physiological Society, 1981, p. 345.

Caruso, G. (ed.): Electromyography in the Diagnosis and Management of Peripheral Nerve Injuries. Minneapolis, J. K. Burgess, 1983.

Eisenberg, E., and Greene, L. E.: The relation of muscle biochemistry to muscle physiology. *Annu. Rev. Physiol.*, 42:293, 1980.

Fabiato, A., and Fabiato, F.: Calcium and cardiac excitation-contraction coupling. *Annu. Rev. Physiol.*, 41:473, 1979.

Freund, H.-J.: Motor unit and muscle activity in voluntary motor control. *Physiol. Rev.*, 63:387, 1983.

Galley, P. M.: Human Movement. An Introductory Text for Physiotherapy Students. New York, Churchill Livingstone, 1983.

Hasselbach, W., and Oetliker, H.: Energetics and electrogenicity of the sarcoplasmic reticulum calcium pump. *Annu. Rev. Physiol.*, 45:325, 1983.

Hockey, R.: Stress and Fatigue in Human Performance. New York, John Wiley & Sons, 1983.

Homsher, E., and Kean, C. J.: Skeletal muscle energetics and metabolism. *Annu. Rev. Physiol.*, 40:93, 1978.

Huxley, A. F., and Gordon, A. M.: Striation patterns in active and passive shortening of muscle. *Nature (Lond.)*, 193:280, 1962.

Huxley, H. E.: Muscular contraction and cell motility. *Nature*, 243:445, 1973.

Huxley, H. E., and Faruqi, A. R.: Time-resolved x-ray diffraction studies on vertebrate striated muscle. *Annu. Rev. Biophys. Bioeng.*, 12:381, 1983.

Ikemoto, N.: Structure and function of the calcium pump protein of sarcoplasmic reticulum. *Annu. Rev. Physiol.*, 44:297, 1982.

Ingels, N. B., Jr. (ed.): The Molecular Basis of Force Development in Muscle. Palo Alto, Cal., Palo Alto Medical Research Foundation, 1979.

Johnson, E. W. (ed.): Practical Electromyography. Baltimore, Williams & Wilkins, 1979.

Jolesz, F., and Sreter, F. A.: Development, innervation, and activity-pattern induced changes in skeletal muscle. *Annu. Rev. Physiol.*, 43:531, 1981.

Knochel, J. P.: Rhabdomyolysis and myoglobinuria. *Annu. Rev. Med.*, 33:435, 1982.

Korn, E. D.: Actin polymerization and its regulation by proteins from nonmuscle cells. *Physiol. Rev.*, 62:672, 1982.

Lamb, D. R.: Physiology of Exercises. Responses and Adaptations. New York, Macmillan Publishing Co., 1984.

Lymn, R. W.: Kinetic analysis of myosin and actomyosin ATPase. *Annu. Rev. Biophys. Bioeng.*, 8:145, 1979.

Martonosi, A.: The development of sarcoplasmic reticulum membranes. *Annu. Rev. Physiol.*, 44:337, 1982.

Martonosi, A. N.: Mechanisms of Ca^{2+} release from sarcoplasmic reticulum of skeletal muscle. *Physiol. Rev.*, 64:1240, 1984.

McLachlan, A. D.: Structural implications of the myosin amino acid sequence. *Annu. Rev. Biophys. Bioeng.*, 13:167, 1984.

Morgan, D. L., and Proske, U.: Vertebrate slow muscle: Its structure, pattern of innervation, and mechanical properties. *Physiol. Rev.*, 64:103, 1984.

Mortimore, J. T.: Motor prostheses. *In* Brooks, V. B. (ed.): Handbook of Physiology. Sec. 1, Vol. II. Bethesda, American Physiological Society, 1981, p. 155.

Northrip, J. W., *et al.*: Introduction to Biomechanic Analysis of Sport. Dubuque, Iowa, W. C. Brown Co., 1979.

Partridge, L. D., and Benton, L. A.: Muscle, the motor. *In* Brooks, V. B. (ed.): Handbook of Physiology. Sec. 1, Vol. II. Bethesda, American Physiological Society, 1981, p. 43.

Pearson, M. L. (ed.): Muscle Development. Molecular and Cellular Control. Cold Spring Harbor, N.Y., Cold Spring Harbor, 1982.

Pollack, G. H.: The cross-bridge theory. *Physiol. Rev.*, 63:1049, 1983.

Porter, R. (ed.): Human Muscle Fatigue. Woodstock, N.Y., Beekman Publishers, 1981.

Rash, J.: Neuromuscular Atlas. New York, Prager Publishers, 1984.

Rogart, R.: Sodium channels in nerve and muscle membrane. *Annu. Rev. Physiol.*, 43:711, 1981.

Schneider, M. F.: Membrane charge movement and depolarization-contraction coupling. *Annu. Rev. Physiol.*, 43:507, 1981.

Schubert, D.: Developmental Biology of Cultured Nerve, Muscle and Glia. New York, John Wiley & Sons, 1984.

Sjodin, R. A.: Ion Transport in Skeletal Muscle. New York, John Wiley & Sons, 1982.

Stefani, E., and Chiarandini, D. J.: Ionic channels in skeletal muscle. *Annu. Rev. Physiol.*, 44:357, 1982.

Sugi, H., and Pollack, G. H. (eds.): Cross-Bridge Mechanism in Muscle Contraction. Baltimore, University Park Press, 1979.

Taylor, C. R., and Heglund, N. C.: Energetics and mechanics of terrestrial locomotion. *Annu. Rev. Physiol.*, 44:97, 1982.

Tregear, R. T., and Marston, S. B.: The crossbridge theory. *Annu. Rev. Physiol.*, 41:723, 1979.

Walton, J. A.: Disorders of Voluntary Muscle. New York, Churchill Livingstone, 1981.

Wiesendanger, M., and Miles, T. S.: Ascending pathway of low-threshold muscle afferents to the cerebral cortex and its possible role in motor control. *Physiol. Rev.*, 62:1234, 1982.

Winegrad, S.: Regulation of cardiac contractile proteins. Correlations between physiology and biochemistry. *Circ. Res.*, 55:565, 1984.

Wray, J. S., and Holmes, K. C.: X-ray diffraction studies of muscle. *Annu. Rev. Physiol.*, 43:553, 1981.

Zak, R., and Rabinowitz, M.: Molecular aspects of cardiac hypertrophy. *Annu. Rev. Physiol.*, 41:539, 1979.

8

Neuromuscular Transmission; Function of Smooth Muscle

TRANSMISSION OF IMPULSES FROM NERVES TO SKELETAL MUSCLE FIBERS: THE NEUROMUSCULAR JUNCTION

The skeletal muscles are innervated by large myelinated nerve fibers that originate in the large motoneurons of the anterior horns of the spinal cord. It was pointed out in the previous chapter that each nerve fiber normally branches many times and stimulates from three to several hundred skeletal muscle fibers. The nerve ending makes a junction, called the *neuromuscular junction*, with the muscle fiber approximately at the nerve fiber's midpoint so that the action potential in the fiber travels in both directions. With the exception of about 2 per cent of the muscle fibers there is only one such junction per muscle fiber.

Physiological Anatomy of the Neuromuscular Junction. Figure 8–1, Parts A and B, illustrates the neuromuscular junction between a large myelinated nerve fiber and a skeletal muscle fiber. The nerve fiber branches at its end to form a complex of branching nerve *terminals* called the *end-plate*, which invaginates into the muscle fiber but lies entirely outside the muscle fiber plasma membrane. The entire structure is covered by one or more Schwann cells that insulate the end-plate from the surrounding fluids.

Figure 8–1C shows an electronmicrographic sketch of the junction between a single-branch axon terminal and the muscle fiber membrane. The invagination of the membrane is called the *synaptic gutter* or *synaptic trough,* and the space between the terminal and the fiber membrane is called the *synaptic cleft.* The synaptic cleft is 20 to 30 nanometers wide and is occupied by a basal lamina, which is a thin layer of spongy reticular fibers through which diffuses extracellular fluid. At the bottom of the gutter are numerous smaller *folds* of the muscle membrane called *subneural clefts,* which greatly increase the surface area at which the synaptic transmitter can act. In the axon terminal are many mitochondria that supply energy mainly for synthe-

sis of the excitatory transmitter *acetylcholine* that, in turn, excites the muscle fiber. The acetylcholine is synthesized in the cytoplasm of the terminal but is rapidly absorbed into many small synaptic vesicles, approximately 300,000 of which are normally in the terminals of a single end-plate. Attached to the matrix of the basal lamina are large quantities of the enzyme *acetylcholinesterase,* which is capable of destroying acetylcholine, to be explained in further detail.

Secretion of Acetylcholine by the Axon Terminals. When a nerve impulse reaches the neuromuscular junction, about 300 vesicles of acetylcholine are released by the terminals into the synaptic clefts between the terminals and the muscle fiber membrane. This results from movement of calcium ions from the extracellular fluid into the membranes of the terminals when the action potential depolarizes their membranes. The calcium ions cause the vesicles of acetylcholine to rupture through the membrane. In the absence of calcium or in the presence of excess magnesium, the release of acetylcholine is greatly depressed.

Destruction of the Released Acetylcholine by Cholinesterase. Within approximately 1 millisecond after acetylcholine is released by the axon terminal, much of it has already diffused out of the synaptic gutter and no longer acts on the muscle fiber membrane, and virtually all the remainder is destroyed by the acetylcholinesterase in the basal lamina lying between the nerve terminal and the subneural clefts. The very short period of time that the acetylcholine remains in contact with the muscle fiber membrane—about 1 millisecond—is almost always sufficient to excite the muscle fiber, and yet the rapid removal of the acetylcholine prevents re-excitation after the muscle fiber has recovered from the first action potential.

Effect of Acetylcholine in Opening Acetylcholine-Gated Ion Channels. Even though the acetylcholine released into the cleft between the end-plate and the muscle membrane lasts for only a very small fraction of a second, during this time the permeability of the muscle membrane to positive

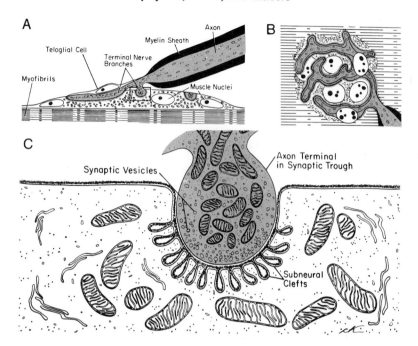

Figure 8–1. Different views of the motor end-plate. *A*, Longitudinal section through the end-plate. *B*, surface view of the end-plate. *C*, Electron micrographic appearance of the contact point between one of the axon terminals and the muscle fiber membrane, representing the rectangular area shown in *A*. (From Bloom and Fawcett, as modified from R. Couteaux: A Textbook of Histology. Philadelphia, W. B. Saunders Company, 1975.)

ions in the cleft increases several thousandfold. This is because of the opening of *acetylcholine-gated ion channels*. These channels are composed basically of a large transmembrane channel protein molecule with a molecular weight of about 240,000. On its external surface is a gate similar to that of the sodium channels discussed in Chapter 6. However, it is a *ligand-activated gate* rather than a voltage-activated gate, responding to acetylcholine as the ligand. The surface-protruding portion of this channel protein acts as a receptor for acetylcholine, and acetylcholine in turn causes a conformational change in the channel molecule to open the gate for about 1 millisecond.

The acetylcholine channels have a diameter of about 0.65 nanometers, which is large enough to allow all the important positive ions—Na^+, K^+, and Ca^{++}—to move easily through the channels. (Negative ions such as chloride ions do not pass through this channel because of strong negative charges in the wall of the channel.)

Yet, from a practical point of view, only sodium ions flow through the channels, for the following reasons: first, the normal resting potential of the muscle fiber membrane is almost equal to the Nernst potential for potassium ions; therefore, opening the channels will not allow significant numbers of potassium ions to flow through the membrane—that is, the potassium concentration gradient is already approximately in equilibrium with the voltage gradient across the channels. On the other hand, both sodium and calcium ions have far greater concentrations outside the nerve fiber than inside, and their Nernst potentials are of opposite polarity to the resting membrane potential. Therefore, opening the acetylcholine channels al-

lows both these ions to flow rapidly to the interior of the muscle fiber. However, the concentration of calcium ions in the extracellular fluid is less than one fiftieth the concentration of sodium ions, and their mobility is also less. Therefore, in essence, opening the acetylcholine channels allows very rapid influx of sodium ions to the interior of the fiber and little else. Nevertheless, even 1 millisecond influx of the sodium ions is still enough to excite an action potential in the muscle fiber.

The "End-Plate Potential" and Excitation of the Skeletal Muscle Fiber. The sudden insurgence of sodium ions into the muscle fiber when the acetylcholine channels open causes the membrane potential in the *local area of the end-plate* to increase in the positive direction as much as 50 to 75 millivolts, creating a *local potential* called the *end-plate potential*. If we recall from the previous chapter that a sudden increase in membrane potential of more than 15 to 30 millivolts is sufficient to initiate the positive feedback effect of sodium channel activation, one can understand that the end-plate potential created by the acetylcholine stimulation is normally far greater than enough to initiate an action potential in the muscle fiber.

Figure 8–2 illustrates the principle of an end-plate potential initiating the action potential. In this figure are shown three separate end-plate potentials. End-plate potentials *A* and *C* are too weak to elicit an action potential, but they do nevertheless give the weak local potentials recorded in the figure. In contrast, end-plate potential *B* is much stronger and causes enough sodium channels to activate so that the self-regenerative effect of more and more sodium ions flowing to the interior of the fiber initiated an action potential. The weak end-plate potential at point *A* was caused by poisoning the muscle fiber with *curare*, a drug that blocks the gating action of acetylcholine on the acetylcholine channels, probably by competing with the acetylcholine for the acetylcholine receptor site. The weak end-plate potential at point *C*

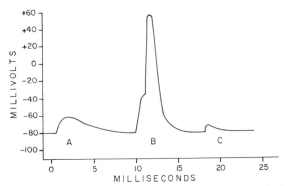

Figure 8–2. End-plate potentials. *A,* A weakened end-plate potential recorded in a curarized muscle, too weak to elicit an action potential; *B,* normal end-plate potential eliciting a muscle action potential; and *C,* weakened end-plate potiental caused by botulinum toxin that decreases end-plate release of acetylcholine, again too weak to elicit a muscle action potential.

resulted from the effect of botulinum toxin, a bacterial toxin that decreases the release of acetylcholine by the nerve terminals.

"Safety Factor" for Transmission at the Neuromuscular Junction; Fatigue of the Junction. Ordinarily, each impulse that arrives at the neuromuscular junction creates an end-plate current flow about three to four times that required to stimulate the muscle fiber. Therefore, the normal neuromuscular junction is said to have a very high *safety factor.* However, artificial stimulation of the nerve fiber at rates greater than 100 times per second for several minutes often diminishes the number of vesicles of acetylcholine released with each impulse so much that impulses then fail to pass into the muscle fiber. This is called *fatigue* of the neuromuscular junction, and it is analogous to fatigue of the synapse in the central nervous system. Under normal functioning conditions, fatigue of the neuromuscular junction probably occurs only at the most exhausting levels of muscular activity.

Molecular Biology of Acetylcholine Formation and Release

The neuromuscular junction is a type of *synapse,* which is defined as a junction between two excitable cells that allows transmission of a signal from the first cell to the next. We shall see in Chapter 10 that literally trillions of synapses occur in the central nervous system between one neuron and the next; these function in much the same way as the neuromuscular junction. However, the central nervous system synapses are so small that it has not been possible to study the precise events of signal transmission in these. On the other hand, the neuromuscular junctions are large enough to be easily studied, and we know much about the formation and release of acetylcholine at this junction. This occurs in the following stages:

1. Very small vesicles, about 40 nanometers in size, are formed by the Golgi apparatus in the cell body of the motor neuron in the spinal cord. These vesicles are then transported by "streaming" of the axoplasm through the core of the axon from the central cell body to the neuromuscular junction at the tips of the nerve fibers. About 300,000 of these small vesicles collect in the nerve terminals of a single end-plate.

2. Acetylcholine is synthesized in the cytosol of the terminal nerve fibers but is then transported through the membranes of the vesicles to their interior, where it is stored in highly concentrated form, with about 10,000 molecules of acetylcholine in each vesicle.

3. Under resting conditions an occasional vesicle fuses with the surface membrane of the nerve terminal and releases its acetylcholine into the synaptic gutter. When this occurs, a so-called *miniature end-plate* potential, about 1 millivolt in intensity and lasting for a few milliseconds, occurs in the local area of the muscle fiber because of the action of this "packet" of acetylcholine.

4. When an action potential arrives at the nerve terminal, this opens many calcium channels in the membrane of the terminal because this terminal has an abundance of voltage-gated calcium channels. As a result, the calcium ion concentration in the terminal increases about a hundredfold, which in turn increases the rate of fusion of the acetylcholine vesicles with the terminal membrane by about 10,000-fold. As each vesicle fuses, its outer surface ruptures through the cell membrane, thus causing *exocytosis* of acetylcholine into the synaptic cleft. Usually about 200 to 300 vesicles rupture with each action potential. This entire sequence of events occurs in approximately 5 milliseconds.

5. After each vesicle has released its acetylcholine, the membrane of the vesicle becomes part of the cell membrane. However, the number of vesicles available in the nerve ending is sufficient only to allow transmission of about 1000 nerve impulses. Therefore, for continued function of the neuromuscular junction, the vesicles need to be retrieved from the nerve membrane. Retrieval is achieved by the process of *pinocytosis.* Within a few seconds after the action potential is over, "coated pits" appear on the surface of the terminal nerve membrane, caused by contractile proteins of the cytosol massing at intermittent points underneath the membrane. The proteins of the original vesicles are attracted to these pits, and within about 20 seconds the contractile proteins contract and cause the pits to break away to the interior of the membrane, thus forming new vesicles. Within another few seconds, acetylcholine is transported to the interior of these vesicles, and they are then ready for a new cycle of acetylcholine release.

Drugs That Affect Transmission at the Neuromuscular Junction

Drugs That Stimulate the Muscle Fiber by Acetylcholine-Like Action. Many different compounds, including *methacholine, carbachol,* and *nicotine,* have the same effect on the muscle fiber as does acetylcholine. The difference between these drugs and acetylcholine is that they are not destroyed by cholinesterase or are destroyed very slowly, so that when once applied to the muscle fiber the action persists for many minutes to several hours. Moderate quantities of the above three drugs applied to a muscle fiber cause localized areas of depolarization, and every time the muscle fiber becomes repolarized elsewhere, these depolarized areas, by virtue of their leaking ions, cause new action potentials, thereby causing a state of spasm. On the other hand, when extreme doses of these drugs are used, two separate effects occur that now cause a state of flaccid paralysis rather than spasm. These effects are: (1) prolonged action of acetylcholine or aceylcholine-like drugs causes the acetylcholine-gated ion channels to become desensitized to these drugs, which is analogous to the inactivation process of sodium channels as discussed in the previous chapter. (2) The moderate degree of depolarization that still persists also causes inactivation of the sodium channels so that they now cannot participate in the initiation of action potentials.

Drugs That Block Transmission at the Neuromuscular Junction. A group of drugs, known as the *curariform drugs,* can prevent passage of impulses from the end-plate into the muscle. Thus, D-tubocurarine affects the membrane, probably by competing with acetylcholine for the receptor sites of the membrane, so that the acetylcholine cannot increase the permeability of the acetylcholine channels sufficiently to initiate a depolarization wave.

Drugs That Stimulate the Neuromuscular Junction by Inactivating Acetylcholinesterase. Three particularly well-known drugs, *neostigmine, physostigmine,* and *diisopropyl fluorophosphate,* inactivate acetylcholinesterase so that the cholinesterase normally in the synapses will not hydrolyze the acetylcholine released at the end-plate. As a result, acetylcholine increases in quantity with successive nerve impulses so that extreme amounts of acetylcholine can accumulate and then repetitively stimulate the muscle fiber. This causes *muscular spasm* when even a few nerve impulses reach the muscle; this can cause death due to laryngeal spasm, which smothers the person.

Neostigmine and physostigmine combine with acetylcholinesterase to inactivate it for several hours, after which they are displaced from the acetylcholinesterase so that it once again becomes active. On the other hand, diisopropyl fluorophosphate, which has military potential as a very powerful "nerve" gas, actually inactivates acetylcholinesterase for several weeks, which makes this a particularly lethal drug.

MYASTHENIA GRAVIS

The disease *myasthenia gravis,* which occurs in about one of every 20,000 persons, causes the person to become paralyzed because of inability of the neuromuscular junctions to transmit signals from the nerve fibers to the muscle fibers. Pathologically, the number of subneural clefts in the synaptic gutter is reduced, and the synaptic cleft itself is widened as much as 50 per cent. Also, antibodies that attack the acetylcholine-gated transport proteins have been demonstrated in the blood of these patients. Therefore, it is believed that myasthenia gravis is an autoimmune disease in which patients have developed antibodies against their own acetylcholine-activated ion channels.

Regardless of the cause, the end-plate potentials developed in the muscle fibers are too weak to stimulate the muscle fibers adequately. If the disease is intense enough, the patient dies of paralysis—in particular, of paralysis of the respiratory muscles. However, the disease can usually be ameliorated with several different drugs, as follows:

Treatment with Drugs. When a patient with myasthenia gravis is treated with a drug, such as neostigmine, that is capable of inactivating acetylcholinesterase, the acetylcholine secreted by the end-plate is not destroyed immediately. If a sequence of nerve impulses arrives at the end-plate, the quantity of acetylcholine present at the membrane increases progressively until finally the end-plate potential caused by the acetylcholine rises above threshold value for stimulating the muscle fiber. Thus, it is sometimes possible by diminishing the quantity of acetylcholinesterase in the muscles of a patient with myasthenia gravis to allow even the inadequate quantities of acetylcholine secreted at the end-plates to effect almost normal muscular activity.

CONTRACTION OF SMOOTH MUSCLE

In the previous chapter and thus far in the present chapter, the discussion has been concerned with skeletal muscle. We now turn to smooth muscle, which is composed of far smaller fibers—usually 2 to 5 microns in diameter and only 50 to 200 microns in length—in contrast to the skeletal muscle fibers that are as much as 20 times as large (in diameter) and thousands of times as long. Nevertheless, many of the principles of contraction apply to smooth muscle the same as to skeletal muscle. Most importantly, essentially the same chemical substances cause contraction in smooth muscle as in skeletal muscle, but the physical arrangement of smooth muscle fibers is entirely different, as we shall see.

TYPES OF SMOOTH MUSCLE

The smooth muscle of each organ is distinctive from that of most other organs in several different ways: physical dimensions, organization into bundles or sheets, response to different types of stimuli, characteristics of innervation, and function. Yet, for the sake of simplicity, smooth muscle can generally be divided into two major types, which are illustrated in Figure 8–3; *multiunit smooth muscle* and *visceral smooth muscle.*

Multiunit Smooth Muscle. This type of smooth muscle is composed of discrete smooth muscle fibers. Each fiber operates entirely independently of the others and is often innervated by a single nerve ending, as occurs for skeletal muscle fibers. Furthermore, the outer surfaces of these fibers, like those of skeletal muscle fibers, are covered by a thin layer of "basement membrane–like" substance, a glycoprotein that helps insulate the separate fibers from each other.

The most important characteristic of multiunit smooth muscle fibers is that their control is exerted mainly by nerve signals (even though they themselves usually do not generate action potentials, as we shall discuss later). This is in contrast to a major share of the control of visceral smooth muscle by non-nervous stimuli. An additional characteristic is that they rarely exhibit spontaneous contractions.

Some examples of multiunit smooth muscle found in the body are the smooth muscle fibers of the ciliary muscle of the eye, the iris of the eye, the nictitating membrane that covers the eyes in some lower animals, the piloerector muscles that cause

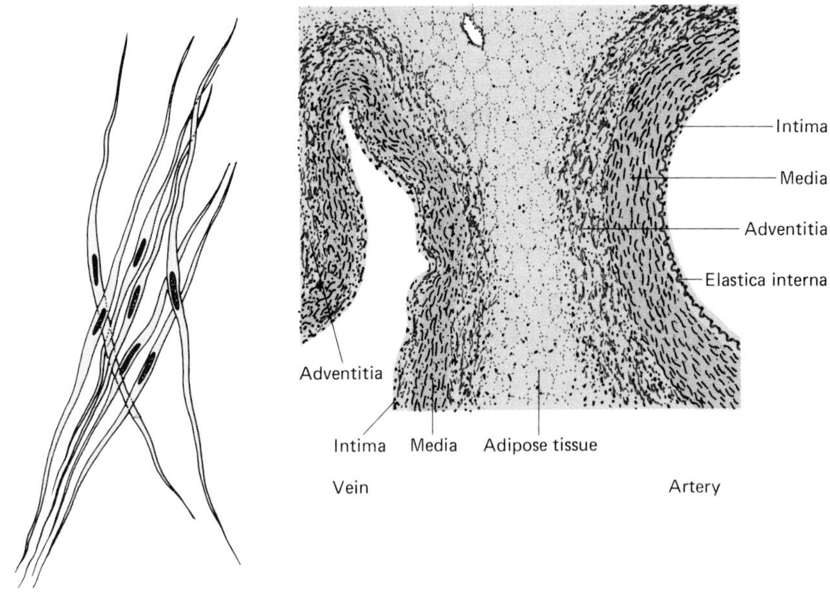

Figure 8–3. Visceral and multiunit smooth muscle fibers.

Multiunit smooth muscle fibers
A

Visceral smooth muscle
B

erection of the hairs when stimulated by the sympathetic nervous system, and the smooth muscle of many of the larger blood vessels.

Visceral Smooth Muscle. Visceral smooth muscle fibers are similar to multiunit fibers except that they are usually arranged in sheets or bundles and the cell membranes contact each other at multiple points to form many *gap junctions* through which ions can flow freely from one cell to the next. Thus the fibers form a *functional syncytium* that usually contracts in large areas at once. For this reason, this type of smooth muscle is also known as *single-unit* or *unitary smooth muscle*. This type of muscle is found in most of the organs of the body, especially in the walls of the gut, the bile ducts, the ureters, the uterus, and so forth.

When one portion of a visceral muscle tissue is stimulated, the action potential is conducted to the surrounding fibers by *direct electrical conduction*. That is, the action potential generated in one area of the muscle electrically excites the adjacent fibers without secretion of any transmitter substance. Instead, electrical current flows through the gap junctions so easily that action potentials spread directly from one smooth muscle fiber to the next almost as though cell membranes did not exist between the fibers.

THE CONTRACTILE PROCESS IN SMOOTH MUSCLE

The Chemical Basis for Smooth Muscle Contraction. Smooth muscle contains both *actin* and *myosin filaments,* having chemical characteristics similar to but not exactly the same as those of the actin and myosin filaments in skeletal muscle. Smooth muscle also contains *tropomyosin,* but it is doubtful whether troponin or a troponin-like substance exists in smooth muscle. This raises a question about the mechanism for control of smooth muscle contraction, which will be discussed in more detail in a subsequent section of this chapter.

Chemical studies have shown that actin and myosin derived from smooth muscle interact with each other in the same way that this occurs for actin and myosin derived from skeletal muscle. Furthermore, the contractile process is activated by calcium ions, and ATP is degraded to ADP to provide the energy for contraction.

On the other hand, there are major differences between the physical organization of smooth muscle and that of skeletal muscle, as well as differences in other aspects of smooth muscle function, such as excitation-contraction coupling, control of the contractile process by calcium ions, duration of contraction, and amount of energy required for the contractile process.

The Physical Basis for Smooth Muscle Contraction. Smooth muscle does not have the same striated arrangement of the actin and myosin filaments as that found in skeletal muscle. And, for a long time, it was impossible to discern even in electron micrographs any specific organization in the smooth muscle cell that could account for contraction. However, recent special electron micrographic techniques suggest the physical organization illustrated in Figure 8–4. This shows large numbers of actin filaments attached to so-called *dense bodies.* Some of these bodies in turn are attached to the cell membrane whereas others are located throughout the cell but are held in place by a scaffold of structural protein cross-attachments from one dense body to another. Interspersed among the actin filaments are a few thick filaments about 2.5 times the diameter of the thin actin

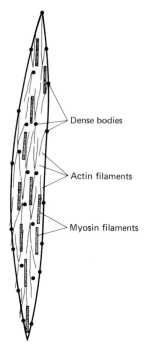

Figure 8–4. Arrangement of actin and myosin filaments in the smooth muscle cell. Note the attachment of the actin filaments to "dense bodies," some of which are themselves attached to the cell membrane.

Dense bodies

Actin filaments

Myosin filaments

filaments. These are assumed to be myosin filaments. However, there are only one twelfth to one fifteenth as many of these "myosin filaments" as actin filaments.

Despite the relative paucity of myosin filaments, it is assumed that they have sufficient cross-bridges to attract the many actin filaments and cause contraction by the sliding filament mechanism in essentially the same way that this occurs in skeletal muscle. And it is especially interesting to note that the maximum strength of contraction of smooth muscle is approximately equal to that of skeletal muscle, about 3 kg per square centimeter of cross-sectional area of the muscle.

Slowness of Contraction and Relaxation of Smooth Muscle. Though each smooth muscle tissue in the body has its own characteristics quite distinct from the others, a typical smooth muscle tissue will begin to contract 50 to 100 milliseconds after it is excited, and will reach full contraction about half a second later. Then the contraction declines in another 1 to 2 seconds, giving a total contraction time of 1 to 3 seconds, which is about 30 times as long as the single-twitch contraction of skeletal muscle. However, smooth muscle contractions as short as 0.2 second and as long as 30 seconds also occur.

A major share of the prolonged contractile state of smooth muscle seems to be caused by slowness of the chemical reactions that cause the contraction. For instance, assuming that smooth muscle contraction occurs by the same "walk-along" mechanism as that proposed for skeletal muscle, it has been calculated that the frequency of power strokes by the heads of the cross-bridges is only one tenth to one hundredth as rapid as in skeletal muscle. This is believed to result from the fact that the

cross-bridge heads have far less ATPase activity than that exhibited by the cross-bridge heads in skeletal muscle.

Energy Required to Sustain Smooth Muscle Contraction. Measurements have shown that only one twentieth to one four-hundredth as much energy is required to sustain the same tension of contraction in smooth muscle as in skeletal muscle. This also is believed to result mainly from the very slow activity of the myosin ATPase but also from the fact that there are far fewer myosin filaments in smooth muscle than in skeletal muscle.

This economy of energy utilization by smooth muscle is exceedingly important to overall function of the body, because organs such as the intestines, the urinary bladder, the gallbladder, and other viscera must maintain moderate degrees of muscle contractile tone day in and day out.

MEMBRANE POTENTIALS AND ACTION POTENTIALS IN SMOOTH MUSCLE

Smooth muscle exhibits membrane potentials and action potentials similar to those that occur in skeletal muscle fibers. Furthermore, smooth muscle contraction can be elicited by depolarization of the membrane in the same way that contraction is initiated by depolarization of skeletal muscle fibers. However, there are both quantitative and qualitative differences in the membrane potentials and action potentials of smooth muscle that require special attention.

Membrane Potentials in Smooth Muscle. The quantitative value of the membrane potential of smooth muscle is variable from one type of smooth muscle to another, and it also depends on the momentary condition of the muscle. However, in the normal resting state, the membrane potential is usually about -50 to -60 millivolts, or about 30 millivolts less negative than in skeletal muscle.

Action Potentials in Visceral Smooth Muscle. Action potentials occur in visceral smooth muscle in the same way that they occur in skeletal muscle. However, action potentials probably do not normally occur in multiunit types of smooth muscle, as will be discussed in a subsequent section.

The action potentials of visceral smooth muscle occur in two different forms: (1) spike potentials and (2) action potentials with plateaus.

Spike Potentials. Typical spike action potentials, such as those seen in skeletal muscle, occur in most types of visceral smooth muscle. The duration of this type of action potential is 10 to 50 milliseconds, as illustrated in Figure 8–5A. Such action potentials can be elicited in many ways, such as by electrical stimulation, by the action of hormones on the smooth muscle, by the action of transmitter substances from nerve fibers, or as a result of spontaneous generation in the muscle fiber itself, as discussed below.

Action Potentials with Plateaus. Figure 8–6 illustrates an action potential with a plateau. The onset of this action potential is similar to that of the typical spike potential. However, instead of rapid

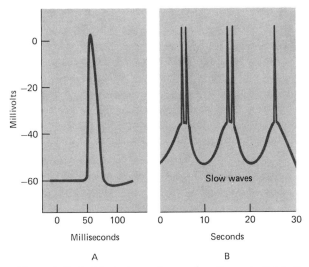

Figure 8–5. *A,* A typical smooth muscle action potential (spike potential) elicited by an external stimulus. *B,* A series of spike action potentials elicited by rhythmic, slow electrical waves occurring spontaneously in the smooth muscle wall of the intestine.

repolarization of the muscle fiber membrane, the repolarization is delayed for several hundred to several thousand milliseconds. The importance of the plateau is that it can account for the prolonged periods of contraction that occur in at least some types of smooth muscle. This type of action potential often occurs in the ureter, in the uterus under some conditions, and in some types of vascular smooth muscle. (Also, this is the type of action potential seen in cardiac muscle fibers that have a prolonged period of contraction, as we shall discuss in the next two chapters.)

Importance of Calcium Channels in Generating the Smooth Muscle Action Potential. The smooth muscle cell membrane has far more voltage-gated calcium channels than does skeletal muscle, but far fewer sodium channels. Therefore, sodium participates to a far less extent in the generation of the action potential in smooth muscle than in skeletal muscle. Instead, the flow of calcium ions to the interior of the fiber is mainly responsible for the action potential. This occurs in the same self-regenerative way as occurs for the sodium channels in nerve fibers and in skeletal muscle fibers. However, calcium channels open many times more slowly than do sodium channels. This accounts in large measure for the slow action potentials of smooth muscle fibers.

Another important feature of calcium entry into the cells during the action potential is that this calcium acts directly on the smooth muscle actin and myosin contractile mechanism to cause contraction, as we shall discuss later. Thus, the calcium performs two tasks at once.

Slow Wave Potentials in Visceral Smooth Muscle and Spontaneous Generation of Action Potentials. Some smooth muscle is self-excitatory. That is, action potentials arise within the smooth muscle itself without an extrinsic stimulus. This is usually associated with a basic *slow wave rhythm* of the membrane potential. A typical slow wave of this type is illustrated in Figure 8–5B. The slow wave itself is not an action potential. It is not a self-regenerative process that spreads progressively over the membranes of the muscle fibers. Instead, it is a local property of the smooth muscle fibers that make up the muscle mass.

The cause of the slow wave rhythm is as yet unknown; one suggestion is that the slow waves are caused by waxing and waning of the pumping of sodium outward through the muscle fiber membrane; the membrane potential becomes more negative when sodium is pumped rapidly and less negative when the sodium pump becomes less active. Another suggestion is that the conductances of the ion channels increase and decrease rhythmically.

The importance of the slow waves lies in the fact that they can initiate action potentials. The slow waves themselves cannot cause muscle contraction, but when the potential of the slow wave rises above the level of approximately −35 millivolts (the approximate threshold for eliciting action potentials in most visceral smooth muscle), an action potential develops and spreads over the visceral smooth muscle mass, and then contraction does occur. Figure 8–5B illustrates this effect, showing that at each peak of the slow wave, one or more action potentials occur. This effect can obviously promote a series of rhythmical contractions of the smooth muscle mass. Therefore, the slow waves are frequently called *pacemaker waves.* This type of activity is especially prominent in tubular types of smooth muscle masses, such as in the gut, the ureter, and so forth. In Chapter 28 we shall see that this type of activity controls the rhythmical contractions of the gut.

Excitation of Visceral Smooth Muscle by Stretch. When visceral smooth muscle is stretched sufficiently, spontaneous action potentials are usually generated. These result from a combination of the normal slow wave potentials plus a decrease in the membrane potential caused by the stretch itself. This response to stretch is an especially important function of visceral smooth muscle because it allows a hollow organ that is excessively stretched to contract automatically and therefore to resist the

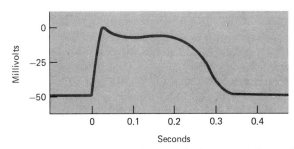

Figure 8–6. Monophasic action potential from a smooth muscle fiber of the rat uterus.

stretch. For instance, when the gut is overstretched by intestinal contents, a local automatic contraction often sets up a peristaltic wave that moves the contents away from the super-stretched intestine.

Depolarization of Multiunit Smooth Muscle Without Action Potentials. The smooth muscle fibers of multiunit smooth muscle normally contract mainly in response to nerve stimuli. The nerve endings secrete acetylcholine in the case of some multiunit smooth muscles and norepinephrine in the case of others. In both instances, these transmitter substances cause depolarization of the smooth muscle membrane, and this response in turn elicits the contraction. However, action potentials most often do not develop. The reason for this is that the fibers are too small to generate an action potential. (When action potentials are elicited in visceral smooth muscle, as many as 30 to 40 smooth muscle fibers must depolarize simultaneously before a self-propagating action potential ensues.) Yet, even without an action potential in the multiunit smooth muscle fibers, the local depolarization caused by the nerve transmitter substance itself spreads "electrotonically" over the entire fiber and is all that is needed to cause the muscle contraction.

EXCITATION-CONTRACTION COUPLING— ROLE OF CALCIUM IONS

In the previous chapter it was pointed out that the actual contractile process in skeletal muscle is activated by calcium ions. This is also true in smooth muscle. However, the source of the calcium ions differs in smooth muscle because the sarcoplasmic reticulum of smooth muscle is poorly developed.

In some types of smooth muscle, almost all the calcium ions that cause contraction enter the muscle cell from the extracellular fluid at the time of the action potential. There is a reasonably high concentration of calcium ions in the extracellular fluid, greater than 10^{-3} molar in comparison with less than 10^{-7} molar in the cell, and as was pointed out in the previous section, the smooth muscle action potential is caused at least partly by influx of calcium ions into the muscle fiber. Because the smooth muscle fibers are extremely small (in contrast to the sizes of the skeletal muscle fibers), these calcium ions can diffuse to all parts of the smooth muscle and elicit the contractile process. The time required for this diffusion to occur is usually 200 to 300 milliseconds and is called the *latent period* before the contraction begins; this latent period is some 50 times as great as that for skeletal muscle contraction.

Yet, in some smooth muscle there is a moderately developed sarcoplasmic reticulum. However, there are no T tubules. Instead, the cisternae of the reticulum abut the cell membrane. Therefore, it is believed that the membrane action potentials in these smooth muscle fibers cause release of calcium ions from these cisternae, thereby providing a greater degree of contraction than would occur on the basis of calcium ions entering through the cell membrane alone.

The Calcium Pump. To cause relaxation of the smooth muscle contractile elements, it is necessary to remove the calcium ions. This removal is achieved by a calcium pump that pumps the calcium ions out of the smooth muscle fiber and back into the extracellular fluid, or pumps the calcium ions into the sarcoplasmic reticulum. However, this pump is very slow-acting in comparison with the fast-acting sarcoplasmic reticulum pump in skeletal muscle. Therefore, the duration of smooth muscle contraction is often in the order of seconds rather than in tens of milliseconds, as occurs for skeletal muscle.

Mechanism by Which Calcium Ions Excite Contraction in Smooth Muscle. The mechanism by which calcium ions excite contraction in smooth muscle fibers is quite different from that in skeletal muscle. In fact, smooth muscle probably does not have an effective troponin complex, the factor that is activated by calcium ions in skeletal muscles to initiate contraction. Instead, the calcium ions excite contraction in smooth muscle fibers by activating the ATPase activity of the myosin heads. When calcium is not present, this ATPase activity in smooth muscle is extremely slight so that ATP cannot be cleaved and the contractile process cannot take place. Calcium ions activate this ATPase activity in the following way:

The first event is the increase in calcium ion concentration as a result of the action potential or of any other stimulus that causes entry of calcium ions into the cell cytosol. Second, the calcium ions bind with a protein, *calmodulin*, that is very similar to the troponin C in skeletal muscle fibers. Third, the bound product of calmodulin and calcium ions in turn binds with or activates one of the light chain polypeptides of the myosin head; this in turn activates the ATPase activity of the myosin head. Fourth, the newly excited ATPase activity of the head then causes cleavage of ATP and the usual conformational changes in the head, leading to the same "walk-along" contractile process in smooth muscle fibers as occurs in skeletal muscle.

However, two other features of this contractile activating process are also considerably different from the activation of skeletal muscle. First, all these events are very slow to take place, which further explains the slowness and long duration of smooth muscle contraction. Second, other factors besides calcium ions can have large effects on the intensity of the contractile process, which usually is not true in skeletal muscle. One of these is the concentration of cyclic AMP in the cell, which, we shall see later, is another means for influencing the strength of smooth muscle contraction.

NEUROMUSCULAR JUNCTIONS OF SMOOTH MUSCLE

Physiological Anatomy of Smooth Muscle Neuromuscular Junctions. Neuromuscular junctions of the type found on skeletal muscle fibers do not occur in smooth muscle. Instead, the nerve fibers generally branch diffusely on top of a sheet of muscle fibers, as illustrated in Figure 8–7. In most instances these fibers do not make direct contact with the smooth muscle fibers at all but instead form so-called *diffuse junctions* that secrete their transmitter substance into the interstitial fluid from a few nanometers to a few microns away from the muscle cells; the transmitter substance then diffuses to the cells. Furthermore, where there are many layers of muscle cells, the nerve fibers often innervate only the outer layer, and the muscle excitation then travels from this outer layer to the inner layers by direct action potential conduction or by subsequent diffusion of the transmitter substance. But, less often, terminal branches of the axons do penetrate into the muscle mass.

The axons innervating smooth muscle fibers also do not have typical branching end-feet, as observed in the end-plate on skeletal muscle fibers. Instead, most of the fine terminal axons have multiple varicosities spread along their axes. At these points the Schwann cells are interrupted so that transmitter substance can be secreted through the walls of the varicosities. In the varicosities are vesicles similar to those present in the skeletal muscle end-plate containing transmitter substance. However, in contrast to the vesicles of skeletal muscle junctions that contain only acetylcholine, the vesicles of the autonomic nerve fiber varicosities contain acetylcholine in some fibers and norepinephrine in others.

In a few instances, particularly in the multiunit type of smooth muscle, the varicosities lie directly on the muscle fiber membrane with a separation from this membrane of as little as 20 nanometers—the same width as the synaptic cleft that occurs in the skeletal muscle junction. These *contact junctions* function in much the same way as the skeletal muscle neuromuscular junction, and the latent period of contraction of these smooth muscle fibers is considerably shorter than of fibers stimulated by the diffuse junctions.

Excitatory and Inhibitory Transmitter Substances at the Smooth Muscle Neuromuscular Junction. Two different transmitter substances known to be secreted by the autonomic nerves innervating smooth muscle are *acetylcholine* and *norepinephrine.* Acetylcholine is an excitatory transmitter substance for smooth muscle fibers in some organs but an inhibitory substance for smooth muscle in other organs. And when acetylcholine excites a muscle fiber, norepinephrine ordinarily inhibits it. Or when acetylcholine inhibits a fiber, norepinephrine usually excites it.

But why these different responses? The answer is that both acetylcholine and norepinephrine excite or inhibit smooth muscle by first binding with a *receptor protein* on the surface of the muscle cell membrane. This receptor in turn controls the opening or closing of ion channels or controls some other means for activating or inhibiting the smooth muscle fiber. Furthermore, some of the receptor proteins are *excitatory receptors* whereas others are *inhibitory receptors.* Thus, it is the type of receptor that determines whether the smooth muscle will be inhibited or excited and also determines which of the two transmitters, acetylcholine or norepinephrine, will be effective in causing the excitation or inhibition. These receptors will be discussed in more detail in Chapter 21 in relation to the function of the autonomic nervous system.

Excitation of Action Potentials in Smooth Muscle Fibers—The Junctional Potential. Transmission of impulses from terminal nerve fibers to smooth muscle fibers occurs in very much the same manner as transmission at the neuromuscular junction of skeletal muscle fibers except for temporal differences. When an action potential reaches the terminal of an excitatory nerve fibril, there is a typical latent period of 50 milliseconds before any change in the membrane potential of the smooth muscle fiber can be detected. Then the potential rises to a maximal level in approximately 100 milliseconds. If an action potential does not occur, this potential gradually disappears at a rate of approximately one half every 200 to 500 milliseconds. This complete sequence of potential changes is called the *junctional potential*; it is analogous to the end-plate potential of the skeletal muscle fibers except that its duration is 20 to 100 times as long.

If the junctional potential rises to the threshold level for discharge of the smooth muscle membrane, an action potential will occur in the smooth muscle fiber in exactly the same way that an action potential occurs in a skeletal muscle fiber. A typical smooth muscle fiber has a normal resting membrane potential of −50 to −60 millivolts, and the threshold potential at which the action potential occurs is about −30 to −35 millivolts.

Inhibition at the Smooth Muscle Neuromuscular Junction. When a transmitter substance at the nerve

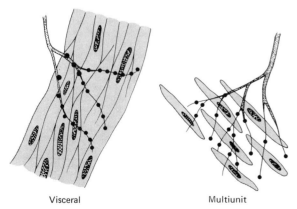

Visceral   Multiunit

Figure 8–7. Innervation of smooth muscle.

ending interacts with an inhibitory receptor instead of an excitatory receptor, the membrane potential of the muscle fiber becomes more negative than ever, for instance down to −70 millivolts; that is, it becomes *hyperpolarized* and therefore becomes much more difficult to excite than is usually the case.

SMOOTH MUSCLE CONTRACTION WITHOUT ACTION POTENTIALS—EFFECT OF LOCAL TISSUE FACTORS AND HORMONES

Though we have thus far discussed smooth muscle contraction elicited only by nervous signals and smooth muscle membrane action potentials, we must quickly disavow the belief that all smooth muscle contraction occurs in this way. In fact, probably half or more of all smooth muscle contraction is initiated not by action potentials but by stimulatory factors acting directly on the smooth muscle contractile machinery. The two types of nonnervous and nonaction potential stimulating factors most often involved are (1) local tissue factors, and (2) various hormones.

Smooth Muscle Contraction in Response to Local Tissue Factors. The very smallest blood vessels have little or no nervous supply. Yet, the smooth muscle is highly contractile, responding rapidly to changes in local conditions in the surrounding interstitial fluid. In this way a powerful local feedback control system controls the blood flow to the local tissue area. Some of the specific control factors are:

(1) Lack of oxygen in the local tissues causes smooth muscle relaxation and therefore vasodilatation.

(2) Excess carbon dioxide causes vasodilatation.

(3) Increased hydrogen ion concentration also causes increased vasodilatation.

And such factors as lactic acid, increased potassium ions, diminished calcium ion concentration, and decreased body temperature will also cause local vasodilatation.

Effects of Hormones on Smooth Muscle Contraction. Most of the circulating hormones in the body affect smooth muscle contraction at least to some degree, and some have very profound effects. Some of the more important bloodborne hormones are norepinephrine, epinephrine, acetylcholine, angiotensin, vasopressin, oxytocin, serotonin, and histamine.

A hormone will cause contraction of smooth muscle when the smooth muscle cells contain an *excitatory receptor* for the respective hormone. However, the hormone will cause inhibition instead of contraction if the cells contain an *inhibitory receptor* rather than an excitatory receptor. Thus, most of the hormones will cause excitation of some smooth muscle but inhibition of other muscle.

Some of the hormones—especially norepinephrine, vasopressin, and angiotensin—have such a powerful excitatory effect that they can cause smooth muscle spasm for hours.

Mechanism of Smooth Muscle Excitation by Local Tissue Factors and Hormones. Most smooth muscle contraction caused by hormones results from an initial increase in calcium ion concentration in the muscle cell, as occurs when an action potential excites the fiber. Each hormone usually binds with a specific receptor protein in the membrane and initiates the contraction, usually by opening calcium ion channels and decreasing the membrane potential a moderate amount—that is, "depolarizing" the membrane—but usually *without causing an action potential*. Nevertheless, the flow of calcium ions to the interior of the cell causes contraction.

In some instances, however, smooth muscle contraction (or relaxation) is initiated by hormones without a change in the membrane potential at all. In these instances it is believed that the exciting hormone binds with a receptor protein that activates a nonvoltage-related mechanism that leads to contraction or relaxation. One such mechanism that usually leads to relaxation is activation of the enzyme *adenylcyclase* in the cell membrane; a portion of this enzyme that protrudes to the interior of the cell then causes the formation of *cyclic AMP*, which is a so-called second messenger. The cyclic AMP in turn promotes intracellular changes that usually cause smooth muscle to relax.

Unfortunately, it is not known how most other local tissue factors besides the hormones, such as oxygen lack, excess CO_2, or changes in hydrogen ion concentration, either excite or inhibit smooth muscle contraction. However, possible mechanisms include changes in the cell membrane potential, changes in the permeability of the membrane to calcium ions, and/or changes in the intracellular contractile machinery.

MECHANICAL CHARACTERISTICS OF SMOOTH MUSCLE CONTRACTION

From the foregoing discussion of the many different types of smooth muscle and the different ways in which contraction can be elicited, one can readily understand why smooth muscle in different parts of the body has many different characteristics of contraction. For instance, the multiunit smooth muscle of the large blood vessels contracts mainly in response to nerve impulses, whereas in many types of visceral smooth muscle—the smaller blood vessels, the ureter, the bile ducts, and other glandular ducts—a self-excitatory process controlled mainly by local factors and by hormones causes continuous rhythmic contraction.

Tone of Smooth Muscle. Smooth muscle can maintain a state of long-term, steady contraction that has been called either *tonus* contraction of smooth muscle or simply *smooth muscle tone*. This is an important feature of smooth muscle contraction because it allows prolonged or even indefinite continuance of the smooth muscle function. For instance, the arterioles are maintained in a state of tonic contraction almost throughout the entire life of the person. Likewise, tonic contraction in the gut wall maintains steady pressure on the contents of the gut, and

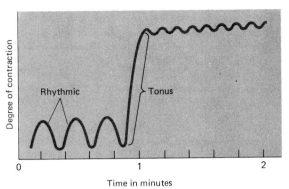

Figure 8–8. Record of rhythmic and tonic smooth muscle contraction.

charges or (2) rhythmical pacemaker slow waves that periodically excite the smooth muscle.

Degree of Shortening of Smooth Muscle During Contraction. A special characteristic of smooth muscle—one that is also different from skeletal muscle—is its ability to shorten a far greater percentage of its length than can skeletal muscle. Skeletal muscle has a useful distance of contraction equal to only 25 to 35 per cent of its length, while smooth muscle can often contract quite effectively to as short as one half or even one fourth its stretched length, giving as much as a fourfold distance of contraction. This allows smooth muscle to perform important functions in the hollow viscera—for instance, allowing the gut, the bladder, blood vessels, and other internal structures of the body to change their lumen diameters from almost zero to very large values.

Stress-Relaxation of Smooth Muscle. Another important characteristic of smooth muscle is its ability to change length greatly without marked changes in tension. This results from a phenomenon called *stress-relaxation*, which may be explained as follows:

If a segment of smooth muscle 1 inch long is suddenly stretched to 2 inches, the tension between the two ends increases tremendously at first, but the extra tension also begins to disappear immediately, and within a few minutes it has returned almost to its level prior to the stretch, even though the muscle is now twice as long. This possibly results from the loose arrangement of the actin and myosin filaments in smooth muscle. Over a period of time, the filaments of the stretched muscle presumably rearrange their bonds and gradually allow the sliding process to take place, thus allowing the tension to return almost to its original amount.

Exactly the converse effect occurs when smooth muscle is shortened. Thus, if the 2 inch segment of smooth muscle is shortened back to 1 inch, essentially all tension will be lost from the muscle immediately. Gradually, over a period of 1 minute or more, much of the tension returns, this again presumably resulting from slow sliding of the filaments. This is called *reverse stress-relaxation*.

tonic contraction of the urinary bladder wall maintains a moderate amount of pressure on the urine in the bladder.

Tonic contractions of smooth muscle can be caused in either of two ways:

1. They are sometimes caused by *summation of individual contractile pulses;* each contractile pulse is initiated by a separate action potential in the same way that tetanic contractions are produced in skeletal muscle.

2. However, most smooth muscle tonic contractions probably result from *prolonged direct smooth muscle excitation* without action potentials, usually caused by local tissue factors or circulating hormones. For instance, prolonged tonic contractions of the blood vessels without the mediation of action potentials are regularly caused by angiotensin, vasopressin, or norepinephrine, and these play an important role in the long-term regulation of arterial pressure, as will be discussed in Chapter 27.

A typical example of a tonic contraction is illustrated in Figure 8–8. This figure also shows that rhythmic contractions can be superimposed onto the tonic contraction because of simultaneous (1) rhythmical nerve dis-

---

REFERENCES

Bennett, M. R.: Development of neuromuscular synapses. *Physiol. Rev.,* 63:915, 1983.

Blaustein, M. P., and Hamlyn, J. M.: Sodium transport inhibition, cell calcium, and hypertension. The natriuretic hormone/Na+ = Ca2+ exchange/hypertension hypothesis. *Am. J. Med., 77:45, 1984.*

Bohr, D. F., and Webb, R. C.: Vascular smooth muscle function and its changes in hypertension. *Am. J. Med., 77:3, 1984.*

Bolton, T. B.: Mechanisms of action of transmitters and other substances on smooth muscle. *Physiol. Rev., 59:606, 1979.*

Borgstrom, P., *et al.:* An evaluation of the metabolic interaction with myogenic vascular reactivity during blood flow autoregulation. *Acta Physiol. Scand., 122:275, 1984.*

Bulbring, E. (ed.): Smooth Muscle. An Assessment of Current Knowledge. Austin, University of Texas Press, 1981.

Bulbring, E., *et al.* (eds.): Physiology of Smooth Muscles; Twenty-sixth International Congress of Physiological Sciences. New York, Raven Press, 1975.

Ceccarelli, B., and Hurlbut, W. P.: Vesicle hypothesis of the release of quanta of acetylcholine. *Physiol. Rev., 60:396, 1980.*

Chamley-Campbell, J., *et al.:* Smooth muscle cell in culture. *Physiol. Rev., 59:1, 1979.*

Changeux, J. P., *et al.:* Acetylcholine receptor: An allosteric protein. *Science, 225:1335, 1984.*

Cotman, C. W., *et al.:* Synapse replacement in the nervous system of adult vertebrates. *Physiol. Rev., 61:684, 1981.*

Daniel, E. E., and Sarna, S.: The generation and conduction of activity in smooth muscle. *Annu. Rev. Pharmacol. Toxicol., 18:145, 1978.*

Dau, P. C. (ed.): Plasmapheresis and the Immunobiology of Myasthenia Gravis. Boston, Houghton Mifflin, 1979.

Dowben, R. M. (ed.): Cell and Muscle Motility. New York, Plenum Publishing Corp., 1983.

Duckles, S. P., and Banner, W., Jr.: Changes in vascular smooth muscle reactivity during development. *Annu. Rev. Pharmacol. Toxicol., 24:65, 1984.*

Eisenberg, E., and Greene, L. E.: The relation of muscle biochemistry to muscle physiology. *Annu. Rev. Physiol., 42:293, 1980.*

Fambrough, D. M.: Control of acetylcholine receptors in skeletal muscle. *Physiol. Rev., 59:165, 1979.*

Fleming, W. W.: The electrogenic Na+,K+-pump in smooth muscle: Physiologic and pharmacologic significance. *Annu. Rev. Pharmacol. Toxicol., 20:129, 1980.*

Furchgott, R. F.: The role of endothelium in the responses of vascular smooth muscle to drugs. *Annu. Rev. Pharmacol. Toxicol., 24:175, 1984.*

Gabella, G.: Structural apparatus for force transmission in smooth muscle. *Physiol. Rev., 64:455, 1984.*

Gage, P. W.: Generation of end-plate potentials. *Physiol. Rev., 56:177, 1976.*

Guyton, A. C., and MacDonald, M. A.: Physiology of botulinus toxin. *Arch. Neurol. Psychiat., 57:578, 1947.*

Guyton, A. C., and Reeder, R. C.: The dynamics of curarization. *J. Pharmacol. Exp. Ther., 97:322, 1949.*

Hartshorne, D. J., and Gorecka, A.: Biochemistry of the contractile proteins of smooth muscle. *In* Bohr, D. F., *et al.* (eds.): Handbook of Physiology. Sec. 2, Vol. II. Baltimore, Williams & Wilkins, 1980, p. 83.

Hartshorne, D. J., and Siemankowski, R. F.: Regulation of smooth muscle actomyosin. *Annu. Rev. Physiol.,* 43:519, 1981.

Hertzberg, E. L., *et al.*: Gap junctional communication. *Annu. Rev. Physiol.,* 43:479, 1981.

Hess, G. P., *et al.*: Acetylcholine receptor-controlled ion translocation: Chemical kinetic investigations of the mechanism. *Annu. Rev. Biophys. Bioeng.,* 12:443, 1983.

Johansson, B.: Vascular smooth muscle reactivity. *Annu. Rev. Physiol.,* 43:359, 1981.

Johansson, B., and Somlyo, A. P.: Electrophysiology and excitation-contraction coupling. *In* Bohr, D. F., *et al.* (eds.): Handbook of Physiology. Sec. 2, Vol. II. Baltimore, Williams & Wilkins, 1980, p. 301.

Klein, W. L.: Biochemistry and regulation of signal transduction by neuronal acetylcholine receptors. *Curr. Top. Cell. Regul.,* 24:129, 1984.

Lambert, J. J., *et al.*: Drug-induced modification of ionic conductance at the neuromuscular junction. *Annu. Rev. Pharmacol. Toxicol.,* 23:505, 1983.

Landmesser, L. T.: The generation of neuromuscular specificity. *Annu. Rev. Neurosci.,* 3:279, 1980.

Lindstrom, J., and Dau, P.: Biology of myasthenia gravis. *Annu. Rev. Pharmacol. Toxicol.,* 20:337, 1980.

Loewenstein, W. R.: Junctional intercellular communication: The cell-to-cell membrane channel. *Physiol. Rev.,* 61:829, 1981.

Loh, H. H., and Law, P. Y.: The role of membrane lipids in receptor mechanisms. *Annu. Rev. Pharmacol. Toxicol.,* 20:201, 1980.

Mark, R. F.: Synaptic repression at neuromuscular junctions. *Physiol. Rev.,* 60:355, 1980.

McKinney, M., and Richelson, E.: The coupling of neuronal muscarinic receptor to responses. *Annu. Rev. Pharmacol. Toxicol.,* 24:121, 1984.

Morgan, D. L., and Proske, U.: Vertebrate slow muscle: Its structure, pattern of innervation, and mechanical properties. *Physiol. Rev.,* 64:103, 1984.

Murphy, R. A.: Filament organization and contractile function in vertebrate smooth muscle. *Annu. Rev. Physiol.,* 41:737, 1979.

Paul, R. J.: Chemical energetics of vascular smooth muscle. *In* Bohr, D. F., *et al.* (eds.): Handbook of Physiology. Sec. 2, Vol. II. Baltimore, Williams & Wilkins, 1980, p. 201.

Peper, K., *et al.*: The acetylcholine receptor at the neuromuscular junction. *Physiol. Rev.,* 62:1271, 1982.

Popot, J.-L., and Changeux, J.-P.: Nicotinic receptor of acetylcholine: Structure of an oligomeric integral membrane protein. *Physiol. Rev.,* 64:1162, 1984.

Prosser, C. L.: Evolution and diversity of nonstriated muscles. *In* Bohr, D. F., *et al.* (eds.): Handbook of Physiology. Sec. 2, Vol. II. Baltimore, Williams & Wilkins, 1980, p. 635.

Pumplin, D. W., and Fambrough, D. M.: Turnover of acetylcholine receptors in skeletal muscle. *Annu. Rev. Physiol.,* 44:319, 1982.

Purves, D., and Lichtman, J. W.: Specific connections between nerve cells. *Annu. Rev. Physiol.,* 45:553, 1983.

Schneider, M. F.: Membrane charge movement and depolarization-contraction coupling. *Annu. Rev. Physiol.,* 43:507, 1981.

Somlyo, A. P.: Ultrastructure of vascular smooth muscle. *In* Bohr, D. F., *et al.* (eds.): Handbook of Physiology. Sec. 2, Vol. II. Baltimore, Williams & Wilkins, 1980, p. 33.

Tauc, L.: Nonvascular release of neurotransmitter. *Physiol. Rev.,* 62:857, 1982.

Vanhoutte, P. M.: Calcium-entry blockers, vascular smooth muscle and systemic hypertension. *Am. J. Cardiol.,* 55:17B, 1985.

9

The Heart: Its Rhythmical Excitation and Nervous Control

The heart is a muscular organ. Like other muscles of the body, it is, in a sense, an extension of the nervous system, for its pumping function is at least partly controlled by nerves.

To perform its pumping function, the heart is divided into four separate chambers. The right and left atria pump blood respectively into the right and left ventricles. The right ventricle then pumps blood through the lungs, and the left ventricle pumps blood through the remainder of the body.

The atria actually function as "primer" pumps for the ventricles. Normally, they contract about one sixth of a second ahead of the ventricles, thus allowing time for extra blood to enter the ventricles prior to their contraction; this greatly increases the effectiveness of ventricular pumping.

The complexity of the heart's pumping cycle requires both rhythmical control of the heart beat and special timing mechanisms for sequential control of the atria and the ventricles. Furthermore, the rate of rhythmicity, as well as the strength of heart beat, can be increased or decreased by signals from the central nervous system. These control mechanisms will be explained later in the chapter. However, first, let us discuss the basic physiology of cardiac muscle itself, especially how it differs from skeletal muscle, which was discussed in Chapter 7.

PHYSIOLOGY OF CARDIAC MUSCLE

The heart is composed of three major types of cardiac muscle: atrial muscle, ventricular muscle, and specialized excitatory and conductive muscle fibers. The atrial and ventricular types contract in much the same way as skeletal muscle, except that the duration of contraction is much longer. On the other hand, the specialized excitatory and conductive fibers contract only feebly because they contain few contractile fibrils; instead, because of their rhythmical properties and their rapidity of conduction, they provide an excitatory system for the heart and a transmission system for rapid conduction of the cardiac excitatory signal throughout the heart.

PHYSIOLOGICAL ANATOMY OF CARDIAC MUSCLE

Figure 9–1 illustrates a typical histological picture of cardiac muscle, showing the cardiac muscle fibers arranged in a latticework, the fibers dividing, then recombining, and then spreading again. One notes immediately from this figure that cardiac muscle is *striated* in the same manner as typical skeletal muscle. Furthermore, cardiac muscle has typical myofibrils that contain *actin* and *myosin filaments* almost identical to those found in skeletal muscle, and these filaments interdigitate and slide along each other during the process of contraction in the same manner as occurs in skeletal muscle. (See Chapter 7.)

Cardiac Muscle as a Syncytium. The angulated dark areas crossing the cardiac muscle fibers in Figure 9–1 are called *intercalated discs;* however, they are actually cell membranes that separate individual cardiac muscle cells from each other. That is, cardiac muscle fibers are made up of many cardiac muscle cells connected in series with each other. Yet electrical resistance through the intercalated disc is only one four-hundredth the resistance through the outside membrane of the cardiac muscle fiber, because the cell membranes fuse with each other and form very permeable junctions that allow relatively free diffusion of ions. Therefore, from a functional point of view, ions move with ease along the axes of the cardiac muscle fibers so that action potentials travel from one cardiac muscle cell to another, past the intercalated discs, with only slight hindrance. Therefore, cardiac muscle is a *syncytium*, in which the cardiac muscle cells are so tightly bound that when one of these cells becomes excited, the action potential spreads to all of them, spreading from cell to cell and spreading throughout the latticework interconnections.

The heart is composed of two separate syncytiums, the *atrial syncytium* that constitutes the walls of the two atria and the *ventricular syncytium* that constitutes the walls of the two ventricles. These are separated from each other by fibrous tissue that surrounds the valvular openings between the atria and ventricles, but action potentials can be conducted from the atrial syncytium into the ventricular syncytium by way of a specialized conductive system, the *A-V bundle,* which will be discussed in detail later in the chapter. This division of the muscle mass of the heart into two separate functional syncytia allows the atria to contract a short time ahead of ventricular contraction, which is important for the effectiveness of heart pumping.

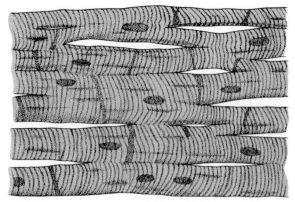

Figure 9–1. The "syncytial," interconnecting nature of cardiac muscle.

All-or-Nothing Principle As Applied to the Heart. Because of the syncytial and interconnecting nature of cardiac muscle, stimulation of any single atrial muscle fiber causes the action potential to travel over the entire atrial muscle mass, and, similarly, stimulation of any single ventricular fiber causes excitation of the entire ventricular muscle mass. If the A-V bundle is intact, the action potential passes also from the atria to the ventricles. This is called the all-or-nothing principle; and it is precisely the same as that discussed in Chapter 6 for nerve fibers. However, because the cardiac muscle fibers all interconnect with each other, the all-or-nothing principle applies to the entire functional syncytium of the heart rather than to single muscle fibers, as in the case of skeletal muscle fibers.

ACTION POTENTIALS IN CARDIAC MUSCLE

The *resting membrane potential* of normal cardiac muscle is approximately −85 to −95 millivolt (mv) and approximately −90 to −100 mv in the specialized conductive fibers, the Purkinje fibers, which are discussed later in the chapter.

The *action potential* recorded in ventricular muscle, shown by the bottom record of Figure 9–2, is 105 mv, which means that the membrane potential rises from its normally very negative value to a slightly positive value of about +20 mv. Because of this change of potential from negative to positive, the positive portion is called the *overshoot potential*. Then, after the initial *spike*, the membrane remains depolarized for about 0.2 second in atrial muscle and about 0.3 second in ventricular muscle, exhibiting a *plateau* as illustrated in Figure 9–2, followed at the end of the plateau by abrupt repolarization. The presence of this plateau in the action potential causes muscle contraction to last 20 to 50 times as long in cardiac muscle as in skeletal muscle.

At this point we must ask the question: Why is the action potential of cardiac muscle so long and why does it have a plateau while that of skeletal muscle does not? The basic biophysical answers to these questions were presented in Chapter 6 but they merit summarizing again.

At least two major differences between the membrane properties of cardiac and skeletal muscle account for the prolonged action potential and the plateau in cardiac muscle.

First, the action potential of skeletal muscle is caused almost entirely by sudden opening of large numbers of so-called fast sodium channels that allow tremendous numbers of sodium ions to enter the skeletal muscle fiber. These channels are called "fast" channels because they remain open for only a few ten-thousandths of a second and then abruptly close. At the end of this closure, the process of repolarization occurs, and the action potential is over within another ten-thousandth of a second or so. In cardiac muscle, on the other hand, the action potential is caused by the opening of two types of channels: (1) the same fast sodium channels as those in skeletal muscle, and (2) another entire population of so-called slow calcium-sodium channels. This second population of channels differs from the fast sodium channels in being slower to open but, more importantly, they remain open for several tenths of a second. During this time large amounts of both calcium and sodium ions continue to flow through the channels to the interior of the cardiac muscle fiber, and this maintains a prolonged period of depolarization. It is this that causes the plateau in the action potential. Furthermore, the calcium ions that enter the muscle during this action potential play an important role in helping excite the muscle contractile process, which is another difference between cardiac muscle and skeletal muscle that we shall discuss later in this chapter.

The second major functional difference between cardiac muscle and skeletal muscle that helps account for both the prolonged action potential and its plateau is this: Immediately after the onset of the action potential, the permeability of the cardiac muscle membrane for potassium *decreases* about fivefold, an effect that does not occur in skeletal muscle. It is possible that this decreased potassium

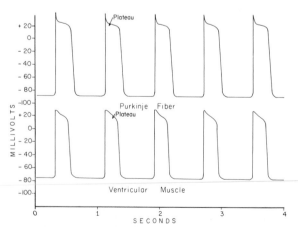

Figure 9–2. Rhythmic action potentials from a Purkinje fiber and from a ventricular muscle fiber, recorded by means of microelectrodes.

permeability is caused in some way by the excess calcium influx through the calcium channels just noted. But, regardless of the cause, the decreased potassium permeability greatly decreases the outflux of potassium ions during the action potential plateau and thereby prevents early recovery. When the slow calcium-sodium channels close at the end of 0.2 to 0.3 second and the influx of calcium and sodium ions ceases, then the membrane permeability for potassium increases very rapidly, and the rapid loss of potassium from the fiber returns the membrane potential to its resting level, thus ending the action potential.

Velocity of Conduction in Cardiac Muscle. The velocity of conduction of the action potential in both atrial and ventricular muscle fibers is about 0.3 to 0.5 meter per second, or about 1/250 the velocity in very large nerve fibers and about one tenth the velocity in skeletal muscle fibers. The velocity of conduction in the specialized conductive system varies from 0.02 to 4 meters per second in different parts of the system, as is explained in the following chapter.

Refractory Period of Cardiac Muscle. Cardiac muscle, like all excitable tissue, is refractory to restimulation during the action potential. An extremely strong electrical stimulus can sometimes initiate a new spike at the very end of the action potential plateau, but this is a very abnormal situation and the spike is not propagated along the muscle. Therefore, the refractory period of the heart is usually stated to be the interval of time, as shown to the left in Figure 9–3, during which a normal cardiac impulse cannot re-excite an already excited area of cardiac muscle. The normal refractory period of the ventricle is 0.25 to 0.3 second, which is approximately the duration of the action potential. There is an additional *relative refractory period* of about 0.05 second during which the muscle is more difficult than normal to excite but nevertheless can be excited, as illustrated by the early premature contraction in Figure 9–3.

The refractory period of atrial muscle is much shorter than that for the ventricles (about 0.15 second), and the relative refractory period is another 0.03 second. Therefore, the rhythmical rate of contraction of the atria can be much faster than that of the ventricles.

CONTRACTION OF CARDIAC MUSCLE

Excitation-Contraction Coupling—Function of Calcium Ions and of the T Tubules. The term excitation-contraction coupling means the mechanism by which the action potential causes the myofibrils of muscle to contract. This was discussed for skeletal muscle in Chapter 7. However, once again there are differences in this mechanism in cardiac muscle that have important effects on the characteristics of cardiac muscle contraction.

As is true for skeletal muscle, when an action potential passes over the cardiac muscle membrane, the action potential also spreads to the interior of the cardiac muscle fiber along the membranes of the T tubules. The T tubule action potentials in turn cause instantaneous release of calcium ions into the muscle sarcoplasm from the cisternae of the sarcoplasmic reticulum. Then the calcium ions diffuse in another few thousandths of a second into the myofibrils where they catalyze the chemical reactions that promote sliding of the actin and myosin filaments along each other; this in turn produces the muscle contraction.

Thus far, this mechanism of excitation-contraction coupling is the same as that for skeletal muscle, but at this point a major difference begins to appear. In addition to the calcium ions that are released into the sarcoplasm from the cisternae of the sarcoplasmic reticulum, large quantities of calcium ions also diffuse into the sarcoplasm from the T tubules at the time of the action potential. Indeed, without this extra calcium from the T tubules, the strength of cardiac muscle contraction would be considerably reduced, because the cisternae of cardiac muscle are less well developed than those of skeletal muscle and do not store enough calcium. On the other hand, the T tubules of cardiac muscle have a diameter five times as great as that of the skeletal muscle tubules and a volume 25 times as great; also, inside the T tubules is a large quantity of mucopolysaccharides that are electronegatively charged and bind an abundant store of calcium ions, keeping this always available for diffusion to the interior of the cardiac muscle fiber when the T tubule action potential occurs.

The strength of contraction of cardiac muscle depends to a great extent on the concentration of calcium ions in the extracellular fluids. The reason for this is that the ends of the T tubules open directly to the outside of the cardiac muscle fibers, allowing the same extracellular fluid that is in the cardiac muscle interstitium to percolate through the

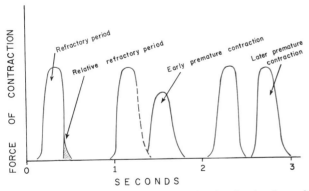

Figure 9–3. Contraction of the heart, showing the durations of the refractory period and the relative refractory period, the effect of an early premature contraction, and the effect of a later premature contraction. Note that the premature contractions do not cause wave summation as occurs in skeletal muscle.

T tubules as well. Consequently, the quantity of calcium ions in the T tubule system, as well as the availability of calcium ions to cause cardiac muscle contraction, depends directly on the extracellular fluid calcium ion concentration.

By way of contrast, the strength of skeletal muscle contraction is hardly affected by the extracellular fluid calcium concentration because its contraction is caused almost entirely by calcium ions released from the sarcoplasmic reticulum inside the skeletal muscle fiber itself.

At the end of the plateau of the action potential the influx of calcium ions to the interior of the muscle fiber is suddenly cut off, and the calcium ions in the sarcoplasm are rapidly pumped back into both the sarcoplasmic reticulum and the T tubules. As a result, the contraction ceases until a new action potential occurs.

Another difference between the tubules of cardiac muscle and those of skeletal muscle is that the T tubules in the skeletal muscle are located adjacent to the actin and myosin filaments where they overlap each other so that there are two T tubule systems to each sarcomere. On the other hand, in cardiac muscle there is only one T tubule system per sarcomere located at the Z line but composed of much larger T tubules. This difference in structure is compatible with the fact that cardiac muscle contracts much more slowly than skeletal muscle so that there is adequate time for calcium ions to diffuse from the Z line to the middle of the sarcomere where the contractile process occurs.

Duration of Contraction. Cardiac muscle begins to contract a few milliseconds after the action potential begins and continues to contract for a few milliseconds after the action potential ends. Therefore, the duration of contraction of cardiac muscle is mainly a function of the duration of the action potential—about 0.2 second in atrial muscle and 0.3 second in ventricular muscle.

Effect of Heart Rate on Duration of Contraction. When the heart rate increases, the duration of each total cycle of the heart, including both the contraction phase and the relaxation phase, obviously decreases. The duration of the action potential and the period of contraction (systole) also decrease but not as great a percentage as does the relaxation phase (diastole). At a normal heart rate of 72 beats per minute, the period of contraction is about 0.40 of the entire cycle. At three times normal heart rate, this period is about 0.65 of the entire cycle, which means that the heart under some conditions does not remain relaxed long enough to allow complete filling of the cardiac chambers prior to the next contraction.

THE SPECIAL EXCITATORY AND CONDUCTIVE SYSTEM OF THE HEART

The adult human heart normally contracts at a rhythmic rate of about 72 beats per minute. Figure 9–4 illustrates the special excitatory and conductive system of the heart that controls these cardiac contractions. The figure shows (1) the *S-A node* in which the normal rhythmic self-excitatory impulse

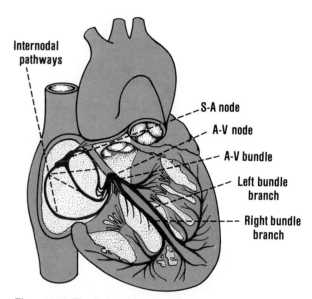

Figure 9–4. The S-A node and the Purkinje system of the heart, showing also the A-V node, the atrial internodal pathways, and the ventricular bundle branches.

is generated, (2) the *internodal pathways* that conduct the impulse from the S-A node to the A-V node, (3) the *A-V node* in which the impulse from the atria is delayed before passing into the ventricles, (4) the *A-V bundle*, which conducts the impulse from the atria into the ventricles, and (5) the *left* and *right bundles of Purkinje fibers*, which conduct the cardiac impulse to all parts of the ventricles.

THE SINOATRIAL NODE

The sinoatrial (S-A) node is a small, flattened, ellipsoid strip of specialized muscle approximately 3 mm wide, 15 mm long, and 1 mm thick; it is located in the anterosuperior wall of the right atrium immediately anterior and lateral to the opening of the superior vena cava. The fibers of this node are each 3 to 5 microns in diameter, in contrast to a diameter of 15 to 20 microns for the surrounding atrial muscle fibers. However, the S-A fibers are continuous with the atrial fibers so that any action potential that begins in the S-A node spreads immediately into the atria.

Automatic Rhythmicity of the Sinoatrial Fibers

Most cardiac fibers have the capability of *self-excitation*, a process that can cause automatic rhythmical contraction. This is especially true of the fibers of the heart's specialized conducting system; the portion of this system that displays self-excitation to the greatest extent is the fibers of the S-A node. For this reason, the sinoatrial node ordinarily controls the rate of beat of the entire heart, as will be discussed in detail later in this chapter. First, however, let us describe this automatic rhythmicity.

Mechanism of S-A Nodal Rhythmicity. The basic biophysics of self-excitatory rhythmicity of excitable tissues was presented in Chapter 6. However, let us review these principles as they apply to the S-A node.

Figure 9–5 illustrates action potentials recorded from an S-A nodal fiber for three heartbeats and, by comparison, a single ventricular muscle fiber action potential, shown to the right. Note that the "resting" potential of the S-A nodal fiber has a maximum negativity of only -55 to -60 millivolts in comparison with -85 to -90 millivolts for the ventricular fiber.

Before attempting to explain the rhythmicity of the S-A nodal fibers, first recall that in cardiac muscle three different types of membrane ion channels play important roles in causing the voltage changes of the action potential. These are (1) the *fast sodium channels*, (2) the *slow calcium-sodium channels*, and (3) the *potassium channels*. The opening of the fast sodium channels for a few ten-thousandths of a second is responsible for the very rapid spike-like onset of the action potential observed in ventricular muscle because of rapid influx of positive sodium ions to the interior of the fiber. Then the plateau of the ventricular action potential is caused primarily by slower opening of the slow calcium-sodium channels, which lasts for a few tenths of a second. Finally, increased opening of the potassium channels and diffusion of large amounts of positive potassium ions out of the fiber return the membrane potential to its resting level.

But there is a difference in the function of these channels in the S-A nodal fiber. The cause of this difference is the much less negativity of the S-A nodal fiber during the "resting" potential—only -55 millivolts. At this level of negativity, the fast sodium channels have mainly become "inactivated," which means that they have become blocked. The cause of this is that any time the membrane potential remains less negative than about -60 millivolts for a prolonged period of time, the gates on the inside of the cell membrane that close these channels become closed and remain so. Therefore, only the slow calcium-sodium channels

can open (that is, can become "activated") and can thereby cause the action potential. As a result, the action potential is slower to develop than that of the ventricular muscle and also recovers with a slow decrement of the potential rather than the abrupt recovery that occurs for the ventricular fiber.

However, there is still another feature of the S-A nodal fibers that is essential for their rhythmical self-excitation. This is the fact that they are quite leaky to sodium ions. This leakiness makes the "resting" potential of the S-A nodal fibers less negative than the resting potential of the ventricular muscle fibers, because entry of the positive sodium ions to the interior of the fiber neutralizes much of the fiber negativity. This leakiness to sodium ions also causes the "resting" potential gradually to rise between each two heart beats, as illustrated in Figure 9–5, until it finally reaches the *threshold voltage* of about -40 millivolts. At this point, this rising voltage suddenly opens the calcium-sodium channels, thus leading to the action potential. Therefore, basically, the inherent leakiness of the S-A nodal fibers to sodium ions causes their self-excitation.

Next, we must answer why this leakiness of sodium ions does not cause the S-A nodal fiber to remain depolarized all the time. The answer to this is that at the termination of the action potential greatly increased numbers of potassium channels have become opened, and these allow far greater quantities of potassium to diffuse out of the fiber than normally. This carries a great excess of positive charges to the exterior and temporarily causes excess negativity inside the fiber, which is called a state of *hyperpolarization*. This hyperpolarization initially carries the "resting" membrane potential down to about -55 to -60 millivolts at the termination of the action potential.

Lastly, we must explain why the state of hyperpolarization also is not maintained forever. The reason is that during the next few tenths of a second after the action potential is over, progressively more and more of the potassium channels begin to close. Now the inward-leaking positive sodium ions once again overbalance the outward flux of potassium ions, which causes the "resting" potential to drift upward, finally reaching the threshold level for discharge at a potential of about -40 millivolts. Then the entire process begins again: self-excitation, recovery from the action potential, hyperpolarization after the action potential is over, upward drift of the "resting" potential, then re-excitation still again to elicit still another cycle; this process continues indefinitely throughout the life of the person.

INTERNODAL PATHWAYS AND TRANSMISSION OF THE CARDIAC IMPULSE THROUGH THE ATRIA

The ends of the S-A nodal fibers fuse with the surrounding atrial muscle fibers, and action potentials originating in the S-A node travel outward into

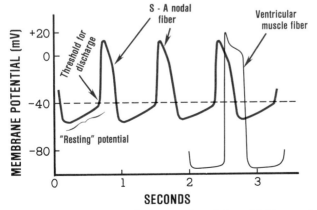

Figure 9–5. Rhythmic discharge of an S-A nodal fiber, and comparison of the S-A nodal action potential with that of a ventricular muscle fiber.

these fibers. In this way, the action potential spreads through the entire atrial muscle mass and eventually also to the A-V node. The velocity of conduction in the atrial muscle is approximately 0.3 meter per second. However, conduction is somewhat more rapid in several small bundles of atrial muscle fibers. One of these, called the *anterior interatrial band*, passes through the anterior walls of the atria to the left atrium and conducts the cardiac impulse at a velocity of about 1 meter per second. In addition, three other small bundles curve through the atrial walls and terminate in the A-V node, also conducting the cardiac impulse at this rapid velocity. These three small bundles are illustrated in Figure 9–4 and are called respectively the *anterior, middle,* and *posterior internodal pathways.* The cause of the more rapid velocity of conduction in these bundles is the presence of a number of specialized conduction fibers mixed with the atrial muscle. These fibers are similar to the very rapidly conducting Purkinje fibers of the ventricles, which will be discussed subsequently.

THE ATRIOVENTRICULAR (A-V) NODE AND THE PURKINJE SYSTEM

Delay in Transmission at the A-V Node. Fortunately, the conductive system is organized so that the cardiac impulse will not travel from the atria into the ventricles too rapidly; this allows time for the atria to empty their contents into the ventricles before ventricular contraction begins. It is primarily the A-V node and its associated conductive fibers that delay this transmission of the cardiac impulse from the atria into the ventricles.

The A-V node is located in the septal wall of the right atrium immediately posterior to the tricuspid valve, as illustrated in Figure 9–4. Figure 9–6 shows diagrammatically the different parts of this node and its connections with the atrial internodal pathway fibers and the A-V bundle. The figure also

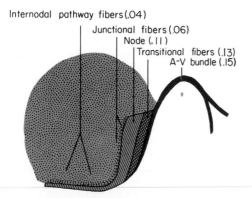

Internodal pathway fibers (.04)
Junctional fibers (.06)
Node (.11)
Transitional fibers (.13)
A-V bundle (.15)

Figure 9–6. Organization of the A-V node. The numbers represent the interval of time from the origin of the impulse in the S-A node. The values have been extrapolated to the human being. (This figure is based on studies in lower animals discussed and illustrated in Hoffman and Cranefield: Electrophysiology of the Heart. New York, McGraw-Hill Book Company, 1960.)

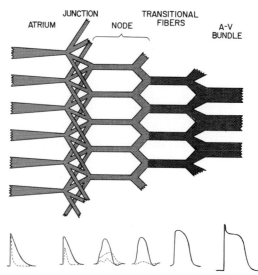

ATRIUM JUNCTION NODE TRANSITIONAL FIBERS A-V BUNDLE

Figure 9–7. Functional diagram of the anatomical relationships in the region of the atrioventricular node. The action potentials at the bottom were recorded under normal conditions (solid lines) and under the influence of acetylcholine (dashed lines), showing blockage of conduction by this substance. (From Hoffman and Cranefield: Electrophysiology of the Heart. New York, McGraw-Hill Book Company, 1960.)

shows the approximate intervals of time in fractions of a second between the genesis of the cardiac impulse in the S-A node and its appearance at different points in the A-V nodal system. Note that the impulse, after traveling through the internodal pathway, reaches the A-V node approximately 0.04 second after its origin in the S-A node. However, between this time and the time that the impulse emerges in the A-V bundle, another 0.11 second elapses. About one half of this time lapse occurs in the *junctional fibers*, which are very small fibers that connect the normal atrial fibers with the fibers of the node itself (illustrated in Figures 9–6 and 9–7). The velocity of conduction in these fibers is as little as 0.02 meter per second (about one twentieth that in normal cardiac muscle), which greatly delays entrance of the impulse into the A-V node. After entering the node proper, the velocity of conduction in the *nodal fibers* is still quite low, only 0.1 meter per second, about one fourth the conduction velocity in normal cardiac muscle. Therefore, a further delay in transmission occurs as the impulse travels through the A-V node into the *transitional fibers* and finally into the *A-V bundle* (also called the *bundle of His*).

Figure 9–7 illustrates a functional diagram of the A-V nodal region, showing the atrial fibers leading into the minute junctional fibers, then progressive enlargement of the fibers again as they spread through the node, through the transitional region, and into the A-V bundle.

Cause of the Delay. The cause of the extremely slow conduction in the junctional and some other A-V nodal fibers is partly their small size. The resistance to conduction of ionic currents both inside and outside small fibers is far greater in relation to the surface membrane area than is true for large fibers, and this makes it a general characteristic of small fibers that they conduct impulses at a slower velocity than do large fibers.

However, another feature of conduction at the A-V node probably accounts for most of the slow conduction. This is the fact that the junctional and A-V nodal fibers, like the S-A nodal fibers, have resting membrane potentials that are much less negative than the normal resting potential of other cardiac muscle. Therefore, the junctional and A-V nodal fibers, also like the S-A nodal fibers, have many if not most of their fast sodium channels blocked, as explained earlier in the chapter for the S-A fibers. As a consequence, the action potentials of these fibers must be initiated by the slow calcium-sodium channels, which are slow to open (to "activate") at the onset of the action potential, causing slow development of the action potential itself.

TRANSMISSION IN THE PURKINJE SYSTEM

The *Purkinje fibers* that lead from the A-V node through the A-V bundle and into the ventricles have functional characteristics quite the opposite of those of the A-V nodal fibers; they are very large fibers, even larger than the normal ventricular muscle fibers, and they transmit impulses at a velocity of 1.5 to 4.0 meters per second, a velocity about six times that in the usual cardiac muscle and 150 times that in the junctional fibers. This allows almost immediate transmission of the cardiac impulse throughout the entire ventricular system.

The very rapid transmission of action potentials by Purkinje fibers is probably caused by increased numbers of nexuses between the successive cardiac cells that make up the Purkinje fibers. At these nexuses, ions are transmitted easily from one cell to the next, thus enhancing the velocity of transmission. The Purkinje fibers also have very few myofibrils, which means that they barely contract during the course of impulse transmission.

Distribution of the Purkinje Fibers in the Ventricles. The Purkinje fibers, after originating in the A-V node, form the A-V bundle, which then threads through the fibrous tissue between the valves of the heart and thence into the ventricular septum, as shown in Figure 9–4. The A-V bundle divides almost immediately into the *left* and *right bundle branches* that lie beneath the endocardium of the respective sides of the septum. Each of these branches spreads downward toward the apex of the respective ventricle but also divides into small branches that spread around each ventricular chamber and finally back toward the base of the heart. The terminal Purkinje fibers penetrate about one third of the way into the muscle mass to terminate on the muscle fibers.

From the time that the cardiac impulse first enters the A-V bundle until it reaches the terminations of the Purkinje fibers, the total time that elapses averages about 0.03 second; therefore, once a cardiac impulse enters the Purkinje system, it spreads almost immediately to the entire endocardial surface of the ventricular muscle.

CONTROL OF EXCITATION AND CONDUCTION IN THE HEART

THE S-A NODE AS THE PACEMAKER OF THE HEART

In the above discussion of the genesis and transmission of the cardiac impulse through the heart, it was stated that the impulse normally arises in the S-A node. However, this need not be the case under abnormal conditions, for other parts of the heart can exhibit rhythmic contraction in the same way that the fibers of the S-A node can; this is particularly true of the A-V nodal and Purkinje fibers.

The A-V nodal fibers, when not stimulated from some outside source, discharge at an intrinsic rhythmic rate of 40 to 60 times per minute, and the Purkinje fibers discharge at a rate of somewhere between 15 and 40 times per minute. These rates are in contrast to the normal rate of the S-A node of 70 to 80 times per minute.

Therefore, the question that we must ask is: Why does the S-A node control the heart's rhythmicity rather than the A-V node or the Purkinje fibers? The answer to this is simply that the rate of the S-A node is considerably greater than that of either the A-V node or the Purkinje fibers. Each time the S-A node discharges, its impulse is conducted into both the A-V node and the Purkinje fibers, discharging their excitable membranes. Then these tissues, as well as the S-A node, recover from the action potential and become hyperpolarized. But the S-A node loses this hyperpolarization much more rapidly than does either of the other two and emits a new impulse before either one of them can reach its own threshold for self-excitation. The new impulse again discharges both the A-V node and Purkinje fibers. This process continues on and on, the S-A node always exciting these other potentially self-excitatory tissues before self-excitation can actually occur.

Thus, the S-A node controls the beat of the heart because its rate of rhythmic discharge is greater than that of any other part of the heart. Therefore, the S-A node is the normal *pacemaker* of the heart.

Abnormal Pacemakers—The Ectopic Pacemaker. Occasionally some other part of the heart develops a rhythmic discharge rate that is more rapid than that of the S-A node. For instance, this often occurs in the A-V node or in the Purkinje fibers. In either of these cases, the pacemaker of the heart shifts from the S-A node to the A-V node or to the excitable Purkinje fibers. Under rare conditions a point in the atrial or ventricular muscle develops excessive excitability and becomes the pacemaker.

A pacemaker elsewhere than the S-A node is called an *ectopic pacemaker*. Obviously, an ectopic pacemaker causes an abnormal sequence of contraction of the different parts of the heart.

ROLE OF THE PURKINJE SYSTEM IN CAUSING SYNCHRONOUS CONTRACTION OF THE VENTRICULAR MUSCLE

It is clear from the previous description of the Purkinje system that the cardiac impulse arrives at almost all portions of the ventricles within a very narrow span of time, exciting the first ventricular muscle fiber only 0.06 second ahead of excitation of the last ventricular muscle fiber. Since the ventricular muscle fibers normally remain contracted for a total period of 0.3 second, one can see that this rapid spread of excitation throughout the entire ventricular muscle mass causes all portions of the ventricular muscle in both ventricles to contract at almost exactly the same time. Effective pumping by the two ventricular chambers requires this synchronous type of contraction. If the cardiac impulse traveled through the ventricular muscle very slowly, then much of the ventricular mass would contract prior to contraction of the remainder, in which case the overall pumping effect would be greatly depressed. Indeed, in some types of cardiac debilities, such slow transmission does indeed occur, and the pumping effectiveness of the ventricles is decreased perhaps as much as 20 to 30 per cent.

CONTROL OF HEART RHYTHMICITY AND CONDUCTION BY THE AUTONOMIC NERVES

The heart is supplied with both sympathetic and parasympathetic nerves, as illustrated in Figure 9–8. The parasympathetic nerves are distributed mainly to the S-A and A-V nodes, to a lesser extent

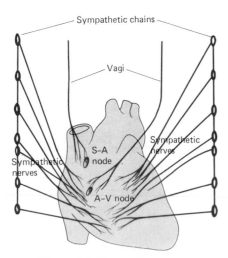

Figure 9–8. The cardiac nerves.

to the muscle of the two atria, and even less to the ventricular muscle. The sympathetic nerves, on the other hand, are distributed to all parts of the heart, with a strong representation to the ventricular muscle as well as to all the other areas.

Effect of Parasympathetic (Vagal) Stimulation on Cardiac Rhythm and Conduction—Ventricular Escape. Stimulation of the parasympathetic nerves to the heart (the vagi) causes the hormone acetylcholine to be released at the vagal endings. This hormone has two major effects on the heart. First, it decreases the rate of rhythm of the S-A node, and, second, it decreases the excitability of the A-V junctional fibers between the atrial musculature and the A-V node, thereby slowing transmission of the cardiac impulse into the ventricles. Very strong stimulation of the vagi can completely stop the rhythmic contraction of the S-A node or completely block transmission of the cardiac impulse through the A-V junction. In either case, rhythmic impulses are no longer transmitted into the ventricles. The ventricles stop beating for 4 to 10 seconds, but then some point in the Purkinje fibers, usually in the A-V bundle, develops a rhythm of its own and causes ventricular contraction at a rate of 15 to 40 beats per minute. This phenomenon is called *ventricular escape.*

Mechanism of the Vagal Effects. The acetylcholine released at the vagal nerve endings greatly increases the permeability of the fiber membranes to potassium, which allows rapid leakage of potassium to the exterior. This causes increased negativity inside the fibers, an effect called *hyperpolarization*, which makes excitable tissue much less excitable, as was explained in Chapter 6.

In the S-A node, the state of hyperpolarization decreases the "resting" membrane potential of the S-A nodal fibers to a level considerably more negative than the normal value, to a level as low as −65 to −75 millivolts rather than the normal level of −55 to −60 millivolts. Therefore, the upward drift of the resting membrane potential caused by sodium leakage requires much longer to reach the threshold potential for excitation. Obviously, this greatly slows the rate of rhythmicity of these nodal fibers. And, if the vagal stimulation is strong enough, it is possible to stop completely the rhythmical self-excitation of this node.

Effect of Sympathetic Stimulation on Cardiac Rhythm, Conduction, and Contractile Strength. Sympathetic stimulation causes essentially the opposite effects on the heart to those caused by vagal stimulation as follows: first, it increases the rate of S-A nodal discharge. Second, it increases the rate of conduction and the excitability in all portions of the heart. Third, it increases greatly the force of contraction of all the cardiac musculature, both atrial and ventricular.

In short, sympathetic stimulation increases the overall activity of the heart. Maximal stimulation can almost triple the rate of heartbeat and can increase the strength of heart contraction as much as twofold.

Mechanism of the Sympathetic Effect. Stimulation of the sympathetic nerves releases the hormone norepinephrine at the sympathetic nerve endings. The precise mechanism by which this hormone acts on cardiac muscle fibers is still somewhat doubtful, but the present belief is that it increases the permeability of the fiber membrane to sodium and calcium. In the S-A node, an increase of sodium permeability would cause increased tendency for the resting membrane potential to drift upward to the threshold level for self-excitation, which ob-

viously would accelerate the onset of self-excitation after each successive heartbeat and therefore increase the heart rate.

In the A-V node, increased sodium permeability would make it easier for each fiber to excite the succeeding fiber, thereby decreasing the conduction time from the atria to the ventricles.

The increase in permeability to calcium ions is at least partially responsible for the increase in contractile strength of the cardiac muscle under the influence of sympathetic stimulation because calcium ions play a powerful role in exciting the contractile process of the myofibrils.

REFERENCES

Akera, T., and Brody, T. M.: Myocardial membranes: Regulation and function of the sodium pump. *Annu. Rev. Physiol.*, 44:375, 1982.

Brown, H. F.: Electrophysiology of the sinoatrial node. *Physiol. Rev.*, 62:505, 1982.

Brutsaert, D. L., and Paulus, W. J.: Contraction and relaxation of the heart as muscle and pump. *In* Guyton, A. C., and Young, D. B. (eds.): International Review of Physiology: Cardiovascular Physiology III. Vol. 18. Baltimore, University Park Press, 1979, p. 1.

Chung, E. K. (ed.): Artificial Cardiac Pacing: Practical Approach. Baltimore, Williams & Wilkins, 1978.

Cobbs, L. A., et al.: Community cardiopulmonary resuscitation. *Annu. Rev. Med.*, 31:453, 1980.

Del Negro, A. A., and Fletcher, R. D.: Indications for and Use of Artificial Cardiac Pacemakers. Chicago, Year Book Medical Publishers, 1978.

DiFrancesco, D., and Noble, D.: A model of cardiac electrical activity incorporating ionic pumps and concentration changes. *Phil. Trans. R. Soc. Lond. (Biol)*, 307:353, 1985.

Durrer, D., et al.: Human cardiac electrophysiology. *In* Dickinson, C. J., and Marks, J. (eds.): Developments in Cardiovascular Medicine. Lancaster, England, MTP Press, 1978, p. 53.

Ellis, D.: Na-Ca exchange in cardiac tissues. *Adv. Myocardiol.*, 5:295, 1985.

Farah, A. E., Alousi, A. A., and Schwartz, R. P., Jr.: Positive inotropic agents. *Annu. Rev. Pharmacol. Toxicol.*, 24:275, 1984.

Fozzard, H. A.: Heart: Excitation-contraction coupling. *Annu. Rev. Physiol.*, 39:201, 1977.

Geddes, L. A.: Cardiovascular Medical Devices. New York, John Wiley & Sons, 1984.

Gilmour, R. F., Jr., and Zipes, D. P.: Slow inward current and cardiac arrhythmias. *Am. J. Cardiol.*, 55:89B, 1985.

Glitsch, H. G.: Electrogenic Na pumping in the heart. *Annu. Rev. Physiol.*, 44:389, 1982.

Guyton, A. C., and Satterfield, J.: Factors concerned in electrical defibrillation of the heart, particularly through the unopened chest. *Am. J. Physiol.*, 167:81, 1951.

Herbette, L., et al.: The interaction of drugs with the sarcoplasmic reticulum. *Annu. Rev. Pharmacol. Toxicol.*, 22:413, 1982.

Hondeghem, L. M., and Katzung, B. G.: Antiarrhythmic agents: The modulated receptor mechanism of action of sodium and calcium channel-blocking drugs. *Annu. Rev. Pharmacol. Toxicol.*, 24:387, 1984.

Irisawa, H.: Comparative physiology of the cardiac pacemaker mechanism. *Physiol. Rev.*, 58:461, 1984.

Jacobson, L.: Cardiac Pacing. Principles and Case Studies. New Hyde Park, New York, Medical Examination Publishing Co., 1981.

Jones, P.: Cardiac Pacing. New York, Appleton-Century-Crofts, 1980.

Josephson, M. E., and Seides, S. F.: Clinical Cardiac Electrophysiology; Techniques and Interpretations. Philadelphia, Lea & Febiger, 1979.

Josephson, M. E., and Singh, B. N.: Use of calcium antagonists in ventricular dysfunction. *Am. J. Cardiol.*, 55:81B, 1985.

Langer, G. A.: Sodium-calcium exchange in the heart. *Annu. Rev. Physiol.*, 44:435, 1982.

Latorre, R., et al.: K^+ channels gated by voltage and ions. *Annu. Rev. Physiol.*, 46:485, 1984.

Lazdunski, M., and Renaud, J. F.: The action of cardiotoxins on cardiac plasma membranes. *Annu. Rev. Physiol.*, 44:463, 1982.

Levy, M. N., et al.: Neural regulation of the heart beat. *Annu. Rev. Physiol.*, 43:443, 1981.

Levy, M. N., and Martin, P. J.: Neural control of the heart. *In* Berne, R. M., et al. (eds.): Handbook of Physiology. Sec. 2, Vol. I. Baltimore, Williams & Wilkins, 1979, p. 581.

Loewenstein, W. R.: Junctional intercellular communication: The cell-to-cell membrane channel. *Physiol. Rev.*, 61:829, 1981.

McAnulty, J., and Rahimtoola, S.: Prognosis in bundle branch block. *Annu. Rev. Med.*, 32:499, 1981.

McDonald, T. F.: The slow inward calcium current in the heart. *Annu. Rev. Physiol.*, 44:425, 1982.

Meijler, F. L.: Atrioventricular conduction versus heart size from mouse to whale. *J. Am. Coll. Cardiol.*, 5:363, 1985.

Nobel, D.: The Initiation of the Heartbeat. New York, Oxford University Press, 1979.

Orrego, F.: Calcium and the mechanism of action of digitalis. *Gen. Pharmacol.*, 15:273, 1984.

Pick, A., and Langendorf, R.: Interpretation of Complex Arrhythmias. Philadelphia, Lea & Febiger, 1980.

Reuter, H.: Properties of two inward membrane currents in the heart. *Annu. Rev. Physiol.*, 41:413, 1979.

Reuter, H.: Ion channels in cardiac cell membranes. *Annu. Rev. Physiol.*, 44:473, 1984.

Sanguinetti, M. C., and Kass, R. S.: Regulation of cardiac calcium channel current and contractile activity by the dihydropyridine Bay K 8644 is voltage-dependent. *J. Mol. Cell. Cardiol.*, 16:667, 1984.

Spear, J. F., and Moore, E. N.: Mechanisms of cardiac arrhythmias. *Annu. Rev. Physiol.*, 44:485, 1982.

Sperelakis, N.: Origin of the cardiac resting potential. *In* Berne, R. M., et al. (eds.): Handbook of Physiology. Sec. 2, Vol. I. Baltimore, Williams & Wilkins, 1979, p. 187.

Sperelakis, N.: Propagation mechanisms in heart. *Annu. Rev. Physiol.*, 41:441, 1979.

Sperelakis, N.: Hormonal and neurotransmitter regulation of Ca^{++} influx through voltage-dependent slow channels in cardiac muscle membrane. *Membr. Biochem.*, 5:131, 1984.

Stull, J. T., and Mayer, S. E.: Biochemical mechanisms of adrenergic and cholinergic regulation of myocardial contractility. *In* Berne, R. M., et al. (eds.): Handbook of Physiology. Sec. 2, Vol. I. Baltimore, Williams & Wilkins, 1979, p. 741.

Vasselle, M.: Electrogenesis of the plateau and pacemaker potential. *Annu. Rev. Physiol.*, 41:425, 1979.

Verrier, R. L., and Lown, B.: Behavioral stress and cardiac arrhythmias. *Annu. Rev. Physiol.*, 46:155, 1984.

IV

THE CENTRAL NERVOUS SYSTEM

10

Organization of the Nervous System; Basic Functions of Synapses

The nervous system, along with the endocrine system, provides most of the control functions for the body. In general, the nervous system controls the rapid activities of the body, such as muscular contractions, rapidly changing visceral events, and even the rates of secretion of some endocrine glands. The endocrine system, by contrast, regulates principally the metabolic functions of the body.

The nervous system is unique in the vast complexity of the control actions that it can perform. It receives literally millions of bits of information from the different sensory organs and then integrates all these to determine the response to be made by the body. The purpose of this chapter is to present, first, a general outline of the overall mechanisms by which the nervous system performs such functions. Then we will discuss the function of central nervous system synapses, the basic structures that control the passage of signals into, through, and then out of the nervous system. In succeeding chapters we will analyze in detail the functions of the individual parts of the nervous system. Before beginning this discussion, however, the reader should refer to Chapters 6 and 8, which present, respectively, the principles of membrane potentials and transmission of signals through neuromuscular junctions.

GENERAL DESIGN OF THE NERVOUS SYSTEM

THE SENSORY DIVISION— SENSORY RECEPTORS

Most activities of the nervous system are initiated by sensory experience emanating from *sensory receptors*, whether these be visual receptors, auditory receptors, tactile receptors on the surface of the body, or other kinds of receptors. This sensory experience can cause an immediate reaction, or its memory can be stored in the brain for minutes, weeks, or years and then can help determine the bodily reactions at some future date.

Figure 10–1 illustrates a portion of the sensory system, the *somatic* portion that transmits sensory information from the receptors of the entire surface of the body and deep structures. This information enters the central nervous system through the spinal nerves and is conducted to multiple "primary" sensory areas in (1) the spinal cord at all levels, (2) the reticular substance of the medulla, pons, and mesencephalon, (3) the cerebellum, (4) the thalamus, and (5) the somesthetic areas of the cerebral cortex. But in addition to these primary sensory areas, signals are then relayed to essentially all other parts of the nervous system as well.

THE MOTOR DIVISION— THE EFFECTORS

The most important ultimate role of the nervous system is control of bodily activities. This is achieved by controlling (1) contraction of skeletal muscles throughout the body, (2) contraction of smooth muscle in the internal organs, and (3) secretion by both exocrine and endocrine glands in many parts of the body. These activities are collectively called *motor functions* of the nervous system, and the muscles and glands are called *effectors* because they perform the functions dictated by the nerve signals.

Figure 10–2 illustrates the *motor axis* of the nervous system for controlling skeletal muscle contraction. Operating parallel to this axis is another similar system for control of the smooth muscles and glands; it is the *autonomic nervous system*, which will be presented in Chapter 21. Note in Figure 10–2 that the skeletal muscles can be controlled from many different levels of the central nervous system, including (1) the spinal cord, (2) the reticular substance of the medulla, pons, and mesencephalon, (3) the basal ganglia, (4) the cerebellum, and (5) the

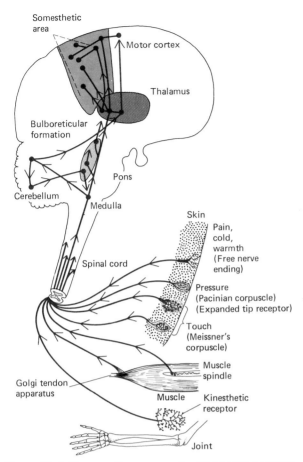

Figure 10–1. The somatic sensory axis of the nervous system.

After the important sensory information has been selected, it is then channeled into proper motor regions of the brain to cause the desired responses, which is called the *integrative function* of the nervous system. Thus, if a person places a hand on a hot stove, the desired response is to lift the hand, plus other associated responses such as moving the entire body away from the stove and perhaps even shouting with pain. Yet even these responses represent activity by only a small fraction of the total motor system of the body.

Role of Synapses in Processing Information. The synapse is the junction point from one neuron to the next and, therefore, is an advantageous site for control of signal transmission. Later in this chapter we will discuss the details of synaptic function. However, it is important to point out here that the synapses determine the directions that the nervous signals spread in the nervous system. Some synapses transmit signals from one neuron to the next with ease, while others transmit signals only with difficulty. Also, facilitatory and inhibitory signals from other areas in the nervous system can control synaptic activity, sometimes opening the synapses for transmission and other times closing them. In addition, some postsynaptic neurons respond with large numbers of impulses, while others respond with only a few. Thus, the synapses perform a selective action, often blocking the weak signals while allowing the strong signals to pass, often selecting and amplifying certain weak signals, and often channeling the signal in many different directions rather than simply in one direction.

motor cortex. Each of these different areas plays its own specific role in the control of body movements, the lower regions being concerned primarily with automatic, instantaneous responses of the body to sensory stimuli and the higher regions with deliberate movements controlled by the thought processes of the cerebrum.

PROCESSING OF INFORMATION— "INTEGRATIVE" FUNCTION OF THE NERVOUS SYSTEM

The nervous system would not be at all effective in controlling bodily functions if each bit of sensory information caused some motor reaction. Therefore, one of the major functions of the nervous system is to process incoming information in such a way that *appropriate* motor responses occur. Indeed, more than 99 per cent of all sensory information is discarded by the brain as irrelevant and unimportant. For instance, one is ordinarily totally unaware of the parts of the body that are in contact with clothing and is also unaware of the seat pressure when sitting. Likewise, attention is drawn only to an occasional object in one's field of vision, and even the perpetual noise of our surroundings is usually relegated to the background.

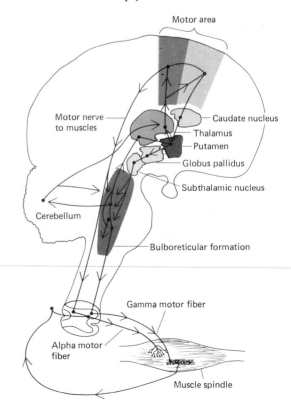

Figure 10–2. The motor axis of the nervous system.

STORAGE OF INFORMATION—MEMORY

Only a small fraction of the important sensory information causes an immediate motor response. Much of the remainder is stored for future control of motor activities and for use in the thinking processes. Most of this storage occurs in the *cerebral cortex*, but not all, for even the basal regions of the brain and perhaps even the spinal cord can store small amounts of information.

The storage of information is the process we call *memory*, and this too is a function of the synapses. That is, each time certain types of sensory signals pass through sequences of synapses, these synapses become more capable of transmitting the same signals the next time, which process is called *facilitation*. After the sensory signals have passed through the synapses a large number of times, the synapses become so facilitated that signals generated within the brain itself can also cause transmission of impulses through the same sequences of synapses even though the sensory input has not been excited. This gives the person a perception of experiencing the original sensations, though in effect they are only memories of the sensations.

Unfortunately, we do not know the precise mechanism by which facilitation of synapses occurs in the memory process, but what is known about this and other details of the memory process will be discussed in Chapter 18.

Once memories have been stored in the nervous system, they become part of the processing mechanism. The thought processes of the brain compare new sensory experiences with the stored memories; the memories help to select the important new sensory information and to channel this into appropriate storage areas for future use or into motor areas to cause bodily responses.

THE THREE MAJOR LEVELS OF CENTRAL NERVOUS SYSTEM FUNCTION

The human nervous system has inherited specific characteristics from each stage of evolutionary development. From this heritage, three major levels of the central nervous system have specific functional attributes: (1) the *spinal cord level*, (2) the *lower brain level*, and (3) the *higher brain* or *cortical level*.

The Spinal Cord Level

We often think of the spinal cord as being only a conduit for signals from the periphery of the body to the brain or in the opposite direction from the brain back to the body. However, this is far from the truth. Even after the spinal cord has been cut in the high neck region, many spinal cord functions still occur. For instance, neuronal circuits in the cord can cause walking movements, and reflexes that withdraw portions of the body from objects, that stiffen the legs to support the body against gravity, that control local blood vessels, gastrointestinal movements, and many other functions.

In fact, the upper levels of the nervous system often operate not by sending signals directly to the periphery of the body but instead by sending signals to the control centers of the cord, simply "commanding" the cord centers to perform their functions.

The Lower Brain Level

Many, if not most of what we call subconscious activities of the body are controlled in the lower areas of the brain—in the medulla, pons, mesencephalon, hypothalamus, thalamus, cerebellum, and basal ganglia. Subconscious control of arterial pressure and respiration is achieved mainly in the medulla and pons. Control of equilibrium is a combined function of the older portions of the cerebellum and the reticular substance of the medulla, pons, and mesencephalon. Feeding reflexes, such as salivation in response to the taste of food and the licking of the lips, are controlled by areas in the medulla, pons, mesencephalon, amygdala, and hypothalamus; and many emotional patterns, such as anger, excitement, sexual activities, reaction to pain, or reaction of pleasure, can occur in animals without a cerebral cortex.

The Higher Brain or Cortical Level

After recounting all the nervous system functions that can occur at the cord and lower brain levels, what is left for the cerebral cortex to do? The answer to this is a complex one, but it begins with the fact that the cerebral cortex is an extremely large memory storehouse. The cortex never functions alone but always in association with the lower centers of the nervous system.

Without the cerebral cortex, the functions of the lower brain centers are often very imprecise. The vast storehouse of cortical information usually converts these functions to very determinative and precise operations.

Finally, the cerebral cortex is essential for most of our thought processes even though it also cannot function alone in this. In fact, it is the lower centers that cause *wakefulness* in the cerebral cortex, thus opening its bank of memories to the thinking machinery of the brain.

Thus, each portion of the nervous system performs specific functions. Many integrative functions are well developed in the spinal cord, and many of the subconscious functions of the brain are originated and executed entirely in the lower regions of the brain. But it is the cortex that opens the world up for one's mind.

COMPARISON OF THE NERVOUS SYSTEM WITH AN ELECTRONIC COMPUTER

When electronic computers were first developed in many different laboratories of the world by as many different scientists, it soon became apparent that all these machines have many features in common with the nervous system. First, they all have input circuits that are comparable to the sensory portion of the nervous system and output circuits that are comparable to the motor portion of the nervous system. In the conducting pathway between the inputs and the outputs are the mechanisms for performing the different types of computations.

In simple computers, the output signals are controlled directly by the input signals, operating in a manner similar to that of the simple reflexes of the spinal cord. But, in the more complex computers, the output is determined both by the input signals and by information that has already been stored in memory in the computer, which is analogous to the more complex reflex and processing mechanisms of our higher nervous system. Furthermore, as the computers become even more complex it is necessary to add still another unit, called the *central programming unit,* which determines the sequence of all operations. This unit is analogous to the mechanism in our brain that allows us to direct our attention first to one thought or sensation or motor activity, then to another, and so forth, until complex sequences of thought or action take place.

Figure 10–3 illustrates a simple block diagram of a modern computer. Even a rapid study of this diagram will demonstrate its similarity to the nervous system. The fact that the basic components of the general purpose computer are analogous to those of the human nervous system demonstrates that the brain is basically a computer that continuously collects sensory information and uses this along with stored information to compute the daily course of bodily activity.

THE CENTRAL NERVOUS SYSTEM SYNAPSES

Every medical student is aware that information is transmitted in the central nervous system mainly in the form of nerve impulses through a succession of neurons, one after another. However, it is not immediately apparent that each impulse (1) may be blocked in its transmission from one neuron to the next, (2) may be changed from a single impulse into repetitive impulses, or (3) may be integrated with impulses from other neurons to cause highly intricate patterns of impulses in successive neurons. All these functions can be classified as *synaptic functions of neurons.*

Types of Synapses—Chemical and Electrical

Nerve signals are transmitted from one neuron to the next through interneuronal junctions called *synapses.* In the animal world there are basically two different types of synapses, the *chemical synapse* and the *electrical synapse.*

From a practical view, almost all the synapses utilized for signal transmission in the central nervous system are chemical synapses. In these, the first neuron secretes a chemical substance called a *neurotransmitter* at the synapse, and this transmitter in turn acts on receptor proteins in the membrane of the next neuron to excite the neuron, to inhibit it, or to modify its sensitivity in some other way. Over 30 different transmitter substances have been discovered thus far.

Electrical synapses are characterized by direct channels that conduct electricity from one cell to the next. Most of these consist of small protein tubular structures called *gap junctions* that allow free movement of ions from the interior of one cell to the next. Only a few gap junctions have been found in the central nervous system, and their significance is not known. On the other hand, it is by way of gap junctions and other similar junctions that action potentials are transmitted from one smooth muscle fiber to the next in visceral smooth muscle (Chapter 8) and also from one cardiac muscle cell to the next in cardiac muscle (Chapter 9).

One-Way Conduction Through Chemical Synapses. Chemical synapses have one exceedingly important characteristic that makes them highly desirable as the form of transmission of nervous system signals: they always transmit the signals in one direction—that is, from the neuron that secretes the transmitter, called the *presynaptic neuron,* to the neuron on which the transmitter acts, called the *postsynaptic neuron.* This is the principle of *one-way conduction* through chemical synapses, and it is quite different from conduction through electrical synapses that can transmit signals in either direction.

Think for a moment about the extreme importance of the one-way conduction mechanism. It allows signals to be directed toward specific goals. Indeed, it is this specific transmission of signals to discrete and highly focused areas in the nervous system that allows the nervous system to perform its myriad functions of sensation, motor control, memory, and many others.

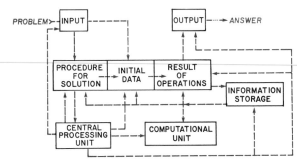

Figure 10–3. Block diagram of a general purpose electronic computer, showing the basic components and their interrelationships.

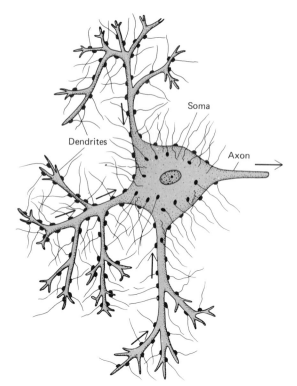

Figure 10–4. A typical motor neuron, showing presynaptic terminals on the neuronal soma and dendrites. Note also the single axon.

PHYSIOLOGICAL ANATOMY OF THE SYNAPSE

Figure 10–4 illustrates a typical *motor neuron* in the anterior horn of the spinal cord. It is composed of three major parts: the *soma*, which is the main body of the neuron; a single *axon*, which extends from the soma into the peripheral nerve; and the *dendrites*, which are thin projections of the soma that extend up to 1 mm into the surrounding areas of the cord.

An average of about 6000 small knobs called *presynaptic terminals* lie on the surfaces of the dendrites and soma of the motor neuron, approximately 80 to 90 per cent of them on the dendrites and only 10 to 20 per cent on the soma. These terminals are the ends of nerve fibrils that originate in many other neurons, and usually not more than a few of the terminals are derived from any single previous neuron. Later it will become evident that many of these presynaptic terminals are *excitatory* and secrete a substance that excites the postsynaptic neuron, whereas others are *inhibitory* and secrete a substance that inhibits the neuron.

Neurons in other parts of the cord and brain differ markedly from the motor neuron in (1) the size of the cell body, (2) the length, size, and number of dendrites, ranging in length from almost none at all up to as long as many centimeters, (3) the length and size of the axon, and (4) the number of presynaptic terminals, which may range from only a few to more than a hundred thousand. These

differences make neurons in different parts of the nervous system react differently to incoming signals and therefore perform different functions.

The Presynaptic Terminals. Electron microscopic studies of the presynaptic terminals show that they have varied anatomical forms, but most resemble small round or oval knobs and therefore are frequently called *terminal knobs, boutons, end-feet,* or *synaptic knobs.*

Figure 10–5 illustrates the basic structure of the presynaptic terminal. It is separated from the neuronal soma by a *synaptic cleft* having a width usually of 200 to 300 angstroms. The terminal has two internal structures important to the excitatory or inhibitory functions of the synapse: the *synaptic vesicles* and the *mitochondria.* The synaptic vesicles contain a *transmitter substance* which, when released into the synaptic cleft, either *excites* or *inhibits* the neurons—excites if the neuronal membrane contains *excitatory receptors,* inhibits if it contains *inhibitory receptors.* The mitochondria provide ATP, which is required to synthesize new transmitter substance. The transmitter must be synthesized extremely rapidly because the amount stored in the vesicles is sufficient to last for only a few seconds to a few minutes of maximum activity.

When an action potential spreads over a presynaptic terminal, the membrane depolarization causes emptying of a small number of vesicles into the cleft; and the released transmitter in turn causes an immediate change in the permeability characteristics of the postsynaptic neuronal membrane, which leads to excitation or inhibition of the neuron, depending on its receptor characteristics.

Mechanism by Which Action Potentials Cause Transmitter Release at the Presynaptic Terminals—Role of Calcium Ions. The synaptic membrane of the presynaptic terminals contains large numbers of *voltage-gated calcium channels.* This is quite different from the other areas of the nerve fiber, which contain very few of these channels. When the action potential depolarizes the terminal, large numbers of calcium ions, along with the sodium ions that

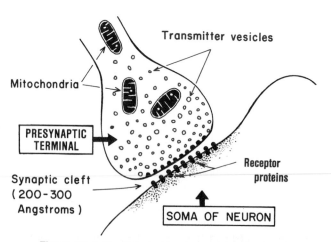

Figure 10–5. Physiological anatomy of the synapse.

cause the action potential, flow into the terminal. And the quantity of transmitter substance that is released into the synaptic cleft is directly related to the number of calcium ions that enter the terminal. The precise mechanism by which the calcium ions cause this release is not known, but it is believed to be the following:

When the calcium ions enter the synaptic terminal, it is believed that they bind with protein receptors on the inside surfaces of the synaptic membrane called *release sites*. This in turn causes the transmitter vesicles in the local vicinity to bind with the membrane and actually to fuse with it, and finally to open to the exterior by the process called *exocytosis*, that is, simply spilling the contents to the exterior. Often several hundred vesicles release their transmitter into the cleft following a single action potential.

Because of the requirement for calcium ions to cause release of the synaptic transmitter, any condition that reduces the quantity of calcium ions entering the presynaptic terminal also will decrease the amount of transmitter released. Some conditions that can cause this are (1) a weak action potential caused by preliminary partial depolarization of the presynaptic terminal, (2) decrease in concentration of calcium ions in the extracellular fluid, or (3) any factor that reduces the permeability of the presynaptic terminal to calcium ions.

One transmitter substance that occurs in certain parts of the nervous system is acetylcholine, as is discussed later. It has been calculated that about 3000 molecules of acetylcholine are present in each vesicle, and enough vesicles are present in the presynaptic terminal on a neuron to transmit a few thousand impulses.

Synthesis of New Transmitter Substance. Fortunately, the presynaptic terminals have the capability of continually synthesizing new transmitter substance. Were it not for this, synaptic transmission would become completely ineffective within a few minutes. The synthesis occurs either partially or totally in the cytoplasm of the presynaptic terminals, and then the newly synthesized transmitter is immediately absorbed into the vesicles and stored until needed.

As an example, acetylcholine is synthesized from acetyl-CoA and choline in the presence of the enzyme *choline acetyltransferase,* an enzyme that is present in abundance in the cytoplasm of the cholinergic type of presynaptic terminal. When acetylcholine is released from the terminal into the synaptic cleft, it is rapidly split again to acetate and choline by the enzyme *cholinesterase* that is adherent to the proteoglycon reticulum that fills the space of the synaptic cleft. Then the choline is actively transported back into the terminal to be used once more for synthesis of new acetylcholine.

Recycling of the Vesicles. Not only are some of the transmitter substances recycled, such as recycling of choline, but the vesicles themselves are also recycled. When they fuse with the synaptic membrane and open up to the exterior, the extra membrane supplied by the vesicles at first simply enlarges the synaptic membrane. However, shortly thereafter, the vesicle portions of the synaptic membrane invaginate back toward the inside of the terminal and then pinch off to form new vesicles. Furthermore, these new vesicles still contain the appropriate transport proteins that are required for concentrating new transmitter substance in the vesicles.

Thus the vesicles are used again and again. But even so, both the vesicles and the mitochondria that supply the energy for transmitter synthesis eventually disintegrate. Fortunately, new vesicles and mitochondria are continually transported from the cell soma down the axon to the presynaptic terminal, moving along the axon at a velocity of about 40 cm per day, thus replenishing the supply in the terminals.

Action of the Transmitter Substance on the Postsynaptic Neuron—The Function of Receptors. At the synapse, the membrane of the postsynaptic neuron contains large numbers of *receptor proteins*, illustrated in Figure 10–5. These receptors have two important components: a *binding component* that protrudes outward from the membrane into the synaptic cleft—it binds with the neurotransmitter from the presynaptic terminal, and an *ionophore component* that protrudes through the membrane to the interior of the postsynaptic neuron. The ionophore in turn is one of two types: a *chemically activated ion channel* or an *enzyme that activates an internal metabolic system of the cell.*

The chemically activated ion channels (also called ligand-activated channels) are mainly of three types: (1) *sodium channels* that allow mainly sodium ions (but some potassium ions as well) to pass through, (2) *potassium channels* that allow mainly potassium ions to pass, and (3) *chloride channels* that allow chloride and a few other anions to pass. We shall learn later that opening the sodium channels excites the postsynaptic neuron. Therefore, a transmitter substance that opens the sodium channels is called an *excitatory transmitter.* On the other hand, opening of potassium and chloride channels inhibits the neuron, and transmitters that open either or both of these are called *inhibitory transmitters.*

Activation of an enzymatic type of receptor causes other effects on the postsynaptic neuron. One effect is to *activate cellular genes,* which in turn manufacture additional receptors for the postsynaptic membrane. Another effect is to *activate protein kinases* that decrease the numbers of receptors. Changes such as these can alter the reactivity of the synapse for minutes, days, months, or even years. Therefore, transmitter substances that cause such effects are called synaptic *modulators* rather than excitatory or inhibitory transmitters. Recent experiments have demonstrated that such modulators are important in at least some of the memory processes, which we shall discuss in Chapter 18.

Duration of Action of the Transmitter, and Removal of the Transmitter from the Synapse. When either an excitatory or an inhibitory transmitter is released into the synaptic cleft, it binds almost instantly with its specific chemically activated ion channels and opens these either to the flow of sodium ions in the case of the excitatory transmitter or the flow of potassium or chloride ions in the case of the inhibitory transmitter. However, after these channels have remained open for only 1 to 2 milliseconds, in most instances, they close equally as rapidly. The reason for this is that the transmitter agent itself is rapidly removed from the synaptic cleft. This is achieved in three different ways:

(1) By *diffusion* of the transmitter out of the cleft into the surrounding fluids.

(2) By *enzymatic destruction* within the cleft itself. For instance, in the case of acetylcholine, the enzyme *cholinesterase* is present in the cleft, bound in the proteoglycan matrix that fills the space. Each molecule of this enzyme can split as many as ten molecules of acetylcholine each millisecond, thus inactivating this transmitter substance. Similar effects occur for other transmitters.

(3) Many of the transmitters are *actively transported back into the presynaptic terminal itself* and are then reused again and again. This is called *transmitter re-uptake*. It occurs especially prominently at the presynaptic terminals of the sympathetic nervous system for the re-uptake of norepinephrine, as we shall discuss in Chapter 21.

The degree to which each of these methods of removal is utilized is different for each type of transmitter.

CHEMICAL AND PHYSIOLOGICAL NATURES OF THE TRANSMITTER SUBSTANCES

Excitation and Inhibition. Whether a transmitter will cause excitation or inhibition is determined not only by the nature of the transmitter but also by the nature of the receptor in the postsynaptic membrane. To give an example, the same neuron might be excited at a synapse that releases acetylcholine but inhibited at still another synapse that releases glycine. Thus, the neuronal membrane at the first synapse contains an *excitatory receptor* for acetylcholine and at the second synapse an *inhibitory receptor* for glycine. To give another example, norepinephrine released at some synapses in the central nervous system causes inhibition whereas at other synapses it causes excitation. In the first case, the postsynaptic neuronal membranes contain an inhibitory receptor for norepinephrine while the others contain an excitatory receptor for the same transmitter.

Chemical Substances That Function As Neurotransmitters

More than 30 different chemical substances have either been proved or postulated to be synaptic transmitters; most are listed in Table 10–1. In gen-

Table 10–1. NEUROTRANSMITTERS

Class I:
 Acetylcholine

Class II: The Amines
 Norepinephrine
 Epinephrine
 Dopamine
 Serotonin

Class III: Amino Acids
 γ-Aminobutyric acid (GABA)
 Glycine
 Glutamate

Class IV: Peptides
 A. Hypothalamic-releasing hormones
  Thyrotropin-releasing hormone
  Luteinizing hormone–releasing hormone
  Somatostatin (growth hormone–inhibitory factor)
 B. Pituitary peptides
  ACTH
  β-Endorphin
  α-Melanocyte-stimulating hormone
  Vasopressin
  Oxytocin
 C. Peptides that act on gut and brain
  Leucine enkephalin
  Methionine enkephalin
  Substance P
  Cholecystokinin
  Vasoactive intestinal polypeptide (VIP)
  Neurotensin
  Insulin
  Glucagon
 D. From other tissues
  Angiotensin II
  Bradykinin
  Carnosine
  Bombesin

eral, there are four different classes of transmitter substances:

 Class 1: Acetylcholine in a class by itself.
 Class 2: Several different amines.
 Class 3: Several different amino acids.
 Class 4: Neuroactive peptides.

The different neurotransmitters have been identified or postulated in a number of different ways: by actually isolating the transmitter substance from the neuronal tissue; by showing that the appropriate enzymes are available for synthesis of the specific transmitter; by demonstrating that injection of the transmitter substance into local neuronal areas will cause excitation or inhibition; by demonstrating specific enzymes for removing the transmitter substance after it is released; and in several other ways.

Some of the more important of the transmitters are the following:

Acetylcholine is secreted by neurons in many areas of the brain, but specifically by the large pyramidal cells of the motor cortex, by many different neurons in the basal ganglia, by the motor neurons that innervate the skeletal muscles, by the preganglionic neurons of the autonomic nervous system, by the postganglionic neurons of the parasympathetic nervous system, and by some of the postganglionic neurons of the sympathetic nervous system. In most instances acetylcholine has an excitatory effect; however, it is known to have inhibitory effects at some of the peripheral parasympathetic nerve endings, such as inhibition of the heart by the vagus nerves.

Norepinephrine is secreted by many neurons whose cell bodies are located in the brain stem and hypothalamus. Specifically, norepinephrine-secreting neurons located in the *locus ceruleus* in the pons send nerve fibers to widespread areas of the brain and help control the overall activity and mood of the mind. In many of these areas it probably causes excitation but in others inhibition. Norepinephrine is also secreted by most of the postganglionic neurons of the sympathetic nervous system, where it excites some organs but inhibits others.

Dopamine is secreted by neurons that originate in the substantia nigra. The terminations of these neurons are mainly in the striatal region of the basal ganglia. The effect of dopamine is usually inhibition.

Glycine is secreted mainly at synapses in the spinal cord. It probably always acts as an inhibitory transmitter.

Gamma-aminobutyric acid (GABA) is secreted by nerve terminals in the spinal cord, the cerebellum, the basal ganglia, and many areas of the cortex. It is believed always to cause inhibition.

Glutamate is probably secreted by the presynaptic terminals in many of the sensory pathways as well as in many areas of the cortex. It probably always causes excitation.

Substance P is probably released by pain fiber terminals in the dorsal horns of the spinal cord. And it is also found in the basal ganglia and hypothalamus. In general, it causes excitation.

Enkephalins are probably secreted by nerve terminals in the spinal cord, in the brain stem, in the thalamus, and in the hypothalamus. These probably act as excitatory transmitters to excite other systems that inhibit the transmission of pain.

Serotonin is secreted by nuclei that originate in the median raphe of the brain stem and project to many brain areas, especially to the dorsal horns of the spinal cord and to the hypothalamus. Serotonin acts as an inhibitor of pain pathways in the cord, and it is also believed to help control the mood of the person, perhaps even to cause sleep.

Despite the length of this list of transmitter substances, it is only a partial list. Other substances that have been proved or suggested include peptides, other amino acids, histamine, prostaglandins, cyclic AMP, and many others.

Release of Only a Single Type of Transmitter Substance by Each Neuron. Except in special cases, it is believed that each neuron releases only one type of transmitter, and it releases this same transmitter at all of its separate terminals. This is frequently called the *Dale principle* in honor of the physiologist most instrumental in developing this concept.

However, like all good theories, a number of exceptions have now been found in which the same nerve terminal might secrete a transmitter that acts as an excitatory or inhibitory transmitter and yet another that acts as a modulator. For instance the excitatory transmitter might be glutamate, which causes immediate excitation, but at the same time one of the neuropeptides might be secreted as a modulator to increase the number of glutamate receptors, in this way increasing the sensitivity of the same synapse for days or weeks. Unfortunately, little is yet known about the modulator mechanisms. Therefore, in the remainder of this chapter we will discuss principally the excitatory and inhibitory effects of the neurotransmitters.

ELECTRICAL EVENTS DURING NEURONAL EXCITATION

The electrical events in neuronal excitation have been studied in the large motor neurons of the anterior horn of the spinal cord. Therefore, the events to be described in the following few sections pertain essentially to these neurons. However, except for some quantitative differences, they apply to most other neurons of the nervous system as well.

The Resting Membrane Potential of the Neuronal Soma. Figure 10–6 illustrates the soma of a motor neuron, showing the resting membrane potential to be about −65 millivolts. This is somewhat less than the −80 to −90 millivolts found in large peripheral nerve fibers and in skeletal muscle fibers; the lower voltage is important, however, because it allows both positive and negative control of the degree of excitability of the neuron. That is, decreasing the voltage to a less negative value makes the membrane of the neuron more excitable, whereas increasing this voltage to a more negative value makes the neuron less excitable. This is the basis of the two modes of function of the neuron—either excitation or inhibition—as we will explain in detail in the following sections.

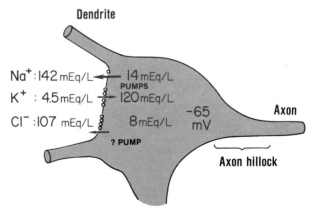

Figure 10–6. Distribution of sodium, potassium, and chloride ions across the neuronal somal membrane; origin of the intrasomal membrane potential.

Concentration Differences of Ions Across the Neuronal Somal Membrane. Figure 10–6 also illustrates the concentration differences across the neuronal somal membrane of the three ions that are most important for neuronal function: sodium ions, potassium ions, and chloride ions.

At the top, the sodium ion concentration is shown to be very great in the extracellular fluid but low inside the neuron. This sodium concentration gradient is caused by a strong sodium pump that continually pumps sodium out of the neuron.

The figure also shows that the potassium ion concentration is large inside the neuronal soma but very low in the extracellular fluid. It illustrates that there is also a potassium pump (the other half of the Na^+-K^+ pump, as described in Chapter 5) that tends to pump potassium to the interior while there is a very high degree of permeability to potassium. The potassium ions leak through the neuronal somal pores so readily that this nullifies most but not all of the effectiveness of the pump.

Figure 10–6 shows the chloride ion to be of high concentration in the extracellular fluid but low concentration inside the neuron. It also shows that the membrane is highly permeable to chloride ions and that there may be a weak chloride pump. But whether there is or is not a chloride pump, most of the reason for the low concentration of chloride ions inside the neuron is the − 65 millivolts in the neuron. That is, this negative voltage repels the negatively charged chloride ions, forcing them outward through the pores until the concentration difference is much greater outside the membrane than on the inside.

Let us recall at this point what we learned in Chapters 5 and 6 about the relationship of ionic concentration differences to membrane potentials. It will be recalled that an electrical potential across the membrane can exactly oppose the movement of ions through a membrane despite concentration differences between the outside and inside of the membrane if the potential is of the proper polarity and magnitude. Such a potential that exactly opposes movement of each type of ion is called the Nernst potential; the equation for this is the following:

$$EMF(mV) = \pm 61 \times \log \left(\frac{\text{Concentration outside}}{\text{Concentration inside}} \right)$$

where EMF is the Nernst potential in millivolts on the *inside of the membrane*. The potential will be positive (+) for a positive ion and negative (−) for a negative ion.

Now, let us calculate the Nernst potential that will exactly oppose the movement of each of the three separate ions: sodium, potassium, and chloride.

For the sodium concentration difference shown in Figure 10–6, 142 mEq/liter on the exterior and 14 mEq/liter on the interior, the membrane potential that would exactly oppose sodium ion movement through the sodium channels would be + 61 millivolts. However, the actual membrane potential is − 65 millivolts, not + 61 millivolts. Therefore, sodium ions normally diffuse inward through the sodium channels; however, not many sodium ions will diffuse because most of the sodium channels are normally closed. Furthermore, those sodium ions that do diffuse to the interior are normally pumped immediately back to the exterior by the sodium pump.

For potassium ions, the concentration gradient is 120 mEq/liter inside the neuron and 4.5 mEq/liter outside. This gives a Nernst potential of − 86 millivolts inside the neuron, which is more negative than the − 65 that actually exists. Therefore there is a tendency for potassium ions to diffuse to the outside of the neuron, but this is opposed by the continual pumping of these potassium ions back to the interior.

Finally, the chloride ion gradient, 107 mEq/liter outside and 8 mEq/liter inside, yields a Nernst potential of − 70 millivolts inside the neuron, which is slightly more negative than the actual value measured. Therefore, chloride ions tend normally to leak to the interior of the neuron, but those that do diffuse are moved back to the exterior, perhaps by an active chloride pump.

Keep these three Nernst potentials in mind and also remember the direction in which the different ions tend to diffuse, for this information will be important in understanding both excitation and inhibition of the neuron by synaptic transmission.

Origin of the Resting Membrane Potential of the Neuronal Soma. The basic cause of the − 65 millivolt resting membrane potential of the neuronal soma is the sodium-potassium pump. This pump causes the extrusion of more positively charged sodium ions to the exterior than potassium to the interior— 3 sodium ions for each 2 potassium ions. Since there are large numbers of negatively charged ions inside the soma that cannot diffuse through the membrane—protein ions, phosphate ions, and many others—extrusion of the excess positive ions to the exterior leaves all these nondiffusible negative ions inside the cell unbalanced by positive ions. Therefore, the interior of the neuron becomes negatively charged as the result of the sodium-potassium pump. This principle was discussed in more detail in Chapter 6 in relation to the resting membrane potential of nerve fibers. In addition, as also explained in Chapter 6, diffusion of potassium ions outward through the membrane is another cause of intracellular negativity.

Uniform Distribution of the Potential Inside the Soma. The interior of the neuronal soma contains a very highly conductive electrolytic solution, the intracellular fluid of the neuron. Furthermore, the diameter of the neuronal soma is very large (from 10 to 80 microns in diameter), causing there to be almost no resistance to conduction of electrical cur-

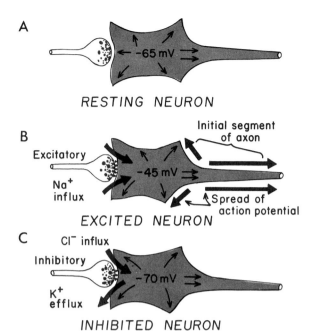

A

—65 mV

RESTING NEURON

B

Initial segment
of axon

Excitatory

—45 mV

Na⁺
influx

Spread of
action potential

EXCITED NEURON

C

Cl⁻ influx

Inhibitory

—70 mV

K⁺
efflux

INHIBITED NEURON

Figure 10–7. Three states of a neuron. *A*, A resting neuron. *B*, A neuron in an excited state, with increased intraneuronal potential caused by sodium influx. *C*, A neuron in an inhibited state, with decreased intraneuronal membrane potential caused by potassium ion influx and chloride ion influx.

rent from one part of the somal interior to another part. Therefore, any change in potential in any part of the intrasomal fluid causes an almost exactly equal change in potential at all other points inside the soma. This is an important principle because it plays a major role in the summation of signals entering the neuron from multiple sources, as we shall see in subsequent sections of this chapter.

Effect of Synaptic Excitation on the Postsynaptic Membrane—The Excitatory Postsynaptic Potential. Figure 10–7A illustrates the resting neuron with an unexcited presynaptic terminal resting upon its surface. The resting membrane potential everywhere in the soma is −65 millivolts.

Figure 10–7B illustrates a presynaptic terminal that has secreted a transmitter into the cleft between the terminal and the neuronal somal membrane. This transmitter acts on a membrane excitatory receptor *to increase the membrane's permeability to both Na⁺ and K⁺*. However, because of the large electrochemical gradient that tends to move sodium inward and because the potassium concentration gradient is not far from equilibrium with the electrical potential, this large opening of the membrane pores mainly allows sodium ions to rush to the inside of the membrane.

The rapid influx of the positively charged sodium ions to the interior of the neuron neutralizes part of the negativity of the resting membrane potential. Thus, in Figure 10–7B the resting membrane potential has been increased from −65 millivolts to −45 millivolts. This increase in voltage above the normal resting neuronal potential—that is, to a less nega-

tive value—is called the *excitatory postsynaptic potential* (or EPSP) because when this potential rises high enough it will elicit an action potential in the neuron, thus exciting it. In this case the EPSP is + 20 millivolts.

However, we must issue a word of warning at this point. Discharge of a single presynaptic terminal can never increase the neuronal potential from −65 millivolts up to −45 millivolts. Instead, an increase of this magnitude requires the simultaneous discharge of many terminals—about 70 for the usual anterior motor neuron—at the same time or in rapid succession. This occurs by a process called *summation*, which will be discussed in detail in the following sections.

Generation of Action Potentials in the Initial Segment of the Axon—Threshold for Excitation. When the membrane potential inside the neuron rises high enough, there comes a point at which this initiates an action potential in the neuron. However, the action potential does not begin on the somal membrane adjacent to the excitatory synapses. Instead, it begins in the initial segment of the axon where it originates from the neuronal soma. The main reason for this point of origin of the action potential is that the soma has relatively few voltage-gated sodium channels in its membrane, which makes it difficult to open the required number of channels to elicit an action potential. On the other hand, the membrane of the initial segment of the axon has seven times as great a concentration of voltage-gated sodium channels and therefore can generate an action potential with much greater ease than can the soma. The excitatory postsynaptic potential that will elicit an action potential in the initial segment is between + 15 and + 20 millivolts. This is in contrast to approximately + 30 millivolts required on the soma.

Once the action potential begins, it travels both peripherally along the axon and also backward over the soma. In many instances, it travels backward into the dendrites, too, but not into all of them because they, like the neuronal soma, also have very few voltage-gated sodium channels.

Thus, in Figure 10–7B, it is shown that under normal conditions the *threshold* for excitation of the neuron is about −45 millivolts, which represents an excitatory postsynaptic potential of + 20 millivolts—that is, 20 millivolts more positive than the normal resting neuronal potential of −65 millivolts.

ELECTRICAL EVENTS IN NEURONAL INHIBITION

Effect of Inhibitory Synapses on the Postsynaptic Membrane—The Inhibitory Postsynaptic Potential. It was pointed out earlier that the excitatory synapses open "sodium" channels in the postsynaptic membrane, and these allow easy passage mainly of sodium ions. And, because of the very large difference between the resting membrane potential and the Nernst potential for sodium, especially large numbers of sodium ions move into the neuron and cause the excitatory postsynaptic potential. The inhibitory synapses, by contrast, open the potassium and chloride channels, allowing easy passage of both these ions. Now, to understand how the inhibitory synapses inhibit the postsynaptic neuron, we must recall what we learned about the Nernst potentials for both the potassium ions and the chloride ions. We calculated this potential for potassium ions to be about -86 millivolts and for chloride ions about -70 millivolts. Both these potentials are more negative than the -65 millivolts normally present inside the resting neuronal membrane. Therefore, opening the potassium and the chloride channels will allow potassium ions to move to the exterior, which will make the membrane potential more negative than normal and will allow the chloride ions to move to the interior, which also will make the membrane potential more negative than usual. This increases the degree of intracellular negativity, which is called *hyperpolarization*. It obviously inhibits the neuron because the membrane potential is now farther away than ever from the threshold for excitation. Therefore, the increase in negativity beyond the normal resting membrane potential level is called the *inhibitory postsynaptic potential* (IPSP).

Thus, Figure 10–7C illustrates the effect on the membrane potential caused by excitation of inhibitory synapses, allowing chloride influx into the cell and potassium efflux from the cell, with the membrane potential decreasing from its normal value of -65 millivolts to the more negative value of -70 millivolts. This membrane potential that is 5 millivolts more negative is the inhibitory postsynaptic potential. Thus the IPSP in this instance is -5 millivolts.

Inhibition of Neurons Without Causing an Inhibitory Postsynaptic Potential—"Short Circuiting" of the Membrane. Sometimes activation of the inhibitory synapses causes little or no inhibitory postsynaptic potential but nevertheless still inhibits the neuron.

The reason that the potential often does not change is that in some neurons the concentration differences across the membrane for the potassium and chloride ions are only able to cause a diffusion potential equal to the normal resting potential. Therefore, when the inhibitory pores open, there is no net flow of ions to cause an inhibitory postsynaptic potential. Yet both the potassium and the chloride ions do diffuse bidirectionally through the wide-open pores many times as rapidly as normally, and this high flux of these two ions inhibits the neuron in the following way. When excitatory synapses fire and sodium ions flow into the neuron, this now causes far less excitatory postsynaptic potential than usual because any tendency for the membrane potential to change away from the resting potential is immediately opposed by rapid flux

of potassium and chloride ions through the inhibitory pores to bring the potential back to the negative equilibrium potential for these two ions. Therefore, the influx of sodium ions required to cause excitation may be as much as 5 to 20 times normal.

This tendency for the potassium and chloride ions to maintain the membrane potential near the resting value when the inhibitory pores are wide open is called "short circuiting" of the membrane, thus making the sodium current flow caused by excitatory synapses ineffective in exciting the cell.

To express the phenomenon of short circuiting more mathematically, one needs to recall the Goldman equation from Chapter 6. This equation shows that the membrane potential is determined by summation of the tendencies for the different ions to carry electrical charges through the membrane in the two directions. The membrane potential will approach the Nernst equilibrium potential for those ions that permeate the membrane to the greatest extent. When the inhibitory channels are wide open, the chloride and potassium ions permeate the membrane greatly. Therefore, when the excitatory channels open, it is difficult to raise the neuronal potential up to the threshold value for excitation.

Presynaptic Inhibition

In addition to the inhibition caused by inhibitory synapses operating at the neuronal membrane, called *postsynaptic inhibition*, another type of inhibition often occurs before the signal reaches the synapse. This type of inhibition, called *presynaptic inhibition*, is believed to occur in the following way.

In presynaptic inhibition, the inhibition is caused by "presynaptic" synapses that lie on the terminal nerve fibrils before they themselves terminate on the following neuron. It is believed that these presynaptic synapses secrete a transmitter substance that in some way not yet understood depresses the voltage of the action potential that occurs at the synaptic membrane of the terminal and, as has already been pointed out, this greatly decreases the amount of calcium ions that enter the terminal and therefore also the amount of transmitter released by the terminal. Therefore, the degree of excitation of the neuron is also greatly suppressed, or inhibited.

Presynaptic inhibition occurs in many of the sensory pathways in the nervous system. That is, the adjacent nerve fibers inhibit each other, which minimizes the spread of signals from one fiber to the next. We will discuss this phenomenon more fully in the following chapter.

The precise mechanism by which the presynaptic synapses function is not known. However, since most of the nerve fibers involved are excitatory types of fibers, it has been suggested that presynaptic inhibition might be caused by excitatory synapses that cause partial depolarization of the terminal nerve fibrils on which they lie. This in turn would reduce the intensity of the action potential passing into this terminal fibril and thereby reduce the release of transmitter substance because even a slight reduction of the magnitude of the action potential reduces calcium entry into the presynaptic terminal and this reduction causes an even far greater reduction in the amount of transmitter released.

Presynaptic inhibition is different from postsynaptic inhibition in its time sequence. It requires many milliseconds to develop, but once it does occur, it can last for as long as minutes or even hours. Postsynaptic inhibition, at least of the anterior motor neurons, lasts for only 10 to 15 milliseconds.

SUMMATION OF POSTSYNAPTIC POTENTIALS

Time Course of Postsynaptic Potentials. When a synapse excites the anterior motor neuron, the neuronal membrane becomes highly permeable for only 1 to 2 milliseconds. During this time sodium ions diffuse rapidly to the interior of the cell to increase the intraneuronal potential, thus creating the *excitatory postsynaptic potential*. This potential then persists for about 15 milliseconds, because this is the time required for the positive charges to flow into the dendrites and axon or for potassium ions to leak out or chloride ions to leak in to re-establish the normal resting membrane potential.

Precisely the opposite effect occurs for the inhibitory postsynaptic potential. That is, the inhibitory synapse increases the permeability of the membrane to potassium and chloride ions for 1 to 2 milliseconds, and this usually decreases the intraneuronal potential to a more negative value than normal, thereby creating the *inhibitory postsynaptic potential*. This potential also persists for about 15 milliseconds.

However, other types of transmitter substances acting on other neurons can perhaps excite or inhibit for hundreds of milliseconds or even for seconds, minutes, or hours.

Spatial Summation of the Postsynaptic Potentials. It has already been pointed out that excitation of a single presynaptic terminal on the surface of a neuron will almost never excite the neuron. The reason for this is that sufficient transmitter substance is released by a single terminal to cause an excitatory postsynaptic potential usually no more than a millivolt at most, instead of the required 15 to 20 millivolts to reach the usual threshold for excitation. However, during excitation in a neuronal pool of the nervous system, many presynaptic terminals are usually stimulated at the same time, and even though these terminals are spread over wide areas of the neuron, their effects can still summate. The reason for this summation is the following: It has already been pointed out that a change in the potential at any single point within the soma will

cause the potential to change everywhere in the soma almost exactly equally. Therefore, for each excitatory synapse that discharges simultaneously, the intrasomal potential becomes more positive by as much as a small fraction of a millivolt up to about 1 millivolt. When the excitatory postsynaptic potential becomes great enough, the threshold for firing will be reached, and an action potential will generate at the initial segment of the axon. This effect is illustrated in Figure 10–8, which shows several excitatory postsynaptic potentials. The bottom postsynaptic potential in the figure was caused by stimulation of only four excitatory synapses; then the next higher potential was caused by stimulation of two times as many synapses; finally, a still higher excitatory postsynaptic potential was caused by stimulation of four times as many synapses. This time an action potential was generated at the initial segment of the axon.

This effect of summing simultaneous postsynaptic potentials by excitation of multiple terminals on widely spaced areas of the membrane is called *spatial summation*.

Temporal Summation. Most presynaptic terminals can fire repetitively in rapid succession only a few milliseconds apart. Each time a terminal fires, the released transmitter substance opens the membrane channels for a millisecond or so. Since the postsynaptic potential lasts up to 15 milliseconds, a second opening of the same channel can increase the postsynaptic potential to a still greater level so that the more rapid the rate of terminal stimulation, the greater the effective postsynaptic potential. Thus, successive postsynaptic potentials of individual presynaptic terminals, if they occur rapidly enough, can summate in the same way that postsynaptic potentials can summate from widely distributed terminals over the surface of the neuron. This summation is called *temporal summation*.

Simultaneous Summation of Inhibitory and Excitatory Postsynaptic Potentials. Obviously, if an inhibitory postsynaptic potential is tending to de-

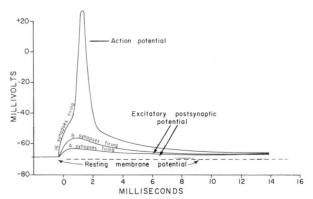

Figure 10–8. Excitatory postsynaptic potentials, showing that simultaneous firing of only a few synapses will not cause sufficient summated potential to elicit an action potential, but that simultaneous firing of many synapses will raise the summated potential to the threshold for excitation and cause a superimposed action potential.

crease the membrane potential to a more negative value while an excitatory postsynaptic potential is tending to increase the potential at the same time, these two effects can either completely nullify each other or partially nullify each other. Also, inhibitory "short circuiting" of the membrane potential can nullify much of an excitatory potential. Thus, if a neuron is currently being excited by an excitatory postsynaptic potential, then an inhibitory signal from another source can easily reduce the postsynaptic potential to less than the threshold value for excitation, thus turning off the activity of the neuron.

Facilitation of Neurons. Often the summated postsynaptic potential is excitatory in nature but has not risen high enough to reach the threshold for excitation. When this happens the neuron is said to be *facilitated*. That is, its membrane potential is nearer the threshold for firing than normally but not yet to the firing level. Nevertheless, a signal entering the neuron from some other source can then excite the neuron very easily. Diffuse signals in the nervous system often facilitate large groups of neurons so that they can respond quickly and easily to signals arriving from second sources.

SPECIAL FUNCTIONS OF DENDRITES IN EXCITING NEURONS

The Large Spatial Field of Excitation of the Dendrites. The dendrites of the anterior motor neurons extend for 0.5 to 1 millimeter in all directions from the neuronal soma. Therefore, these dendrites can receive signals from a large spatial area around the motor neuron. This provides vast opportunity for summation of signals from many separate presynaptic neurons.

It is also important that between 80 and 90 per cent of all the presynaptic terminals terminate on the dendrites of the anterior motor neuron in contrast to only 10 to 20 per cent terminating on the neuronal soma. Therefore, the preponderant share of the excitation of the neuron is provided by signals transmitted over the dendrites.

Failure of Many Dendrites to Transmit Action Potentials. Many dendrites fail to transmit action potentials because their membranes have relatively few voltage-gated sodium channels, so that their thresholds for excitation are very high. Yet they do transmit *electrotonic current* down the dendrites to the soma. (Transmission of electrotonic current means the direct spread of current by electrical conduction in the fluids of the dendrites with no generation of action potentials.) Stimulation of the neuron by this current has special characteristics, as follows:

Decrement of Electrotonic Conduction in the Dendrites—Greater Excitation by Synapses Near the Soma. In Figure 10–9 a number of excitatory and inhibitory synapses are shown stimulating the den-

drites of a neuron. On the two dendrites to the left in the figure are shown excitatory effects near the ends of the dendrites; note the high levels of the excitatory postsynaptic potentials at these ends—that is, the less negative membrane potentials. However, a large share of the excitatory postsynaptic potential is lost before it reaches the soma. The reason for this is that the dendrites are long and thin, and their membranes are also leaky to electrical current. Therefore, before the excitatory potentials can reach the soma, a large share of the potential is lost by leakage through the membrane. This decrease in membrane potential as it spreads electrotonically along dendrites toward the soma is called *decremental conduction.*

It is also obvious that the nearer the excitatory synapse is to the soma of the neuron, the less will be the decrement of conduction. Therefore, those synapses that lie near the soma have far more excitatory effect than those that lie far away from the soma.

Rapid Re-Excitation of the Neuron by the Dendrites After the Neuron Fires. When an action potential is generated in a neuron, this action potential spreads back over the soma but not always over the dendrites. Therefore, the excitatory postsynaptic potentials in the dendrites often are only partially disturbed by the action potential, so that just as soon as the action potential is over, the potentials still existing in the dendrites are ready and waiting to excite the neuron again. Thus, the dendrites have a "holding capacity" for the excitatory signal from presynaptic sources.

Summation of Excitation and Inhibition in Dendrites. The uppermost dendrite of Figure 10–9 is shown to be stimulated by both excitatory and inhibitory synapses. At the tip of the dendrite is a strong excitatory postsynaptic potential, but nearer to the soma are two inhibitory synapses acting on the same dendrite. These inhibitory synapses pro-

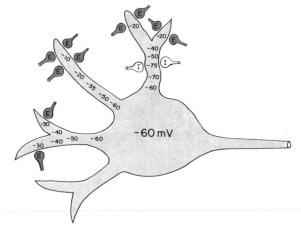

Figure 10–9. Stimulation of a neuron by presynaptic terminals located on dendrites, showing, especially, decremental conduction of excitatory electrotonic potentials in the two dendrites to the left and inhibition of dendritic excitation in the dentrite that is uppermost.

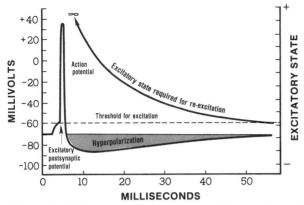

Figure 10–10. A neuronal potential followed by a prolonged period of neuronal hyperpolarization. Also shown is the "excitatory state" required for re-excitation of the neuron at given intervals after the action potential is over.

vide a hyperpolarizing voltage that completely nullifies the excitatory effect and indeed transmits a small amount of inhibition by electrotonic conduction toward the soma. Thus, dendrites can summate excitatory and inhibitory postsynaptic potentials in the same way that the soma can.

RELATION OF STATE OF EXCITATION OF THE NEURON TO THE RATE OF FIRING

The "Excitatory State." The "excitatory state" of a neuron is defined as the degree of excitatory drive to the neuron. If there is a higher degree of excitation than inhibition of the neuron at any given instant, then it is said that there is an *excitatory state*. On the other hand, if there is more inhibition than excitation, then it is said that there is an *inhibitory state*.

When the excitatory state of a neuron rises above the threshold for excitation, then the neuron will fire repetitively as long as the excitatory state remains at this level. However, the *rate* at which it will fire is determined by *how much* the excitatory state is above threshold. To explain this, we must first consider what happens to the neuronal somal potential during and following the action potential.

Changes in Neuronal Somal Potential During and Following the Action Potential. Figure 10–10 illustrates an action potential spreading backward over the neuronal soma after being initiated at the axon hillock by an excitatory postsynaptic potential. Following the spike portion of the action potential, there is a very long *positive after-potential*—that is, a state of "hypolarization"—lasting for many milliseconds. During this interval the somal membrane potential falls below the normal resting membrane potential of −65 millivolts. This is probably caused by a high degree of permeability of the neuronal membrane to potassium ions that persists for many milliseconds after the action potential is over. And, in addition, the high membrane conductivity for

potassium ions also "short circuits" excitatory potentials.

The importance of this state of hyperpolarization and short circuiting after the spike potential is that the neuron remains in an *inhibited state* during this period of time. Therefore, a far greater excitatory state is required during this time than normally to cause re-excitation of the neuron.

Relationship of Excitatory State to Frequency of Firing. The curve shown at the top of Figure 10–10, labeled "Excitatory state required for re-excitation," depicts the relative level of the excitatory state required at each instant after an action potential is over to re-excite the neuron. Note that very soon after an action potential is over, a very high excitatory state is required. That is, a very large number of excitatory synapses must be firing simultaneously. Then, after many milliseconds have passed and the state of hyperpolarization and the short circuiting of the neuron have begun to disappear, the excitatory state required becomes greatly reduced.

Therefore, it is immediately evident that when the excitatory state is high, a second action potential will appear very soon after the previous one. Then still a third action potential will appear soon after the second, and this process will continue indefinitely. Thus, at a very high excitatory state the frequency of firing of the neuron is great.

On the other hand, when the excitatory state is only barely above threshold, the neuron must recover almost completely from the hyperpolarization and short circuiting, which requires many milliseconds, before it will fire again. Therefore, the frequency of neuronal firing is low.

Response Characteristics of Different Neurons to Increasing Levels of Excitatory State. Histological study of the nervous system immediately convinces one of the widely varying types of neurons in different parts of the nervous system. And, physiologically, the different types of neurons perform different functions. Therefore, as would be expected, the ability to respond to stimulation by the synapses varies from one type of neuron to another.

Figure 10–11 illustrates theoretical responses of three different types of neurons to varying levels of excitatory state. Note that neuron #1 has a low threshold for excitation while neuron #3 has a high threshold. But note also that neuron #2 has the lowest maximum frequency of discharge, while neuron #3 has the highest maximum frequency.

Some neurons in the central nervous system fire continuously because even the normal excitatory state is above the threshold level. Their frequency of firing can usually be increased still more by further increasing their excitatory state. Or, the frequency may be decreased, or firing even be stopped, by superimposing an inhibitory state on the neuron.

Thus, different neurons respond differently, have different thresholds for excitation, and have widely

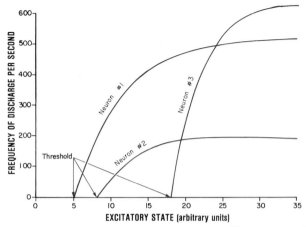

Figure 10–11. Response characteristics of different types of neurons to progressively increasing levels of excitatory state.

differing maximal frequencies of discharge. With a little imagination one can readily understand the importance of having neurons with many different types of response characteristics to perform the widely varying functions of the nervous system.

SOME SPECIAL CHARACTERISTICS OF SYNAPTIC TRANSMISSION

Fatigue of Synaptic Transmission. When excitatory synapses are repetitively stimulated at a rapid rate, the number of discharges by the post-synaptic neuron is at first very great, but it becomes progressively less in succeeding milliseconds or seconds. This is called *fatigue* of synaptic transmission.

Fatigue is an exceedingly important characteristic of synaptic function, for when areas of the nervous system become overexcited, fatigue causes them to lose this excess excitability after a while. For example, fatigue is probably the most important means by which the excess excitability of the brain during an epileptic convulsion is finally subdued so that the convulsion ceases. Thus, the development of fatigue is a protective mechanism against excess neuronal activity. This will be discussed further in the description of reverberating neuronal circuits in the following chapter.

The mechanism of fatigue is mainly exhaustion of the stores of transmitter substance in the synaptic terminals, particularly since it has been calculated that the excitatory terminals can store enough excitatory transmitter for only 10,000 normal synaptic transmissions, an amount that can be exhausted in only a few seconds to a few minutes. However, part of the fatigue process probably also results from two other factors as well: progressive inactivation of many of the postsynaptic membrane receptors and slow buildup of calcium ions inside the postsynaptic neuronal cell caused by the successive action potentials—these calcium ions in turn open calcium-activated potassium channels, which cause an inhibitory effect on the postsynaptic neuron.

Post-Tetanic Facilitation. When a rapidly repetitive series of impulses stimulates an excitatory synapse for a period of time and then a rest period is allowed, the postsynaptic neuron will usually be even more responsive to subsequent stimulation than normally. This is called *post-tetanic facilitation.*

Experiments have shown that post-tetanic facilitation is caused mainly by the buildup of excess calcium ions in the presynaptic terminals, caused by the successive influx of more calcium ions with each action potential because the calcium pump pumps too slowly to remove all of these immediately. These accumulated calcium ions add to the effects of the action potentials themselves in causing more and more vesicular release of transmitter substance. Occasionally the effect can be great enough to cause the release of transmitter at a rate two times normal.

The physiological significance of post-tetanic facilitation is still very doubtful, and it may have no real significance at all. However, since post-tetanic facilitation can last from a few seconds in some neurons to several hours in others, it is immediately apparent that neurons could possibly store information by this mechanism. Therefore post-tetanic facilitation might well be a mechanism of "short-term" memory in the central nervous system. This possibility will be discussed further in Chapter 18 in relation to the memory function of the cerebral cortex.

Effect of Acidosis and Alkalosis on Synaptic Transmission. The neurons are highly responsive to changes in pH of the surrounding interstitial fluids. *Alkalosis greatly increases neuronal excitability.* For instance, a rise in arterial pH from the normal of 7.4 to about 7.8 often causes cerebral convulsions because of increased excitability of the neurons. This can be demonstrated especially well by having a person who is predisposed to epileptic convulsions hyperventilate. The hyperventilation elevates the pH of the blood only momentarily, but even this short interval can often precipitate an epileptic attack.

On the other hand, *acidosis greatly depresses neuronal activity;* a fall in pH from 7.4 to below 7.0 usually causes a comatose state. For instance, in very severe diabetic or uremic acidosis, coma always develops.

Effect of Hypoxia on Synaptic Transmission. Neuronal excitability is also highly dependent on an adequate supply of oxygen. Cessation of oxygen supply for only a few seconds can cause complete inexcitability of the neurons. This is often seen when the cerebral circulation is temporarily interrupted, for within 3 to 5 seconds the person becomes unconscious.

Effect of Drugs on Synaptic Transmission. Many different drugs are known to increase the excitability of neurons, and others are known to decrease the excitability. For instance, caffeine, theophylline, and theobromine, which are found in coffee, tea, and cocoa, respectively, all increase neuronal excitability, presumably by reducing the threshold for excitation of the neurons. However, strychnine, which is one of the best known of all the agents that increase the excitability of neurons, does not reduce the threshold for excitation of the neurons at all but, instead, *inhibits the action of at least some of the inhibitory transmitters* on the neurons, probably especially the inhibitory effect of glycine in the spinal cord. In consequence, the effects of the excitatory transmitters become overwhelming, and the neurons become so excited that they go into rapidly repetitive discharge, resulting in severe convulsions.

Most anesthetics increase the membrane threshold for excitation and thereby decrease synaptic transmission at many points in the nervous system. Because most of the anesthetics are lipid-soluble, it has been reasoned that they might change the physical characteristics of the neuronal membranes, making them less responsive to excitatory agents.

Synaptic Delay. In transmission of an action potential from a presynaptic neuron to a postsynaptic neuron, a certain amount of time is consumed in the process of (1) discharge of the transmitter substance by the presynaptic terminal, (2) diffusion of the transmitter to the postsynaptic neuronal membrane, (3) action of the transmitter on the membrane receptor, (4) action of the receptor to increase the membrane permeability, and (5) inward diffusion of sodium to raise the excitatory postsynaptic potential to a high enough value to elicit an action potential. The *minimal* period of time required for all these events to take place, even when large numbers of presynaptic terminals are stimulated simultaneously, is about 0.5 millisecond. This is called the *synaptic delay*. It is important for the following reason: neurophysiologists can measure the *minimal* delay time between an input volley of impulses and an output volley and from this can estimate the number of series neurons in the circuit.

REFERENCES

Addink, A. D. (ed.): Exogenous and Endogenous Influences on Metabolic and Neural Control. New York, Pergamon Press, 1982.

Barde, Y. A., et al.: New neurotrophic factors. *Annu. Rev. Physiol.*, 45:601, 1983.

Berg, D. K.: New neuronal growth factors. *Annu. Rev. Neurosci.*, 7:149, 1984.

Buchtel, H. A.: The Conceptual Nervous System. New York, Pergamon Press, 1982.

Changeux, J. P., *et al.*: Acetylcholine receptor: An allosteric protein. *Science*, 225:1335, 1984.

Creese, I., *et al.*: The classification of dopamine receptors: Relationship to radioligand binding. *Annu. Rev. Neurosci.*, 6:43, 1983.

Eccles, J. C.: My scientific odyssey. *Annu. Rev. Physiol.*, 39:1, 1977.

Eyzaguirre, C.: Physiology of the Nervous System. Chicago, Year Book Medical Publishers, 1985.

Fernstrom, J. D.: Dietary precursors and brain neurotransmitter formation. *Annu. Rev. Med.*, 32:413, 1981.

Ganong, W. F.: The brain renin-angiostensin system. *Annu. Rev. Physiol.*, 46:17, 1984.

Hanin, I. (ed.): Dynamics of Neurotransmitter Function. New York, Raven Press, 1984.

Iversen, L. L.: Nonopioid neuropeptides in mammalian CNS. *Annu. Rev. Pharmacol. Toxicol.*, 23:1, 1983.

Kehoe, J., and Marty, A.: Certain slow synaptic responses: Their properties and possible underlying mechanisms. *Annu. Rev. Biophys. Bioeng.*, 9:437, 1980.

Kennedy, M. B.: Experimental approaches to understanding the role of protein phosphorylation in the regulation of neuronal function. *Annu. Rev. Neurosci.*, 6:493, 1983.

Kostyuk, P. G.: Intracellular perfusion of nerve cells and its effects on membrane currents. *Physiol. Rev.*, 64:435, 1984.

Krnjevic, K.: Transmitters in motor systems. *In* Brooks, V. B. (ed.): Handbook of Physiology. Sec. 1, Vol. II. Bethesda, American Physiological Society, 1981, p. 107.

Laduron, P. M.: Presynaptic heteroreceptors in regulation of neuronal transmission. *Biochem. Pharmacol.*, 34:467, 1985.

Landis, S. C.: Neuronal growth cones. *Annu. Rev. Physiol.*, 45:567, 1983.

Loh, H. H., and Law, P. Y.: The role of membrane lipids in receptor mechanisms. *Annu. Rev. Pharmacol. Toxicol.*, 20:201, 1980.

Lynch, G., and Schubert, P.: The use of in vitro brain slices for multidisciplinary studies of synaptic function. *Annu. Rev. Neurosci.*, 3:1, 1980.

McKay, R. D. G.: Molecular approach to the nervous system. *Annu. Rev. Neurosci.*, 6:527, 1983.

McKerns, K. W. (ed.): Hormonally Active Brain Peptides. Structure and Function. New York, Plenum Publishing Corp., 1982.

Nicoll, R. A., *et al.*: Substance P as a transmitter candidate. *Annu. Rev. Neurosci.*, 3:227, 1980.

Popot, J.-L., and Changeux, J.-P.: Nicotinic receptor of acetylcholine: Structure of an oligomeric integral membrane protein. *Physiol. Rev.*, 64:1162, 1984.

Purves, D., and Lichtman, J. W.: Specific connections between nerve cells. *Annu. Rev. Physiol.*, 45:553, 1983.

Reichardt, L. F.: Immunological approaches to the nervous system. *Science*, 225:1294, 1984.

Schubert, D.: Developmental Biology of Cultured Nerve, Muscle and Glia. New York, John Wiley & Sons, 1984.

Silverman, A.-J.: Magnocellular neurosecretory system. *Annu. Rev. Neurosci.*, 6:357, 1983.

Stein, J. F.: Introduction to Neurophysiology. St. Louis, C. V. Mosby, 1982.

Su, C.: Purinergic neurotransmission and neuromodulation. *Annu. Rev. Pharmacol. Toxicol.*, 23:397, 1983.

Tucek, S.: Regulation of acetylcholine synthesis in the brain. *J. Neurochem.*, 44:11, 1985.

Wright, E. M.: Electrophysiology of plasma membrane vesicles. *Am. J. Physiol.*, 246:F363, 1984.

11

Neuronal Mechanisms and Circuits for Processing Information

Certain types of neuronal mechanisms and neuronal circuits are used again and again throughout the nervous system. The purpose of this chapter is to characterize some of these and to preview some of their important uses.

INFORMATION, SIGNALS, AND IMPULSES

The term *information*, as it applies to the nervous system, means a variety of different things, such as knowledge, facts, quantitative values, intensity of pain, intensity of light, temperature, and any other aspect of the body or its immediate surroundings that has meaning. Thus, pain from a pin prick is information, pressure on the bottom of the feet is information, degree of angulation of the joints is information, and a stored memory in the brain is information.

However, information cannot be transmitted in its original form but only in the form of action potentials, also called *nerve impulses*. Thus, a part of the body that is subjected to pain must first convert this information into nerve impulses; specific areas of the brain convert abstract thoughts also into nerve impulses that are then transmitted either elsewhere in the brain or into peripheral nerves to motor effectors throughout the body. The retina of the eye converts vision into nerve impulses, the nerve endings of the joints convert degree of angulation of the joints into nerve impulses, and so forth.

Signals. In the transmission of information, it is frequently not desirable to speak in terms of the individual impulses but instead of the overall pattern of impulses; this pattern is called a *signal*. As an example, when pressure is applied to a large area of skin, impulses are transmitted by large numbers of parallel nerve fibers, and the total pattern of impulses transmitted by all these fibers is a signal. Thus, we can speak of visual signals, auditory signals, somesthetic sensory signals, motor signals, and so forth.

TRANSMISSION OF SIGNALS IN NERVE TRACTS

SIGNAL STRENGTH

One of the characteristics of information that always must be conveyed is its quantitative intensity, for instance the intensity of pain. The different gradations of intensity can be transmitted either by utilizing increasing numbers of parallel fibers or by sending more impulses along a single fiber. These two mechanisms are called respectively, spatial summation and temporal summation.

Spatial Summation (Multiple Fiber Summation). Figure 11–1 illustrates the phenomenon of spatial summation, whereby increasing signal strength is transmitted by using progressively greater numbers of fibers. This figure shows a section of skin innervated by a large number of parallel pain nerve fibers. Each of these arborizes into hundreds of minute *free nerve endings* that serve as pain receptors. The entire cluster of fibers from one pain fiber frequently covers an area of skin as large as 5 cm in diameter, and this area is called the *receptive field* of that fiber. The number of endings is large in the center of the field but diminishes toward the periphery. One can also see from the figure that the arborizing nerve fibrils overlap those from other pain fibers. Therefore, a pin prick of the skin usually stimulates endings from many different pain fibers simultaneously. But, if the pin prick is in the center of the receptive field of a particular pain fiber, the degree of stimulation of that fiber is far greater than if it is in the periphery of the field.

Thus, in the lower part of Figure 11–1 is shown three separate views of the cross-section of the nerve bundle leading from the skin area. To the left is shown the effect of a weak stimulus, with only a single nerve fiber in the middle of the bundle stimulated very strongly (represented by the solid fiber), whereas several adjacent fibers are stimulated weakly (half-solid fibers). The other two views of the nerve cross-section show the effect respec-

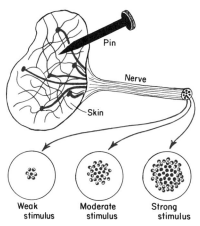

Figure 11–1. Pattern of stimulation of pain fibers in a nerve trunk leading from an area of skin pricked by a pin.

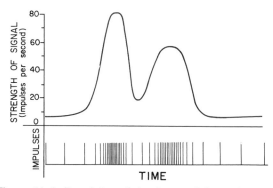

Figure 11–2. Translation of signal strength into a frequency-modulated series of nerve impulses, showing *above* the strength of signal and *below* the separate nerve impulses.

tively of a moderate stimulus and a strong stimulus, with progressively more fibers being stimulated. Thus, the stronger signals spread to more and more fibers. This phenomenon is called *spatial summation*, which means simply that one of the means by which signals of increasing strength are transmitted in the nervous system is by utilizing progressively greater numbers of fibers.

Temporal Summation. A second means for transmitting signals of increasing strength is by increasing the *frequency* of nerve impulses in each fiber, which is called *temporal summation.* Figure 11–2 illustrates this type of summation, showing in the upper part a changing strength of signal and in the lower part the actual impulses transmitted by the nerve fiber.

TRANSMISSION AND PROCESSING OF SIGNALS IN NEURONAL POOLS

The central nervous system is made up of literally hundreds or even thousands of separate neuronal pools, some of which contain very few neurons while others hold vast numbers. For instance, the entire cerebral cortex could be considered to be a single large neuronal pool. It has many separate fiber tracts coming to it (afferent fibers) and others leaving it (efferent fibers). Furthermore, it maintains the same quality of spatial orientation as that found in the nerve bundles, individual points of the cortex connecting with specific points elsewhere in the nervous system or connecting through the peripheral nerves with specific points in the body. However, within this pool of neurons are large numbers of short nerve fibers whereby signals spread horizontally from neuron to neuron within the pool itself.

Other neuronal pools include the different basal ganglia and the specific nuclei in the thalamus, cerebellum, mesencephalon, pons, and medulla.

Also, the entire dorsal gray matter of the spinal cord could be considered to be one long pool of neurons, and the entire anterior gray matter another long neuronal pool. Each pool has its own special characteristics of organization which cause it to process signals in its own special way, thus allowing these special characteristics to achieve the multitude of functions of the nervous system. Yet, despite their differences in function, the pools also have many similarities that are described in the following pages.

RELAYING OF SIGNALS THROUGH NEURONAL POOLS

Organization of Neurons for Relaying Signals. Figure 11–3 is a schematic diagram of several neurons in a neuronal pool, showing "input" fibers to the left and "output" fibers to the right. Each input

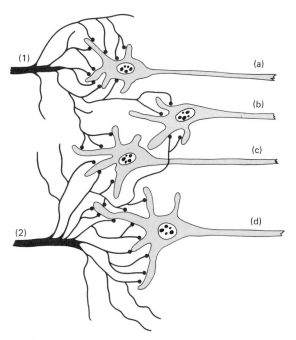

Figure 11–3. Basic organization of a neuronal pool.

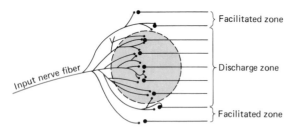

Figure 11–4. "Discharge" and "facilitated" zones of a neuronal pool.

fiber divides hundreds to thousands of times, providing an average of a thousand or more terminal fibrils that spread over a large area in the pool to synapse with the dendrites or cell bodies of the neurons in the pool. The dendrites of some of the neurons also arborize and spread in the pool. The neuronal area stimulated by each incoming nerve fiber is called its *stimulatory field.* Note that each input fiber arborizes so that large numbers of its terminals lie on the centermost neurons in its "field," but progressively fewer terminals lie on the neurons farther from the center of the field.

Threshold and Subthreshold Stimuli—Facilitation. From the discussion of synaptic function in the previous chapter, it will be recalled that discharge of a single excitatory presynaptic terminal almost never stimulates the postsynaptic neuron. Instead, large numbers of terminals must discharge on the same neuron either simultaneously or in rapid succession to cause excitation. For instance, in Figure 11–3, let us assume that six separate terminals must discharge simultaneously to excite any one of the neurons. If the student will count the number of terminals on each one of the neurons from each input fiber, he or she will see that input fiber (*1*) has more than enough terminals to cause neuron (*a*) to discharge. Therefore, the stimulus from input fiber (*1*) to this neuron is said to be an *excitatory stimulus,* or it is also called a *threshold stimulus* because it is above the threshold required for excitation.

Input fiber (*1*) also contributes terminals to neurons (*b*) and (*c*) but not enough to cause excitation. Nevertheless, discharge of these terminals makes both these neurons more excitable to signals arriving through other incoming nerve fibers. Therefore, the stimulus to these neurons is said to be *subthreshold,* and the neurons are said to be *facilitated.*

Similarly for input fiber (*2*) the stimulus to neuron (*d*) is a threshold stimulus and to neurons (*b*) and (*c*) a subthreshold, but facilitating, stimulus.

It must be recognized that Figure 11–3 represents a highly condensed version of a neuronal pool, for each input nerve fiber usually provides terminals to hundreds or thousands of separate neurons in its distribution "field," as illustrated in Figure 11–4. In the central portion of the field, almost all the neurons are stimulated by the in-coming fiber, designated in Figure 11–4 by the darkened circle area.

Therefore, this is said to be the *discharge zone* of the incoming fiber, also called *excited zone* or *liminal zone.* To either side, the neurons are facilitated but not excited, and these areas are called the *facilitated zone,* or also called *subthreshold zone* or *subliminal zone.*

Inhibition of a Neuronal Pool. We must also remember that some incoming fibers inhibit neurons rather than excite them. This is exactly the opposite of facilitation, and the entire field of the inhibitory branches is called the *inhibitory zone.* However, the degree of inhibition in the center of this zone is very great because of large numbers of endings in the center while it becomes progressively less toward its edges.

Divergence of Signals Passing Through Neuronal Pools

Often it is important for signals entering a neuronal pool to excite far greater numbers of nerve fibers leaving the pool. This phenomenon is called *divergence.* Two major types of divergence occur and have entirely different purposes. These are illustrated in Figure 11–5 and may be described as follows.

An *amplifying* type of divergence often occurs, illustrated in Figure 11–5A. This means simply that an input signal spreads to an increasing number of neurons as it passes through successive pools of a nervous pathway. This type of divergence is characteristic of the corticospinal pathway in its control of skeletal muscles. Stimulation of a single large pyramidal cell in the motor cortex transmits a single impulse into the spinal cord. Yet, under appropriate conditions of very strong cord facilitation, this impulse can stimulate perhaps several hundred interneurons and anterior motor neurons. Each of the motor neurons then stimulates as many as a hundred or more muscle fibers. Thus, there is a total divergence, or amplification, of as much as 10,000-fold.

The second type of divergence, illustrated in

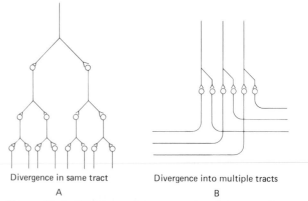

Divergence in same tract

A

Divergence into multiple tracts

B

Figure 11–5. "Divergence" in neuronal pathways. *A,* Divergence within a pathway to cause "amplification" of the signal. *B,* Divergence into multiple tracts to transmit the signal to separate areas.

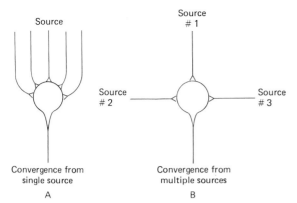

Figure 11–6. "Convergence" of multiple input fibers on a single neuron. *A*, Input fibers from a single source. *B*, Input fibers from multiple sources.

Figure 11–5B, is *divergence into multiple tracts.* In this case, the signal is transmitted in two separate directions from the pool to different parts of the nervous system where it is needed. For instance, information transmitted in the dorsal columns of the spinal cord takes two courses in the lower part of the brain: into the cerebellum and on through the lower regions of the brain to the thalamus and cerebral cortex. Likewise, in the thalamus almost all sensory information is relayed both into deep structures of the thalamus and to discrete regions of the cerebral cortex.

Convergence of Signals

Often it is important for signals from multiple incoming neurons to excite the same neuron. That is, these incoming fibers *converge* on this same neuron. Like divergence, there are also two basic types of convergence, illustrated in Figure 11–6.

Section A of this figure shows *convergence from a single source.* That is, multiple terminals from an incoming fiber tract terminate on the same neuron. The importance of this is that neurons are almost never excited by an action potential from a single input terminal. But action potentials from multiple input terminals will provide enough "summation" to bring the neuron to the threshold required for discharge.

However, *convergence can also result from input signals* (excitatory or inhibitory) *from several different sources,* which is illustrated in Figure 11–6B. For instance, the interneurons of the spinal cord receive converging signals from (1) peripheral nerve fibers entering the cord, (2) propriospinal fibers passing from one segment of the cord to another, (3) corticospinal fibers from the cerebral cortex, and (4) several other long pathways descending from the brain into the spinal cord. Then the signals from the interneurons converge on the anterior motor neurons to control muscle function.

Such convergence allows summation of information from different sources, and the resulting response is a summated effect of all the different types of information. Obviously, therefore, convergence is one of the important means by which the central nervous system correlates, summates, and sorts different types of information.

Neuronal Circuit Causing Both Excitatory and Inhibitory Output Signals

Sometimes an incoming signal to a neuronal pool causes an output excitatory signal going in one direction and at the same time an inhibitory signal going elsewhere. For instance, at the same time that an excitatory signal is transmitted by one set of neurons in the spinal cord to cause forward movement of a leg, an inhibitory signal is transmitted simultaneously through a separate set of neurons to inhibit the muscles on the back of the leg so that they will not oppose the forward movement. This type of circuit is characteristic of control of all antagonistic pairs of muscles, and it is called the *reciprocal inhibition circuit.*

Figure 11–7 illustrates the means by which the inhibition is achieved. The input fiber directly excites the excitatory output pathway, but it stimulates an intermediate *inhibitory neuron* (neuron 2) which then inhibits the second output pathway from the pool. This type of circuit is probably also important in preventing overactivity in many parts of the brain.

TRANSMISSION OF SPATIAL PATTERNS THROUGH SUCCESSIVE NEURONAL POOLS

Most information is transmitted from one part of the nervous system to another through several successive neuronal pools. For instance, sensory information from the skin passes first through the peripheral nerve fibers, then through second order neurons that originate either in the spinal cord or in the cuneate and gracile nuclei of the medulla, and finally through third order neurons originating in the thalamus to the cerebral cortex. Such a pathway is illustrated at the top of Figure 11–8. Note that the sensory nerve endings in the skin overlap each other tremendously; and the terminal fibrils of each nerve fiber, on entering each neuronal pool, spread to many adjacent neurons, innervating perhaps a hundred or more separate neurons. On first thought, one would expect signals from the skin to become completely mixed up by this hap-

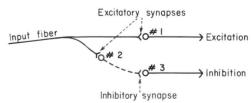

Figure 11–7. Inhibitory circuit. Neuron 2 is an inhibitory neuron.

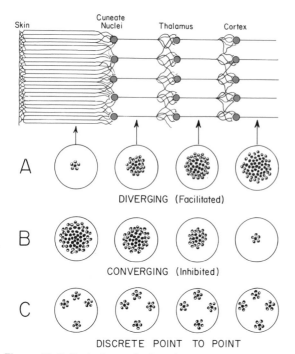

Figure 11–8. Typical organization of a sensory pathway from the skin to the cerebral cortex. *Below*: The patterns of fiber stimulation at different points in the pathway following stimulation by a pinprick when the pathway is *A*, facilitated; *B*, inhibited; and *C*, normally excitable.

hazard arrangement of terminal fibrils in each neuronal pool. For statistical reasons, however, this does not occur, which can be explained as follows:

First, if a single point is stimulated in the skin, the nerve fiber with the most nerve endings in that particular spot becomes stimulated to the strongest extent, while the immediately adjacent nerve fibers become stimulated less strongly, and the nerve fibers still farther away become stimulated only weakly. When this signal arrives at the first neuronal pool, the stimulus spreads in many directions in the terminal fibrils of the neuronal pool. Yet the *greatest number* of *excited presynaptic terminals* lies very near the point of entry of the most excited input nerve fiber. Therefore, the neuron closest to this central point is the one that becomes stimulated to the greatest extent. Exactly the same effect occurs in the second neuronal pool in the thalamus and again when the signal reaches the cerebral cortex.

Yet, it is true that a signal passing through *highly facilitated neuronal pools* could diverge so much that the spatial pattern at the terminus of the pathway would be completely obscured. This effect is illustrated in Figure 11–8A, which shows successively expanding spatial patterns of neuron stimulation in such a facilitated, diverging pathway.

However, the degree of facilitation of the different neuronal pools varies from time to time. Under some conditions the degree of facilitation is so low that the pathway becomes converging, as illustrated in Figure 11–8B. In this case, a broad area of the skin is stimulated, but the signal loses part of its

fringe stimuli as it passes through each successive pool until the breadth of the stimulus becomes contracted at the opposite end. One can achieve this type of stimulation by pressing ever so lightly with a flat object on the skin. The signal converges to give the person a sensation of almost a point contact.

In Figure 11–8C, four separate points are simultaneously stimulated on the skin, and the degree of excitability in each neuronal pool is exactly that amount required to prevent either divergence or convergence. Therefore, a reasonably true spatial pattern of each of the four points of stimulation is transmitted through the entire pathway.

Centrifugal Control of Neuronal Facilitation in the Sensory Pathways. It is obvious from the preceding discussion that the degree of facilitation of each neuronal pool must be maintained at exactly the proper level if faithful transmission of the spatial pattern is to occur. Recent discoveries have demonstrated that the degrees of inhibition or facilitation of most—indeed, probably all—neuronal pools in the different sensory pathways are controlled by *centrifugal nerve fibers* that pass from the respective sensory areas of the cortex downward to the separate sensory relay neuronal pools. Thus, these nerve fibers undoubtedly help to control the faithfulness of signal transmission.

Lateral Inhibition to Provide Contrast in the Spatial Pattern. When a single point of the skin or other sensory area is stimulated, not only is a single fiber excited but a number of "fringe" fibers are excited less strongly at the same time, as already explained. Therefore, the spatial pattern is blurred even before the signal begins to be transmitted through the pathway. However, in almost all pathways that transmit very exact information, such as the critical sensory pathways, lateral *inhibitory circuits* inhibit the fringe neurons and re-establish a truer spatial pattern.

Figure 11–9A illustrates one type of lateral inhibitory circuit, showing that the nerve fibers of a pathway give off collateral fibers that excite inhibitory neurons. These inhibitory neurons in turn

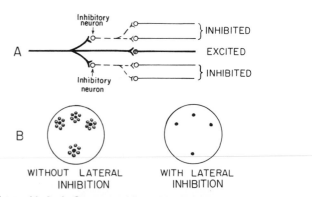

Figure 11–9. *A*, One type of lateral inhibitory circuit by which an excited fiber of a neuronal pool can cause inhibition of adjacent fibers. *B*, Increase in contrast of the stimulus pattern caused by the inhibitory circuit.

inhibit the less excited fringe neurons in the signal pathway. The effect of this on transmission of the spatial pattern is illustrated in Figure 11–9B, which shows the same point-to-point transmission pattern that was illustrated in Figure 11–8C. The left-hand pattern illustrates four strongly excited fibers (the solid fibers) with penumbras of fringe excitation surrounding each of these. In the illustration to the right, the penumbras have been removed by the lateral inhibitory circuits; obviously, this increases the *contrast* in the signal and helps in the *faithfulness* of transmission of the spatial pattern.

Unfortunately, we still know little about all the capabilities of the lateral inhibition mechanism, but the more we learn the more it becomes clear that this is one of the most useful of all the neuronal circuits of the nervous system to differentiate and analyze sensory signals. We shall discuss this much more fully in the following chapters.

PROLONGATION OF A SIGNAL BY A NEURONAL POOL—"AFTER-DISCHARGE"

Thus far, we have considered signals that are merely relayed through neuronal pools. However, in many instances, a signal entering a pool causes a prolonged output discharge, called *after-discharge*, even after the incoming signal is over, and lasting from a few milliseconds to as long as many minutes. The three basic mechanisms by which after-discharge occurs are the following:

Synaptic After-Discharge. When excitatory synapses discharge on the surfaces of dendrites or the soma of a neuron, a postsynaptic potential develops in the neuron and lasts for many milliseconds—in the anterior motor neuron for up to 15 milliseconds, though perhaps much longer in other neurons—especially so when some of the long-acting synaptic transmitter substances are involved. As long as this potential lasts it can continue to excite the neuron, causing it to transmit a continuous train of output impulses, as was explained in the previous chapter. Thus, as a result of this synaptic after-discharge mechanism alone, it is possible for a single instantaneous input to cause a sustained signal output (a series of repetitive discharges) lasting as long as 15 or more milliseconds.

The Parallel Circuit Type of After-Discharge. Figure 11–10 illustrates a second type of neuronal circuit that can cause intermediate periods of after-discharge. In this case, the input signal spreads through a series of neurons in the neuronal pool, and from many of these neurons impulses keep converging on an output neuron. It will be recalled that a signal is delayed at each synapse for about 0.5 millisecond, which is called the *synaptic delay*. Therefore, signals passing through a succession of intermediate neurons reach the output neuron one by one after varying periods of delay. Therefore, the output neuron continues to be stimulated for many milliseconds.

It is doubtful that more than a few dozen successive neurons ordinarily enter into a parallel after-discharge circuit. Therefore, one would suspect that this type of after-discharge circuit could cause after-discharges that last for no more than perhaps 25 to 50 milliseconds. Yet, this circuit does represent a means by which a single input signal, lasting less than 1 millisecond, can be converted into a sustained output signal lasting for a rather precise period of time.

The Reverberatory (Oscillatory) Circuit as a Cause of After-Discharge. Many neurophysiologists believe that one of the most important of all circuits in the entire nervous system is the *reverberatory*, or *oscillatory*, *circuit*. Such circuits are caused by positive feedback within the neuronal pool. That is, the output of a neuronal circuit feeds back to re-excite the same circuit. Consequently, once stimulated, the circuit discharges repetitively for a long time.

Several different postulated varieties of reverberatory circuits are illustrated in Figure 11–11, the simplest—in Figure 11–11A—involving only a single neuron. In this case, the output neuron simply sends a collateral nerve fiber back to its own dendrites or soma to restimulate itself; therefore, once the neuron should discharge, the feedback stimuli could theoretically help keep the neuron discharging for a long time thereafter.

Figure 11–11B illustrates a few additional neurons in the feedback circuit, which would give a longer period of time between the initial discharge and the feedback signal. Figure 11–11C illustrates a still more complex system in which both facilitatory and inhibitory fibers impinge on the reverberating pool. A facilitatory signal increases the ease with which reverberation takes place, whereas an inhibitory signal decreases the ease of reverberation.

Figure 11–11D illustrates that most reverberating pathways are constituted of many parallel fibers, and at each cell station the terminal fibrils diffuse widely. In such a system the total reverberating signal can be either weak or strong, depending on how many parallel nerve fibers are momentarily involved in the reverberation.

Finally, reverberation need not occur only in a single neuronal pool, for it can occur through a circuit involving two or more successive pools in the positive feedback pathway.

Characteristics of After-Discharge from a Rever-

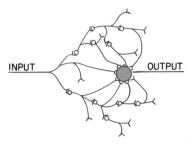

Figure 11–10. The parallel after-discharge circuit.

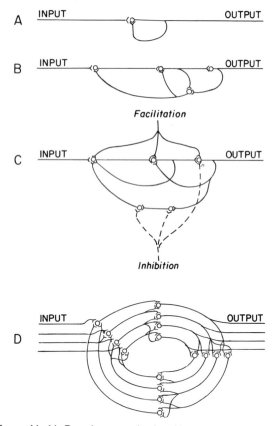

Figure 11–11. Reverberatory circuits of increasing complexity.

On the other hand, the greater the number of successive stages of neurons in the reverberatory pathway and the greater the number of collateral feedback fibrils, the easier would it be to keep the reverberation going.

Some Reverberatory Systems of the Nervous System and Their Durations of Reverberation. Even though neurophysiologists are not certain which functions of the nervous system can rightfully be ascribed to reverberatory circuits, some of those that have been postulated have reverberatory durations as short as 10 milliseconds or as long as several minutes, or perhaps even hours. Some examples include: (1) In an animal whose spinal cord is transected in the neck, a sudden painful stimulus to the animal's paw will cause the flexor muscles to contract and remain contracted from a fraction of a second to as much as several seconds after the stimulus ends. It is believed that this is caused by an after-discharge of the reverberatory type. (2) During respiration the inspiratory neuronal pool in the medulla becomes excited for about 2 seconds during each respiratory cycle. One theory suggests that this is caused by reverberation within the inspiratory neuronal pool. And (3) one theory of wakefulness is that continual reverberation occurs somewhere within the brain stem to keep a wakefulness area excited during the waking hours. If this be true, then this would represent a 14 to 18 hour period of reverberation.

Continuous Signal Output From Neuronal Pools

Some neuronal pools emit output signals continuously even without excitatory input signals. At least two different mechanisms theoretically can cause this effect: intrinsic neuronal discharge and reverberatory signals.

Continuous Discharge Caused by Intrinsic Neuronal Excitability. Neurons, like other excitable tissues, discharge repetitively if their membrane potentials rise above certain threshold levels. The membrane potentials of many neurons even normally are high enough to cause them to emit impulses continually. This occurs especially in large numbers of the neurons of the cerebellum as well as in most of the interneurons of the spinal cord.

beratory Circuit. Figure 11–12 illustrates postulated output signals from a reverberatory after-discharge circuit. The input stimulus need last only 1 millisecond or so, and yet the output can last for many milliseconds or even minutes. The figure demonstrates that the intensity of the output signal increases to a reasonably high value early in the reverberation, then decreases to a critical point, and at that point suddenly ceases entirely. Furthermore, the duration of the after-discharge is determined by the degree of inhibition or facilitation of the neuronal pool. In this way, signals from other parts of the brain can control the reaction of the pool to the input stimulus.

Almost these exact patterns of output signals can be recorded from the motor nerves exciting a muscle involved in the flexor reflex (discussed in Chapter 15), which is believed to be caused by a reverberating type of after-discharge following stimulation of pain fibers.

Importance of Synaptic Fatigue in Determining the Duration of Reverberation. It was pointed out in the previous chapter that synapses fatigue if stimulated for prolonged periods of time. Therefore, one of the most important factors that determines the duration of the reverberatory type of after-discharge is undoubtedly the rapidity with which the involved synapses fatigue. Rapid fatigue would obviously tend to shorten the period of after-discharge.

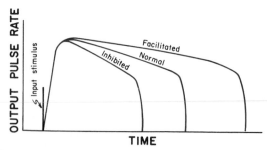

Figure 11–12. Typical pattern of the output signal from a reverberatory circuit following a single input stimulus, showing the effects of facilitation and inhibition.

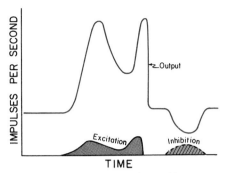

Figure 11–13. Continuous output from either a reverberating circuit or from a pool of intrinsically discharging neurons. This figure also shows the effect of excitatory or inhibitory input signals.

The rates at which these cells emit impulses can be increased by facilitatory signals or decreased by inhibitory signals; the latter can sometimes decrease the rate to extinction.

Continuous Signals Emitted from Reverberating Circuits as a Means for Transmitting Information. Obviously, a reverberating circuit that never fatigues to extinction could also be a source of continual impulses. Facilitatory impulses entering the reverberating pool, as illustrated in Figure 11–11C, could increase the output signal, and inhibition could decrease or even extinguish the output signal.

Figure 11–13 illustrates a continual output signal from a pool of neurons, whether it be a pool emitting impulses because of intrinsic neuronal excitability or as a result of reverberation. Note that an excitatory (or facilitatory) input signal greatly increases the output signal, whereas an inhibitory input signal greatly decreases the output. Those students who are familiar with radio transmitters will recognize this to be a *carrier wave* type of information transmission. That is, the excitatory and inhibitory control signals are not the *cause* of the output signal, but they do *control* it. Note that this carrier wave system allows decrease in signal intensity as well as increase, whereas, up to this point, the types of information transmission that we have discussed have been only positive information rather than negative information. This type of information transmission is used by the autonomic nervous system to control such functions as vascular tone, gut tone, degree of constriction of the iris, heart rate, and others.

RHYTHMIC SIGNAL OUTPUT

Many neuronal circuits emit rhythmic output signals—for instance, the rhythmic respiratory signal originating in the reticular substance of the medulla and pons. This repetitive rhythmic signal continues throughout life, while other rhythmic signals, such as those that cause scratching movements by the hind leg of a dog or the walking movements in an animal, require input stimuli into the respective circuits to initiate the signals.

Many rhythmic signals are postulated to result from reverberating circuits or successive reverberating circuits that feed excitatory or inhibitory signals from one to the next. However, many other more complex mechanisms could also be responsible for rhythmic signals.

Obviously, facilitatory or inhibitory signals can affect rhythmic signal output in the same way that they can affect continuous signal outputs. Figure 11–14, for instance, illustrates the rhythmic respiratory signal in the phrenic nerve. However, when the carotid body is stimulated by arterial oxygen deficiency, the frequency and amplitude of the rhythmic signal pattern increase progressively.

INSTABILITY AND STABILITY OF NEURONAL CIRCUITS

Almost every part of the brain connects either directly or indirectly with every other part, and this creates a serious problem. If the first part excites the second, the second the third, the third the fourth, and so on until finally the signal re-excites the first part, it is clear that an excitatory signal entering any part of the brain would set off a continuous cycle of re-excitation of all parts. If this should occur, the brain would be inundated by a mass of uncontrolled reverberating signals—signals that would be transmitting no information but, nevertheless, would be consuming the circuits of the brain so that none of the informational signals could be transmitted. Such an effect actually occurs in widespread areas of the brain during *epileptic convulsions*.

How does the central nervous system prevent this from happening all the time? The answer seems to lie in two basic mechanisms that function throughout the central nervous system: inhibitory circuits and fatigue of synapses.

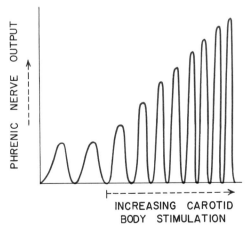

Figure 11–14. The rhythmical output from the respiratory center, showing that progressively increasing stimulation of the carotid body increases both the intensity and frequency of oscillation.

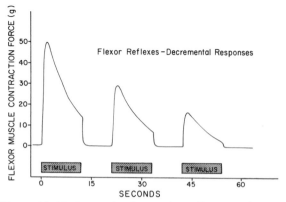

Figure 11–15. Successive flexor reflexes illustrating fatigue of conduction through the reflex pathway.

INHIBITORY CIRCUITS AS A MECHANISM FOR STABILIZING NERVOUS SYSTEM FUNCTION

The phenomenon of lateral inhibition that was discussed earlier in the chapter prevents signals in an informational pathway from spreading diffusely everywhere. In addition, two other types of inhibitory circuits in widespread areas of the brain help prevent excessive spread: (1) inhibitory feedback circuits that return from the termini of pathways back to the initial excitatory neurons of the same pathways—these are believed to occur in all the sensory nervous pathways, and they inhibit the input neurons when the termini become overly excited, and (2) some neuronal pools that exert gross inhibitory control over widespread areas of the brain—for instance, many of the basal ganglia exert inhibitory influences throughout the motor control system.

SYNAPTIC FATIGUE AS A MEANS FOR STABILIZING THE NERVOUS SYSTEM

Synaptic fatigue means simply that the signal becomes progressively weaker the more prolonged the period of excitation. Figure 11–15 illustrates three successive records of a flexor reflex elicited in an animal caused by inflicting pain in the footpad of the paw. Note in each record that the strength of contraction progressively "decrements"–that is, its strength diminishes; this is believed to be caused by *fatigue* of the synapses in the flexor reflex circuit. Furthermore, the shorter the interval between the successive flexor reflexes, the less becomes the intensity of the reflex response. Thus, in most neuronal circuits that are overused, the sensitivities of the circuits become depressed.

Automatic Short-Term Adjustment of Pathway Sensitivity by the Fatigue Mechanism. Now let us apply this phenomenon of fatigue to multiple pathways in the brain. Those that are overused usually become fatigued so that their sensitivities will be reduced. On the other hand, those that are underused will become rested and their sensitivities will increase. Thus, fatigue and recovery from fatigue constitute an important short-term means for moderating the sensitivities of the different nervous system circuits, helping to keep them operating in a range of sensitivity that allows effective function.

Long-Term Changes in Synaptic Sensitivity Caused by Automatic Downgrading or Upgrading of Synaptic Receptors. Recently it has been learned that the long-term sensitivities of synapses can be changed tremendously by downgrading the number of receptor proteins at the synaptic sites when there is overactivity and upgrading the receptors when there is underactivity. The mechanism for this is believed to be the following: Receptor proteins are being formed constantly by the endoplasmic reticular–Golgi apparatus system and are constantly being inserted into the synaptic membrane. However, when the synapses are overused and excesses of transmitter substance combine with the receptor proteins, many of these proteins are inactivated permanently and presumably removed from the synaptic membrane. This is especially true when some of the "modulator" transmitter substances are released at the synapses.

Therefore, in many if not most cases, overusage of a circuit will lead to gradually decreasing sensitivity of the synapses because of decreased receptor proteins, whereas underusage will cause prolonged increase in sensitivity. This is still another mechanism for continually adjusting the sensitivities of the respective neuronal circuits. It is indeed fortunate that fatigue and downgrading or upgrading of receptors, as well as other control mechanisms of the nervous system, continually adjust the sensitivity in each circuit to almost the exact level required for proper function. Think for a moment how serious it would be if the sensitivities of only a few of these circuits should be abnormally high; one might then expect almost continual muscle cramps, convulsions, psychotic disturbances, hallucinations, tension, or many other nervous disorders. But the automatic controls normally readjust the sensitivities of the circuits back to a controllable range of reactivity any time the circuits begin to be too active.

REFERENCES

American Physiological Society: Sensory Processes. Washington, D.C., American Physiological Society, 1984.

An der Heiden, U.: Analysis of Neural Networks. New York, Springer-Verlag, 1980.

Anderson, H., *et al.*: Developmental neurobiology of invertebrates. *Annu. Rev. Neurosci.*, 3:97, 1980.

Asanuma, H., and Wilson, V. J. (eds.): Integration in the Nervous System. New York, Igaku-Shoin, 1979.

Baldissera, F., Hultborn, H., and Illert, M.: Integration in spinal neuronal systems. *In* Brooks, V. B. (ed.): Handbook of Physiology. Sec. 1, Vol. II. Bethesda, American Physiological Society, 1981, p. 509.

Bennett, M. V. L. (ed.): Synaptic Transmission and Neuronal Interaction. New York, Raven Press, 1975.

Björklund, A., and Stenevi, U.: Regeneration of monoaminergic and cholinergic neurons in the mammalian central nervous system. *Physiol. Rev.,* 59:62, 1979.

Björklund, A., and Stenevi, U.: Intracerebral neural implants: Neuronal replacement and reconstruction of damaged circuitries. *Annu. Rev. Neurosci.,* 7:279, 1984.

Blumenthal, R., *et al.* (eds.): Dynamic Patterns of Brain Cell Assemblies. Neurosciences Research Program Bulletin. Vol. 12, No. 1. Cambridge, Mass., Massachusetts Institute of Technology, 1974.

Cotman, C. W., *et al.*: Synapse replacement in the nervous system of adult vertebrates. *Physiol. Rev.,* 61:684, 1981.

Cowan, W. M.: The development of the brain. *Sci. Am. 241*(3):112, 1979.

Darian, S. I.: The Nervous System. Section 1, Vol. III: Sensory Processes. Baltimore, Waverly Press, 1984.

Freides, D.: Human information processing and sensory modality: Cross-modal functions, information complexity, memory, and deficit. *Psychol. Bull.,* 81:284, 1974.

Friesen, W. O., and Stent, G. S.: Neural circuits for generating rhythmic movements. *Annu. Rev. Biophys. Bioeng.,* 7:37, 1978.

Gilbert, C. D.: Microcircuitry of the visual cortex. *Annu. Rev. Neurosci.,* 6:217, 1983.

Grinnell, A. D.: Specificity of neurons and their interconnections. *In* Brookhart, J. M., and Mountcastle, V. B. (eds.): Handbook of Physiology. Sec. 1, Vol. 1. Baltimore, Williams & Wilkins, 1977, p. 803.

Henneman, E., and Mendell, L. M.: Functional organization of motoneuron pool and its inputs. *In* Brooks, V. B. (ed.): Handbook of Physiology. Sec. 1, Vol. II. Bethesda, American Physiological Society, 1981, p. 423.

Kalia, M. P.: Anatomical organization of central respiratory neurons. *Annu. Rev. Physiol.,* 43:105, 1981.

Kandel, E. R.: Small systems of neurons. *Sci. Am. 241*(3):66, 1979.

Karlin, A., *et al.* (eds.): Neuronal Information Transfer. New York, Academic Press, 1978.

Kennedy, D., and Davis, W. J.: Organization of invertebrate motor systems. *In* Brookhart, J. M., and Mountcastle, V. B. (eds.): Handbook of Physiology. Sec. 1, Vol. 1. Baltimore, Williams & Wilkins, 1977, p. 1023.

Laduron, P. M.: Presynaptic heteroreceptors in regulation of neuronal transmission. *Biochem. Pharmacol.,* 34:467, 1985.

Levi-Montalcini, R., and Calissano, P.: The nerve-growth factor. *Sci. Am. 240*(6):68, 1979.

Mendell, L. M.: Modifiability of spinal synapses. *Physiol. Rev.,* 64:260, 1984.

Mountcastle, V. B.: Central nervous mechanisms in mechanoreceptive sensibility. *In* Darian-Smith, I. (ed.): Handbook of Physiology. Sec. 1, Vol. III. Bethesda, American Physiological Society, 1984, p. 789.

Nicholls, J. C., and Van Essen, D.: The nervous system of the leech. *Sci. Am.,* 230:38, 1974.

Pinsker, H. M., and Willis, W. D., Jr. (eds.): Information Processing in the Nervous System. New York, Raven Press, 1980.

Purves, D., and Lichtman, J. W.: Formation and maintenance of synaptic connections in autonomic ganglia. *Physiol. Rev.,* 58:821, 1978.

Purves, D., and Lichtman, J. W.: Specific connections between nerve cells. *Annu. Rev. Physiol.,* 45:553, 1983.

Rovainen, C. M.: Neurobiology of lampreys. *Physiol. Rev.,* 59:1007, 1979.

Sachs, M. B.: Neural coding of complex sounds: Speech. *Annu. Rev. Physiol.,* 46:261, 1984.

Shepherd, B. M.: The Synaptic Organization of the Brain: an Introduction. New York, Oxford University Press, 1974.

Shepherd, G. M.: Microcircuits in the nervous system. *Sci. Am.,* 238(2):92, 1978.

Sherman, S. M., and Spear, P. D.: Organization of visual pathways in normal and visually deprived cats. *Physiol. Rev.,* 62:738, 1982.

Sobel, I., *et al.*: Special techniques for the automatic computer reconstruction of neuronal structures. *Annu. Rev. Biophys. Bioeng.,* 9:347, 1980.

Stein, J. F.: Introduction to Neurophysiology. St. Louis, C. V. Mosby, 1982.

Sterling, P.: Microcircuitry of the cat retina. *Annu. Rev. Neurosci.,* 6:149, 1983.

Su, C.: Purinergic neurotransmission and neuromodulation. *Annu. Rev. Pharmacol. Toxicol.,* 23:397, 1983.

Szentagothai, J., *et al.* (eds.): Conceptual Models of Neural Organization. Neurosciences Research Program. Cambridge, Mass., Massachusetts Institute of Technology, 1974.

Uttley, A. M.: Information Transmission in the Nervous System. New York, Academic Press, 1979.

Wong, R. K., *et al.*: Local circuit interactions in synchronization of cortical neurones. *J. Exp. Biol.,* 112:169, 1984.

Wooldridge, D. E.: Sensory Processing in the Brain: An Exercise in Neuroconnective Modeling. New York, John Wiley & Sons, 1979.

12

Sensory Receptors and Their Basic Mechanisms of Action

Input to the nervous system is provided by the sensory receptors that detect such sensory stimuli as touch, sound, light, pain, cold, warmth, and so forth. The purpose of this chapter is to discuss the basic mechanisms by which these receptors change sensory stimuli into nerve signals and, also, how both the type of sensory stimulus and its strength are detected by the brain.

TYPES OF SENSORY RECEPTORS AND THE SENSORY STIMULI THEY DETECT

The student of physiology will have already studied many different anatomical types of nerve endings, and Table 12–1 gives a list and classification of most of the body's sensory receptors. This table shows that there are basically five different types of sensory receptors: (1) *mechanoreceptors*, which detect mechanical deformation of the receptor or of cells adjacent to the receptor; (2) *thermoreceptors*, which detect changes in temperature, some receptors detecting cold and others warmth; (3) *nociceptors*, which detect damage in the tissues, whether it be physical damage or chemical damage; (4) *electromagnetic receptors*, which detect light on the retina of the eye; and (5) *chemoreceptors*, which detect taste in the mouth, smell in the nose, oxygen level in the arterial blood, osmolality of the body fluids, carbon dioxide concentration, and perhaps other factors that make up the chemistry of the body.

This chapter will discuss the function of a few specific types of receptors, primarily peripheral mechanoreceptors, to illustrate some of the basic principles by which receptors in general operate. Other receptors will be discussed in relation to the sensory systems that they subserve. Figure 12–1 illustrates some of the different types of mechanoreceptors found in the skin or in the deep structures of the body, and Table 12–1 gives their respective sensory functions. All these receptors will be discussed in the following chapters in relation to the respective sensory systems. However, the functions

of some of these are described for illustrative purposes in this chapter as well.

DIFFERENTIAL SENSITIVITY OF RECEPTORS

The first question that must be answered is, how do two types of sensory receptors detect different types of sensory stimuli? The answer is by virtue of differential sensitivities. That is, each type of receptor is very highly sensitive to one type of stimulus for which it is designed and yet is almost nonresponsive to normal intensities of the other types of sensory stimuli. Thus, the rods and cones are highly responsive to light but are almost completely nonresponsive to heat, cold, pressure on the eyeballs, or chemical changes in the blood. The osmoreceptors of the supraoptic nuclei in the hypothalamus detect minute changes in the osmolality of the body fluids but have never been known to respond to sound. Finally, pain receptors in the skin are almost never stimulated by usual touch or pressure stimuli but do become highly active the moment tactile stimuli become severe enough to damage the tissues.

Modality of Sensation— The "Labeled Line" Principle

Each of the principal types of sensation that we can experience—pain, touch, sight, sound, and so forth—is called a *modality* of sensation. Yet, despite the fact that we experience these different modalities of sensation, nerve fibers transmit only impulses. Therefore, how is it that different nerve fibers transmit different modalities of sensation?

The answer to this is that each nerve tract terminates at a specific point in the central nervous system and the type of sensation felt when a nerve fiber is stimulated is determined by this point in the nervous system to which the fiber leads. For instance, if a pain fiber is stimulated, the person perceives pain regardless of what type of stimulus excites the fiber. The stimulus can be electricity,

Table 12–1. CLASSIFICATION OF SENSORY
RECEPTORS

Mechanoreceptors
Skin tactile sensibilities (epidermis and dermis)
   Free nerve endings
   Expanded tip endings
      Merkel's discs
      Plus several other variants
   Spray endings
      Ruffini's endings
   Encapsulated endings
      Meissner's corpuscles
      Krause's corpuscles
   Hair end-organs
Deep tissue sensibilities
   Free nerve endings
   Expanded tip endings
      Plus a few other variants
   Spray endings
      Ruffini's endings
   Encapsulated endings
      Pacinian corpuscles
      Plus a few other variants
   Muscle endings
      Muscle spindles
      Golgi tendon receptors
Hearing
   Sound receptors of cochlea
Equilibrium
   Vestibular receptors
Arterial pressure
   Baroreceptors of carotid sinuses and aorta

Thermoreceptors
Cold
   Cold receptors
Warmth
   Warm receptors

Nociceptors
Pain
   Free nerve endings

Electromagnetic Receptors
Vision
   Rods
   Cones

Chemoreceptors
Taste
   Receptors of taste buds
Smell
   Receptors of olfactory epithelium
Arterial oxygen
   Receptors of aortic and carotid bodies
Osmolality
   Probably neurons of supraoptic nuclei
Blood CO_2
   Receptors in or on surface of medulla and in aortic and carotid
      bodies
Blood glucose, amino acids, fatty acids
   Receptors in hypothalamus

heat, crushing, or stimulation of the pain nerve ending by damage to the tissue cells. Yet, whatever the means of stimulation, the person still perceives pain. Likewise, if a touch fiber is stimulated by exciting a touch receptor electrically or in any other way, the person perceives touch because touch fibers lead to specific touch areas in the brain. Similarly, fibers from the retina of the eye terminate in the vision areas of the brain, fibers from the ear terminate in the auditory areas of the brain, and temperature fibers terminate in the temperature areas.

This specificity of nerve fibers for transmitting only one modality of sensation is called the *"labeled line"* principle.

TRANSDUCTION OF SENSORY STIMULI INTO NERVE IMPULSES

LOCAL CURRENTS AT NERVE ENDINGS— RECEPTOR POTENTIALS

All sensory receptors have one feature in common. Whatever the type of stimulus that excites the receptor, its immediate effect is to change the potential across the receptor membrane. This change in potential is called a *receptor potential*.

Mechanisms of Receptor Potentials. Different receptors can be excited in several different ways to cause receptor potentials: (1) by mechanical deformation of the receptor, which stretches the membrane and opens ion channels; (2) by application of a chemical to the membrane, which also opens ion channels; (3) by change of the temperature of the membrane, which alters the permeability of the membrane; or (4) by the effects of electromagnetic radiation such as light on the receptor, which either directly or indirectly changes the membrane characteristics and allows ions to flow through membrane channels. It will be recognized that these four different means for exciting receptors correspond in general with the different types of known sensory

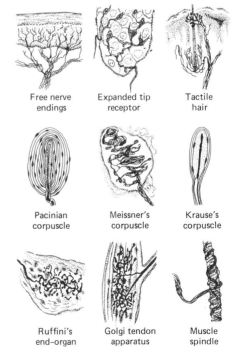

Figure 12–1. Several types of somatic sensory nerve endings.

Free nerve endings   Expanded tip receptor   Tactile hair

Pacinian corpuscle   Meissner's corpuscle   Krause's corpuscle

Ruffini's end-organ   Golgi tendon apparatus   Muscle spindle

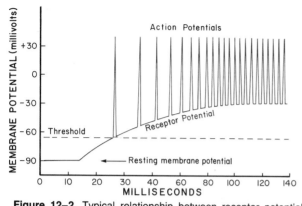

Figure 12–2. Typical relationship between receptor potential and action potentials when the receptor potential rises above the threshold level.

receptors. In all instances, the basic cause of the change in membrane potential is a change in receptor membrane permeability, which allows ions to diffuse more or less readily through the membrane and thereby change the transmembrane potential.

Relationship of the Receptor Potential to Action Potentials. When the receptor potential rises above the threshold for eliciting action potentials in the nerve fiber attached to the receptor, then action potentials begin to appear. This is illustrated in Figure 12–2. Note also that the more the receptor potential rises above the threshold level, the greater becomes the action potential frequency. Thus, the receptor potential stimulates the terminal nerve fiber in the same way that the excitatory postsynaptic potential stimulates neurons in the central nervous system.

Illustrative Examples of Receptor Function

The Receptor Potential of the Pacinian Corpuscle. The pacinian corpuscle is a very large and easily dissected sensory receptor. For this reason, one can study in detail the mechanism by which tactile stimuli excite it and by which it causes action potentials in the sensory nerve fiber leading from it. Note in Figure 12–3 that the pacinian corpuscle has a central nonmyelinated tip of a nerve fiber

extending through its core. Surrounding this fiber are many concentric capsule layers, as shown in Figure 12–1, so that compression on the outside of the corpuscle tends to elongate, indent, or otherwise deform the central core of the fiber, depending on how the compression is applied. This deformation causes sudden opening of ion channels that mainly carry positively charged sodium ions to the interior of the fiber. This in turn creates more positivity in the fiber, which is the receptor potential. The receptor potential in turn induces a local circuit of current flow that spreads along the nerve fiber. At the first node of Ranvier, which itself lies inside the capsule of the pacinian corpuscle, the local current flow initiates action potentials in the fiber. That is, the current flow through the node depolarizes it, and this then sets off a typical action potential that is transmitted along the nerve fiber toward the central nervous system.

Relationship Between Stimulus Strength and the Receptor Potential. Figure 12–4 illustrates the effect on the amplitude of the receptor potential caused by progressively stronger mechanical compression applied experimentally to the central core of the pacinian corpuscle. Note that the amplitude increases rapidly at first but then progressively less rapidly at high stimulus strengths. The maximum amplitude that can be achieved by receptor potentials is around 100 millivolts. That is, a receptor potential can have almost as high a voltage as an action potential.

Relationship of Amplitude of Receptor Potential to Nerve Impulse Rate. The frequency of action potentials in the nerve fiber (impulse rate) is almost directly proportional to the amplitude of the receptor potential. This relationship is illustrated in Figure 12–5, which shows the impulse rate corresponding to different receptor potential amplitudes recorded from a muscle spindle; there is an almost exact proportional relationship. This same relationship between receptor potential and impulse rate is approximately true for most sensory receptors.

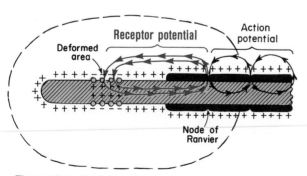

Figure 12–3. Excitation of a sensory nerve fiber by a receptor potential produced in a pacinian corpuscle. (Modified from Loëwenstein: *Ann. N.Y. Acad. Sci., 94:*510, 1961.)

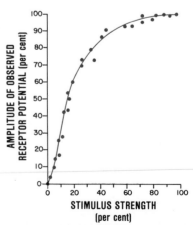

Figure 12–4. Relationship of amplitude of receptor potential to strength of a stimulus applied to a pacinian corpuscle. (From Loëwenstein: *Ann. N.Y. Acad. Sci., 94:*510, 1961.)

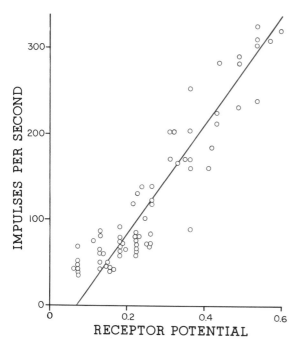

Figure 12–5. Relationship between the receptor potential of a muscle spindle and the frequency of sensory impulses transmitted from the spindle. (From Katz: *J. Physiol. [Lond.]. 111*:261, 1950.)

ADAPTATION OF RECEPTORS

A special characteristic of all sensory receptors is that they *adapt* either partially or completely to their stimuli after a period of time. That is, when a continuous sensory stimulus is applied, the receptors respond at first with a very high impulse rate, then at a progressively lower rate until finally many of them no longer respond at all.

Figure 12–6 illustrates typical adaptation of certain types of receptors. Note that the pacinian corpuscle adapts extremely rapidly and hair receptors adapt within a second or so, while joint capsule and muscle spindle receptors adapt very slowly.

Furthermore some sensory receptors adapt to a far greater extent than others. For example, the pacinian corpuscles adapt to "extinction" within a few thousandths to a few hundredths of a second, and the hair base receptors adapt to extinction within a second or more. It is probable that all other *mechanoreceptors* also adapt completely eventually, but some require hours or days to do so, for which reason they are frequently called "nonadapting" receptors. The longest measured time for complete adaptation of a mechanoreceptor is about two days for the carotid and aortic baroreceptors.

Some of the other types of receptors, the chemoreceptors and pain receptors for instance, probably never adapt completely. Each of these will be discussed in turn in subsequent chapters.

Mechanisms by Which Receptors Adapt. Adaptation of receptors is an individual property of each type of receptor in much the same way that development of a receptor potential is an individual

property. For instance, in the eye, the rods and cones adapt by changing their chemical compositions (which will be discussed in Chapter 23). In the case of the mechanoreceptors, the receptor that has been studied for adaptation in greatest detail is the pacinian corpuscle. Adaptation occurs in this receptor in two ways. First, the corpuscular structure itself very rapidly adapts to the deformation of the tissue. This can be explained as follows: The pacinian corpuscle is a viscoelastic structure, so that when a distorting force is suddenly applied to one side of the corpuscle this force is instantly transmitted by the viscous component of the corpuscle directly to the same side of the central core, thus eliciting the receptor potential. However, within a few thousandths to a few hundredths of a second the fluid within the corpuscle redistributes so that the pressure becomes essentially equal all through the corpuscle; this now applies an even pressure on all sides of the central core fiber, so that the receptor potential is no longer elicited. Thus, the receptor potential appears at the onset of compression but then disappears within a small fraction of a second even though the compression continues.

Then, when the distorting force is removed from the corpuscle, essentially the reverse events occur. The sudden removal of the distortion from one side of the corpuscle allows rapid expansion on that side, and a corresponding distortion of the central core occurs once more. Again, within milliseconds, the pressure becomes equalized all through the corpuscle and the stimulus is lost. Nevertheless, this disturbance of the central core fiber signals the termination of compression as well as the onset of compression.

The second mechanism of adaptation of the pacinian corpuscle, but a much slower one, results from a process called *accommodation* that occurs in the nerve fiber itself. That is, even if by chance the central core fiber should continue to be excited, as can be achieved after the capsule has been removed and the core is compressed with a stylus, the tip of the nerve fiber itself gradually becomes "accommodated" to the stimulus. This probably results

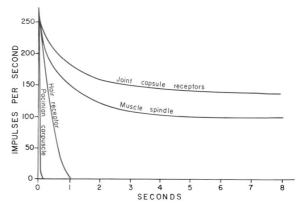

Figure 12–6. Adaptation of different types of receptors, showing rapid adaptation of some receptors and slow adaptation of others.

from "inactivation" of the sodium channels in the nerve fiber membrane, which means that the current flow itself through the channels in some way causes them gradually to close, as was explained in Chapter 6.

Presumably, these same two general mechanisms of adaptation apply to other types of mechanoreceptors. That is, part of the adaptation results from readjustments in the structure of the receptor itself, and part results from accommodation in the terminal nerve fibril.

Function of the Slowly Adapting and Nonadapting Receptors to Detect Continuous Stimulus Strength—The "Tonic" Receptors. The slowly adapting receptors continue to transmit impulses to the brain as long as the stimulus is present (or at least for many minutes or hours). Therefore, they keep the brain constantly apprised of the status of the body and its relation to its surroundings. For instance, impulses from the slowly adapting joint capsule receptors allow the person to "know" at all times the degree of bending of the joints and therefore the positions of the different parts of the body. And impulses from the muscle spindles and Golgi tendon apparatuses allow the central nervous system to know respectively the status of muscle contraction and the load on the muscle tendon at each instant.

Other types of slowly adapting receptors include the receptors of the macula in the vestibular apparatus, the pain receptors, the baroreceptors of the arterial tree, the chemoreceptors of the carotid and aortic bodies, and some of the tactile receptors, such as the Ruffini endings and the Merkel's discs.

Because the slowly adapting receptors can continue to transmit information for many hours, they are also called *tonic* receptors. Many of these slowly adapting receptors will adapt to extinction if the intensity of the stimulus remains absolutely constant for several hours or days. Fortunately, because of our continually changing bodily state, these receptors almost never reach a state of complete adaptation.

Function of the Rapidly Adapting Receptors to Detect Change in Stimulus Strength—The "Rate Receptors" or "Movement Receptors" or "Phasic Receptors." Obviously, receptors that adapt rapidly cannot be used to transmit a continuous signal because these receptors are stimulated only when the stimulus strength changes. Yet they react strongly *while a change is actually taking place*. Furthermore, the number of impulses transmitted is directly related to the *rate at which the change takes place*. Therefore, these receptors are called *rate* receptors, *movement* receptors, or *phasic* receptors. Thus, in the case of the pacinian corpuscle, sudden pressure applied to the skin excites this receptor for a few milliseconds, and then its excitation is over even though the pressure continues. But then it transmits a signal again when the pressure is released. In other words, the pacinian corpuscle is

exceedingly important for transmitting information about rapid changes in pressure against the body, but it is useless for transmitting information about constant pressure applied to the body.

Importance of the Rate Receptors—Their Predictive Function. If one knows the rate at which some change in bodily status is taking place, one can predict the state of the body a few seconds or even a few minutes later. For instance, the receptors of the semicircular canals in the vestibular apparatus of the ear detect the rate at which the head begins to turn when one runs around a curve. Using this information, a person can predict a turn of 10, 30, or some other number of degrees within the next 10 seconds and can adjust the motion of the limbs *ahead of time* to keep from losing balance. Likewise, pacinian corpuscles and other receptors located in or near the joint capsules help detect the rates of movement of the different parts of the body. Therefore, when one is running, information from these receptors allows the nervous system to predict where the feet will be during any precise fraction of a second, and appropriate motor signals can be transmitted to the muscles of the legs to make any necessary anticipatory corrections in limb position so that the person will not fall. Loss of this predictive function makes it impossible for the person to run.

PSYCHIC INTERPRETATION OF STIMULUS STRENGTH

The ultimate goal of most sensory stimulation is to apprise the psyche of the state of the body and its surroundings. Therefore, it is important that we discuss briefly some of the principles related to the transmission of sensory stimulus strength to the higher levels of the nervous system.

The first question that comes to mind is: How is it possible for the sensory system to transmit sensory experiences of tremendously varying intensities? For instance, the auditory system can detect the weakest possible whisper but can also discern the meanings of an explosive sound only a few feet away, even though the sound intensities of these two experiences can vary more than ten billion fold; the eyes can see visual images with light intensities that vary as much as a half million fold; or the skin can detect pressure differences of ten thousand to one hundred thousand fold.

As a partial explanation of these effects, note in Figure 12–4 the relationship of the receptor potential produced by the pacinian corpuscle to the strength of stimulus. At low stimulus strength, very slight changes in stimulus strength increase the potential markedly, whereas at high levels of stimulus strength further increases in receptor potential are very slight. Thus, the pacinian corpuscle is capable of accurately measuring extremely minute changes in stimulus strength at low intensity levels, but at high intensity levels the change in stimulus strength must be much greater to cause the same amount of change in receptor potential.

The transduction mechanism for detecting sound by the cochlea of the ear illustrates still another method for separating gradations of stimulus intensity. When sound causes vibration at a specific point on the basilar membrane, weak vibration stimulates only those hair cells at the point of maximum vibration. But, as the vibration intensity increases, not only do these hair cells become more intensely stimulated, but still many more hair cells in each direction farther away from the maximum vibratory point also become stimulated. Thus, signals transmitted over progressively increasing numbers of cochlear nerve fibers is another mechanism by which stimulus strength is transmitted into the central nervous system. This mechanism plus the direct effect of stimulus strength on impulse rate in each nerve fiber, as well as several other mechanisms, makes it possible for the ear to operate reasonably faithfully at stimulus intensity levels changing more than ten billionfold.

Importance of the Tremendous Intensity Range of Sensory Reception. Were it not for the tremendous intensity range of sensory reception that we can experience, the various sensory systems would more often than not operate in the wrong range. This is illustrated by the attempts of most persons to adjust the light exposure on a camera without using a light meter. Left to intuitive judgment of light intensity, a person almost always overexposes the film on very bright days and greatly underexposes the film at twilight. Yet, that person's eyes are capable of discriminating with great detail the surrounding objects in both very bright sunlight and at twilight; the camera cannot do this because of the narrow critical range of light intensity required for proper exposure of film.

JUDGMENT OF STIMULUS STRENGTH

Physiopsychologists have evolved numerous methods for testing one's judgment of sensory stimulus strength, but only rarely do the results from the different methods agree with each other. For instance, one testing method requests the subject to select a weight that is exactly 100 per cent heavier than another. But the person usually selects a weight that is about 50 per cent heavier instead of 100 per cent heavier. Thus, the weak stimulus is underestimated and the strong stimulus is overestimated. In still another test procedure, a person is given a weight to hold and is then required to select the minimum amount of additional weight that must be added to detect a difference. In this case the person might be holding a 30 gram weight and finds that an additional 1 gram is needed to detect a difference. Then the person holds a 300 gram weight and finds that 10 grams of additional weight are required. In this instance the discriminatory ability is far greater at the low intensity level than at the high intensity level. Thus, the results of these two different types of tests are exactly opposite to each other, which means that the real argument lies in the meaning of the tests themselves. Therefore, at present no real agreement exists as to a proper method for measuring one's judgment of stimulus strength. Yet, two principles are widely discussed in the physiopsychology field of sensory interpretation: the *Weber-Fechner principle* and the *power principle*.

The Weber-Fechner Principle—Detection of ''Ratio'' of Stimulus Strength. In the mid-1800s, Weber first and Fechner later proposed the principle that *gradations of stimulus strength are discriminated approximately in proportion to the logarithm of stimulus strength*. This principle is based

primarily on one's ability to judge minimal *changes* in stimulus strength. That is, in the second test described in the previous section the person could barely detect a 1 gram increase in weight when holding 30 grams, or a 10 gram increase when holding 300 grams. Thus, the *ratio* of the change in stimulus strength required for detection of a change remained essentially constant, about 1 to 30, which is what the logarithmic principle means. To express this mathematically,

Interpreted signal strength = log (Stimulus) + Constant

Because the Weber-Fechner principle offers a ready explanation for the tremendous range of stimulus strength that our nervous system can discern, it unfortunately became widely accepted for all types of sensory experience and for all levels of background sensory intensity. More recently it has become evident that this principle applies mainly to higher intensities of visual, auditory, and cutaneous sensory experience and it applies only poorly to most other types of sensory experience.

Yet, the Weber-Fechner principle is still a good one to remember because it emphasizes that the greater the background sensory stimulus, the greater also must be the additional change in stimulus strength in order for the psyche to detect the change.

The Power Law. Another attempt by physiopsychologists to find a good mathematical relationship between actual stimulus strength and interpretation of stimulus strength is the following formula, known as the power law:

Interpreted signal strength = K · (Stimulus − k) ^{y}

In this formula K and k are constants, and y is the power to which the stimulus strength is raised. The exponent y and the constants K and k are different for each type of sensation.

When this power law relationship is plotted on a graph using double logarithmic coordinates, as illustrated in Figure 12–7, a linear relationship can be attained between interpreted stimulus strength and actual stimulus strength over a large range for almost any type of sensory

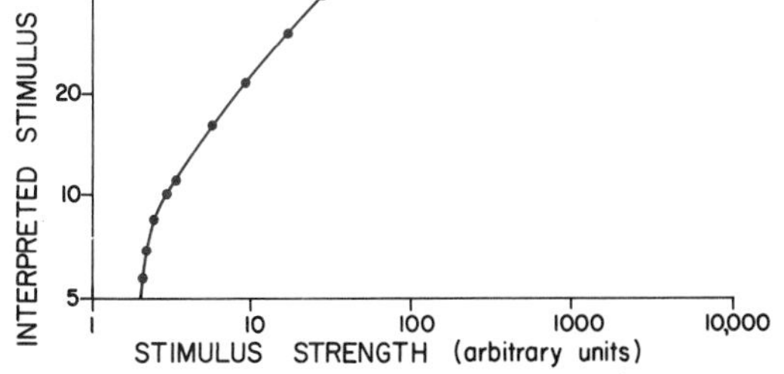

Figure 12–7. Graphical demonstration of the "power law" relationship between actual stimulus strength and strength that the psyche interprets it to be. Note that the power law does not hold at either very weak or very strong stimulus strengths.

perception. However, as illustrated in the figure, even this power law relationship fails to hold satisfactorily at both very low and very high stimulus strengths.

PHYSIOLOGICAL CLASSIFICATION OF NERVE FIBERS

Some sensory signals need to be transmitted to the central nervous system extremely rapidly, or otherwise the information would be useless. An example of this is the sensory signals that apprise the brain of the momentary positions of the limbs at each fraction of a second during running. It is important that this information be transmitted by way of extremely rapidly conducting nerve fibers. At the other extreme, some types of sensory information, such as that depicting prolonged, aching pain, do not need to be transmitted rapidly at all, so that very slowly conducting fibers will suffice. Fortunately, nerve fibers come in all sizes between 0.2 and 20 microns in diameter—the larger the diameter, the greater the conducting velocity. The range of conducting velocities is between 0.5 and 120 meters per second.

Figure 12–8 gives two different classifications of nerve fibers that are in general use. One of these is a general classification that includes both sensory and motor fibers, including the autonomic nerve fibers as well. The other is a classification of sensory nerve fibers that is used primarily by sensory neurophysiologists.

In the general classification, the fibers are divided into types A and C, and the type A fibers are further subdivided into α, β, γ, and δ fibers.

Type A fibers are the typical myelinated fibers of spinal nerves. Type C fibers are the very small, unmyelinated nerve fibers that conduct impulses at low velocities. These constitute more than half the sensory fibers in most peripheral nerves and also all of the post-ganglionic autonomic fibers.

The sizes, velocities of conduction, and functions of the different nerve fiber types are given in the figure. Note that the very large fibers can transmit impulses at velocities as great as 120 meters per second, a distance in one second that is longer than a football field. On the other hand, the smallest fibers transmit impulses as slowly as 0.5 meter per second, requiring about 2 seconds to go from the big toe to the spinal cord.

Over two thirds of all the nerve fibers in peripheral nerves are type C fibers. Because of their great number, these can transmit tremendous amounts of information from the surface of the body, even though their velocities of transmission are very slow. Utilization of type C fibers for transmitting this great mass of information represents an important economy of space in the nerves, for use of the larger type A fibers for transmitting all information would require peripheral nerves the size of large ropes and a spinal cord almost as large as the body itself.

Alternate Classification Used by Sensory Physiologists. Certain recording techniques have made it possible to separate the type Aα fibers into two subgroups, yet these same recording techniques cannot distinguish easily

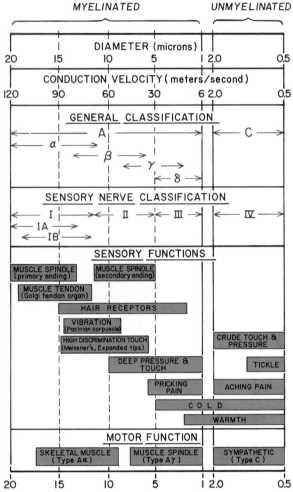

Figure 12–8. Physiological classifications and functions of nerve fibers.

between Aβ and Aγ fibers. Therefore, the following classification is frequently used by sensory physiologists:

Group Ia. Fibers from the annulospiral endings of muscle spindles. (Average about 17 microns in diameter. These are alpha type A fibers in the general classification.)

Group Ib. Fibers from the Golgi tendon organs. (Average about 16 microns in diameter; these also are alpha type A fibers.)

Group II. Fibers from the discrete cutaneous tactile receptors and also from the flower-spray endings of the muscle spindles. (Average about 8 microns in diameter; these are beta and gamma type A fibers in the other classification.)

Group III. Fibers carrying temperature, crude touch, and pricking pain sensations. (Average about 3 microns in diameter; these are delta type A fibers in the other classification.)

Group IV. Unmyelinated fibers carrying pain, itch, temperature, and crude touch sensations. (These are 0.5 to 2 microns in diameter; called type C fibers in the other classification.)

REFERENCES

American Physiological Society: Sensory Processes. Washington, D.C., American Physiological Society, 1984.

Anderson, D. J., *et al.*: Sensory mechanisms in mammalian teeth and their supporting structures. *Physiol. Rev., 50*:171, 1970.

Anstis, S. M., *et al.*: Perception. New York, Springer-Verlag, 1978.

Babel, J., *et al.*: Ultrastructure of the Peripheral Nervous System and Sense Organs. New York, Churchill Livingstone, 1971.

Bate, C. M., *et al.*: Development of Sensory System. New York, Springer-Verlag, 1978.

Bennett, T. L.: The Sensory World: An Introduction to Sensation and Perception. Monterey, Cal., Brooks/Cole Publishing Co., 1978.

Brown, E., and Deffenbacher, K.: Perception and the Senses. New York, Oxford University Press, 1979.

Brown, M.: Touch Will Tell. New York, Franklin Watts, 1979.

Catton, W. T.: Mechanoreceptor function. *Physiol. Rev., 50*:297, 1970.

Coren, S., *et al.*: Sensation and Perception. New York, Academic Press, 1979.

Darian-Smith, I.: The sense of touch: Performance and peripheral neural processes. *In* Darian-Smith, I. (ed.): Handbook of Physiology. Sec. 1, Vol. III. Bethesda, American Physiological Society, 1984, p. 739.

Friedhoff, A. J., and Miller, J. C.: Clinical implications of receptor sensitivity modification. *Annu. Rev. Neurosci., 6*:121, 1983.

Goldstein, E. B.: Sensation and Perception. Belmont, Cal., Wadsworth Publishing Co., 1980.

Granit, R.: Receptors and Sensory Perception. New Haven, Conn., Yale University Press, 1955.

Gray, J. A. B.: Initiation of impulses at receptors. *In* Magoun, H. W. (ed.): Handbook of Physiology. Sec. 1, Vol. I. Baltimore, Williams & Wilkins, 1959.

Halata, Z.: The Mechanoreceptors of the Mammalian Skin. New York, Springer-Verlag, 1975.

Hochberg, J.: Perception. *In* Darian-Smith, I. (ed.): Handbook of Physiology. Sec. 1, Vol. III. Bethesda, American Physiological Society, 1984, p. 75.

Jung, R.: Sensory research in historical perspective: Some philosophical foundations of perception. *In* Darian-Smith, I. (ed.): Handbook of Physiology. Sec. 1, Vol. III. Bethesda, American Physiological Society, 1984, p. 1.

Loewenstein, W. R.: The generation of electrical activity in a nerve ending. *Ann. N.Y. Acad. Sci., 81*:367, 1959.

Loewenstein, W. R.: Excitation and inactivation in a receptor membrane. *Ann. N.Y. Acad. Sci., 94*:510, 1961.

Lynn, B.: Somatosensory receptors and their CNS connections. *Annu. Rev. Physiol., 37*:105, 1975.

McCloskey, D. I.: Kinesthetic sensibility. *Physiol. Rev., 58*:763, 1978.

Neff, W. D. (ed.): Contributions to Sensory Physiology. New York, Academic Press, 1982.

Paintal, A. A. (ed.): Morphology and Mechanisms of Chemoreceptors. Delhi, India, Vallabhbhai Patel Chest Institute, University of Delhi, 1976.

Porter, R. (ed.): Studies in Neurophysiology. New York, Cambridge University Press, 1978.

Schmidt, R. F. (ed.): Fundamentals of Sensory Physiology. New York, Springer-Verlag, 1978.

Somjen, G.: Sensory Coding in the Mammalian Nervous System. New York, Appleton-Century-Crofts, 1972.

Stebbins, W. C., Brown, C. H., and Petersen, M. R.: Sensory function in animals. *In* Darian-Smith, I. (ed.): Handbook of Physiology. Sec. 1, Vol. III. Bethesda, American Physiological Society, 1984, p. 123.

Thompson, R. F., and Patterson, M. (eds.): Bioelectric Recording Techniques, Part C. Receptor and Effector Processes. New York, Academic Press, 1974.

Weiss, T. F.: Relation of receptor potentials of cochlear hair cells to spike discharges of cochlear neurons. *Annu. Rev. Physiol., 46*:247, 1984.

Wiederhold, M. L.: Mechanosensory transduction in "sensory" and "motile" cilia. *Annu. Rev. Biophys. Bioeng., 5*:39, 1976.

Wiersma, C. A. G., and Roach, J. L. M.: Principles in the organization of invertebrate sensory systems. *In* Brookhart, J. M., and Mountcastle, V. B. (eds.): *Handbook of Physiology*. Sec. 1, Vol. 1. Baltimore, Williams & Wilkins, 1977, p. 1089.

Zimmermann, M.: Neurophysiology of nociception. *Int. Rev. Physiol., 10*:179, 1976.

13

Somatic Sensations: I. The Mechanoreceptive Sensations

The *somatic senses* are the nervous mechanisms that collect sensory information from the body. These senses are in contradistinction to the *special senses*, which mean specifically vision, hearing, smell, taste, and equilibrium.

CLASSIFICATION OF SOMATIC SENSES

The somatic senses can be classified into three different physiological types: (1) the *mechanoreceptive somatic senses*, stimulated by mechanical displacement of some tissue of the body, (2) the *thermoreceptive senses*, which detect heat and cold, and (3) the *pain sense*, which is activated by any factor that damages the tissues. This chapter deals with the mechanoreceptive somatic senses, and the following chapter discusses the thermoreceptive and pain senses.

The mechanoreceptive senses include *touch, pressure, vibration,* and *tickle* senses (which are frequently called the *tactile senses*) and the *position sense*, which determines the relative positions and rates of movement of the different parts of the body.

Other Classifications of Somatic Sensations. Different types of somatic sensations are also grouped together in special classes that are not necessarily mutually exclusive, as follows:

Exteroreceptive sensations are those from the surface of the body. *Proprioceptive sensations* are those having to do with the physical state of the body, including position sensations, tendon and muscle sensations, pressure sensations from the bottom of the feet, and even the sensation of equilibrium, which is generally considered to be a "special" sensation rather than a somatic sensation.

Visceral sensations are those from the viscera of the body; in using this term one usually refers specifically to sensations from the internal organs.

The *deep sensations* are those that come from the deep tissues, such as from fasciae, muscles, bone, and so forth. These include mainly "deep" pressure, pain, and vibration.

DETECTION AND TRANSMISSION OF TACTILE SENSATIONS

Interrelationship Between the Tactile Sensations of Touch, Pressure, and Vibration. Though touch, pressure, and vibration are frequently classified as separate sensations, they are all detected by the same types of receptors. The only differences among these three are (1) touch sensation generally results from stimulation of tactile receptors in the skin or in tissues immediately beneath the skin, (2) pressure sensation generally results from deformation of deeper tissues, and (3) vibration sensation results from rapidly repetitive sensory signals, but some of the same types of receptors as those for touch and pressure are utilized—specifically the very rapidly adapting types of receptors.

The Tactile Receptors. At least six entirely different types of tactile receptors are known, but many more similar to these also exist. Some of these receptors were illustrated in Figure 12–1 of Chapter 12, and their special characteristics are the following:

First, some *free nerve endings*, which are found everywhere in the skin and in many other tissues, can detect touch and pressure. For instance, even light contact with the cornea of the eye, which contains no other type of nerve ending besides free nerve endings, can nevertheless elicit touch and pressure sensations.

Second, a touch receptor of special sensitivity is *Meissner's corpuscle*, an encapsulated nerve ending that excites a large (type Aβ) myelinated sensory nerve fiber. Inside the capsulation are many whorls of terminal nerve filaments. These receptors are present in the nonhairy parts of the skin (called *glabrous skin*) and are particularly abundant in the fingertips, lips, and other areas of the skin where one's ability to discern spatial characteristics of touch sensations is highly developed. They, along with the expanded tip receptors described subsequently, are mainly responsible for the ability to recognize exactly what point of the body is touched and to recognize the texture of objects touched. Meissner's corpuscles adapt in a fraction of a second after they are stimulated, which means that they are particularly sensitive to movement of very light objects over the surface of the skin and also to low frequency vibration.

Third, the fingertips and other areas that contain large numbers of Meissner's corpuscles also contain large numbers of *expanded tip tactile receptors*, one type of which is *Merkel's discs*. The hairy parts of the skin also contain moderate numbers of expanded tip receptors, even though they have almost no Meissner's corpuscles. These receptors differ from Meissner's corpuscles in that they transmit an initially strong but partially adapting signal and then a continuing weaker signal that adapts only slowly. Therefore, they are responsible for giving steady state signals that allow one to determine continuous touch of objects against the skin. Merkel's discs are often grouped together in a single receptor organ called the *Iggo dome receptor*, which projects upward against the underside of the epithelium of the skin, as illustrated in Figure 13–1. This causes the epithelium at this point to protrude outward, thus creating a dome. Also note that the entire group of Merkel's discs is innervated by a single large type of myelinated nerve fiber (type Aβ). Each dome receptor has a diameter averaging only 0.2 mm, and these receptors are extremely sensitive. They probably play an important role in localizing touch sensations to the specific surface areas of the body.

Fourth, slight movement of any hair on the body stimulates the nerve fiber entwining its base. Thus, each hair and its basal nerve fiber, called the *hair end-organ*, is also a touch receptor. This receptor adapts readily and, therefore, like Meissner's corpuscles, detects mainly movement of objects on the surface of the body or initial contact with the body.

Fifth, located in the deeper layers of the skin and also in deeper tissues are many *Ruffini's end-organs*, which are multibranched, encapsulated endings, as described and illustrated in the previous chapter. These endings adapt very little and, therefore, are important for signaling continuous states of deformation of the skin and deeper tissues, such as heavy and continuous touch signals and pressure signals. They are also found in joint capsules and help signal the degree of joint rotation.

Sixth, *pacinian corpuscles*, which were discussed in detail in Chapter 12, lie both immediately beneath the skin and also deep in the fascial tissues of the body. These are stimulated only by very rapid movement of the tissues because they adapt in a few thousandths or a few hundredths of a second. Therefore, they are particularly important for detecting tissue vibration or other extremely rapid changes in the mechanical state of the tissues.

Transmission of Tactile Sensations in Peripheral Nerve Fibers. Almost all the specialized sensory receptors, such as Meissner's corpuscles, Iggo dome receptors, hair receptors, pacinian corpuscles, and Ruffini's endings, transmit their signals in type Aβ nerve fibers that have transmission velocities of 30 to 70 meters per second. On the other hand, free nerve ending tactile receptors transmit signals mainly via the small type Aδ myelinated fibers that conduct at velocities of 5 to 30 meters per second. Some tactile free nerve endings transmit via type C unmyelinated fibers at velocities from a fraction of a meter up to 2 meters per second; these send signals into the spinal cord and lower brain stem, probably subserving mainly the sensation of tickle. Thus, the more critical types of sensory signals— those that help to determine precise localization on the skin, minute gradations of intensity, or rapid changes in sensory signal intensity—are all transmitted in the rapidly conducting types of sensory nerve fibers. On the other hand, the cruder types

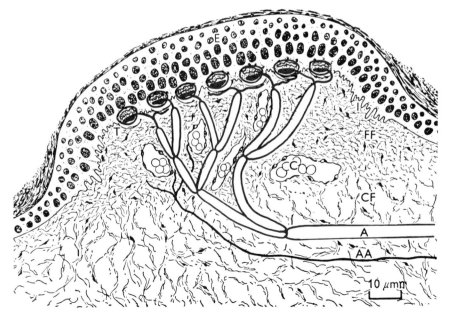

Figure 13–1. The Iggo dome receptor. Note the multiple numbers of Merkel's discs innervated by a single large myelinated fiber and abutting tightly the undersurface of the epithelium. (From Iggo and Muir: *J. Physiol.*, 200:763, 1969.)

of signals, such as crude pressure, poorly localized touch, and especially tickle, are transmitted via much slower nerve fibers that require much less space than the faster fibers.

DETECTION OF VIBRATION

All the different tactile receptors are involved in detection of vibration, though different receptors detect different frequencies of vibration. Pacinian corpuscles can signal vibrations from 60 to 500 cycles per second, because they respond extremely rapidly to minute and rapid deformations of the tissues, and they also transmit their signals over type Aβ nerve fibers, which can transmit more than 1000 impulses per second.

Low frequency vibrations up to 80 cycles per second, on the other hand, stimulate other tactile receptors—especially Meissner's corpuscles, which are less rapidly adapting than pacinian corpuscles.

TICKLING AND ITCH

Recent neurophysiological studies have demonstrated the existence of very sensitive, rapidly adapting mechanoreceptive free nerve endings that elicit only the tickle and itch sensation. Furthermore, these endings are found almost exclusively in the superficial layers of the skin, which is also the only tissue from which the tickle and itch sensation usually can be elicited. This sensation is transmitted by very small type C unmyelinated fibers similar to those that transmit the aching type of pain.

The purpose of the itch sensation is presumably to call attention to mild surface stimuli such as a flea crawling on the skin or a fly about to bite, and the elicited signals then excite the scratch reflex or other maneuvers that rid the host of the irritant.

The relief of itch by the process of scratching occurs only when the irritant is removed or when the scratch is strong enough to elicit pain. The pain signals are believed to suppress the itch signals in the cord by the process of inhibition that will be described in the following chapter.

THE DUAL SYSTEM FOR TRANSMISSION OF MECHANORECEPTIVE SOMATIC SENSORY SIGNALS INTO THE CENTRAL NERVOUS SYSTEM

Either all or almost all sensory information from the somatic segments of the body enters the spinal cord through the dorsal roots of the spinal nerves. However, from this point to the brain the sensory signals are carried through one of two alternate sensory pathways: the *dorsal column–lemniscal system*

and the *anterolateral system*. These two systems come together again at the level of the thalamus.

The dorsal column–lemniscal system, as its name implies, carries signals mainly in the *dorsal columns* of the cord and then upward through the brain stem to the thalamus by way of the *medial lemniscus*. On the other hand, signals of the anterolateral system, after originating in the dorsal horns of the spinal gray matter, cross to the opposite side of the cord and ascend through the cord in the anterior and lateral white columns to terminate at all levels of the lower brain stem and also in the thalamus.

The dorsal column–lemniscal system is composed of large myelinated nerve fibers that transmit signals to the brain at velocities of 30 to 110 meters per second, whereas the anterolateral system is composed of much smaller myelinated fibers (averaging 4 microns in diameter) that transmit signals at velocities ranging between 8 and 40 meters per second.

Another difference between the two systems is that the dorsal column–lemniscal system has a very high degree of spatial orientation of the nerve fibers with respect to their origin on the surface of the body, whereas the anterolateral system has a much smaller degree of spatial orientation, with some fibers seeming to have very little orientation at all.

These differences immediately characterize the types of sensory information that can be transmitted by the two systems. First, sensory information that must be transmitted rapidly and with temporal fidelity is transmitted in the dorsal column–lemniscal system, while that which does not need to be transmitted rapidly is transmitted mainly in the anterolateral system. Second, those sensations that detect fine gradations of intensity are transmitted in the dorsal column–lemniscal system, while those that lack the fine gradations are transmitted in the anterolateral system. And, third, sensations that are discretely localized to exact points in the body are transmitted in the dorsal system, while those transmitted in the anterolateral system can be localized much less exactly. On the other hand, the anterolateral system has a special capability that the dorsal system does not have: the ability to transmit a broad spectrum of sensory modalities—pain, warmth, cold, and crude tactile sensations; the dorsal system is limited to mechanoreceptive sensations alone. With this differentiation in mind we can now list the types of sensations transmitted in the two systems.

The Dorsal Column–Lemniscal System

1. Touch sensations requiring a high degree of localization of the stimulus.
2. Touch sensations requiring transmission of fine gradations of intensity.
3. Phasic sensations, such as vibratory sensations.
4. Sensations that signal movement against the skin.
5. Position sensations.

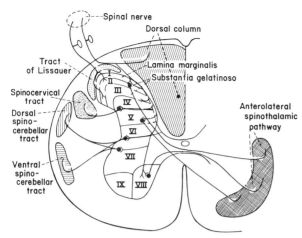

Figure 13–2. Cross-section of the spinal cord showing the anatomical laminae I through IX of the cord gray matter and the ascending sensory tracts in the white columns of the spinal cord.

6. Pressure sensations having to do with fine degrees of judgment of pressure intensity.

The Anterolateral System

1. Pain.
2. Thermal sensations, including both warm and cold sensations.
3. Crude touch and pressure sensations capable of only crude localizing ability on the surface of the body and having little capability for intensity discrimination.
4. Tickle and itch sensations.
5. Sexual sensations.

TRANSMISSION IN THE DORSAL COLUMN–LEMNISCAL SYSTEM

ANATOMY OF THE DORSAL COLUMN– LEMNISCAL SYSTEM

On entering the spinal cord from the spinal nerve dorsal roots, the large myelinated fibers from specialized mechanoreceptors first pass medially into the lateral margin of the dorsal white columns. However, almost immediately each of these fibers divides to form a *medial* and a *lateral branch*, as illustrated by the medial dorsal root fiber in Figure 13–2. The medial branch turns upward in the dorsal column and proceeds by way of the dorsal column pathway to the brain.

The lateral branch proceeds laterally and anteriorly in the same segment of the cord and divides many times to give off multiple terminals to almost all parts of the intermediate and anterior portions of the cord gray matter. These terminals serve two purposes. Some of them elicit local spinal cord reflexes, which will be discussed in Chapter 15. Others excite relay neurons that give rise to the spinocerebellar and spinocervical tracts. We will discuss the spinocerebellar tracts in Chapter 17 in relation to the function of the cerebellum. The spinocervical tract is an accessory pathway for transmission of somatosensory information upward in the spinal cord and functions

in close association with the dorsal column–lemniscal system, as we shall discuss subsequently.

Anatomy of the Dorsal Column Pathway. Note in Figure 13–3 that the nerve fibers entering the dorsal columns pass up these columns to the medulla, where they synapse in the *dorsal column nuclei* (the *cuneate* and *gracile nuclei*). From here, *second order neurons* decussate immediately to the opposite side and then pass upward to the thalamus through bilateral pathways called the *medial lemnisci*. Each medial lemniscus terminates in a *ventrobasal complex of nuclei* that includes the ventral posterior lateral nucleus of the thalamus and the posterior nuclear group located slightly farther posteriorly. In its pathway through the brain stem, the medial lemniscus is joined by additional fibers from the *main sensory nucleus of the trigeminal nerve* and from the *upper portion of its descending nuclei*; these fibers subserve the same sensory functions for the head that the dorsal column fibers subserve for the body.

From the ventrobasal complex, *third order nerve fibers* project, as shown in Figure 13–4, mainly to the *postcentral gyrus* of the *cerebral cortex*, which is called *somatic sensory area I*. In addition, fewer fibers project to the lowermost lateral portion of each parietal lobe, an area called *somatic sensory area II*.

Anatomy of the Spino-Cervical Pathways. Until re-

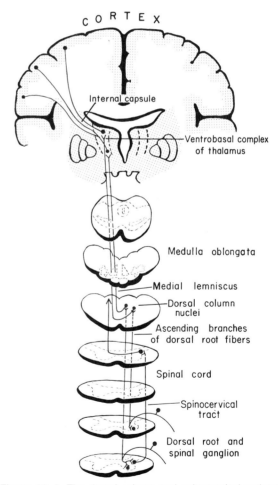

Figure 13–3. The dorsal column and spinocervical pathways for transmitting critical types of tactile signals. (Modified from Ranson and Clark: Anatomy of the Nervous System. Philadelphia, W. B. Saunders Company, 1959.)

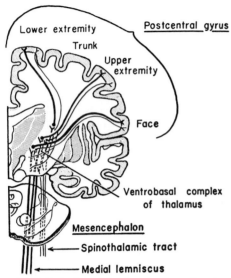

Figure 13–4. Projection of the dorsal column–lemniscal system from the thalamus to the somatic sensory cortex. (Modified from Brodal: Neurological Anatomy in Relation to Clinical Medicine. New York, Oxford University Press, 1969.)

cently it was believed that all the dorsal column–lemniscal system signals were trasmitted only through the dorsal columns. However, complete transection of the dorsal column does not cause total loss of transmission in this system. Instead, many signals that can partially substitute for the dorsal columns can still be transmitted through the *spinocervical pathway*.

The anatomy of the spinocervical pathway is much less well known than that of the dorsal column pathway. However, many collateral terminals from the large sensory fibers synapse in lamina IV and adjacent laminae of the cord gray matter and give rise to second order fibers that enter the dorsal portion of the *lateral white column* and ascend in the spinocervical tract to the cervical region of the cord or even to the medulla. Here the fibers again synapse either in the dorsal horn of the cord or in medullary nuclei adjacent to or part of the *dorsal column nuclei*. Then third order neurons decussate to the opposite side and pass along with the second order neurons of the dorsal column pathway upward to the thalamus through the *medial lemnisci*. Thus, the pathway within the brain parallels that of the dorsal column–lemniscal pathway.

Separation of Sensory Modalities Between the Dorsal Column–Lemniscal Pathway and the Spinocervical Pathway

The way in which the nervous system distinguishes among the different modalities of sensation is to transmit the signals of different modalities to separate central nervous system areas. This separation of modality begins in the spinal cord. It has already been noted that only mechanoreceptor modalities are transmitted in the dorsal column–lemniscal system whereas all the other somatic modalities are transmitted in the anterolateral system. However, even within the dorsal column–lemniscal system there is an additional degree of separation. The dorsal column tract transmits mainly signals from rapidly adapting sensory receptors. For instance, it is only through the

dorsal columns that signals are transmitted from the extremely rapidly adapting pacinian corpuscles. Also, most of the signals from the Meissner's corpuscles and from the hair receptors, both of which are rapidly adapting receptors, are transmitted through this pathway.

On the other hand, some of the more slowly adapting signals from the Merkel's discs, from the deep tissue Ruffini end-organs, and from the slowly adapting Ruffini position sense receptors of the joint capsules seem to be transmitted through the spinocervical pathway.

Spatial Orientation of the Nerve Fibers in the Dorsal Column–Lemniscal System

One of the distinguishing features of the dorsal column–lemniscal system is a distinct spatial orientation of nerve fibers from the individual parts of the body that is maintained throughout. For instance, in the dorsal columns, the fibers from the lower parts of the body lie toward the center, while those that enter the spinal cord at progressively higher segmental levels form successive layers laterally.

The spatial orientation in the spinocervical pathway is less well known. However, stimulation experiments of single fibers within this pathway have shown that the sensory signals diverge very little, indicating a high degree of spatial orientation in this pathway as well.

In the thalamus, the distinct spatial orientation is still maintained, with the tail end of the body represented by the most lateral portions of the ventrobasal complex and the head and face represented in the medial component of the complex. However, because of the crossing of the medial lemnisci in the medulla, the left side of the body is represented in the right side of the thalamus, and the right side of the body is represented in the left side of the thalamus.

THE SOMATIC SENSORY CORTEX

The area of the cerebral cortex to which the sensory signals are projected is called the *somatic sensory cortex*. In the human being, this area lies mainly in the anterior portions of the parietal lobes. Two distinct and separate areas are known to receive direct afferent nerve fibers from the relay nuclei of the thalamus; these, called *somatic sensory area I* and *somatic sensory area II*, are illustrated in Figure 13–5. However, somatic sensory area I is so much more important to the sensory functions of the body than is somatic sensory area II that in popular usage, the term somatic sensory cortex is almost always used to mean area I exclusive of area II. Yet, to keep these two areas distinct we will henceforth refer to them separately as somatic sensory area I and somatic sensory area II.

Projection of the Body in Somatic Sensory Area I. Somatic sensory area I lies in the postcentral gyrus of the human cerebral cortex (in Brodmann areas 1, 2, and 3 immediately behind the central

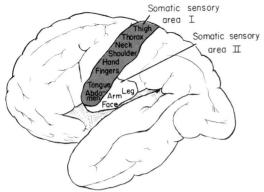

Figure 13–5. The two somatic sensory cortical areas, somatic sensory areas I and II.

sulcus—see map of the cerebral cortex in Figure 18–1 in Chapter 18). A distinct spatial orientation exists in this area for reception of nerve signals from the different areas of the body. Figure 13–6 illustrates a cross-section through the brain at the level of the postcentral gyrus, showing the representations of the different parts of the body in separate regions of somatic sensory area I. Note, however, that each side of the cortex receives sensory information exclusively from the opposite side of the body (with the exception of a small amount of sensory information from the same side of the face).

Some areas of the body are represented by large areas in the somatic cortex—the lips by far the greatest of all, followed by the face and thumb—whereas the entire trunk and lower part of the body are represented by relatively small areas. The sizes of these areas are directly proportional to the number of specialized sensory receptors in each respective peripheral area of the body. For instance, a great number of specialized nerve endings are

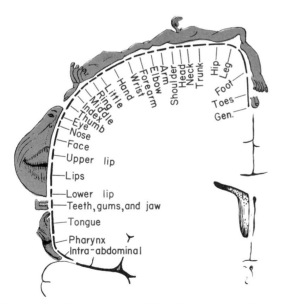

Figure 13–6. Representation of the different areas of the body in the somatic sensory area I of the cortex. (From Penfield and Rasmussen: Cerebral Cortex of Man: A Clinical Study of Localization of Function. New York, Macmillan Company, 1968.)

found in the lips and thumb, while only a few are present in the skin of the trunk.

Note also that the head is represented in the most lateral portion of somatic sensory area I, whereas the lower part of the body is represented in the medial portion of the area.

Somatic Sensory Area II. The second cortical area to which somatic afferent fibers project, somatic sensory area II, is a much smaller area that lies posterior and inferior to the lateral end of somatic sensory area I, as shown in Figure 13–5. The degree of localization of the different parts of the body is very poor in this area compared with somatic sensory area I. The face is represented anteriorly, the arms centrally, and the legs posteriorly.

So little is known about the function of somatic sensory area II that it cannot be discussed intelligently. It is known that signals enter this area from both sides of the body and also from other sensory areas of the brain, such as visual and auditory signals. Also, stimulation of somatic sensory area II in some instances causes complex body movements, for which reason it is possibly it plays a role in sensory control of motor functions.

The Layers of the Somatic Sensory Cortex and Their Function

The cerebral cortex contains *six* separate layers of neurons, beginning with layer I next to the surface and extending progressively deeper to layer VI. As would be expected, the neurons in each layer perform functions different from those in other layers. Some of these functions are:

1. The incoming sensory signal excites mainly neuronal layer IV first; then the signal spreads toward the surface of the cortex and also toward the deeper layers.

2. Layers I and II receive a diffuse, nonspecific input from the reticular activating system that can facilitate the whole brain at once; this system will be described in Chapter 19. This input perhaps controls the overall level of excitability of the cortex.

3. The neurons in layers II and III send axons to other closely related portions of the cerebral cortex.

4. The neurons in layers V and VI send axons to more distant parts of the nervous system. Those in layer V are generally larger and project to more distant areas. For instance, many of these pass all the way into the brain stem and spinal cord to provide control signals to these areas. From layer VI especially large numbers of axons extend to the thalamus, providing feedback signals from the cerebral cortex to the thalamus.

Representation of the Different Sensory Modalities in the Somatic Sensory Cortex—The Vertical Columns of Neurons

Functionally, the neurons of the somatic sensory cortex are arranged in vertical columns extending all the way through the six layers of the cortex, each column having a diameter of 0.33 to 1 mm and containing some 100,000 neuronal cell bodies. Each of these columns serves a single specific sensory modality, some responding to stretch receptors around joints, some to stimulation of tactile hairs, others to discrete localized pressure points on the skin, and so forth. Furthermore, the columns for the different modalities are interspersed among each other. At layer IV, where the signals first enter the cord, the columns of neurons function almost entirely separately from each other. However, at other levels of the columns interactions occur that allow beginning analysis of the meanings of the sensory signals.

In the most anterior portion of the postcentral gyrus, located deep in the central sulcus in Brodmann's area 3a (see Chapter 18 for a map of Brodmann's areas), a disproportionately large share of the vertical columns respond to muscle, tendon, or joint stretch receptors. The signals from these in turn impact mainly on the motor cortex located immediately anterior to the central sulcus and help control muscle function. As one proceeds more posteriorly in somatic sensory cortex I, more and more of the vertical columns respond to the slowly adapting cutaneous receptors, and then still farther posteriorly greater numbers of the columns are sensitive to deep pressure.

In the most posterior portion of somatic sensory area I, about 6 per cent of the vertical columns respond only when a stimulus moves across the skin in a particular direction. Thus, this is a still higher order of interpretation of sensory signals; and the process becomes even more complex still farther posteriorly in the parietal cortex, which is called the *somatic association area* as we shall discuss subsequently.

Functions of Somatic Sensory Area I

The functional capabilities of different areas of the somesthetic cortex have been determined by selective excision of the different portions. Widespread excision of somatic sensory area I causes loss of the following types of sensory judgment:

1. The person is unable to localize discretely the different sensations in the different parts of the body. However, he or she can localize these sensations very crudely, such as to a particular hand, which indicates that the thalamus or parts of the cerebral cortex not normally considered to be concerned with somatic sensations can perform some degree of localization.

2. He is unable to judge critical degrees of pressure against his body.

3. He is unable to judge exactly the weights of objects.

4. He is unable to judge shapes or forms of objects. This is called *astereognosis.*

5. He is unable to judge texture of materials, for this type of judgment depends on highly critical sensations caused by movement of the skin over the surface to be judged.

Note in the list that nothing has been said about loss of pain and temperature sense. However, in the absence of somatic sensory area I, the appreciation of these sensory modalities may be altered either in quality or in intensity. But more important, the pain and temperature sensations that do occur are poorly localized, indicating that both pain and temperature localization probably depend mainly upon simultaneous stimulation of tactile stimuli that use the topographical map of the body in somatic sensory area I to localize the source.

SOMATIC ASSOCIATION AREAS

Brodmann's areas 5 and 7 of the cerebral cortex, which are located in the parietal cortex behind somatic sensory area I and above somatic sensory area II, play important roles in deciphering the sensory information that enters the somatic sensory areas. Therefore, these areas are called the *somatic association areas.*

Electrical stimulation in the somatic association area can occasionally cause a person to experience a complex somatic sensation, sometimes even the "feeling" of an object such as a knife or a ball. Therefore, it seems clear that the somatic association area combines information from multiple points in the somatic sensory area to decipher its meaning. This also fits with the anatomical arrangement of the neuronal tracts that enter the somatic association area, for it receives signals from (1) somatic sensory area I, (2) the ventrobasal complex of the thalamus, (3) other areas of the thalamus which themselves receive input from the ventrobasal complex, (4) the visual cortex, and (5) the auditory cortex.

Effect of Removing the Somatic Association Area—Amorphosynthesis. When the somatic association area is removed, the person especially loses the ability to recognize complex objects and complex forms by the process of feeling them. In addition, the person loses most of the sense of form of his or her own body. An especially interesting fact is that loss of the somatic association area on one side of the brain causes the person sometimes to be oblivious of the opposite side of the body—that is, to forget that it is there. Likewise, when feeling objects, the person will tend to feel only one side of the object and to forget that the other side even exists. This complex sensory deficit is called *amorphosynthesis.*

CHARACTERISTICS OF TRANSMISSION IN THE DORSAL COLUMN– LEMNISCAL SYSTEM

Faithfulness of Transmission. The most important functional characteristic of the dorsal column–lemniscal system is its *faithfulness* of transmission. That is, each time a point in the periphery is stimulated, a signal ordinarily is transmitted all the way to the somatic sensory cortex. Also, if this peripheral stimulus increases in intensity, the intensity of the signal at the cerebral cortex increases approximately proportionately. And, finally, when a discrete area of the body is stimulated, the signal from this area is transmitted to a discrete area of the cerebral cortex. Thus, the dorsal system is adequately organized for transmission of accurate information from the periphery to the sensorium. Furthermore, the responsiveness of this system can be altered only moderately by stimuli from other areas of the nervous system, and it is not depressed to a significant extent even by moderate degrees of general anesthesia; this is quite different for most portions of the anterolateral sensory system.

Basic Neuronal Circuit and Discharge Pattern in the Dorsal Column–Lemniscal System. The lower part of Figure 13–7 illustrates the basic organization of the neuronal circuit of the dorsal column pathway, showing that at each synaptic stage divergence occurs. However, the upper part of the figure shows that a single receptor stimulus on the skin does not cause all the cortical neurons with which that receptor connects to discharge at the same rate. Instead, the cortical neurons that discharge to the greatest extent are those in a central part of the cortical "field" for each respective receptor. Thus, a weak stimulus causes only the centralmost neurons to

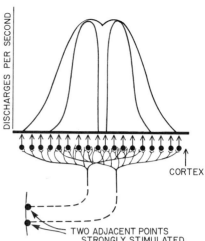

Figure 13–8. Transmission of signals to the cortex from two adjacent pinpoint stimuli. The solid black curve represents the pattern of cortical stimulation without "surround" inhibition, and the two colored curves represent the pattern with "surround" inhibition.

fire. A stronger stimulus causes still more neurons to fire, but those in the center still discharge at a considerably more rapid rate than do those farther away from the center.

Two-Point Discrimination. A method frequently used to test tactile capabilities is to determine a person's so-called "two-point discriminatory ability." In this test, two needles are pressed against the skin, and the subject determines whether two points of stimulus are felt or one point. On the tips of the fingers a person can distinguish two separate points even when the needles are as close together as 1 to 2 mm. However, on the person's back, the needles must usually be as far apart as 30 to 70 mm before one can detect two separate points. The reason for this is that there are many specialized tactile receptors in the tips of the fingers in comparison with a small number in the skin of the back. Referring back to Figure 13–6, we can see also that the portions of the body that have a high degree of two-point discrimination have a correspondingly large cortical representation in somatic sensory area I.

Figure 13–8 illustrates the mechanism by which the dorsal column pathway, and the other sensory pathways as well but to a less critical degree, transmit two-point discriminatory information. This figure shows two adjacent points on the skin that are strongly stimulated, and it also shows the small area of the somatic sensory cortex (greatly enlarged) that is excited by signals from the two stimulated points. The solid black curve shows the spatial pattern of cortical excitation when both skin points are stimulated simultaneously. Note that the resultant zone of excitation has two separate peaks. It is these two peaks separated by a valley that allow the sensory cortex to detect the presence of two stimulatory points rather than a single point. However, the capability of the sensorium to distinguish between two points of stimulation is strongly influ-

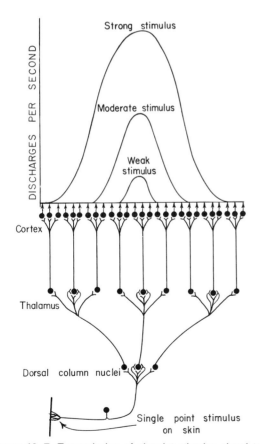

Figure 13–7. Transmission of pinpoint stimulus signal to the cortex.

enced by another mechanism, the mechanism of *lateral inhibition*, as explained in the following section.

Increase in Contrast in the Perceived Spatial Pattern Caused by Lateral Inhibition. In Chapter 11 it was pointed out that contrast in sensory patterns is increased by inhibitory signals transmitted laterally in the sensory pathway. This effect was illustrated in Figure 11–9 of that chapter.

In the case of the dorsal column system, an excited sensory receptor in the skin transmits not only excitatory signals to the somatic sensory cortex but also inhibitory signals laterally to adjacent fiber pathways. These inhibitory signals occur at each synaptic level, for instance in the dorsal column nuclei and in the ventrobasal complex of the thalamus, and they help block lateral spread of the excitatory signal, a process called *lateral inhibition* or *surround inhibition*. As a result, the peak of excitation stands out, and much of the surrounding diffuse stimulation is blocked. This effect is illustrated by the two colored curves in Figure 13–8, showing complete separation of the peaks when the intensity of the surround inhibition is very great. Obviously, this mechanism accentuates the contrast between the areas of peak stimulation and the surrounding areas, thus greatly increasing the contrast or sharpness of the perceived spatial pattern.

Transmission of Rapidly Changing and Repetitive Sensations. The dorsal column system is of particular value for apprising the sensorium of rapidly changing peripheral conditions. This system can "follow" changing stimuli up to at least 400 cycles per second and can "detect" changes as high as 700 cycles. Obviously, very rapid response to a sudden stimulus on the skin allows one to direct attention immediately to any point of contact, which, in turn, allows one to make necessary corrections before damage can be done.

Vibratory Sensation. Vibratory signals are rapidly repetitive and can be detected as vibration up to 700 cycles per second. These signals are transmitted only in the dorsal column pathway and not in the more slowly conducting pathways. For this reason, application of vibration with a tuning fork to different peripheral parts of the body is an important tool used by the neurologist for testing functional integrity of the dorsal columns.

THE POSITION SENSE

The term position sense can be divided into two subtypes: *static position*, which means conscious recognition of the orientation of the different parts of the body with respect to each other, and *kinesthesia*, which means conscious recognition of rates of movement of the different parts of the body. The position sensations are transmitted to the sensorium almost entirely through the dorsal column–lemniscal system. However, special features of the position sense require further explanation.

The Position Sense Receptors. Sensory information from many different types of receptors is used to determine both static position and kinesthesia. These include the extensive sensory endings in the joint capsules and ligaments, the receptors in the skin and deep tissues near the joints, and probably also the muscle spindles that detect muscle stretch, as we shall discuss in Chapter 15.

Three major types of nerve endings have been described in the joint capsules and ligaments about the joints. (1) By far the most abundant of these are spray-type *Ruffini endings*, one of which was illustrated in Figure 12–1 of Chapter 12. These endings are stimulated strongly when the joint is suddenly moved; they adapt slightly at first but then transmit a steady signal thereafter. (2) A second type of ending resembling the stretch receptors found in muscle tendons (called *Golgi tendon receptors*) is found particularly in the ligaments about the joints. Though far less numerous than the Ruffini endings, they have essentially the same response properties. (3) A few *pacinian corpuscles* are also found in the tissues around the joints. These adapt extremely rapidly and presumably help to detect *rate of rotation* at the joint.

Detection of Static Position by the Joint Receptors. Figure 13–9 illustrates the excitation of seven different nerve fibers leading from separate joint receptors in the capsule of a cat's knee joint. Note that at 180 degrees of joint rotation one of the receptors is stimulated; then at 150 degrees still another is stimulated; at 140 degrees two are stimulated, and so forth. The information from these joint receptors continually apprises the central nervous system of the momentary rotation of the joint. That is, the rotation determines *which* receptor is stimulated and how much it is stimulated, and from this the brain knows how far the joint is bent.

Detection of Rate of Movement (Kinesthesia) at the Joint. Because pacinian corpuscles are especially adapted for detecting movement of tissues, it is tempting to suggest that rate of movement at the joints is detected by the pacinian corpuscles. However, the number of pacinian corpuscles in the joint tissues is small, for which reason rate of movement at the joint is probably detected mainly in the following way: the Ruffini and Golgi endings in the

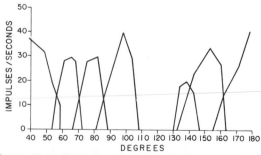

Figure 13–9. Response of seven different nerve fibers from knee joint receptors in a cat at different degrees of rotation. (Modified from Skoglund: *Acta Physiol. Scand.*, Suppl. 124, 36:1, 1956.)

joint tissues are stimulated very strongly at first by the joint movement, but within a fraction of a second this strong level of stimulation fades to a lower, steady state rate of firing. Nevertheless, this early overshoot in receptor stimulation is directly proportional to the rate of joint movement and is believed to be the signal used by the brain to discern the rate of movement.

Transmission of Position Sense Signals in the Dorsal Column–Lemniscal Pathway. In the past it had been believed that essentially all the position sense signals were transmitted in the dorsal columns. However, on the basis of studies in animals, there is now much reason to believe that some of these signals are transmitted in the spinocervical pathway as well. This is probably especially true of the static position signals, that is, those signals that are slowly adapting and that transmit information about the relative positions of the different parts of the body when the person is not moving.

Processing of Position Sense Information in the Dorsal Column–Lemniscal Pathway. Despite the faithfulness of transmission of signals from the periphery to the sensory cortex in the dorsal column–lemniscal system, there nevertheless seems to be some processing of position sense signals before they reach the cerebral cortex. For instance, Figure 13–9 showed that individual joint receptors are stimulated maximally at specific degrees of rotation of the joint, with the intensity of stimulation decreasing on either side of the maximal point for each receptor. However, the static position signal for joint rotation is quite different at the level of the ventrobasal complex of the thalamus, as can be seen by referring to Figure 13–10. This figure shows that the ventrobasal neurons that respond to the joint rotation signal are of two types: those that are maximally stimulated when the joint is at full rotation and those that are maximally stimulated when the joint is at minimal rotation. In each case, as the degree of rotation changes, the rate of stimulation of the neuron either decreases or increases, de-

pending on the direction in which the joint is being rotated. Furthermore, the intensity of neuronal excitation changes over angles of 40 to 60 degrees of angulation in contrast to 20 to 30 degrees for the individual receptors, as was illustrated in Figure 13–9. Thus, the signals from the individual joint receptors have been integrated in the space domain by the time they reach the thalamic neurons, giving a progressively stronger signal as the joint moves in only one direction rather than giving a peaked signal as occurs in stimulation of individual receptors.

TRANSMISSION IN THE ANTEROLATERAL SYSTEM

It was pointed out earlier in the chapter that the anterolateral system transmits sensory signals that do not require highly discrete localization of the signal source and also do not require discrimination of fine gradations of intensity. These include pain, heat, cold, crude tactile, tickle and itch, and sexual sensations. In the following chapter pain and temperature sensations will be discussed; the present chapter is concerned principally with transmission of the tactile sensations.

ANATOMY OF THE ANTEROLATERAL PATHWAY

The anterolateral fibers originate mainly in laminae I, IV, V, and VI in the dorsal horns where many of the dorsal root sensory nerve fibers terminate after entering the cord (see Figure 13–2). Then, as illustrated in Figure 13–11, the fibers cross in the anterior commissure of the cord to the opposite anterolateral white column where they turn upward toward the brain. These fibers ascend rather diffusely throughout the anterolateral columns. However, anatomical studies have shown that there is at least a partial differentiation of this pathway into an anterior division, called the *anterior spinothalamic tract,* and a lateral division, called the *lateral spinothalamic tract.* Also encompassed in the anterolateral pathway are a *spinoreticular pathway* (to the reticular substance of the brain stem) and a *spinotectal tract* (to the tectum of the mesencephalon). However, it has been difficult to make these differentiations using electrical recording techniques.

The upper terminus of the anterolateral pathway is mainly twofold: (1) throughout the *reticular nuclei of the brain stem* and (2) in two different nuclear complexes of the thalamus, the *ventrobasal complex* and the *intralaminar nuclei.* In general, the tactile signals are transmitted mainly into the ventrobasal complex, terminating in the same thalamic nuclei as the dorsal column–lemniscal system, and this is probably also true for the temperature signals. From here, the tactile signals are transmitted to the somatosensory cortex along with the signals from the dorsal columns. On the other hand, only part of the pain signals project to this complex. Instead, most of these enter the reticular nuclei of the brain stem and intralaminar nuclei of the thalamus, as will be discussed in greater detail in the following chapter.

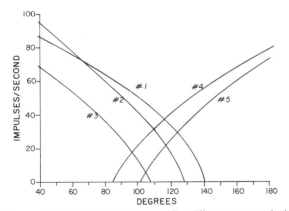

Figure 13–10. Typical responses of five different neurons in the knee joint receptor field of the ventrobasal complex when the knee joint is moved through its range of motion. (The curves were constructed from data in Mountcastle et al.: *J. Neurophysiol.,* 26:807, 1963.)

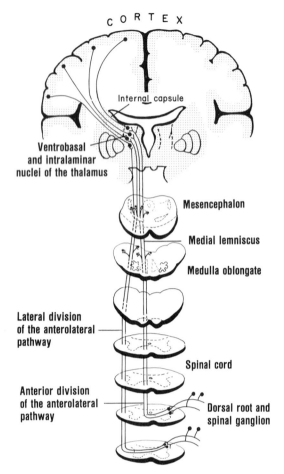

Figure 13–11. The anterior and lateral divisions of the antero-lateral pathway.

Characteristics of Transmission in the Anterolateral Pathway. In general, the same principles apply to transmission in the anterolateral pathway as in the dorsal column–lemniscal system except for the following differences: (1) the velocities of transmission are only one half to one third those in the dorsal column–lemniscal system, ranging between 8 and 40 meters per second; (2) the degree of spatial localization of signals is poor, especially in the pain pathways; (3) the gradations of intensities are also far less acute, most of the sensations being recognized in 10 to 20 gradations of strength rather than in as many as 100 gradations for the dorsal column system; and (4) the ability to transmit rapidly repetitive sensations is poor.

Thus, it is evident that the anterolateral system is a cruder type of transmission system than the dorsal column–lemniscal system. Even so, certain modalities of sensation are transmitted in this system only and not at all in the dorsal column–lemniscal system. These are pain, thermal, tickle and itch, and sexual sensations in addition to crude touch and pressure.

SOME SPECIAL ASPECTS OF SENSORY FUNCTION

Function of the Thalamus in Somatic Sensation. When the somatosensory cortex of a human being is destroyed, that person loses most critical tactile sensibilities, but a slight degree of crude tactile sensibility does return. Therefore, it must be assumed that the thalamus (as well as other lower centers) has a slight ability to discriminate tactile sensation even though the thalamus normally functions mainly to relay this type of information to the cortex.

On the other hand, loss of the somatosensory cortex has little effect on one's perception of pain sensation and only a moderate effect on the perception of temperature. Therefore, there is much reason to believe that the thalamus and other associated basal regions of the brain play perhaps the dominant role in discrimination of these sensibilities; it is interesting that these sensibilities appeared very early in the phylogenetic development of animalhood while the critical tactile sensibilities were a late development.

Cortical Control of Sensory Sensitivity. Almost all sensory information that enters the cerebrum, except that from the olfactory system, but including sensory information from the eyes, the ears, the taste receptors, and all the somatic receptors, is relayed through one or another of the thalamic nuclei. Furthermore, the conscious brain is capable of directing its attention to different segments of the sensory system. This function is believed

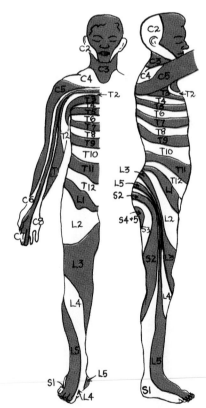

Figure 13–12. The dermatomes. (Modified from Grinker and Sahs: Neurology. Charles C Thomas, 1966.)

to be mainly achieved through facilitation or inhibition of the cortical receptive areas, perhaps as a result of signals from the thalamus.

But, in addition, "corticofugal" signals are transmitted from the cortex to the lower relay stations in the sensory pathways to *inhibit* transmission. For instance, corticofugal pathways control the sensitivity of the synapses at all levels of the sensory pathways—in the thalamus, in the brain stem reticular nuclei, in the dorsal column nuclei, and especially in the dorsal horn relay station of the anterolateral system. Also, similar inhibitory mechanisms are known for the visual, auditory, and olfactory systems, which are discussed in later chapters. Each corticofugal pathway begins in the cortex where the sensory pathway that it controls terminates. Thus, a feedback control loop exists for each sensory pathway.

Obviously, corticofugal control of sensory input could allow the cerebral cortex to alter the threshold for different sensory signals. Also, it might help the brain focus its attention on specific types of information, which is an important and necessary characteristic of nervous system function.

Automatic Gain Control in the Sensory Pathways and Enhancement of Contrast. One of the byproducts of corticofugal inhibition is believed to be automatic gain control in many if not most of the sensory pathways. That is, when excess sensory signals pass to the brain, recurrent inhibition back to the cord decreases the sensitivity of the sensory pathway. This obviously prevents overloading of the pathway with signals. Also, it helps to preserve contrast in the perception of sensory signals because an excess of signals in the pathway would deluge both the relay nuclei and the cerebral cortex with such a high degree of excitation that it would be impossible to distinguish the highlights from the chaff.

Segmental Fields of Sensation—The Dermatomes. Each spinal nerve innervates a "segmental field" of the skin called a *dermatome*. The different dermatomes are illustrated in Figure 13–12. However, these are shown as if there were distinct borders between the adjacent dermatomes, which is far from true because much overlap exists from segment to segment. Indeed, because of the great overlap, the posterior roots from an entire segment of the spinal cord can be destroyed without causing significant loss of sensation in the skin.

Figure 13–12 shows that the anal region of the body lies in the dermatome of the most distal cord segment. In the embryo, this is the tail region and is the most distal portion of the body. The legs develop from the lumbar and upper sacral segments rather than from the distal sacral segments, which is evident from the dermatomal map. Obviously, one can use a dermatomal map such as that illustrated in Figure 13–12 to determine the level in the spinal cord at which various cord injuries may have occurred when the peripheral sensations are disturbed.

REFERENCES

See bibliographies of Chapters 12 and 14.

14

Somatic Sensations: II. Pain, Visceral Pain, Headache, and Thermal Sensations

Many, if not most, ailments of the body cause pain. Furthermore, the ability to diagnose different diseases depends to a great extent on a doctor's knowledge of the different qualities of pain. For these reasons, the present chapter is devoted mainly to pain and to the physiological basis of some of the associated clinical phenomena.

The Purpose of Pain. Pain is a protective mechanism for the body; it occurs whenever any tissues are being damaged, and it causes the individual to react to remove the pain stimulus. Even such simple activities as sitting for a long time on the ischia can cause tissue destruction because of lack of blood flow to the skin where the skin is compressed by the weight of the body. When the skin becomes painful as a result of the ischemia, the person shifts weight unconsciously. A person who has lost the pain sense, such as after spinal cord injury, fails to feel the pain and therefore fails to shift weight. This eventually results in ulceration at the areas of pressure unless special measures are taken to move the person from time to time.

THE TWO TYPES OF PAIN AND THEIR QUALITIES—ACUTE PAIN AND SLOW PAIN

Pain has been classified into two different major types: *acute pain* and *slow pain*. Acute pain occurs within about 0.1 second when a pain stimulus is applied, whereas slow pain begins only after a second or more and then increases slowly over a period of many seconds and sometimes even minutes. During the course of this chapter we shall see that the conduction pathways for these two types of pain are different and that each of them has specific qualities.

Acute pain is also described by many alternate names, such as *sharp pain, pricking pain, fast pain, electric pain,* and others. This type of pain is felt when a needle is stuck into the skin or when the

skin is cut with a knife, and this pain is also felt when the skin is subjected to electric shock. Acute, sharp pain is not felt in most of the deeper tissues of the body.

Slow pain goes by multiple additional names such as *burning pain, aching pain, throbbing pain, nauseous pain,* and *chronic pain*. This type of pain is usually associated with *tissue destruction*. It can become excruciating and can lead to prolonged, unbearable suffering. It can occur both in the skin and in almost any internal tissue or organ.

We will learn later that the acute type of pain is transmitted through type $A\delta$ pain fibers, whereas the slow type of pain results from stimulation of the more primitive type C fibers.

METHODS FOR MEASURING THE PERCEPTION OF PAIN

The intensity of a stimulus necessary to cause pain can be measured in many different ways, but the mostused methods have been pricking the skin with a pin at measured pressures, pressing a solid object against a protruding bone with measured force, pinching the skin, or heating the skin with measured amounts of heat. The last method has proved to be especially accurate from a quantitative point of view.

Figure 14–1 illustrates the basic principles of a heat apparatus used for measuring pain threshold. An intense light is focused by a large condenser lens onto a black spot painted on the forehead of the subject, and the heat intensity delivered by the light is controlled by a rheostat. In determining the subject's threshold for pain, the intensity of the heat is increased in progressive steps, and the length of time required for the forehead to heat sufficiently to elicit pain is recorded for each heat intensity. These data are then plotted in the form of a "strength-duration curve" to express pain threshold, as shown in Figure 14–2. The lowest intensity of stimulus, illustrated by the dashed line in the figure, that will excite the sensation of pain when the stimulus is applied for a prolonged period of time is called the *pain threshold*.

The Pain Threshold. Figure 14–3 shows graphically the skin temperature at which pain is first perceived by

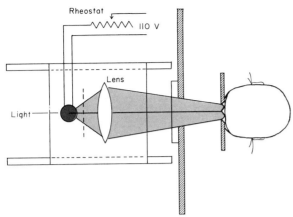

Figure 14–1. Heat apparatus for measuring pain threshold. (From Hardy, Wolff, and Goodell: *J. Clin. Invest., 19*:649, 1940.)

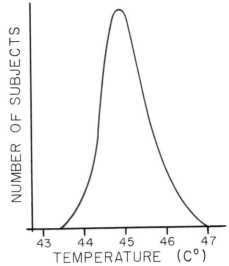

Figure 14–3. Distribution curve obtained from a large number of subjects of the minimal skin temperature that causes pain. (Modified from Hardy: *J. Chronic Dis., 4*:22, 1956.)

different persons. By far the greatest number perceive pain when the skin temperature reaches almost exactly 45° C, and almost everyone perceives pain before the temperature reaches 47° C. Indeed, measurements in people as widely different as Eskimos, Indians, and whites have shown little differences in their *thresholds for pain*. However, different people do *react* very differently to pain, as is discussed later.

THE PAIN RECEPTORS AND THEIR STIMULATION

Free Nerve Endings as Pain Receptors. The pain receptors in the skin and other tissues are all free nerve endings. They are widespread in the superficial layers of the *skin* and also in certain internal tissues, such as the *periosteum*, the *arterial walls*, the *joint surfaces*, and the *falx* and *tentorium* of the cranial vault. Most of the other deep tissues are not extensively supplied with pain endings but are weakly supplied; nevertheless, any widespread tissue damage can still summate to cause the slow-chronic-aching type of pain in these areas.

Types of Stimuli That Excite Pain Receptors— Mechanical, Thermal, and Chemical. Some pain fibers are excited almost entirely by excessive mechanical stress or mechanical damage to the tissues; these are called *mechanosensitive pain receptors*. Others are sensitive to extremes of heat or cold and therefore are called *thermosensitive pain receptors*.

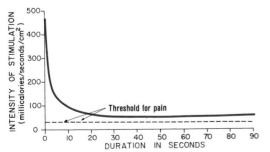

Figure 14–2. Strength-duration curve for depicting pain threshold. (From Hardy: *J. Chronic Dis., 4*:20, 1956.)

And still others are sensitive to various chemical substances and are called *chemosensitive pain receptors*. Some of the different chemicals that excite the chemosensitive receptors include *bradykinin, serotonin, histamine, potassium ions, acids, prostaglandins, acetylcholine,* and *proteolytic enzymes.*

Though some pain receptors are mainly sensitive to only one of the above types of stimuli, most are sensitive to more than one of the types.

Nonadapting Nature of Pain Receptors. In contrast to most other sensory receptors of the body, the pain receptors adapt either not at all or almost not at all. In fact, under some conditions, the threshold for excitation of the pain fibers becomes progressively lower and lower as the pain stimulus continues, thus allowing these receptors to become progressively more activated with time. This increase in sensitivity of the pain receptors is called *hyperalgesia.*

One can readily understand the importance of this failure of pain receptors to adapt, for it allows them to keep the person apprised of a damaging stimulus that causes the pain as long as it persists.

RATE OF TISSUE DAMAGE AS A CAUSE OF PAIN

The average critical temperature of 45° C at which a person first begins to perceive pain is also the temperature at which the tissues begin to be damaged by heat; indeed, the tissues are eventually completely destroyed if the temperature remains at this level indefinitely. Therefore, it is immediately apparent that pain resulting from heat is closely correlated with the ability of heat to damage the tissues.

Furthermore, the intensity of pain has also been closely correlated with the rate of tissue damage caused by other effects besides heat, whether this be damage caused by bacterial infection, tissue ischemia, tissue contusion, or otherwise.

Special Importance of Chemical Pain Stimuli During Tissue Damage. Extracts from damaged tissues cause intense pain when injected beneath the normal skin. Among the substances in such extracts that are especially painful are *bradykinin, histamine, prostaglandins, acids, excesses of potassium ions, serotonin,* and *proteolytic enzymes,* which are the same substances that are known from electrophysiological data to excite the pain nerve endings. Obviously, many of these substances could cause direct damage to the pain nerve endings, especially the proteolytic enzymes. But some of the other substances, such as bradykinin and some of the prostaglandins, can cause direct extreme stimulation of pain nerve fibers without necessarily damaging them.

Release of the various substances listed above not only stimulates the chemosensitive pain endings but also greatly decreases the threshold for stimulation of the mechanosensitive and thermosensitive pain receptors as well. A widely known example of this is the extreme pain caused by slight mechanical or heat stimuli following tissue damage by sunburn.

Tissue Ischemia as a Cause of Pain. When blood flow to a tissue is blocked, the tissue becomes very painful within a few minutes. And the greater the rate of metabolism of the tissue, the more rapidly the pain appears. For instance, if a blood pressure cuff is placed around the upper arm and inflated until the arterial blood flow ceases, exercise of the forearm muscles can cause severe muscle pain within 15 to 20 seconds. In the absence of muscle exercise, the pain will not appear for three to four minutes. Cessation of blood flow to the skin, in which the metabolic rate is very low, usually does not cause pain for about 20 to 30 minutes.

One of the suggested causes of pain in ischemia is accumulation of large amounts of lactic acid in the tissues, formed as a consequence of the anaerobic metabolism (metabolism without oxygen) that occurs during ischemia. However, it is also possible that other chemical agents, such as bradykinin, proteolytic enzymes, and so forth, are formed in the tissues because of cell damage and that these, rather than lactic acid, stimulate the pain nerve endings.

Muscle Spasm as a Cause of Pain. Muscle spasm is also a very common cause of pain, and it is the basis of many clinical pain syndromes. This pain probably results partially from the direct effect of muscle spasm in stimulating mechanosensitive pain receptors. However, it possibly results also from the indirect effect of muscle spasm in causing ischemia and thereby stimulating chemosensitive pain receptors. The muscle spasm not only compresses the blood vessels and diminishes blood flow but also increases the rate of metabolism in the muscle tissue at the same time, thus making the

relative ischemia even greater, creating ideal conditions for release of chemical pain-inducing substances.

THE DUAL PATHWAY FOR TRANSMISSION OF PAIN SIGNALS INTO THE CENTRAL NERVOUS SYSTEM

Even though all pain endings are free nerve endings, these endings utilize two separate pathways for transmitting pain signals into the central nervous system. The two pathways correspond to the two different types of pain, an *acute-sharp pain pathway* and a *slow-chronic pain pathway.*

The Peripheral Pain Fibers—"Fast" and "Slow" Fibers. The acute-sharp pain signals are transmitted in the peripheral nerves to the spinal cord by small type Aδ fibers at velocities of between 6 and 30 meters per second. On the other hand, the slow-chronic type of pain is transmitted by type C fibers at velocities of between 0.5 and 2 meters per second. When the type Aδ fibers are blocked without blocking the C fibers by moderate compression of the nerve trunk, the acute-sharp pain disappears. On the other hand, when the type C fibers are blocked without blocking the delta fibers by low concentrations of local anesthetic, the slow-chronic-aching type of pain disappears.

Because of this double system of pain innervation, a sudden onset of painful stimulus gives a "double" pain sensation: a fast, sharp pain followed a second or so later by a slow, burning pain. The sharp pain apprises the person very rapidly of a damaging influence and, therefore, plays an important role in making the person react immediately to remove himself or herself from the stimulus. On the other hand, the slow, burning sensation tends to become more and more painful over a period of time. This sensation gives one the intolerable suffering of long-continued pain.

Dual Processing of the Pain Signals in the Spinal Cord. On entering the spinal cord from the dorsal spinal roots, the pain fibers ascend or descend one to three segments in the *tract of Lissauer* that lies immediately posterior to the dorsal horn of the cord gray matter. Then they terminate on neurons in the dorsal horns. However, here again, there are two systems for processing the pain signals prior to relaying the signals to the brain, as illustrated in Figure 14–4.

Processing of the "fast" pain signals: The "fast" type Aδ pain fibers terminate at two points in the dorsal horns, in lamina I (lamina marginalis) and lamina V, as shown by the medialmost dorsal root fiber in the figure. In both of these laminae the incoming pain fibers excite second order neurons that send long fibers immediately to the opposite side of the cord in the anterior commissure and then upward

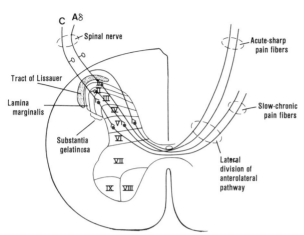

Figure 14-4. Transmission of both "acute-sharp" and "slow-chronic" pain signals into and through the spinal cord on the way to the brain stem.

to the brain in the lateral division of the anterolateral sensory pathway, as described in the previous chapter.

Processing of the "slow" signals: The type C fibers that transmit the "slow" pain signals terminate almost entirely in laminae II and III of the dorsal horns, an area called the *substantia gelatinosa* as shown by the lateralmost dorsal root fiber in the figure. Most of the signals then pass through one or more additional short-fiber neurons, eventually terminating mainly in lamina V. Here the last neuron in the series gives rise to long axons, most of which join the fibers from the fast pathway and pass through the anterior commissure to the opposite side of the cord, then upward to the brain via the lateral division of the anterolateral sensory pathway. However, a few of these fibers do not cross but instead pass ipsilaterally to the brain.

In the lateral division of the anterolateral pathway, the fast pain fibers and the slow fibers remain differentiated from each other, the fast fibers having diameters of 3 to 5 microns and the slow fibers 1 to 3 microns, and with correspondingly faster transmission in the fast fibers.

Termination of the Fast-Acute Pain Pathway in the Brain Stem and Thalamus. Figure 14–5 illustrates the pain pathways entering the brain stem from the spinal cord. About three quarters to nine tenths of all pain fibers terminate in the reticular formation of the medulla, pons, and mesencephalon. From these areas, higher order neurons are transmitted to the thalamus, hypo-thalamus, and other areas of the diencephalon and cerebrum.

However, a small proportion of the pain fibers, especially those that transmit the fast-acute type of pain, pass directly to the thalamus and terminate in the ventrobasal complex and posterior nuclear group of the thalamus, along with the sensory fibers from the dorsal column–lemniscal pathway. From here signals are transmitted into other areas of the thalamus and also to the somatic sensory cortex.

These signals to the cortex are probably important mainly for localizing the pain, not for interpreting it.

Termination of the Slow-Chronic Pain Fibers in the Brain Stem and Thalamus. In contrast to the fibers of the acute-fast pain pathway, those of the slow-chronic pathway terminate almost entirely in the reticular formation of the brain stem. However, great numbers of signals are relayed upward through this formation and finally into the intralaminar nuclei of the thalamus. Both the reticular area of the brain stem and the intralaminar nuclei are parts of the reticular activating system. In Chapter 19 we will discuss in detail the functions of this system; briefly, it transmits activating signals into essentially all parts of the brain, especially upward through the thalamus to all areas of the cerebral cortex and also laterally into the basal regions of the brain around the thalamus, including very importantly the hypothalamus.

Thus, the slow-burning-aching pain fibers, because they do excite the reticular activating system, have a very potent effect in activating essentially the entire nervous system—that is, to arouse one from sleep, to create a state of excitement, to create a sense of urgency, and to promote defense and aversion reactions designed to rid the person or animal of the painful stimulus.

The signals that are transmitted through the slow-burning-aching pain pathway can be localized only to very gross areas of the body. Therefore, these signals are designed almost entirely for the single purpose of calling one's attention to injurious processes in the body. They create suffering that is sometimes intolerable. Their gradation of intensity

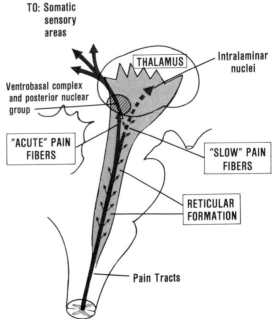

Figure 14-5. Transmission of pain signals into the hindbrain, thalamus, and cortex via the "pricking pain" pathway and the "burning pain" pathway.

is poor; instead, even weak pain signals can summate over a period of time by a process of temporal summation to create an unbearable feeling even though the same pain for short periods of time may be relatively mild.

Function of the Reticular Formation, Thalamus, and Cerebral Cortex in the Appreciation of Pain. Complete removal of the somatic sensory areas of the cerebral cortex does not destroy one's ability to perceive pain. Therefore, it is believed that pain impulses entering only the reticular formation, thalamus, and other lower centers can cause conscious perception of pain. However, this does not mean that the cerebral cortex has nothing to do with normal pain appreciation; indeed, electrical stimulation of the cortical somatic sensory areas causes a person to perceive mild pain in approximately 3 per cent of the stimulations. It is believed that the cortex plays an important role in interpreting the quality of pain even though pain perception might be a function of lower centers.

Localization of Pain in the Body. Most localization of pain probably results from simultaneous stimulation of tactile receptors along with the pain stimulation. However, the acute type of pain, transmitted through type Aδ fibers, can be localized perhaps within 10 to 20 cm of the stimulated area. On the other hand, the slow-burning-aching type of pain, transmitted through C fibers, is localizable only very grossly, perhaps to a major part of the body such as a limb but certainly not to small areas. This is in keeping with the fact that these fibers terminate extremely diffusely in the brain stem and thalamus.

Surgical Interruption of Pain Pathways. Often a person has such severe and intractable pain (this often results from rapidly spreading cancer) that it is necessary to relieve the pain. To do this the pain pathway can be destroyed at any one of several different points. If the pain is in the lower part of the body, a *cordotomy* in the upper thoracic region often relieves the pain for a few weeks to a few months. To do this, the spinal cord on the side opposite the pain is sectioned almost entirely through its anterolateral quadrant, which interrupts the anterolateral sensory pathway.

Unfortunately, though, the cordotomy is not always successful in relieving the pain for two reasons. First, many of the pain fibers from the upper part of the body do not cross to the opposite side of the spinal cord until they have reached the brain so that the cordotomy does not transect these fibers. Second, pain frequently returns several months later; indeed, the new pain is often even more objectionable than the original pain. This pain presumably is transmitted in the dorsal half of the cord, but the locus and destination of the fiber pathways are unknown.

An experimental operative procedure to relieve pain is to place lesions in or around the pain-receptive areas of the thalamus to block the pain pathway at this point. It has been claimed that destruction of portions of the intralaminar nuclei in the thalamus can relieve the suffering elicited by pain while still leaving intact one's appreciation of "acute" pain, which remains an important protective mechanism.

A PAIN CONTROL ("ANALGESIA") SYSTEM IN THE BRAIN AND SPINAL CORD

The degree to which each person reacts to pain varies tremendously. This results partly from the capability of the brain itself to control the degree of input of pain signals to the nervous system by activation of a pain control system, called an *analgesia system.*

The analgesia system is illustrated in Figure 14–6. It consists of three major components (plus other accessory components). (1) The *periaqueductal gray area* of the mesencephalon and upper pons surrounding the aqueduct of Sylvius. Neurons from this area send their signals to (2) the *raphe magnus nucleus,* a thin midline nucleus located in the lower pons and upper medulla. From here the signals are transmitted down the spinal cord to (3) a *pain inhibitory complex located in the dorsal horns of the spinal cord.* At this point the pain signals can be blocked before they are relayed on to the brain.

Electrical stimulation in either the periaqueductal gray area or in the raphe magnus nucleus can almost completely suppress many very strong pain signals entering by way of the dorsal spinal roots. Also, stimulation of areas at still higher levels of the brain that in turn excite the periaqueductal gray, especially the *periventricular nuclei in the hypothalamus* lying adjacent to the third ventricle and to a lesser extent the *medial forebrain bundle* also in the hypo-

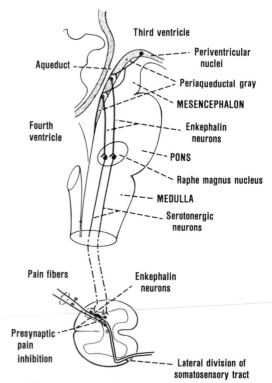

Figure 14–6. The analgesia system of the brain stem and spinal cord, showing inhibition of incoming pain signals at the cord level.

thalamus, can suppress pain though perhaps not quite so much so.

Several different transmitter substances are involved in the analgesia system; especially involved are *enkephalin* and *serotonin.* Many of the nerve fibers derived from both periventricular nuclei and the periaqueductal gray area secrete enkephalin at their endings. Thus, as shown in Figure 14–6, the endings of many of the fibers in the raphe magnus nucleus release enkephalin. The fibers originating in this nucleus but terminating in the dorsal horns of the spinal cord secrete serotonin at their endings. The serotonin in turn acts on still another set of local cord neurons that are believed to secrete enkephalin. The enkephalin, in some way not presently understood, is believed to cause presynaptic inhibition of the incoming pain fibers to laminae I through V in the dorsal horns.

Thus, the analgesia system can block pain signals at the initial entry point to the spinal cord. In fact, it can also block many of the local cord reflexes that result from pain signals, especially the withdrawal reflexes that will be described in the following chapter.

It is probable that this analgesia system can also inhibit pain transmission at other points in the pain pathway, especially in the reticular nuclei in the brain stem and in the intralaminar nuclei of the thalamus.

Most important, it must be noted that this pain analgesia system is capable of blocking both the fast-sharp type of pain and also the slow-burning-aching type of pain.

The Brain's Opiate System— The Endorphins and Enkephalins

More than 20 years ago it was discovered that injection of extremely minute quantities of morphine into either the periventricular nucleus around the third ventricle of the diencephalon or into the periaqueductal gray area of the brain stem will cause an extreme degree of analgesia. In subsequent studies, it has now been found that morphine acts at still many other points in the analgesia system, including both in the raphe magnus nucleus and in the dorsal horns of the spinal cord. Because most drugs that alter the excitability of neurons do so by acting on synaptic receptors, it was assumed that the "morphine-receptors" of the analgesia system must in fact be receptors for some morphine-like neurotransmitter that is naturally secreted in the brain. Therefore, 20 years ago an extensive search was set into motion for a natural opiate of the brain. At least nine such opiate-like substances have now been found at different points of the nervous system. Furthermore, multiple areas of the brain have been shown to have opiate receptors, especially the areas in the analgesia system. Among the more important of the opiate substances are: (1) β-*endor-*phin, (2) *met-enkephalin,* (3) *leu-enkephalin,* and (4) *dynorphin.*

The two enkephalins are found in the portions of the analgesia system described earlier, and β-endorphin is present both in the hypothalamus and in the pituitary gland. In addition, the pituitary gland contains a large peptide, β-*lipotropin,* that includes within its molecule β-endorphin; and β-endorphin includes within its molecule met-enkephalin and presumably can release this enkephalin slowly over a prolonged period of time. Dynorphin, though found in only minute quantities in nervous tissue, is important because it is an extremely powerful opiate, having 200 times as much pain-killing effect as morphine when injected directly into the analgesia system.

Thus, although all the fine details of the brain's opiate system are not yet entirely understood, nevertheless activation of the analgesia system either by nervous signals entering the periaqueductal gray area or by morphine-like drugs can totally or almost totally suppress many pain signals entering through the peripheral nerves.

INHIBITION OF PAIN TRANSMISSION AT THE CORD LEVEL BY TACTILE SIGNALS

Another important landmark in the saga of pain control was the discovery that stimulation of large sensory fibers from the peripheral tactile receptors depresses the transmission of pain signals either from the same area of the body or even from areas sometimes located many segments away. This explains why such simple maneuvers as rubbing the skin near painful areas is often very effective in relieving pain. And it probably also explains why liniments are often useful in the relief of pain. This mechanism and simultaneous psychogenic excitation of the central analgesia system are probably also the basis of pain relief by acupuncture.

Treatment of Pain by Electrical Stimulation. Several clinical procedures have been developed recently for suppressing pain by stimulating large sensory nerve fibers. The stimulating electrodes are placed on selected areas of the skin, or on occasion they have been implanted over the spinal cord to stimulate the dorsal sensory columns. And, in a few patients, electrodes have even been placed stereotaxically in the periventricular or periaqueductal area of the diencephalon. The patient can then personally control the degree of stimulation. Dramatic relief has been reported in some instances.

REFERRED PAIN

Often a person feels pain in a part of his or her body that is considerably removed from the tissues causing the pain. This pain is called *referred pain.* Usually the pain is initiated in one of the visceral organs and referred to an area on the body surface. Also, pain may be referred to another deep area of the body not exactly coincident with the location of the viscus producing the pain. A knowledge of these different types of referred pain is extremely

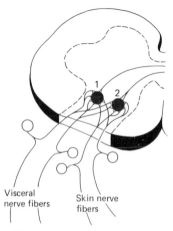

Figure 14–7. Mechanism of referred pain and referred hyperalgesia.

important in clinical diagnosis because many visceral ailments cause no other signs except referred pain.

Mechanism of Referred Pain. Figure 14–7 illustrates the most likely mechanism by which most pain is referred. In the figure, branches of visceral pain fibers are shown to synapse in the spinal cord with some of the same second order neurons that receive pain fibers from the skin. When the visceral pain fibers are stimulated, pain signals from the viscera are then conducted through at least some of the same neurons that conduct pain signals from the skin, and the person has the feeling that the sensations actually originate in the skin itself.

REFERRED PAIN CAUSED BY REFLEX MUSCULAR SPASM

Some types of referred pain are caused secondarily by reflex muscular spasm. For instance, pain in a ureter can cause reflex spasm of the lumbar muscles. Often the pain from the ureter itself is hardly felt at all, but instead almost all the pain results from spasm of the muscles.

Many back pains and some types of headache also appear to be caused by muscular spasm, the spasm being excited reflexly from much weaker pain signals originating elsewhere in the body.

VISCERAL PAIN

In clinical diagnosis, pain from the different viscera of the abdomen and chest is one of the few criteria that can be used for diagnosing visceral inflammation, disease, and other ailments. In general, the viscera have sensory receptors for no other modalities of sensation besides pain. Also, visceral pain differs from surface pain in several important aspects.

One of the most important differences between surface pain and visceral pain is that highly localized types of damage to the viscera rarely cause severe pain. For instance, a surgeon can cut the gut entirely in two in a patient who is awake without causing significant pain. On the other hand, any stimulus that causes *diffuse stimulation of pain nerve endings* throughout a viscus causes pain that can be extremely severe. For instance, ischemia

caused by occluding the blood supply to a large area of gut stimulates many diffuse pain fibers at the same time and can result in extreme pain.

CAUSES OF TRUE VISCERAL PAIN

Any stimulus that excites pain nerve endings in diffuse areas of the viscera causes visceral pain. Such stimuli include ischemia of visceral tissue, chemical damage to the surfaces of the viscera, spasm of the smooth muscle in a hollow viscus, distention of a hollow viscus, or stretching of the ligaments.

Essentially all the true visceral pain originating in the thoracic and abdominal cavities is transmitted through sensory nerve fibers that run in the sympathetic nerves. These fibers are small type C fibers and, therefore, can transmit only the chronic-burning-aching type of pain. The pathways for transmitting true visceral pain will be discussed in more detail later in this chapter.

Ischemia. Ischemia causes visceral pain in exactly the same way that it does in other tissues, presumably because of the formation of acidic metabolic end-products or tissue degenerative products, such as bradykinin, proteolytic enzymes, or others that stimulate the pain nerve endings.

Chemical Stimuli. On occasion, damaging substances leak from the gastrointestinal tract into the peritoneal cavity. For instance, proteolytic acidic gastric juice often leaks through a ruptured gastric or duodenal ulcer. This juice causes widespread digestion of the visceral peritoneum, thus stimulating extremely broad areas of pain fibers. The pain is usually extremely severe.

Spasm of a Hollow Viscus. Spasm of the gut, the gallbladder, a bile duct, the ureter, or any other hollow viscus can cause pain in exactly the same way that spasm of skeletal muscle causes pain. This possibly results from mechanical stimulation of the pain endings. Or its cause might be diminished blood flow to the muscle combined with increased metabolic need of the muscle for nutrients. Thus, *relative* ischemia could develop, which causes severe pain.

Often, pain from a spastic viscus occurs in the form of *cramps*, the pain increasing to a high degree of severity and then subsiding, this process continuing rhythmically once every few minutes. The rhythmic cycles result from rhythmic contraction of smooth muscle. For instance, each time a peristaltic wave travels along an overly excitable spastic gut, a cramp occurs. The cramping type of pain frequently occurs in gastroenteritis, constipation, menstruation, parturition, gallbladder disease, or ureteral obstruction.

Overdistension of a Hollow Viscus. Extreme overfilling of a hollow viscus also results in pain, presumably because of overstretch of the tissues themselves. However, overdistension can also collapse the blood vessels that encircle the viscus, or that pass into its wall, thus perhaps promoting ischemic pain.

Insensitive Viscera

A few visceral areas are almost entirely insensitive to pain of any type. These include the parenchyma of the liver and the alveoli of the lungs. Yet the liver *capsule* is extremely sensitive to both direct trauma and stretch, and the *bile ducts* are also sensitive to pain. In the lungs, even though the alveoli are insensitive, the bronchi and the parietal pleura are both very sensitive to pain.

"PARIETAL" PAIN CAUSED BY VISCERAL DAMAGE

In addition to true visceral pain, some pain sensations are also transmitted from the viscera through nonvisceral nerve fibers that innervate the parietal peritoneum, pleura, or pericardium.

Characteristics of Parietal Visceral Pain. When a disease affects a viscus, it often spreads to the parietal wall of the visceral cavity. This wall, like the skin, is supplied with extensive innervation from the spinal nerves, not from the sympathetic nerves, including the "fast" delta fibers which are different from the "slow" type C fibers in the true visceral pain pathways of the sympathetic nerves. Therefore, pain from the parietal wall of the visceral cavity is frequently very sharp and pricking in quality, though it can also have burning and aching qualities as well if the pain stimulus is diffuse. To emphasize the difference between this pain and true visceral pain: a knife incision through the *parietal* peritoneum is very painful, even though a similar cut through the visceral peritoneum or through a gut is not painful.

LOCALIZATION OF VISCERAL PAIN— THE "VISCERAL" AND THE "PARIETAL" TRANSMISSION PATHWAYS

Pain from the different viscera is frequently difficult to localize for a number of reasons. First, the brain does not know from firsthand experience that the different organs exist, and, therefore, any pain that originates internally can be localized only generally. Second, sensations from the abdomen and thorax are transmitted by two separate pathways to the central nervous system—the *true visceral pathway* and the *parietal pathway*. The true visceral pain is transmitted via sensory fibers of the autonomic nervous system, and the sensations are *referred* to surface areas of the body often far from the painful organ. On the other hand, parietal sensations are conducted *directly* into the local spinal nerves from the parietal peritoneum, pleura, or pericardium, and the sensations are usually *localized directly over the painful area.*

The True Visceral Pathway for Transmission of Pain. Most of the internal organs of the body are supplied by type C pain fibers that pass along the visceral sympathetic nerves into the spinal cord and thence up the lateral division of the anterolateral sensory pathway along with the pain fibers from the body's surface. A few visceral pain fibers—those from the distal portion of the colon, from the rectum, and from the bladder—enter the spinal cord through the sacral parasympathetic nerves, and some enter the central nervous system through various cranial nerves. These include fibers in the glossopharyngeal and vagus nerves which transmit pain from the pharynx, trachea, and upper esophagus. Some fibers from the surfaces of the diaphragm as well as from the lower esophagus are also carried in the phrenic nerves.

Localization of Referred Pain Transmitted by the Visceral Pathways. The position in the cord to which visceral afferent fibers pass from each organ, as well as the position on the surface of the body to which pain is

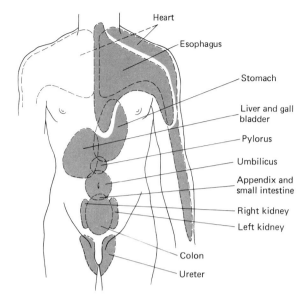

Figure 14–8. Surface areas of referred pain from different visceral organs.

referred, as illustrated in Figure 14–8, depends on the segment of the body from which the organ developed embryologically. For instance, the heart originated in the neck and upper thorax. Consequently, the heart's visceral pain fibers enter the cord all the way from segment C-3 down to T-5. The stomach had its origin approximately from the seventh to the ninth thoracic segments of the embryo, and consequently the visceral afferents from the stomach enter the spinal cord between these levels. The gallbladder had its origin almost entirely in the ninth thoracic segment, so that the visceral afferents from the gallbladder enter the spinal cord at T-9.

Because the visceral afferent pain fibers are responsible for transmitting referred pain from the viscera, the location of the referred pain on the surface of the body is in the dermatome of the segment from which the visceral organ was originally derived in the embryo. Some of the areas of referred pain on the surface of the body are shown in Figure 14–8.

The Parietal Pathway for Transmission of Abdominal and Thoracic Pain. A second set of pain fibers penetrates inward from the spinal nerves that supply the external body surfaces to innervate as well the parietal peritoneum, parietal pleura, and parietal pericardium. Also, retroperitoneal visceral organs and perhaps portions of the mesentery are innervated to some extent by parietal pain fibers. The kidney, for instance, is supplied by both visceral and parietal fibers.

Pain from the viscera is frequently localized to two surface areas of the body at the same time because of the dual pathways for transmission of pain. Figure 14–9 illustrates dual transmission of pain from an inflamed appendix. Impulses pass from the appendix through the sympathetic visceral pain fibers into the sympathetic chain and then into the spinal cord at approximately T-10 or T-11; this pain is referred to an area around the umbilicus and is of the aching, cramping type. On the other hand, pain impulses also often originate in the parietal peritoneum where the inflamed appendix touches the abdominal wall, and these impulses pass through the spinal nerves into the spinal cord at a level of approximately L-1 or L-2. This pain is localized directly over the

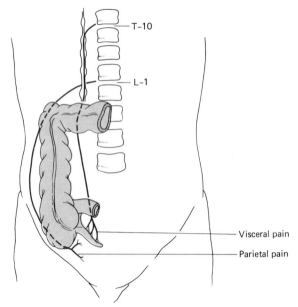

Figure 14–9. Visceral and parietal transmission of pain from the appendix.

irritated peritoneum in the right lower quadrant of the abdomen and is of the sharp type.

VISCERAL PAIN FROM VARIOUS ORGANS

Cardiac Pain. Almost all pain that originates in the heart results from ischemia secondary to coronary sclerosis, usually resulting from atherosclerosis. This pain is referred mainly to the base of the neck, over the shoulders, over the pectoral muscles, and down the arms. Most frequently, the referred pain is on the left side rather than on the right—probably because the left side of the heart is much more frequently involved in coronary disease than is the right side—but occasionally referred pain occurs on the right side of the body as well as on the left.

The pain impulses are conducted through sympathetic nerves passing to the middle cervical ganglia, to the stellate ganglia, and to the first four or five thoracic ganglia of the sympathetic chains. Then the impulses pass into the spinal cord through the second, third, fourth, and fifth thoracic spinal nerves.

Direct Parietal Pain from the Heart. When coronary ischemia is extremely severe, such as immediately after a coronary thrombosis, intense cardiac pain frequently occurs directly underneath the sternum simultaneously with pain referred to other areas. This direct pain from underneath the sternum is difficult to explain on the basis of the visceral nerve connections. Therefore, it is highly probable that sensory nerve endings passing from the heart through the pericardial reflections around the great vessels conduct this direct pain.

In addition to pain from the heart, other sensations may accompany coronary thrombosis. One of these is a tight, oppressive sensation beneath the sternum. The exact cause of this is unknown, but a possible cause is reflex spasm of blood vessels, bronchioles, or muscles in the chest region.

Esophageal Pain. Pain from the esophagus is usually referred to the pharynx, to the lower neck, to the arms, or to midline chest regions beginning at the upper portion of the sternum and ending approximately at the lower level of the heart. Irritation of the gastric end of the esophagus may cause pain directly over the heart, though the pain has nothing whatever to do with the heart. Such pain may be caused by spasm of the lower esophageal sphincter, or it may result from chemical, bacterial, or other types of inflammatory irritations.

Gastric Pain. Pain arising in the fundus of the stomach—usually caused by gastritis—is referred to the anterior surface of the chest or upper abdomen, from slightly below the heart to an inch or so below the xyphoid process. This pain is frequently characterized as burning pain; it, or pain from the lower esophagus, causes the condition known as "heartburn."

Most peptic ulcers occur within 1 to 2 inches on either side of the pylorus in the stomach or in the duodenum, and pain from such ulcers is usually referred to a surface point approximately midway between the umbilicus and the xiphoid process. The cause of ulcer pain is almost undoubtedly chemical, because when the acid juices of the stomach are not allowed to reach the pain fibers in the ulcer crater the pain does not exist. This pain is characteristically intensely burning.

Biliary and Gallbladder Pain. Pain from the bile ducts and gallbladder is localized in the midepigastrium in almost the same place as pain caused by peptic ulcers. Also, biliary and gallbladder pain is often burning, like that from ulcers, though cramps often occur too.

Biliary disease, in addition to causing pain on the abdominal surface, frequently refers pain to a small area on the back at the tip of the right scapula. This pain is transmitted through sympathetic afferent fibers that enter the ninth thoracic segment of the spinal cord.

Pancreatic Pain. Lesions of the pancreas, such as acute or chronic pancreatitis in which the pancreatic enzymes eat away the pancreas and surrounding structures, promote intense pain in areas both anterior to and behind the pancreas. It should be remembered that the pancreas is located beneath the parietal peritoneum and that it receives many parietal sensory fibers from the posterior abdominal wall. Therefore, the pain is usually localized directly behind the pancreas in the back and is severe and burning in character.

Renal Pain. The kidney, kidney pelvis, and ureters are all retroperitoneal structures and receive most of their pain fibers directly from skeletal nerves. Therefore, pain is usually felt directly behind the ailing structure. However, pain occasionally is referred via visceral afferents to the anterior abdominal wall below and about 2 inches to the side of the umbilicus.

Pain from the bladder is felt directly over the bladder, presumably because the bladder is well innervated by parietal pain fibers. However, pain also is sometimes referred to the groin and testicles because some nerve fibers from the bladder apparently synapse in the cord in association with fibers from the genital areas.

Uterine Pain. Both parietal and visceral afferent pain may be transmitted from the uterus. The low abdominal cramping pains of dysmenorrhea are mediated through the sympathetic afferents, and an operation to cut the hypogastric nerves between the hypogastric plexus and the uterus will in many instances relieve this pain. On the other hand, lesions of the uterus that spread into the adnexa around the uterus, or lesions of the fallopian tubes and broad ligaments, usually cause pain in the lower back or side. This pain is conducted over parietal nerve fibers and is usually sharper in nature than the diffuse cramping pain of true dysmenorrhea.

SOME CLINICAL ABNORMALITIES OF PAIN AND OTHER SENSATIONS

HYPERALGESIA

A pain pathway may become excessively excitable; this gives rise to *hyperalgesia,* which means hypersensitivity to pain. The basic causes of hyperalgesia are excessive sensitivity of the pain receptors themselves, which is called *primary hyperalgesia,* or facilitation of sensory transmission, which is called *secondary hyperalgesia.*

An example of primary hyperalgesia is the extreme sensitivity of sunburned skin. Secondary hyperalgesia frequently results from lesions in the spinal cord or in the thalamus. Several of these will be discussed in subsequent sections.

THE THALAMIC SYNDROME

Occasionally the posterolateral branch of the posterior cerebral artery, a small artery supplying the postero-ventral portion of the thalamus, becomes blocked by thrombosis so that the nuclei of this area of the thalamus degenerate, while the medial and anterior nuclei of the thalamus remain intact. The patient suffers a series of abnormalities. First, loss of almost all sensations from the opposite side of the body occurs because of destruction of the relay nuclei. Second, ataxia (inability to control movements precisely) may be evident because of loss of position and kinesthetic signals normally relayed through the thalamus to the cortex. Third, after a few weeks to a few months some sensory perception in the opposite side of the body returns, but strong stimuli are usually necessary to elicit this. When the sensations do occur, they are poorly—if at all—localized, almost always very painful, sometimes lancinating, regardless of the type of stimulus applied to the body. Fourth, the person is likely to perceive many affective sensations of extreme unpleasantness or, rarely, extreme pleasantness; the unpleasant ones are often associated with emotional tirades.

The medial nuclei of the thalamus are not destroyed by thrombosis of the artery. Therefore, it is believed that these nuclei become facilitated and give rise to the enhanced sensitivity to pain transmitted through the reticular system as well as to the affective perceptions.

HERPES ZOSTER

Occasionally a herpes virus, which is believed to be identical to the chickenpox virus, infects a dorsal root ganglion. This causes severe pain in the dermatomal segment normally subserved by the ganglion, thus eliciting a segmental type of pain that circles halfway around the body. The disease is called *herpes zoster,* and the pain is commonly called "shingles."

There are two possible causes of the pain of herpes zoster. One is that the disease destroys mainly the large mechanoreceptor afferent sensory fibers. This theoretically could reduce the normal inhibitory effect of these fibers on the pain pathway in the substantia gelatinosa of the dorsal horn. Therefore, pain signals could become exacerbated in the absence of this inhibition.

A second possibility is that the irritated neuronal cell bodies of the root ganglion are stimulated to excessive activity and thereby cause the pain.

TIC DOULOUREUX

Lancinating pains occur in some persons over one side of the face in part of the sensory distribution area of the fifth or ninth nerves; this phenomenon is called *tic douloureux* (or *trigeminal neuralgia* or *glossopharyngeal neuralgia*). The pains feel like sudden electric shocks, and they may appear for only a few seconds at a time or they may be almost continuous. Often, they are set off by exceedingly sensitive "trigger areas" on the surface of the face, in the mouth or in the throat—almost always by a mechanoreceptive stimulus instead of a pain stimulus. For instance, when the patient swallows a bolus of food, as the food touches a tonsil it might set off a severe lancinating pain in the mandibular portion of the fifth nerve.

The pain of tic douloureux can usually be blocked by cutting the peripheral nerve from the hypersensitive area. The sensory portion of the fifth nerve is often sectioned immediately inside the cranium, where the motor and sensory roots of the fifth nerve can be separated so that the motor portions, which are needed for many of the jaw movements, are spared while the sensory elements are destroyed. Obviously, this operation leaves the side of the face anesthetic, which in itself may be annoying. Furthermore, it is sometimes unsuccessful, indicating that the lesion might be more central than the nerves themselves.

THE BROWN-SEQUARD SYNDROME

Obviously, if the spinal cord is transected entirely, all sensations and motor functions distal to the segments of transection are blocked, but if only one side of the spinal cord is transected, the so-called Brown-Séquard syndrome occurs. The following effects of such a transection occur, and these can be predicted from a knowledge of the cord fiber tracts illustrated in Figure 14–10: All motor functions are blocked on the side of the transection in all segments below the level of the transection, yet only some of the modalities of sensation are lost on the transected side and others are lost on the opposite side. The sensations of pain, heat, and cold are lost on the opposite side of the body in all dermatomes two to six segments below the level of the transection. The sensations that are transmitted only in the dorsal and dorsolateral columns—kinesthetic and position sensations, vibration sensation, discrete localization, and two-point discrimination—are lost entirely on the side of the transection in all dermatomes below the level of the transection. Touch is impaired on the side of the transection because the principal pathway for transmission of light touch, the dorsal columns, is transected. Yet, "crude touch," which is poorly localized, still persists because of transmission in the opposite ventral spinothalamic tract.

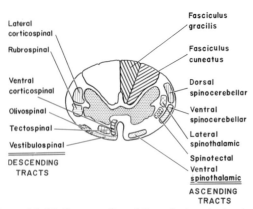

Figure 14–10. Cross-section of the spinal cord, showing principal ascending tracts on the right and principal descending tracts on the left.

HEADACHE

Headaches are actually referred pain to the surface of the head from the deep structures. Many headaches result from pain stimuli arising inside the cranium, but equally as many probably result from pain arising outside the cranium.

HEADACHE OF INTRACRANIAL ORIGIN

Pain-Sensitive Areas in the Cranial Vault. The brain itself is almost totally insensitive to pain. Even cutting or electrically stimulating the somatic sensory areas of the cortex only occasionally causes pain; instead, it causes tactile pins and needles types of paresthesias on the area of the body represented by the portion of the sensory cortex stimulated. Therefore, it is obvious from the outset that much or most of the pain of headache probably is not caused by damage within the brain itself.

On the other hand, *tugging on the venous sinuses, damaging the tentorium,* or *stretching the dura at the base of the brain* can all cause intense pain that is recognized as headache. Also, almost any type of traumatizing, crushing, or stretching stimulus to the *blood vessels of the dura* can cause headache. A very sensitive structure is the middle meningeal artery, and neurosurgeons are careful to anesthetize this artery specifically when performing brain operations under local anesthesia.

Areas of the Head to Which Intracranial Headache Is Referred. Stimulation of pain receptors in the intracranial vault above the tentorium, including the upper surface of the tentorium itself, initiates impulses in the fifth nerve and, therefore, causes referred headache to the front half of the head in the area supplied by the fifth cranial nerve, as illustrated in Figure 14–11.

On the other hand, pain impulses from beneath the tentorium enter the central nervous system mainly through the second cervical nerve, which also supplies the scalp behind the ear. Therefore, subtentorial pain stimuli cause "occipital headache" referred to the posterior part of the head as shown in Figure 14–11.

Types of Intracranial Headache. *Headache of Meningitis.* One of the most severe headaches of all is that resulting from meningitis, which causes inflammation of all the meninges, including the sensitive areas of the dura

and the sensitive areas around the venous sinuses. Such intense damage as this can cause extreme headache pain referred over the entire head.

Headache Resulting from Direct Meningeal Trauma. Following a brain operation the patient ordinarily has intense headache for several days to several weeks. Though part of this headache may result from the brain trauma, experiments indicate that most of it results from meningeal irritation.

Another type of meningeal trauma that almost invariably causes headache is the meningeal irritation resulting from brain tumor. Usually, tumor headache is referred to a localized area of the head, the exact area depending on the portion of the meninges affected by the tumor. Since a tumor above the tentorium is likely to refer its pain to the front half of the head and any tumor below the tentorium to the occipital region of the skull, the general location of an intracranial tumor can often be predicted from the area of the headache.

Headache Caused by Low Cerebrospinal Fluid pressure. Removing as little as 20 ml of fluid from the spinal canal, particularly if the person remains in the upright position, often causes intense intracranial headache. Removing this quantity of fluid removes the flotation for the brain that is normally provided by the cerebrospinal fluid. Therefore, the weight of the brain stretches the various dural surfaces and thereby elicits the pain which causes the headache.

Migraine Headache. Migraine headache is a special type of headache that is thought to result from abnormal vascular phenomena, though the exact mechanism is unknown.

Migraine headaches often begin with various prodromal sensations, such as nausea, loss of vision in part of the field of vision, visual aura, or other types of sensory hallucinations. Ordinarily, the prodromal symptoms begin half an hour to an hour prior to the beginning of the headache itself. Therefore, any theory that explains migraine headache must also explain these prodromal symptoms.

One of the *theories* of the cause of migraine headaches is that prolonged emotion or tension causes reflex vasospasm of some of the arteries of the head, including arteries that supply the brain itself. The vasospasm the-

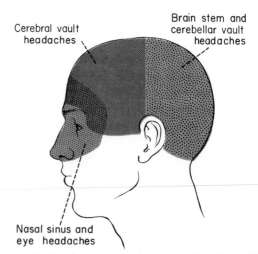

Figure 14–11. Areas of headache resulting from different causes.

oretically produces ischemia of portions of the brain, and this is responsible for the prodromal symptoms. Then, as a result of the intense ischemia, something happens to the vascular wall to allow it to become flaccid and incapable of maintaining vascular tone for 24 to 48 hours. The blood pressure in the vessels causes them to dilate and pulsate intensely, and it is postulated that the excessive stretching of the walls of the arteries—including the extracranial arteries such as the temporal artery—causes the actual pain of migraine headaches. However, it is possible that diffuse aftereffects of ischemia in the brain itself are at least partially if not mainly responsible for this type of headache.

Alcoholic Headache. As many people have experienced, a headache usually follows an alcoholic binge. It is most likely that alcohol, because it is toxic to tissues, directly irritates the meninges and causes intracranial pain.

Headache Caused by Constipation. Constipation causes headache in many persons. Because it has been shown that constipation headache can occur in persons whose spinal cords have been cut, we know that this headache is not caused by nervous impulses from the colon. Therefore, it possibly results from absorbed toxic products or from changes in the circulatory system resulting from loss of fluid into the gut.

EXTRACRANIAL TYPES OF HEADACHE

Headache Resulting from Muscular Spasm. Emotional tension often causes many of the muscles of the head, including especially those muscles attached to the scalp and the neck muscles attached to the occiput, to become spastic, and it is postulated that this is one of the common causes of headache. The pain of the spastic head muscles supposedly is referred to the overlying areas of the head and gives one the same type of headache as do intracranial lesions.

Headache Caused by Irritation of the Nasal and Accessory Nasal Structures. The mucous membranes of the nose and also of all the nasal sinuses are sensitive to pain, but not intensely so. Nevertheless, infection or other irritative processes in widespread areas of the nasal structures usually cause headache that is referred behind the eyes or, in the case of frontal sinus infection, to the frontal surfaces of the forehead and scalp, as illustrated in Figure 14–11. Also, pain from the lower sinuses—such as the maxillary sinuses—can be felt in the face.

Headache Caused by Eye Disorders. Difficulty in focusing one's eyes clearly may cause excessive contraction of the ciliary muscles in an attempt to gain clear vision. Even though these muscles are extremely small, tonic contraction of them can be the cause of retro-orbital headache. Also, excessive attempts to focus the eyes can result in reflex spasm in various facial and extraocular muscles, which is also a possible cause of headache.

A second type of headache originating in the eyes occurs when the eyes are exposed to excessive irradiation by ultraviolet light rays. Watching the sun or the arc of an arc-welder for even a few seconds may result in headache that lasts from 24 to 48 hours. The headache sometimes results from "actinic" irritation of the conjunctivae, and the pain is referred to the surface of the head or retro-orbitally. However, focusing intense light from an arc or the sun on the retina can actually burn the retina, and this could result in headache.

THERMAL SENSATIONS

THERMAL RECEPTORS AND THEIR EXCITATION

The human being can perceive different gradations of cold and heat, progressing from *freezing cold* to *cold* to *cool* to *indifferent* to *warm* to *hot* to *burning hot.*

Thermal gradations are discriminated by at least three different types of sensory receptors: the cold receptors, the warmth receptors, and pain receptors. The pain receptors are stimulated only by extreme degrees of heat or cold and therefore are responsible, along with the cold and warmth receptors, for "freezing cold" and "burning hot" sensations.

The cold and warmth receptors are located immediately under the skin at discrete but separated points, each having a stimulatory diameter of about 1 mm. In most areas of the body there are three to ten times as many cold receptors as warmth receptors, and the number in different areas of the body varies from as great as 15 to 25 cold points per square centimeter in the lips, to 3 to 5 cold points per square centimeter in the finger, to less than 1 cold point per square centimeter in some broad surface areas of the trunk. There are correspondingly fewer numbers of warmth points.

Though it is quite certain on the basis of psychological tests that there are distinctive warmth nerve endings, these have not yet been identified histologically. They are presumed to be free nerve endings because warmth signals are transmitted mainly over type C nerve fibers at transmission velocities of only 0.4 to 2 meters per second.

On the other hand, a definitive cold receptor has been identified. It is a special, small, type Aδ myelinated nerve ending that branches a number of times, the tips of which protrude into the bottom surfaces of basal epidermal cells. Signals are transmitted from these receptors via delta nerve fibers at velocities of up to about 20 meters per second. However, some cold sensations are also transmitted in type C nerve fibers, which suggests that some free nerve endings also might function as cold receptors.

Stimulation of Thermal Receptors—Sensations of Cold, Cool, Indifferent, Warm, and Hot. Figure 14–12 illustrates the effects of different temperatures on the responses of four different nerve fibers: (1) a pain fiber stimulated by cold, (2) a cold fiber, (3) a warmth fiber, and (4) a pain fiber stimulated by heat. Note especially that these fibers respond differently at different levels of temperature. For instance, in the *very* cold region only the pain fibers are stimulated (if the skin becomes even colder so that it nearly freezes or actually does freeze, even these fibers cannot be stimulated). As the temperature rises to 10 to 15° C, pain impulses cease, but

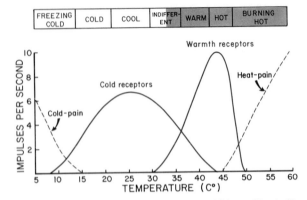

Figure 14–12. Frequencies of discharge of (1) a cold-pain fiber, (2) a cold fiber, (3) a warmth fiber, and (4) a heat-pain fiber. (The responses of these fibers are drawn from original data collected in separate experiments by Zotterman, Hensel, and Kenshalo.)

the cold receptors begin to be stimulated. Then, above about 30° C the warmth receptors become stimulated while the cold receptors fade out at about 43° C. Finally, at around 45° C, pain fibers begin to be stimulated by heat.

One can understand from Figure 14–12, therefore, that a person determines the different gradations of thermal sensations by the relative degrees of stimulation of the different types of endings. For instance, at 20° C only cold endings are stimulated, whereas at 44° C only warm endings are stimulated; at 35° C both cold and warm endings are stimulated; at 60° C pain endings are again stimulated. One can understand also from this figure why extreme degrees of cold or heat can both be painful and why both these sensations, when intense enough, may give almost exactly the same quality of sensations—that is, freezing cold and burning hot sensations feel almost alike; they are both very painful. (Also, not shown in the figure is the fact that high temperatures, as well as cold temperatures, excite the cold endings, which also makes hot temperatures often feel cold and painful.)

Stimulatory Effects of Rising and Falling Temperature—Adaption of Thermal Receptors. When a cold receptor is suddenly subjected to an abrupt fall in temperature, it becomes strongly stimulated at first, but this stimulation fades rapidly during the first few seconds and progressively more slowly during the next half hour or more. In other words, the receptor adapts to a very great extent; this is illustrated in Figure 14–13, which shows that the frequency of discharge of a cold receptor rose approximately fourfold when the temperature fell suddenly from 32° to 30° C, but in less than a minute the frequency fell about five sixths of the way back to the original control value. Later, the temperature was suddenly raised from 30° to 32° C. The cold receptor stopped firing entirely for a short time but after adapting returned to its original control level.

Thus, it is evident that the thermal senses re-

spond markedly to *changes in temperature* in addition to being able to respond to steady states of temperature, as was depicted in Figure 14–12. This means, therefore, that when the temperature of the skin is actively falling, a person feels much colder than when the temperature remains at the same level. Conversely, if the temperature is actively rising the person feels much warmer than he or she would at the same temperature if it were constant.

The response to changes in temperature explains the extreme degree of heat that one feels on first entering a tub of hot water and the extreme degree of cold felt on going from a heated room to the out-of-doors on a cold day.

Mechanism of Stimulation of the Thermal Receptors. It is believed that the thermal receptors are stimulated by changes in their metabolic rates, these changes resulting from the fact that temperature alters the rates of intracellular chemical reactions more than twofold for each 10° C change. In other words, thermal detection probably results not from direct physical stimulation but instead from chemical stimulation of the endings as modified by the temperature.

Spatial Summation of Thermal Sensations. Because the number of cold or warmth endings in any one surface area of the body is very slight, it is difficult to judge gradations of temperature when small areas are stimulated. However, when a large area of the body is stimulated all at once, the thermal signals from the entire area summate. Indeed, one reaches the maximum ability to discern minute temperature variations when the entire body is subjected to a temperature change all at once. For instance, rapid changes in temperature of as little as 0.01° C can be detected if this change affects the entire surface of the body simultaneously. On the other hand, temperature changes 100 times this great might not be detected when the skin surface affected is only a square centimeter or so in size.

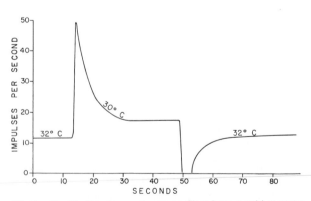

Figure 14–13. Response of a nerve fiber from a cold receptor following, first, instantaneous change in skin temperature from 32° to 30° C and, second, instantaneous change back to 32° C. Note the adaptation of the receptor and also the higher steady state level of discharge at 30° than at 32°.

TRANSMISSION OF THERMAL SIGNALS IN THE NERVOUS SYSTEM

In general, thermal signals are transmitted in almost parallel, but not the same, pathways as pain signals. On entering the spinal cord, the signals travel for a few segments upward or downward in the *tract of Lissauer* and then terminate mainly in laminae I, II, and III of the dorsal horns. After a small amount of processing by one or more cord neurons, the signals enter long, ascending thermal fibers that cross to the lateral division of the opposite anterolateral sensory tract and terminate in the reticular areas of the brain stem and the ventrobasal complex of the thalamus. A few thermal signals are also relayed to the somatic sensory cortex from the ventrobasal complex. Occasionally, a neuron in somatic sensory area I has been found by microelectrode studies to be directly responsive to either cold or warm stimuli in specific areas of the skin. Furthermore, it is known that removal of the postcentral gyrus in the human being reduces the ability to distinguish gradations of temperature.

REFERENCES

Akil, H., *et al*.: Endogenous opioids: Etiology and function. *Annu. Rev. Neurosci.*, 7:223, 1984.

American Physiological Society: Sensory Processes. Washington, D.C., American Physiological Society, 1984.

Basbaum, A. I., and Fields, H. L.: Endogenous pain control systems: Brainstem spinal pathways and endorphin circuitry. *Annu. Rev. Neurosci.*, 7:309, 1984.

Berger, P. A., *et al*.: Behavioral pharmacology of the endorphins. *Annu. Rev. Med.*, 33:397, 1982.

Bond, M. R.: Pain—Its Nature, Analysis, and Treatment. New York, Churchill Livingstone, 1984.

Brainard, J. B.: Control of Migraine. New York, W. W. Norton & Co., 1979.

Coren, S., *et al*.: Sensation and Perception. New York, Academic Press, 1979.

Currie, D. J.: Abdominal Pain. Washington, D.C., Hemisphere Publishing Corporation, 1979.

Darian-Smith, I.: The sense of touch: Performance and peripheral neural process. *In* Darian-Smith, I. (ed.): Handbook of Physiology. Sec. 1, Vol. III. Bethesda, American Physiological Society, 1984, p. 739.

Darian-Smith, I.: Thermal sensibility. *In* Darian-Smith, I. (ed.): Handbook of Physiology. Sec. 1, Vol. III. Bethesda, American Physiological Society, 1984, p. 879.

Darian-Smith, I., *et al*.: Posterior parietal cortex: Relations of unit activity to sensorimotor function. *Annu. Rev. Physiol.*, 41:141, 1979.

Dubner, R., and Bennett, G. J.: Spinal and trigeminal mechanisms of nociception. *Annu. Rev. Neurosci.*, 6:381, 1983.

Fields, H. L., and Basbaum, A. I.: Brainstem control of spinal pain-transmission neurons. *Annu. Rev. Physiol.*, 40:217, 1978.

Friedhoff, A. J., and Miller, J. C.: Clinical implications of receptor sensitivity modification. *Annu. Rev. Neurosci.*, 6:121, 1983.

Gelmers, H. J.: Calcium-channel blockers in the treatment of migraine. *Am. J. Cardiol.*, 55:139B, 1985.

Goldstein, E. B.: Sensation and Perception. Belmont, Cal., Wadsworth Publishing Co., 1980.

Graham, M. (ed.): Disorders of the Facial Nerve. Anatomy, Diagnosis and Management. New York, Raven Press, 1982.

Guyton, A. C., and Reeder, R. C.: Pain and contracture in poliomyelitis. *Arch. Neurol. Psychiatr.*, 63:954, 1950.

Haft, J. I. (ed.): Differential Diagnosis of Chest Pain and Other Cardiac Symptoms. Mt. Kisco, N.Y., Futura Publishing Co., 1983.

Han, J. S., and Terenius, L.: Neurochemical basis of acupuncture analgesia. *Annu. Rev. Pharmacol. Toxicol.*, 22:193, 1982.

Hardy, J. D.: The nature of pain. *J. Chronic Dis.*, 4:22, 1956.

Hardy, J. D., *et al*.: Pain Sensations and Reactions. Baltimore, Williams & Wilkins, 1952.

Health and Public Policy Committee, American College of Physicians: Biofeedback for headaches. *Ann. Intern. Med.*, 102:128, 1985.

Hochberg, J.: Perception. *In* Darian-Smith, I. (ed.): Handbook of Physiology. Sec. 1, Vol. III. Bethesda, American Physiological Society, 1984, p. 75.

Hyvarinen, J.: Posterior parietal lobe of the primate brain. *Physiol. Rev.*, 62:1060, 1982.

Ischia, S. (ed.): Pain Treatment. Pituitary Neuroadenolysis in the Treatment of Cancer Pain and Hormone-Dependent Tumors. New York, Raven Press, 1983.

Jacob, J. (ed.): Receptors. New York, Pergamon Press, 1979.

Jung, R.: Sensory research in historical perspective: Some philosophical foundations of perception. *In* Darian-Smith, I. (ed.): Handbook of Physiology. Sec. 1, Vol. III. Bethesda, American Physiological Society, 1984, p. 1.

Kaas, J. H.: What, if anything, is SI? Organization of first somatosensory area of cortex. *Physiol. Rev.*, 63:206, 1983.

Kaas, J. J., *et al*.: The reorganization of the somatosensory cortex following peripheral nerve damage in adult and developing mammals. *Annu. Rev. Neurosci.*, 6:325, 1983.

Kenshalo, D. R. (ed.): Sensory Function of the Skin of Humans. New York, Plenum Press, 1979.

Kruger, L. (ed.): Neural Mechanisms of Pain. New York, Raven Press, 1984.

Lewis, R. V., and Stern, A. S.: Biosynthesis of the enkephalins and enkephalin-containing polypeptides. *Annu. Rev. Pharmacol. Toxicol.*, 23:353, 1983.

Mountcastle, V. B.: Central nervous mechanisms in mechanoreceptive sensibility. *In* Darian-Smith, I. (ed.): Handbook of Physiology. Sec. 1, Vol. III. Bethesda, American Physiological Society, 1984, p. 789.

Neff, W. D. (ed.): Contributions to Sensory Physiology. New York, Academic Press, 1982.

Norrsell, U.: Behavioral studies of the somatosensory system. *Physiol. Rev.*, 60:327, 1980.

Olton, D. S.: Spatial memory. *Sci. Am.*, 236(6):82, 1977.

Perl, E. R.: Pain and nociception. *In* Darian-Smith, I. (ed.): Handbook of Physiology. Sec. 1, Vol. III. Bethesda, American Physiological Society, 1984, p. 915.

Perl, E. R., and Boivie, J. G.: Neural substrates of somatic sensations. *In* MTP International Review of Science: Physiology. Vol. 3. Baltimore, University Park Press, 1974, p. 303.

Raj: Practical Management of Pain. Chicago, Year Book Medical Publishers, 1985.

Raskin, N. H.: Chemical headaches. *Annu. Rev. Med.*, 32:63, 1981.

Raskin, N. H., and Appenzeller, O.: Headache. Philadelphia, W. B. Saunders Co., 1980.

Scheibel, A. B.: The brain stem reticular core and sensory function: *In* Darian-Smith, I. (ed.): Handbook of Physiology. Sec. 1, Vol. III. Bethesda, American Physiological Society, 1984, p. 213.

Seltzer, S.: Pain in Dentistry: Diagnosis and Management. Philadelphia, J. B. Lippincott Co., 1978.

Silen, W. (rev.): Cope's Early Diagnosis of the Acute Abdomen. New York, Oxford University Press, 1979.

Stebbins, W. C., Brown, C. H., and Petersen, M. R.: Sensory function in animals. *In* Darian-Smith, I. (ed.): Handbook of Physiology. Sec. 1, Vol. III. Bethesda, American Physiological Society, 1984, p. 123.

Stimmel, B.: Pain, Analgesia, and Addiction. The Pharmacologic Treatment of Pain. New York, Raven Press, 1983.

Weiss, T. F.: Relation of receptor potentials of cochlear hair cells to spike discharges of cochlear neurons. *Annu. Rev. Physiol.*, 46:247, 1984.

Woolsey, C. N. (ed.): Cortical Sensory Organization. Multiple Somatic Areas. Clifton, N.J., Humana Press, 1981.

Zimmerman, M.: Neurophysiology of nociception. *Int. Rev. Physiol.*, 10:179, 1976.

15

Motor Functions of the Spinal Cord; and the Cord Reflexes

In the discussion of the nervous system thus far, we have considered principally the input of sensory information. In the following chapters we will discuss the origin and output of motor signals, the signals that cause muscle contraction and other motor effects throughout the body. Sensory information is integrated at all levels of the nervous system and causes appropriate motor responses, beginning in the spinal cord with relatively simple reflexes, extending into the brain stem with still more complicated responses, and, finally, extending to the cerebrum where the most complicated responses are controlled. The present chapter discusses the control of motor function especially in response to spinal cord reflexes.

Experimental Preparations for Studying Cord Reflexes—The Spinal Animal and the Decerebrate Animal. Normally, most functions of the spinal cord are strongly influenced by signals from the brain. Therefore, to study the isolated cord reflexes it is necessary to separate the cord from the higher centers. This is usually done in one of two different types of preparations, the *spinal animal* or the *decerebrate animal*.

The spinal animal is prepared by cutting the spinal cord at any level above the region in which the cord reflexes are to be studied. For a variable period of time, depending upon the phylogenetic level of the animal, as will be discussed later in the chapter, the cord reflexes are deeply depressed immediately after removal of the signals from the brain. However, over a period of minutes, hours, or days in animals and over a period of weeks in the human being, the cord reflexes become progressively more active and can then be studied independently of control by the upper levels of the nervous system. Often the cord reflexes become even more excitable under these conditions than normally, as will be discussed later in the chapter.

In the decerebrate preparation, the brain stem is usually transected between the superior and inferior colliculi. Transecting the brain stem at this level removes the voluntary control centers of the forebrain, and it also removes inhibitory influences from the basal ganglia that normally suppress the activities of the lower brain stem and spinal cord; this will be discussed in detail in the following chapter. Removal of this inhibition causes an immediate increase in the activity of many of the cord reflexes, especially the antigravity reflexes that help the animal hold itself up against gravity. This preparation has an advantage over the spinal animal in that many of the cord reflexes are exacerbated even in the acute preparation and, therefore, can be studied immediately, though, of course, lower brain stem reflexes may still interfere with the cord functions.

ORGANIZATION OF THE SPINAL CORD FOR MOTOR FUNCTIONS

The cord gray matter is the integrative area for the cord reflexes and other motor functions. Figure 15–1 shows the typical organization of the cord gray matter in a single cord segment. Sensory signals enter the cord through the sensory roots. After entering the cord, every sensory signal travels to two separate destinations. First, the sensory nerve or its collaterals terminate in the gray matter of the cord and elicit local segmental responses—local excitatory effects, facilitatory effects, reflexes, and so forth. Second, the signals travel to higher levels of the nervous system—to higher levels in the cord itself, to the brain stem, or even to the cerebral cortex, as described in the past few chapters.

Each segment of the spinal cord has several million neurons in its gray matter. Aside from the sensory relay neurons discussed in Chapters 13 and 14, the remainder of these neurons are of two separate types, the *anterior motor neurons* and the *interneurons*.

The Anterior Motor Neurons. Located in each segment of the anterior horns of the cord gray matter are several thousand neurons that are 50 to 100 per cent larger than most of the others and are called *anterior motor neurons*. These give rise to the nerve fibers that leave the cord via the anterior roots and innervate the skeletal muscle fibers. The neurons are of two types, the *alpha motor neurons* and the *gamma motor neurons*.

The Alpha Motor Neurons. The alpha motor neurons give rise to large type A alpha (Aα) nerve fibers ranging from 9 to 20 microns in diameter that innervate the large skeletal muscle fibers. Stimula-

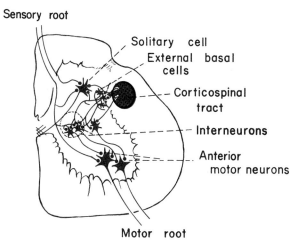

Figure 15–1. Connections of the sensory fibers and cortico-spinal fibers with the interneurons and anterior motor neurons of the spinal cord.

tion of a single nerve fiber excites from as few as three to as many as several hundred skeletal muscle fibers, which are collectively called the *motor unit.* Transmission of nerve impulses into skeletal muscles and their stimulation of the muscle fibers were discussed in Chapters 6 through 8.

The Gamma Motor Neurons. In addition to the alpha motor neurons that excite contraction of the skeletal muscle fibers, about one half as many much smaller gamma motor neurons are located along with the alpha motor neurons in the anterior horns. These transmit impulses through type A gamma (Aγ) fibers, averaging 5 microns in diameter, to very small, special skeletal muscle fibers called *intrafusal fibers.* These are part of the *muscle spindle,* which is discussed later in the chapter.

The Interneurons. The interneurons are present in all areas of the cord gray matter—in the dorsal horns, in the anterior horns, and in the intermediate areas between these two. These cells are numerous—approximately 30 times as numerous as the anterior motor neurons. They are small and highly excitable, often exhibiting spontaneous activity and capable of firing as rapidly as 1500 times per second. They have many interconnections one with the other, and many of them directly innervate the anterior motor neurons, as illustrated in Figure 15–1. The interconnections among the interneurons and anterior motor neurons are responsible for many of the integrative functions of the spinal cord that are discussed in the remainder of this chapter.

Essentially all the different types of neuronal circuits described in Chapter 11 are found in the interneuron pool of cells of the spinal cord, including the *diverging, converging,* and *repetitive-discharge* circuits. In this chapter we will see many applications of these different circuits to the performance of specific reflex acts by the spinal cord.

Only a few incoming sensory signals from the spinal nerves or signals from the brain terminate directly on the anterior motor neurons. Instead, most of them are transmitted first through interneurons where they are appropriately processed. Thus, in Figure 15–1, it is shown that the corticospinal tract terminates almost entirely on interneurons, and it is only after the signals from this tract have been integrated in the interneuron pool with signals from other spinal tracts or from the spinal nerves that they finally impinge on the anterior motor neurons to control muscular function.

The Renshaw Cell Inhibitory System. Located also in the ventral horns of the spinal cord in close association with the motor neurons are a large number of small interneurons called *Renshaw cells.* Almost immediately after the motor axon leaves the motor neuron, collateral branches from the axon pass to the adjacent Renshaw cells. These in turn are inhibitory cells that transmit inhibitory signals to the nearby motor neurons. Thus, stimulation of each motor neuron tends to inhibit the surrounding motor neurons, an effect called *recurrent inhibition.* This effect is probably important for the following major reason:

It shows that the motor system utilizes the principle of lateral inhibition to focus or sharpen its signals in the same way that the sensory system utilizes this principle—that is, to allow unabated transmission of the primary signal while suppressing the tendency for signals to spread to adjacent neurons.

Multisegmental Connections in the Spinal Cord–The Propriospinal Fibers

More than half of all the nerve fibers ascending and descending in the spinal cord are *propriospinal fibers.* These are fibers that run from one segment of the cord to another. In addition, the terminal fibrils of sensory fibers as they enter the cord branch both up and down the spinal cord, some of the branches transmitting signals only a segment or two in each direction, whereas others transmit signals many segments. These ascending and descending fibers of the cord provide pathways for the multisegmental reflexes that will be described later in this chapter, including reflexes that coordinate movements in the forelimbs and hindlimbs simultaneously.

THE MUSCLE RECEPTORS—MUSCLE SPINDLES AND GOLGI TENDON ORGANS—AND THEIR ROLES IN MUSCLE CONTROL

Proper control of muscle function requires not only excitation of the muscle by the anterior motor neurons but also continuous feedback of information from each muscle to the nervous system, giving the status of the muscle at each instant. That is, what is the length of the muscle, what is its instantaneous tension, and how rapidly is its length or tension changing? To provide this information, the muscles and their tendons are supplied abundantly with two special types of sensory receptors: *muscle spindles,* which are distributed throughout the belly of the muscle and which send information to the nervous system about either the muscle length or rate of change of its length, and *Golgi tendon organs,* which transmit information about tension or rate of change of tension.

The signals from these two receptors are either entirely or almost entirely for the purpose of muscle control itself, because they operate almost entirely at a subconscious level. Even so, they transmit tremendous amounts of information into the spinal cord, the cerebellum, and even the cerebral cortex, helping each of these portions of the nervous system in its function for controlling muscle contraction.

RECEPTOR FUNCTION OF THE MUSCLE SPINDLE

Structure and Innervation of the Muscle Spindle. The physiological organization of the muscle spindle is illustrated in Figure 15–2. Each spindle is built around 3 to 12 small *intrafusal muscle fibers* that are pointed at their ends and are attached to the glycocalyx of the surrounding *extrafusal* skeletal muscle fibers. Each intrafusal fiber is a very small skeletal muscle fiber. However, the central region of each of these fibers—that is, the area midway between its two ends—has either no or few actin and myosin filaments. Therefore, this central portion does not contract when the ends do. Instead, it functions as a sensory receptor as we shall describe later. The end portions are excited by the small *gamma motor nerve fibers* originating from the gamma motor neurons that were described earlier. These fibers are frequently also called *gamma efferent fibers*, in contradistinction to the *alpha efferent fibers* that innervate the extrafusal skeletal muscle.

Excitation of the Spindle Receptors

The receptor portion of the muscle spindle is its central portion where the intrafusal muscle fibers have no contractile elements. As illustrated in Figure 15–2, and also in more detail in Figure 15–3, sensory fibers originate in this area, and these are

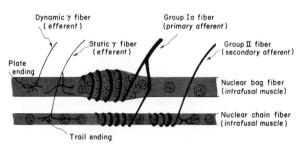

Figure 15–3. Details of nerve connections to the nuclear bag and nuclear chain muscle spindle fibers. (Modified from Stein: *Physiol Rev.*, 54:225, 1974, and Boyd: *Philos. Trans. R. Soc. Lond. [Biol. Sci.]*, 245:81, 1962.)

stimulated by stretch of this midportion of the spindle. One can readily see that the muscle spindle receptor can be excited in two different ways. (1) Lengthening the whole muscle will obviously stretch the midportion of the spindle and therefore excite the receptor. (2) Even if the length of the entire muscle does not change, contraction of the end-portions of the intrafusal fibers will also stretch the midportions of the spindle and therefore excite the receptor.

Two types of sensory endings are found in the receptor area of the muscle spindle.

The Primary Ending. In the very center of the receptor area a large sensory fiber encircles the central portion of each intrafusal fiber, forming the so-called *primary ending* or also called the *annulospiral ending*. This nerve fiber is a type Ia fiber averaging 17 microns in diameter, and it transmits sensory signals to the spinal cord at a velocity of 70 to 120 meters per second, as rapidly as any type of sensory nerve fiber in the entire body.

The Secondary Endings. Usually one, but sometimes two, smaller sensory nerve fiber, a type II fiber with an average diameter of 8 microns, innervates the receptor region on one side of the primary ending, as illustrated in Figures 15–2 and 15–3. This sensory ending is called the *secondary ending*, or sometimes the *flower spray ending* because in some preparations it looks like a flower spray even though it mainly encircles the intrafusal fibers in the same way that the type Ia fiber does.

Division of the Intrafusal Fibers into Nuclear Bag and Nuclear Chain Fibers—Dynamic and Static Responses of the Muscle Spindle. There are also two different types of intrafusal fibers: (1) *nuclear bag fibers* (one to three in each spindle), in which a large number of nuclei are congregated into a bag in the central portion of the receptor area, and (2) *nuclear chain fibers* (three to nine), which are about half as large in diameter and half as long as the nuclear bag fibers and have nuclei aligned in a chain throughout the receptor area. The primary ending innervates both the nuclear bag intrafusal fibers *and* the nuclear chain fibers. On the other hand, the secondary ending usually innervates only the nuclear chain fibers. These relationships are all illustrated in Figure 15–3.

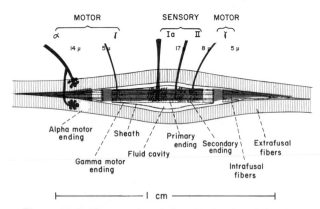

Figure 15–2. The muscle spindle, showing its relationship to the large extrafusal skeletal muscle fibers. Note also both the motor and the sensory innervation of the muscle spindle.

Response of Both the Primary and Secondary Endings to Length of the Receptor—The "Static" Response. When the receptor portion of the muscle spindle is stretched slowly, the number of impulses transmitted from both the primary and the secondary endings increases almost directly in proportion to the degree of stretch, and the endings continue to transmit these impulses for many minutes. This effect is called the *static response* of the spindle receptor, meaning simply that both the primary and the secondary endings continue to transmit their signals for as long as the receptor itself remains stretched. Because only the *nuclear chain* type of intrafusal fiber is innervated by both the primary and the secondary endings, it is believed that these nuclear chain fibers are responsible for the static response.

Response of the Primary Ending (But Not the Secondary Ending) to Rate of Change of Receptor Length—The "Dynamic" Response. When the length of the spindle receptor increases suddenly, the primary ending (but not the secondary ending) is stimulated especially powerfully, much more powerfully than the stimulus caused by the static response. This excess stimulus of the primary ending is called the *dynamic response,* which means that the primary ending responds extremely actively to a rapid *rate of change* in length. When the length of a spindle receptor increases only a fraction of a micron, if this increase occurs in a fraction of a second, the primary receptor transmits tremendous numbers of excess impulses into the Ia fiber, but only *while the length is actually increasing.* As soon as the length has stopped increasing, the rate of impulse discharge returns almost back to its original level, except for the small static response that is still present in the signal.

Conversely, when the spindle receptor shortens, this change momentarily decreases the impulse output from the primary ending; then, as soon as the receptor area has reached its new shortened length, the impulses reappear in the Ia fiber within a fraction of a second. Thus, the primary ending sends extremely strong signals to the central nervous system to apprise it of any change in length of the spindle receptor area.

Since only the primary endings innervate the nuclear bag intrafusal fibers, it is assumed that the nuclear bag fibers are responsible for the powerful dynamic response.

Control of the Static and Dynamic Responses by the Gamma Motor Nerves. Some physiologists believe that the gamma motor nerves to the muscle spindle can be divided into two different types: gamma-dynamic (gamma-d) and gamma-static (gamma-s). The first of these is believed to excite the nuclear bag intrafusal fibers and the second mainly the nuclear chain intrafusal fibers. When the gamma-d fibers excite the nuclear bag fibers, the dynamic response of the muscle spindle becomes tremendously enhanced, whereas the static response is hardly affected. On the other hand, stimulation of the gamma-s fibers, which are believed to excite mainly the nuclear chain fibers, supposedly enhances the static response while having little influence on the dynamic response. We shall see in subsequent paragraphs that these two different types of responses of the muscle spindle are exceedingly important in different types of muscle control.

Continuous Discharge of the Muscle Spindles Under Normal Conditions. Normally, particularly when there is a slight amount of gamma motor excitation, the muscle spindles emit sensory nerve impulses continuously. Stretching the muscle spindles increases the rate of firing, while shortening the spindles decreases this rate of firing. Thus, the spindles can send either *positive signals* to the spinal cord—that is, increased numbers of impulses to indicate increased stretch of a muscle, or they can send *negative signals*—decreased numbers of impulses below the normal level to indicate that the muscle is actually being unstretched.

THE STRETCH REFLEX (ALSO CALLED MYOTATIC REFLEX)

From the prior description of all the intricacies of the muscle spindle, one can readily see that it is a very complex organ. Its function is manifested in the form of the muscle *stretch reflex*—that is, whenever a muscle is stretched, excitation of the spindles causes reflex contraction of the muscle.

Neuronal Circuitry of the Stretch Reflex. Figure 15–4 illustrates the basic circuit of the muscle spindle stretch reflex, showing a type Ia nerve fiber originating in a muscle spindle and entering the dorsal root of the spinal cord. Then, in contrast to most other nerve fibers entering the cord, one branch of it passes directly to the anterior horn of the cord gray matter and synapses directly with anterior motor neurons that send nerve fibers back to the same muscle from whence the muscle spindle fiber originated. Thus, this is a *monosynaptic pathway* that allows a reflex signal to return with almost no delay back to the same muscle after excitation of the spindle.

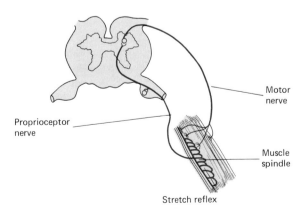

Proprioceptor
nerve

Motor
nerve

Muscle
spindle

Stretch reflex

Figure 15–4. Neuronal circuit of the stretch reflex.

Some of the type II fibers from the secondary spindle endings also terminate monosynaptically with the anterior motor neurons. However, most of the type II fibers (as well as many collaterals from the Ia fibers from the primary endings) terminate on multiple interneurons in the cord gray matter, and these in turn transmit more delayed signals to the anterior motor neurons and also serve other functions.

The Dynamic Stretch Reflex and the Static Stretch Reflex. The stretch reflex can be divided into two separate components called respectively the dynamic stretch reflex and the static stretch reflex. The *dynamic stretch reflex* is elicited by the potent dynamic signal transmitted from the primary endings of the muscle spindles. That is, when a muscle is suddenly stretched, a strong signal is transmitted to the spinal cord, and this causes an instantaneous, very strong reflex contraction of the same muscle from which the signal originated. Thus, the reflex functions to oppose sudden changes in the length of the muscle, because the muscle contraction opposes the stretch.

The dynamic stretch reflex is over within a fraction of a second after the muscle has been stretched to its new length, but then a weaker *static stretch reflex* continues for a prolonged period of time thereafter. This reflex is elicited by the continuous static receptor signals transmitted by both the primary and secondary endings. The importance of the static stretch reflex is that it continues to cause muscle contraction as long as the muscle is maintained at excessive length. The muscle contraction in turn opposes the force that is causing the excess length.

The Negative Stretch Reflex. When a muscle is suddenly shortened, exactly opposite effects occur. If the muscle is already taut, any sudden release of the load on the muscle that allows it to shorten will elicit both dynamic and static reflex muscle inhibition rather than reflex excitation. Thus, this *negative stretch reflex* opposes the shortening of the muscle in the same way that the positive stretch reflex opposes lengthening of the muscle. Therefore, one can begin to see that the stretch reflex tends to maintain the status quo for the length of a muscle.

Feedback Control of Muscle Length— The Load Reflex

Let us assume that a person's biceps is contracted so that the forearm is horizontal to the earth. Then assume that a five-pound weight is put in the hand. The hand will immediately drop. However, the amount that the hand will drop is determined to a great extent by the degree of activity of the muscle spindle reflex. If the gamma-s fibers to the muscle spindles are strongly stimulated so that the static reflex is very active, even slight lengthening of the biceps, and therefore also of the muscle spindles in the biceps, will cause a strong feedback contraction of the extrafusal skeletal muscle fibers of the biceps.

This contraction in turn will limit the degree of fall of the hand, thus automatically maintaining the forearm in a nearly horizontal position. This response is called the *load reflex.*

The Damping Function of the Dynamic and Static Stretch Reflexes

Another important function of the stretch reflex—indeed, probably just as important as, if not more important than, the load reflex—is the ability of the stretch reflex to prevent some types of oscillation and jerkiness of the body movements. This is a *damping* or *smoothing* function.

Use of the Damping Mechanism in Smoothing Muscle Contraction. Occasionally, signals from other parts of the nervous system are transmitted to a muscle in a very unsmooth form, increasing in intensity for a few milliseconds, then decreasing in intensity, then changing to another intensity level, and so forth. When the muscle spindle apparatus is not functioning satisfactorily, the muscle contraction is very jerky during the course of such a signal. This effect is illustrated in Figure 15–5, which shows an experiment in which a sensory nerve signal entering one side of the cord is transmitted to a motor nerve on the other side of the cord to excite a muscle. In curve A the muscle spindle reflex of the excited muscle is intact. Note that the contraction is relatively smooth even though the sensory nerve is excited at a very slow frequency of eight per second. Curve B, on the other hand, is the same experiment in an animal whose muscle spindle sensory nerves from the excited muscle had been sectioned three months earlier. Note the very unsmooth muscle contraction. Thus, curve A illustrates very graphically the ability of the damping mechanism of the muscle spindle to smooth muscle contractions even though the input signals to the muscle motor system may themselves be very jerky. This effect can also be called a *signal averaging* function of the muscle spindle reflex.

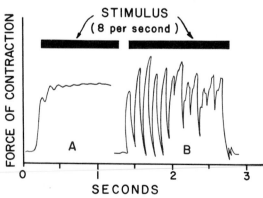

Figure 15–5. Muscle contraction caused by a spinal cord signal under two different conditions: *A*, in a normal muscle, and *B*, in a muscle whose muscle spindles had been denervated by section of the posterior roots of the cord 82 days previously. Note the smoothing effect of the muscle spindle reflex in *A*. (Modified from Creed et al.)

ROLE OF THE MUSCLE SPINDLE IN VOLUNTARY MOTOR ACTIVITY

To emphasize the importance of the gamma efferent system, one needs to recognize that 31 per cent of all the motor nerve fibers to the muscle are gamma efferent fibers rather than large, type A alpha motor fibers. Whenever signals are transmitted from the motor cortex or from any other area of the brain to the alpha motor neurons, almost invariably the gamma motor neurons are stimulated simultaneously, an effect called *co-activation* of the alpha and gamma motor neurons. This causes both the extrafusal and the intrafusal muscle fibers to contract at the same time.

The purpose of contracting the muscle spindle fibers at the same time that the large skeletal muscle fibers contract is probably twofold: First, it keeps the muscle spindle from opposing the muscle contraction. Second, it also maintains proper damping and proper load responsiveness of the muscle spindle regardless of change in muscle length. For instance, if the muscle spindle should not contract and relax along with the large muscle fibers, the receptor portion of the spindle would sometimes be flail and at other times be overstretched, in neither instance operating under optimal conditions for spindle function.

Possible "Servo" Control of Muscle Contraction by Exciting the Gamma Motor Neurons. Several physiologists have suggested that the muscle spindle reflex can also operate as a servo controller of muscle contraction. A "servo" control system is one in which the output of the system is not activated directly by the input signal but instead is activated indirectly in the following way: Suppose that a gamma efferent nerve fiber to a muscle spindle were stimulated. This would contract the intrafusal fibers and excite the muscle spindle receptors. The signals from these receptors would then pass to the cord and thence back to the extrafusal skeletal muscle fibers to cause them to contract also. Thus, an initial contraction of the spindle intrafusal fibers would cause a similar contraction of the surrounding extrafusal fibers.

If such a servo system as this should exist, signals transmitted from the brain downward through the gamma efferent system could cause secondary contractions of the muscles in accordance with the dictates of the muscle spindles. Unfortunately, most of the data indicate that a mechanism such as this probably does not occur to a significant extent. For a system of this type to function properly, it would be necessary to have a static response of the muscle spindles that is very potent and also unchanging. Unfortunately, the static response of the muscle spindles is usually weak—that is, it has a low gain. Also, it decays very slowly over a period of many minutes to an hour so that changes in length of a muscle spindle could cause only temporary changes in length of the surrounding large skeletal muscle fibers. Therefore, despite the attractiveness of this possible type of muscle control, it is doubtful that it does actually occur in normal function.

Probable Servo-Assist Function of the Muscle Spindle Reflex. It is much more likely that the muscle spindle reflex acts as a servo-assist device than as a pure servo controller. But, first, let us explain what is meant by a "servo-assist mechanism."

When both the alpha and gamma motor neurons are stimulated simultaneously, if the intra- and extrafusal fibers contract equal amounts the degree of stimulation of the muscle spindles will not change at all—neither increase nor decrease. However, in case the extrafusal muscle fibers should contract less than the intrafusal fibers (as might occur when the muscle is contracting against a great load), this mismatch would stretch the receptor portions of the spindles and, therefore, elicit a stretch reflex that would provide extra excitation of the extrafusal fibers. Thus, failure of the extrafusal fibers to contract to the same degree as the intrafusal fibers contract would cause an accessory neuronal signal that would increase the degree of stimulation of the extrafusal fibers. This is exactly the same mechanism as that employed by power steering in an automobile. That is, if the front wheels are resistant to following the movement of the steering wheel, a servo-assist device becomes activated that applies additional force to turn the wheels.

The servo-assist type of motor function could have several important advantages, as follows:

1. It would allow the brain to cause a muscle contraction against a load without the brain having to expend much extra nervous energy—instead, the spindle reflex would provide most of the nervous energy.

2. It would make the muscle contract almost the desired length even when the load is increased or decreased between successive contractions. In other words, it would make the length of contraction less load-sensitive.

3. It could compensate for fatigue or other abnormalities of the muscle itself, because any failure of the muscle to provide the proper contraction would elicit an additional muscle spindle reflex stimulus to make the contraction occur.

But, unfortunately, we still do not know how important this probable function of the muscle spindle reflex actually is.

Brain Areas for Control of the Gamma Efferent System

The gamma efferent system is excited primarily by the *bulboreticular facilitatory* region of the brain stem, and secondarily by impulses transmitted into this area from (a) the *cerebellum,* (b) the *basal ganglia,* and even (c) the *cerebral cortex.* Unfortunately, though, little is known about the precise mechanisms of control of the gamma efferent system. However, since the bulboreticular facilitatory area is particularly concerned with antigravity contractions, and also because the antigravity muscles have an especially high density of muscle spindles, emphasis is given to the possible or probable important role of the gamma efferent mechanism in controlling muscle contraction for positioning the different parts of the body and for damping the movements of the different parts.

CLINICAL APPLICATIONS OF THE STRETCH REFLEX

The Knee Jerk and Other Muscle Jerks. Clinically, a method used to determine the sensitivity of the stretch reflexes is to elicit the knee jerk and other muscle jerks. The knee jerk can be elicited by simply striking the patellar tendon with a reflex hammer; this stretches the quadriceps muscle and initiates a *dynamic stretch reflex* that in turn causes the lower leg to jerk forward. The

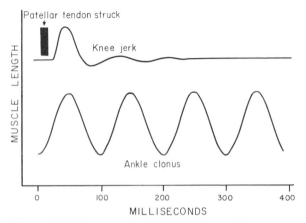

Figure 15–6. Myograms recorded from the quadriceps muscle during elicitation of the knee jerk from the gastrocnemius muscle during ankle clonus.

upper part of Figure 15–6 illustrates a myogram from the quadriceps muscle recorded during a knee jerk.

Similar reflexes can be obtained from almost any muscle of the body either by striking the tendon of the muscle or by striking the belly of the muscle itself. In other words, sudden stretch of muscle spindles is all that is required to elicit a stretch reflex.

The muscle jerks are used by neurologists to assess the degree of facilitation of spinal cord centers. When large numbers of facilitatory impulses are being transmitted from the upper regions of the central nervous system into the cord, the muscle jerks are greatly exacerbated. On the other hand, if the facilitatory impulses are depressed or abrogated, the muscle jerks are considerably weakened or completely absent. These reflexes are used most frequently to determine the presence or absence of muscle spasticity following lesions in the motor areas of the brain. Ordinarily, large lesions in the contralateral motor areas of the cerebral cortex, especially those caused by strokes or brain tumors, cause greatly exacerbated muscle jerks.

Clonus. Under appropriate conditions, the muscle jerks can oscillate, a phenomenon called *clonus* (see lower myogram, Fig. 15–6). Oscillation can be explained particularly well in relation to ankle clonus, as follows:

If a man standing on his tiptoes suddenly drops his body downward to stretch one of his gastrocnemius muscles, impulses are transmitted from the muscle spindles into the spinal cord. These reflexly excite the stretched muscle, which lifts the body back up again. After a fraction of a second, the reflex contraction of the muscle dies out and the body falls again, thus stretching the spindles a second time. Again a dynamic stretch reflex lifts the body, but this too dies out after a fraction of a second, and the body falls once more to elicit still a new cycle. In this way, the stretch reflex of the gastrocnemius muscle continues to oscillate, often for long periods of time; this is clonus.

Clonus ordinarily occurs only if the stretch reflex is highly sensitized by facilitatory impulses from the brain. For instance, in the decerebrate animal, in which the stretch reflexes are highly facilitated, clonus develops readily. Therefore, to determine the degree of facilitation of the spinal cord, neurologists test patients for clonus by suddenly stretching a muscle and keeping a steady stretching force applied to the muscle. If clonus occurs, the degree of facilitation is certain to be very high.

THE TENDON REFLEX

The Golgi Tendon Organ and Its Excitation. Golgi tendon organs, illustrated in Figure 15–7, are encapsulated sensory receptors through which the muscle tendons pass immediately beyond their attachments to the muscle fibers. An average of 10 to 15 muscle fibers are usually connected in series with each Golgi tendon organ, and the organ is stimulated by the tension produced by this small bundle of muscle fibers. Thus, the major difference between the function of the Golgi tendon organ and the muscle spindle is that the spindle detects relative muscle length, while the tendon organ detects muscle *tension*.

The tendon organ, like the primary receptor of the muscle spindle, has both a *dynamic response* and a *static response*, responding very intensely when the muscle tension suddenly increases (the dynamic response), but within a small fraction of a second it settles down to a lower level of steady state firing that is almost directly proportional to the muscle tension (the static response). Thus, the Golgi tendon organs provide the nervous system with instantaneous information of the degree of tension on each small segment of each muscle.

Transmission of Impulses from the Tendon Organ into the Central Nervous System. Signals from the tendon organ are transmitted through large, rapidly conducting type Ib nerve fibers, fibers averaging 16 microns in diameter, only slightly smaller than those from the primary ending of the muscle spindle. These fibers, like those from the primary endings, transmit signals both into local areas of the cord and through the spinocerebellar tracts into the cerebellum and through still other tracts to the cerebral cortex. The local cord signal excites a single inhibitory interneuron that in turn inhibits the anterior alpha motor neuron. This local circuit directly inhibits the individual muscle without affecting adjacent muscles. The signals to the brain will be discussed in Chapter 17.

Inhibitory Nature of the Tendon Reflex. When the Golgi tendon organs of a muscle are stimulated by increased muscle tension, signals are transmitted into the spinal cord to cause reflex effects in the respective muscle. However, this reflex is entirely inhibitory, the exact opposite to the muscle spindle reflex. Thus, this reflex provides a negative feedback mechanism that prevents the development of too much tension on the muscle.

When tension on the muscle and, therefore, on

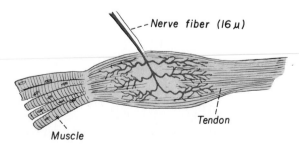

Figure 15–7. Golgi tendon organ.

the tendon becomes extreme, the inhibitory effect from the tendon organ can be so great that it causes sudden relaxation of the entire muscle. (The signals from the secondary endings of the muscle spindles are believed also to help in causing this reaction.) This effect is called the *lengthening reaction;* it is probably a protective mechanism to prevent tearing of the muscle or avulsion of the tendon from its attachments to the bone. We know, for instance, that direct electrical stimulation of muscles in the laboratory, which cannot be opposed by this tension reflex, can frequently cause such destructive effects.

The Tendon Reflex as a Possible Servo Control Mechanism for Muscle Tension. In the same way that the stretch reflex possibly operates as a feedback mechanism to control muscle length, the tendon reflex theoretically can operate as a servo feedback mechanism to control muscle tension. That is, if the tension on the muscle becomes too great, inhibition from the tendon organ decreases this tension back to a lower value. On the other hand, if the tension becomes too little, impulses from the tendon organ cease; and the resulting loss of inhibition allows the alpha motor neurons to become active again, thus increasing muscle tension back toward a higher level.

Very little is known at present about the function or control of this tension servo feedback mechanism, but it is postulated to operate in the following basic manner: Signals from the brain are presumably transmitted to the cord to apprise a neuronal group in the cord of the tension required in each given muscle. At the same time, signals are also transmitted through the alpha motor neurons to cause muscle contraction. Then, as the degree of contraction approaches the tension limit set for the muscle, as detected by the feedback from the Golgi tendon organs, the neuronal group automatically inhibits the muscle contraction to prevent additional tension. In this way, the tension becomes adjusted to the ''set-point'' dictated by the brain.

Yet, a word of caution: Despite this speculation, the measured feedback gains of this muscle tension feedback system have been far too little to prove that it can be very useful as a tension servo controller.

Possible Value of a Servo Mechanism for Control of Tension. An obvious value of a mechanism for setting the degree of muscle tension would be to allow the different muscles to apply a desired amount of force irrespective of how far the muscles contract. An example of this is paddling a boat, in which a person sets the amount of force with which he pulls backward on the paddle and maintains that degree of force throughout the entire movement. Were it not for some type of tension feedback mechanism, the same amount of force would not be maintained throughout the stroke because uncontrolled muscles change their force of contraction as their lengths change. One can imagine hundreds of different patterns of muscle function that might require maintenance of constant tension rather than maintenance of constant lengths of the muscles.

THE FLEXOR REFLEX (THE WITHDRAWAL REFLEXES)

In the spinal or decerebrate animal, almost any type of cutaneous sensory stimulus on a limb is likely to cause the flexor muscles of the limb to contract, thereby withdrawing the limb from the stimulus. This is called the flexor reflex.

In its classic form the flexor reflex is elicited most powerfully by stimulation of pain endings, such as by pinprick, heat, or some other painful stimulus, for which reason it is also frequently called a *nociceptive reflex,* or simply *pain reflex.* However, even stimulation of the touch receptors can also occasionally elicit a weaker and less prolonged flexor reflex.

If some part of the body besides one of the limbs is painfully stimulated, this part, in a similar manner, will be withdrawn from the stimulus, but the reflex may not be confined entirely to flexor muscles even though it is basically the same type of reflex. Therefore, the many patterns of reflexes of this type in the different areas of the body are called the *withdrawal reflexes.*

Neuronal Mechanism of the Flexor Reflex. The left-hand portion of Figure 15–8 illustrates the neuronal pathways for the flexor reflex. In this instance, a painful stimulus is applied to the hand; as a result, the flexor muscles of the upper arm become reflexly excited, thus withdrawing the hand from the painful stimulus.

The pathways for eliciting the flexor reflex do not pass directly to the anterior motor neurons but, instead, pass first into the interneuron pool of neurons and then to the motor neurons. The shortest possible circuit is a three- or four-neuron arc; however, most of the signals of the reflex traverse many more neurons than this and involve the following basic types of circuits: (1) diverging circuits to spread the reflex to the necessary muscles for withdrawal, (2) circuits to inhibit the antagonist muscles, called *reciprocal inhibition circuits,* and (3) circuits to cause a prolonged repetitive after-discharge even after the stimulus is over.

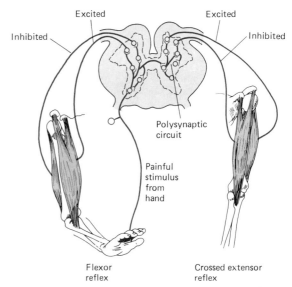

Figure 15–8. The flexor reflex, the crossed extensor reflex, and reciprocal inhibition.

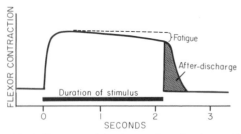

Figure 15–9. Myogram of the flexor reflex, showing rapid onset of the reflex, an interval of fatigue, and finally after-discharge after the stimulus is over.

Figure 15–9 illustrates a typical myogram from a flexor muscle during a flexor reflex. Within a few milliseconds after a pain nerve begins to be stimulated, the flexor response appears. Then, in the next few seconds the reflex begins to *fatigue*, which is characteristic of essentially all of the more complex integrative reflexes of the spinal cord. Then, soon after the stimulus is over, the contraction of the muscle begins to return toward the base line, but, because of *after-discharge*, will not return all the way for many milliseconds. The duration of the after-discharge depends on the intensity of the sensory stimulus that had elicited the reflex; a weak tactile stimulus causes almost no after-discharge in contrast to an after-discharge lasting for several seconds following a very strong pain stimulus.

The after-discharge that occurs in the flexor reflex almost certainly results from all three types of repetitive-discharge circuits that were discussed in Chapter 11. Electrophysiological studies indicate that the immediate after-discharge, lasting for about 6 to 8 milliseconds, results from the interneuron repetitive firing mechanism and from the parallel type of circuit, with impulses being transmitted from one interneuron to another to another and all these in turn transmitting their signals successively to the anterior motor neurons. However, the prolonged after-discharge that occurs following strong pain stimuli presumably involves reverberating circuits in the interneurons, these transmitting impulses to the anterior motor neurons sometimes for several seconds after the incoming sensory signal is completely over.

Thus, the flexor reflex is appropriately organized to withdraw a pained or otherwise irritated part of the body away from the stimulus. Furthermore, because of the after-discharge the reflex can still hold the irritated part away from the stimulus for as long as 1 to 3 seconds after the irritation is over. During this time, other reflexes and actions of the central nervous system can move the entire body away from the painful stimulus.

The Pattern of Withdrawal. The pattern of withdrawal that results when the flexor reflex (or the many other types of withdrawal reflexes) is elicited depends on the sensory nerve that is stimulated. Thus, a painful stimulus on the inside of the arm not only elicits a flexor reflex in the arm but also

contracts the abductor muscles to pull the arm outward. In other words, the integrative centers of the cord cause those muscles to contract that can most effectively remove the pained part of the body from the object that causes pain. This same principle, which is called the principle of "local sign," applies for any part of the body but especially to the limbs, because they have highly developed flexor reflexes.

THE CROSSED EXTENSOR REFLEX

Approximately 0.2 to 0.5 second after a stimulus elicits a flexor reflex in one limb, the opposite limb begins to extend. This is called the *crossed extensor reflex*. Extension of the opposite limb obviously can push the entire body away from the object causing the painful stimulus.

Neuronal Mechanism of the Crossed Extensor Reflex. The right-hand portion of Figure 15–8 illustrates the neuronal circuit responsible for the crossed extensor reflex, showing that signals from the sensory nerves cross to the opposite side of the cord to cause exactly opposite reactions to those that cause the flexor reflex. Because the crossed extensor reflex usually does not begin until 200 to 500 milliseconds following the initial pain stimulus, it is certain that many interneurons are in the circuit between the incoming sensory neuron and the motor neurons of the opposite side of the cord responsible for the crossed extension. Furthermore, after the painful stimulus is removed, the crossed extensor reflex continues for an even longer period of after-discharge than that for the flexor reflex. Therefore, again, it is presumed that this prolonged after-discharge results from reverberatory circuits among the internuncial cells.

Figure 15–10 illustrates a myogram recorded from a muscle involved in a crossed extensor reflex. This shows the relatively long latency before the reflex begins and also the long after-discharge following the end of the stimulus. The prolonged after-discharge obviously would be of benefit in holding the body away from a painful object until other nervous reactions could cause the body to move away.

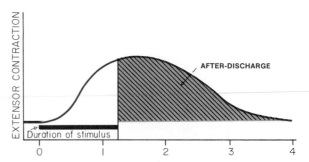

Figure 15–10. Myogram of a crossed extensor reflex, showing slow onset but prolonged after-discharge.

RECIPROCAL INHIBITION AND RECIPROCAL INNERVATION

In the foregoing paragraphs we have pointed out several times that excitation of one group of muscles is often associated with inhibition of another group. For instance, when a stretch reflex excites one muscle, it simultaneously inhibits the antagonist muscles. This is the phenomenon of *reciprocal inhibition,* and the neuronal mechanism that causes this reciprocal relationship is called *reciprocal innervation.* Likewise, reciprocal relationships exist between the two sides of the cord, as exemplified by the flexor and extensor reflexes described above.

Figure 15–11 illustrates a typical example of reciprocal inhibition. In this instance, a moderate but prolonged flexor reflex is elicited from one limb of the body, and while this reflex is still being elicited a still stronger flexor reflex is elicited in the opposite limb, causing reciprocal inhibition of the first limb. Then removal of the strong flexor reflex allows the original reflex to reassume its previous intensity.

FATIGUE OF REFLEXES; REBOUND

Figure 15–9 illustrated that the flexor reflex begins to *fatigue* within a few seconds after its initiation. This is a common effect in most of the cord reflexes as well as many other reflexes of the central nervous system, and it presumably results from progressive fatigue of synaptic transmission in the reflex circuits, a subject that was discussed more fully in Chapter 10.

Another effect closely allied to fatigue is *rebound.* This means that, immediately after a reflex is over, a second reflex of the same type is much more difficult to elicit for a given time thereafter. However, because of reciprocal innervation, reflexes of the antagonist muscles become even more easily elicited during that same period of time. For instance, if a flexor reflex occurs in a left limb, a second flexor reflex is more difficult to establish for a few seconds thereafter, but a crossed extensor reflex in this same limb will be greatly exacerbated. Rebound is probably one of the important mechanisms for coordinating the rhythmic to-and-fro movements required in locomotion, described in more detail later in the chapter.

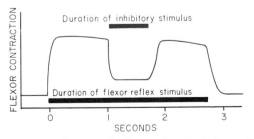

Figure 15–11. Myogram of a flexor reflex, illustrating reciprocal inhibition caused by a stronger flexor reflex in the opposite limb.

THE REFLEXES OF POSTURE AND LOCOMOTION

THE POSTURAL AND LOCOMOTIVE REFLEXES OF THE CORD

The Positive Supportive Reaction. Pressure on the footpad of a decerebrate animal causes the limb to extend against the pressure being applied to the foot. Indeed, this reflex is so strong that an animal whose spinal cord has been transected for several months, when the reflexes have become exacerbated, can often be placed on its feet, and the reflex will stiffen the limbs sufficiently to support the weight of the body—the animal will stand in a rigid position. This reflex is called the *positive supportive reaction.*

The positive supportive reaction involves a complex circuit in the interneurons similar to those responsible for the flexor and the crossed-extensor reflexes. Furthermore, the locus of the pressure on the pad of the foot determines the position to which the limb will extend; pressure on one side causes extension in that direction, an effect called the *magnet reaction.* This obviously helps keep an animal from falling to that side.

The Cord "Righting" Reflexes. When a spinal cat or even a well-recovered young spinal dog is laid on its side, it will make incoordinate movements that indicate that it is trying to raise itself to the standing position. This is called a *cord righting reflex,* and it illustrates that relatively complicated reflexes associated with posture are at least partially integrated in the spinal cord. Indeed, a puppy with a well-healed transected thoracic cord between the cord level for the forelimbs and the hindlimbs can completely right itself from the lying position and can even walk on its hindlimbs. And, in the case of the opossum with a similar transection of the thoracic cord, the walking movements of the hindlimbs are hardly different from those in the normal opossum—except that the hindlimb movements are not synchronized with those of the forelimbs as is normally the case.

Stepping and Walking Movements

Rhythmic Stepping Movements of a Single Limb. Rhythmic stepping movements are frequently observed in the limbs of spinal animals. Indeed, even when the lumbar portion of the spinal cord is separated from the remainder of the cord and a longitudinal section is made down the center of the cord to block neuronal connections between the two limbs, each hind limb can still perform stepping functions. Forward flexion of the limb is followed a second or so later by backward extension. Then flexion occurs again, and the cycle is repeated over and over.

This oscillation back and forth between the flexor and extensor muscles occurs even after the sensory nerves have been cut, and it seems to result mainly from reciprocal inhibition and rebound circuits that oscillate within the matrix of the cord itself. That is, the forward flexion of the limb causes reciprocal inhibition of the cord center controlling the extensor muscles, but shortly thereafter the flexion begins to die out; as it does so, *rebound* inhibition of the flexors and reciprocal *rebound* excitation of the extensors cause the leg to move downward and backward. After extension has continued for a time, it, too, begins to die and is followed by reciprocal rebound excitation of the flexor muscles. And the oscillating cycle continues again and again.

The sensory signals from the footpads and from the position sensors around the joints play a strong role in controlling foot pressure and rate of stepping when the foot is allowed to walk along a surface. In fact, the cord mechanism for control of stepping can be still more complex. For instance, if during the forward thrust of the foot the top of the foot encounters an obstruction, the forward thrust will stop temporarily, the foot will be lifted higher, and then the foot will proceed forward to be placed over the obstruction. Thus, the cord is an intelligent walking controller.

Reciprocal Stepping of Opposite Limbs. If the lumbar spinal cord is not sectioned down its center as noted above, every time stepping occurs in the forward direction in one limb, the opposite limb ordinarily steps backward. This effect results from reciprocal innervation between the two limbs.

Diagonal Stepping of All Four Limbs—The "Mark Time" Reflex. If a well-healed spinal animal, with the spinal transection above the forelimb area of the cord, is held up from the table and its legs are allowed to fall downward as illustrated in Figure 15–12, the stretch on the limbs occasionally elicits stepping reflexes that involve all four limbs. In general, stepping occurs diagonally between the fore- and hindlimbs. That is, the right hindlimb and the left forelimb move backward together while the right forelimb and left hindlimb move forward. This diagonal response is another manifestation of reciprocal innervation, this time occurring the entire

distance up and down the cord between the fore- and hindlimbs. Such a walking pattern is often called a *mark time reflex.*

The Galloping Reflex. Another type of reflex that occasionally develops in the spinal animal is the galloping reflex, in which both forelimbs move backward in unison while both hindlimbs move forward. If stretch or pressure stimuli are applied almost exactly equally to opposite limbs at the same time, a galloping reflex will likely result, whereas unequal stimulation of one side versus the other elicits the diagonal walking reflex. This is in keeping with the normal patterns of walking and of galloping, for, in walking, only one limb at a time is stimulated, and this would predispose to continued walking. Conversely, when the animal strikes the ground during galloping, the limbs on both sides are stimulated approximately equally; this obviously would predispose to further galloping and, therefore, would continue this pattern of motion in contradistinction to the walking pattern.

THE SCRATCH REFLEX

An especially important cord reflex in lower animals is the scratch reflex, which is initiated by the *itch and tickle sensation.* It actually involves two different functions: (1) a *position sense* that allows the paw to find the exact point of irritation on the surface of the body, and (2) a *to-and-fro scratching movement.*

Obviously, the scratch reflex, like the stepping movements of locomotion, involves reciprocal innervation circuits that cause oscillation. One of the important discoveries in relation to the to-and-fro movement of the scratch reflex (and also of the stepping movements as described above) is that it can still occur even when all the sensory roots from the oscillating limb are sectioned. In other words, feedback from the limb itself is not necessary to maintain the neuronal oscillation, which means that the oscillation can occur intrinsically as a result of oscillating circuits within the spinal interneurons themselves.

The *position sense* of the scratch reflex is also a highly developed function, for even though a flea might be crawling as far forward as the shoulder of a spinal animal, the hind paw can find its position. Furthermore, this can be accomplished even though 19 different muscles in the limb must be contracted simultaneously in a precise pattern to bring the paw to the position of the crawling flea. To make the reflex even more complicated, when the flea crosses the midline, the paw stops scratching, but the opposite paw begins the to-and-fro motion and eventually finds the flea.

THE SPINAL CORD REFLEXES THAT CAUSE MUSCLE SPASM

In human beings, local muscle spasm is often observed. The mechanism of this has not been elucidated to complete satisfaction even in experimental animals, but it is known that pain stimuli can cause reflex spasm of local muscles, which presumably is the cause of much if not most of the muscle spasm observed at localized regions of the human body.

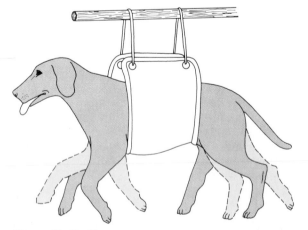

Figure 15–12. Diagonal stepping movements exhibited by a spinal animal.

Muscle Spasm Resulting from a Broken Bone. One type of clinically important spasm occurs in muscles surrounding a broken bone. This seems to result from the pain impulses initiated from the broken edges of the bone, which cause the muscles surrounding the area to contract powerfully and tonically. Relief of the pain by injection of a local anesthetic relieves the spasm; a general anesthetic also relieves the spasm. One of these procedures is often necessary before the spasm can be overcome sufficiently for the two ends of the bone to be set back into appropriate positions.

Abdominal Muscle Spasm in Peritonitis. Another type of local spasm caused by a cord reflex is the abdominal spasm resulting from irritation of the parietal peritoneum by peritonitis. Here, again, relief of the pain caused by the peritonitis allows the spastic muscle to relax. Almost the same type of spasm often occurs during surgical operations; pain impulses from the parietal peritoneum cause the abdominal muscles to contract extensively and sometimes actually to extrude the intestines through the surgical wound. For this reason deep surgical anesthesia is usually required for intra-abdominal operations.

Muscle Cramps. Still another type of local spasm is the typical muscle cramp. Electromyographic studies indicate that the cause of at least some muscle cramps is the following:

Any local irritating factor or metabolic abnormality of a muscle—such as severe cold, lack of blood flow to the muscle, or overexercise of the muscle—can elicit pain or other types of sensory impulses that are transmitted from the muscle to the spinal cord, thus causing reflex muscle contraction. The contraction in turn stimulates the same sensory receptors still more, which causes the spinal cord to increase the intensity of contraction still further. Thus, a positive feedback mechanism occurs so that a small amount of initial irritation causes more and more contraction until a full-blown muscle cramp ensues. Reciprocal inhibition of the muscle can sometimes relieve the cramp. That is, if a person purposefully contracts the muscle on the opposite side of the joint from the cramped muscle while at the same time using another hand or foot to prevent movement of the joint, the reciprocal inhibition that occurs in the cramped muscle can at times relieve the cramp.

THE AUTONOMIC REFLEXES IN THE SPINAL CORD

Many different types of segmental autonomic reflexes occur in the spinal cord, most of which are discussed in other chapters. Briefly, these include (1) changes in vascular tone, resulting from local skin heat and cold, (2) sweating, which results from localized heat on the surface of the body, (3) intestinointestinal reflexes that control some motor functions of the gut, (4) peritoneointestinal reflexes that inhibit gastric motility in response to peritoneal irritation, and (5) evacuation reflexes for emptying the bladder and the colon. Most of these reflexes are discussed in Chapter 28. In addition, all the segmental reflexes can at times be elicited simultaneously in the form of the so-called mass reflex.

The Mass Reflex. In a spinal animal or human being, the spinal cord sometimes suddenly becomes excessively active, causing massive discharge of large portions of the cord. The usual stimulus that causes this is a strong nociceptive stimulus to the skin or excessive filling of a viscus, such as overdistention of the bladder or of the gut. Regardless of the type of stimulus, the resulting reflex, called the *mass reflex*, involves large portions or even all of the cord, and its pattern of reaction is the same. The effects are (1) a major portion of the body goes into strong flexor spasm, (2) the colon and bladder are likely to evacuate, (3) the arterial pressure often rises to maximal values—sometimes to a mean pressure well over 200 mm Hg, and (4) large areas of the body break out into profuse sweating. The mass reflex might be likened to the epileptic seizures that involve the central nervous system in which large portions of the brain become massively activated.

The precise neuronal mechanism of the mass reflex is unknown. However, since it lasts for minutes, it presumably results from activation of great masses of reverberating circuits that excite large areas of the cord at once.

SPINAL CORD TRANSECTION AND SPINAL SHOCK

When the spinal cord is suddenly transected, essentially all cord functions, including the cord reflexes, immediately become depressed to the point of oblivion, a reaction called *spinal shock*. The reason for this is that normal activity of the cord neurons depends to a great extent on continual tonic discharges from higher centers, particularly discharges transmitted through the reticulospinal tracts, vestibulospinal tracts, and corticospinal tracts.

After a few hours to a few days or weeks of spinal shock, the spinal neurons gradually regain their excitability. This seems to be a natural characteristic of neurons everywhere in the nervous system—that is, after they lose their source of facilitatory impulses, they increase their own natural degree of excitability to make up for the loss. But there is also some possibility of sprouting of multiple new nerve endings in the cord, which could also increase excitability. In most nonprimates, the excitability of the cord centers returns essentially to normal within a few hours to a day or so, but in human beings the return is often delayed for several weeks and occasionally is never complete; or, on the other hand, recovery is sometimes excessive, with resultant hyperexcitability of all or most cord functions.

Some of the spinal functions specifically affected during or following spinal shock are: (1) The arterial blood pressure falls immediately—sometimes to as low as 40 mm Hg—thus illustrating that sympathetic activity becomes blocked almost to extinction. However, the pressure ordinarily returns to normal within a few days. (2) All skeletal muscle reflexes integrated in the spinal cord are completely blocked during the initial stages of shock. In lower animals, a few hours to a few days are required for these reflexes to return to normal, and in human beings two weeks to several months are usually required. Sometimes, both in animals and people, some reflexes eventually become hyperexcitable, particularly if a few facilitatory pathways remain intact between the brain and the cord while the remainder of the spinal cord is transected. The first reflexes to return are the stretch reflex, followed in order by the progressively more complex reflexes, the flexor reflexes, the postural antigravity reflexes, and remnants of stepping reflexes. (3) The sacral reflexes for control of bladder and colon evacuation are completely suppressed in human beings for the first few weeks following cord transection, but they eventually return.

REFERENCES

Arbib, M. A.: Perceptual structures and distributed motor control. *In* Brooks, V. B. (ed.): Handbook of Physiology. Sec. 1, Vol. II. Bethesda, American Physiological Society, 1981, p. 1449.

Austin, G.: The Spinal Cord. New York, Igaku Shoin Medical Publishers, 1981.

Baldissera, F., Hultborn, H., and Illert, M.: Integration in spinal neuronal systems. *In* Brooks, V. B. (ed.): Handbook of Physiology. Sec. 1, Vol. II. Bethesda, American Physiological Society, 1981, p. 509.

Burke, R. E.: Motor units: Anatomy, physiology, and functional organization. *In* Brooks, V. B. (ed.): Handbook of Physiology. Sec. 1, Vol. II. Bethesda, American Physiological Society, 1981, p. 345.

Burke, R. E., and Rudomin, P.: Spinal neurons and synapses. *In* Brookhart, J. M., and Mountcastle, V. B. (eds.): Handbook of Physiology. Sec. 1, Vol. 1. Baltimore, Williams & Wilkins, 1977, p. 877.

Creed, R. S., *et al.*: Reflex Activity of the Spinal Cord. New York, Oxford University Press, 1932.

Desmedt, J. E. (ed.): Physiological Tremor, Pathological Tremors and Clonus. New York, S. Karger, 1978.

Easton, T. A.: On the normal use of reflexes. *Am. Sci.*, 60:591, 1972.

Freund, H.-J.: Motor unit and muscle activity in voluntary motor control. *Physiol. Rev.*, 63:387, 1983.

Gallistel, C. R.: The Organization of Action: A New Synthesis. New York, Halsted Press, 1979.

Granit, R.: Muscular tone, *J. Sport Med.*, 2:46, 1962.

Granit, R.: Comments on history of motor control. *In* Brooks, V. B. (ed.): Handbook of Physiology. Sec. 1, Vol. II. Bethesda, American Physiological Society, 1981, p. 1.

Granit, R., and Pompeiano, O. (eds.): Reflex Control of Posture and Movement. New York, Elsevier Scientific Publishing Co., 1979.

Granit, R., *et al.*: First supraspinal control of mammalian muscle spindles: extra- and intrafusal co-activation. *J. Physiol. (Lond.)*, 147:385, 1959.

Grillner, S.: Control of locomotion in bipeds, tetrapods, and fish. *In* Brooks, V. B. (ed.): Handbook of Physiology. Sec. 1, Vol. II. Bethesda, American Physiological Society, 1981, p. 1179.

Grillner, S.: Neurobiological bases of rhythmic motor acts in vertebrates. Science 228:143, 1985.

Halstead, L. S.: Neuroactive Drugs of Choice in Spinal Cord Injury. A Guide for Using Neurologically Active Medications in Spinal Injured Patients. New York, Raven Press, 1981.

Henneman, E., and Mendell, L. M.: Functional organization of motoneuron pool and its inputs. *In* Brooks, V. B. (ed.): Handbook of Physiology. Sec. 1, Vol. II. Bethesda, American Physiological Society, 1981, p. 423.

Houk, J. C.: Regulation of stiffness in skeletomotor reflexes. *Annu. Rev. Physiol.*, 41:99, 1979.

Houk, J. C., and Rymer, W. Z.: Neural control of muscle length and tension. *In* Brooks, V. B. (ed.): Handbook of Physiology. Sec. 1, Vol. II. Bethesda, American Physiological Society, 1981, p. 257.

Hughes, J. T.: Pathology of the Spinal Cord. Philadelphia, W. B. Saunders Co., 1978.

Hunt, C. C., and Perl, E. R.: Spinal reflex mechanisms concerned with skeletal muscle. *Physiol. Rev.*, 40:538, 1960.

Kao, C. C. (ed.): Spinal Cord Reconstruction. New York, Raven Press, 1983.

Kostyuk, P. G., and Vasilenko, D.: Spinal interneurons. *Annu. Rev. Physiol.*, 41:115, 1979.

Le Douarin, N. M., *et al.*: From the neural crest to the ganglia of the peripheral nervous system. *Annu. Rev. Physiol.*, 43:653, 1981.

Matthews, P. B. C.: Mammalian Muscle Receptors and Their Central Actions. Baltimore, Williams & Wilkins, 1972.

Matthews, P. B. C.: Muscle spindles: Their messages and their fusimotor supply. *In* Brooks, V. B. (ed.): Handbook of Physiology. Sec. 1, Vol. II. Bethesda, American Physiological Society, 1981, p. 189.

Mendell, L. M.: Modifiability of spinal synapses. *Physiol. Rev.*, 64:260, 1984.

Merton, P. A.: How we control the contraction of our muscles. *Sci. Am.*, 226:30, 1972.

Orlovsky, G. N., and Shik, M. L.: Control of locomotion: A neurophysiological analysis of the cat locomotor system. *Int. Rev. Physiol.*, 10:281, 1976.

Pearson, K.: The control of walking. *Sci. Am.* 235(6):72, 1976.

Peterson, B. W.: Reticulospinal projections to spinal motor nuclei. *Annu. Rev. Physiol.*, 41:127, 1979.

Porter, R.: The neurophysiology of movement performance. *In* MTP International Review of Science: Physiology. Vol. 3. Baltimore, University Park Press, 1974, p. 151.

Purves, D.: Long-term regulation in the vertebrate peripheral nervous system. *Int. Rev. Physiol.*, 10:125, 1976.

Rack, P. M. H.: Limitations of somatosensory feedback in control of posture and movement. *In* Brooks, V. B. (ed.): Handbook of Physiology. Sec. 1, Vol. II. Bethesda, American Physiological Society, 1981, p. 229.

Rogers, M. A.: Paraplegia, Boston, Faber and Faber, 1978.

Rowell, L. B.: Reflex control of regional circulation in humans. *J. Auton. Nerv. Syst.*, 11:101, 1984.

Sherrington, C. S.: The Integrative Action of the Nervous System. New Haven, Conn., Yale University Press, 1911.

Shik, M. L., and Orlovsky, G. N.: Neurophysiology of Locomotor Automatism. *Physiol. Rev.*, 56:465, 1976.

Stein, P. S. G.: Motor systems with specific reference to the control of locomotion. *Annu. Rev. Neurosci.*, 1:61, 1978.

Stein, R. B.: Peripheral control of movement. *Physiol. Rev.*, 54:215, 1974.

Stein, R. B., and Lee, R. G.: Tremor and clonus. *In* Brooks, V. B. (ed.): Handbook of Physiology. Sec. 1, Vol. II. Bethesda, American Physiological Society, 1981, p. 325.

Wiesendanger, M., and Miles, T. S.: Ascending pathway of low-threshold muscle afferents to the cerebral cortex and its possible role in motor control. *Physiol. Rev.*, 62:1234, 1982.

Young, R.: Spinal Cord Injuries Case Studies. New Hyde Park, N. Y., Medical Examination Publishing Co., 1981.

16

Motor Functions of the Brain Stem and Basal Ganglia—Reticular Formation, Vestibular Apparatus, Equilibrium, and Brain Stem Reflexes

The brain stem is a complex extension of the spinal cord. Collected in it are numerous neuronal circuits to control respiration, cardiovascular function, gastrointestinal function, eye movement, equilibrium, support of the body against gravity, and many special stereotyped movements of the body. Some of these functions—such as control of respiration and cardiovascular functions—are described in special sections of this text. In the present chapter we shall discuss the role of the brain stem in controlling whole body movement and equilibrium.

THE RETICULAR FORMATION, AND SUPPORT OF THE BODY AGAINST GRAVITY

Throughout the entire extent of the brain stem—in the medulla, pons, and mesencephalon—are areas of diffuse neurons collectively known as the *reticular formation*. Figure 16–1 illustrates the extent of the reticular formation, showing it to begin at the upper end of the spinal cord and to extend upward through the medulla, pons, and mesencephalon. Many of the ascending and descending fiber tracts between the brain and spinal cord pass through the reticular formation, and as they do so they also provide collateral nerve endings to all reticular areas. In turn, the reticular formation provides multiple efferent fibers that pass both upward and downward in the axis of the nervous system. The lower end of the reticular formation is continuous with the interneurons of the spinal cord, and, indeed, the reticular formation of the brain stem functions in a manner quite analogous to many of the functions of the interneurons in the cord gray matter.

Interspersed throughout the reticular formation are both motor and sensory neurons; these vary in size from very small to very large. The small neurons, which constitute the greater number, make multiple connections within the reticular formation itself. The large neurons are mainly motor in function, and their axons often bifurcate almost immediately, with one division extending downward to the spinal cord and the other extending upward to the thalamus or other basal regions of the diencephalon or cerebrum. The axons passing into the spinal cord help control the axial and girdle movements—that is, the trunk, neck, shoulder, hip, and proximal limb movements. On the other hand, the nerve fibers extending into the diencephalon and cerebrum play important roles in controlling overall activity of the brain or activity in specific portions of the brain. These especially play prominent roles in the control of wakefulness and sleep, as we shall discuss in Chapter 19.

The input signals to the reticular formation are derived from multiple sources, including: (1) the spinoreticular tracts and collaterals from the spinothalamic tracts, (2) the vestibular nuclei, (3) the cerebellum, (4) the basal ganglia, (5) the cerebral cortex, from both the sensory and the motor regions, and (6) the hypothalamus and other nearby associated areas.

Though most of the neurons in the reticular formation are evenly dispersed, some of them are collected into *specific nuclei*, some of which are labeled in Figure 16–1. In general, these specific nuclei are not considered to be part of the reticular formation per se even though they do operate in association with it. In most instances they are the loci of "preprogrammed" control of stereotyped movements, as we shall discuss later in the chapter. Note especially in Figure 16–1 the location of the

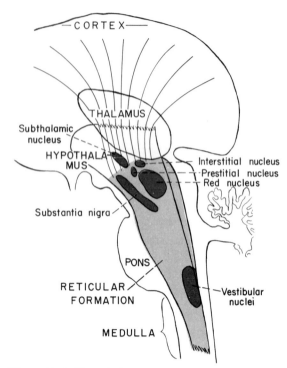

Figure 16–1. The reticular formation and associated nuclei.

vestibular nuclei in the posterior portion of the lower pons and upper medulla. These nuclei provide preprogrammed attitudinal contractions of appropriate muscles for maintaining equilibrium, and they share almost equally with the reticular formation in the control of the other motor functions by the brain stem.

The Motor Pathways from the Brain Stem to the Spinal Cord. Figure 16–2 illustrates the principal motor pathways from the brain stem to the spinal cord. These include:

1. Two vestibulospinal tracts that originate in the vestibular nuclei: a *lateral vestibulospinal tract* and a *medial vestibulospinal tract.* Both these are located in the anteromedial column of the spinal cord, and they excite motor neurons located mainly in the medial portion of the anterior horn. These neurons control the axial and girdle muscles.

2. Two reticulospinal tracts: a *pontine reticulospinal tract* located in the anteromedial column of the cord, and a *medullary reticulospinal tract* located in the lateral column. The pontine tract originates principally in the reticular formation of the pons whereas the medullary tract originates in the medulla. Both terminate on the medial motor neurons of the anterior horn. However, the signals from the pontine reticulospinal tract are mainly excitatory whereas those from the medullary tract are mainly inhibitory.

3. Imbedded within the lateral vestibulospinal tract and the pontine reticulospinal tract are several smaller tracts from the brain stem, including the *tectospinal tract,* which originates in the tectum of the mesencephalon, and the *interstitiospinal* tract, which originates in the interstitial nucleus within the reticular formation of the mesencephalon.

Note that most of the pathways from the brain stem to the spinal cord are located in the anteromedial columns of the cord and that they terminate on the medial motor

neurons of the anterior horn. These motor neurons control the axial musculature of the body and the musculature of the two body girdles—the shoulders and hips and proximal portions of the limbs. This complex of pathways and motor neurons is sometimes called the *medial motor system;* it is important because it is the principal controller of background body and girdle muscle contractions. It especially provides contraction of the antigravity muscles to support the body against gravity, while inhibiting the flexor muscles to prevent their opposition to the antigravity muscles. However, the medullary reticulospinal tract is different from the other tracts originating in the brain stem, for it tends to inhibit the antigravity muscles while providing perhaps some degree of excitation to the flexors.

Excitation of the Antigravity Muscles by the Brain Stem—The Decerebrate Animal

Both the vestibular nuclei and the pontine portion of the reticular formation, the two of which function in very close association with each other, are intrinsically excitable. However, this excitability is usually held in check by inhibitory signals that originate mainly in the basal ganglia but to a lesser extent in the cerebral cortex and cerebellum. When the brain stem is sectioned above the vestibular nuclei at the midpontine level, the intrinsic activity of these nuclei immediately causes a considerable degree of rigidity of all the antigravity muscles in the body. If this section is made still higher in the brain stem, for instance at the midlevel of the mesencephalon, then the intrinsic activity of the pontine portion of the reticular formation adds still more to the rigidity of the antigravity muscles, and the animal can usually even stand on its feet. This is called the *decerebrate animal.* Finally, if the cerebellum is removed at the same time to remove its inhibitory influences, the rigidity becomes still further enhanced.

Thus, the principal role of the brain stem in the control of motor function is to provide background contractions of the trunk and neck musculature and proximal portions of the limbs; and the most im-

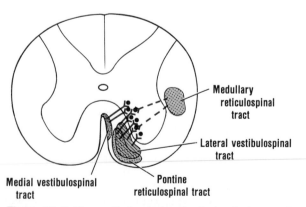

Figure 16–2. The vestibulospinal and reticulospinal tracts descending in the spinal cord to excite (solid lines) or inhibit (dashed lines) the anterior motor neurons that control the body's axial musculature.

portant function of these contractions is to provide support of the body against gravity.

The relative degree of contraction of the individual antigravity muscles is determined by the equilibrium mechanisms. Thus, if an animal begins to fall to one side, the extensor muscles on that side stiffen while those on the opposite side relax. In turn, the equilibrium mechanisms are controlled by signals mainly from the *vestibular apparatuses*, which are the sensory organs for equilibrium that will be discussed fully in subsequent sections of this chapter.

VESTIBULAR SENSATIONS AND THE MAINTENANCE OF EQUILIBRIUM

THE VESTIBULAR APPARATUS

The vestibular apparatus is the organ that detects sensations concerned with equilibrium. It is composed of a system of bony tubes and chambers in the petrous portion of the temporal bone called the *bony labyrinth* and within this a system of membranous tubes and chambers called the *membranous labyrinth,* which is the functional part of the apparatus. The top of Figure 16–3 illustrates the membranous labyrinth; it is composed mainly of the *cochlear duct,* three *semicircular canals,* and two large chambers known as the *utricle* and the *saccule.* The cochlear duct is the major sensory area for hearing and has nothing to do with equilibrium. However, the *utricle,* the *semicircular canals,* and probably the *saccule* are all integral parts of the equilibrium mechanism.

The Macula—The Sensory Organ of the Utricle and the Saccule for Detecting the Orientation of the Head with Respect to Gravity. Located on the inside surface of each utricle and saccule is a small sensory area slightly over two mm in diameter called a *macula.* The macula of the utricle lies in the horizontal plane on the inferior surface of the utricle and plays an important role in determining the normal orientation of the head with respect to the direction of gravitational or acceleratory forces. On the other hand, the macula of the saccule is located in a vertical plane on the medial wall of the saccule. Some research studies suggest that it operates in close association with the cochlear duct for detecting certain types of sounds and therefore may not be very important as an equilibrium apparatus. However, it is possible if not probable that the saccule also operates as an equilibrium apparatus, especially when the head is not in a vertical position.

Each macula is covered by a gelatinous layer in which many small calcium carbonate crystals called *statoconia* (or *otoliths)* are imbedded. Also, in the macula are thousands of *hair cells,* one of which is illustrated in Figure 16–4; these project *cilia* up into the gelatinous layer. The bases and sides of the hair cells synapse with sensory axons of the vestibular nerve.

Even under resting conditions, most of the nerve fibers leading from the hair cells transmit a continuous series of nerve impulses, averaging about 200 per second. Bending the cilia of a hair cell to one side causes the impulse traffic in its nerve fibers to increase markedly; bending the cilia to the opposite side decreases the impulse traffic, often turning it off completely. Therefore, as the orientation of the head in space changes and the weight of the otoconia (whose specific gravity is about three times that of the surrounding tissues) bends the cilia, appropriate signals are transmitted to the brain to control equilibrium.

In each macula the different hair cells are oriented in different directions so that some of them are stimulated when the head bends forward, some when it bends backward, others when it bends to one side, and so forth. Therefore, a different pattern of excitation occurs in the macula for each position

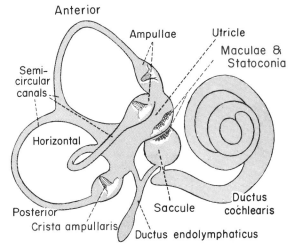

MEMBRANOUS LABYRINTH

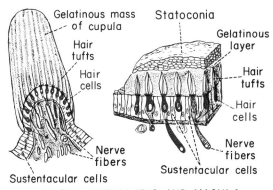

CRISTA AMPULLARIS AND MACULA

Figure 16–3. The membranous labyrinth, and organization of the crista ampullaris and the macula. (Modified from Goss: Gray's Anatomy of the Human Body. Philadelphia, Lea & Febiger; modified from Kolmer by Buchanan: Functional Neuroanatomy. Philadelphia, Lea & Febiger.)

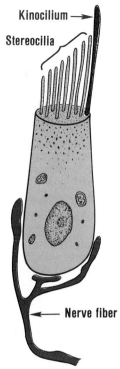

Figure 16–4. A hair cell of the membranous labyrinth of the equilibrium apparatus.

of the head; it is this "pattern" that apprises the brain of the head's orientation.

The Semicircular Canals. The three semicircular canals in each vestibular apparatus, known respectively as the *anterior, posterior,* and *horizontal semicircular canals,* are arranged at right angles to each other so that they represent all three planes in space. When the head is bent forward approximately 30 degrees, the two horizontal semicircular canals are located approximately horizontal with respect to the surface of the earth. The anterior canals are then located in vertical planes that project *forward and 45 degrees outward,* and the posterior canals are also then in vertical planes but project *backward and 45 degrees outward.* Thus, the anterior canal on each side of the head is in a plane parallel to that of the posterior canal on the opposite side of the head, whereas the two horizontal canals on the two sides are located in approximately the same plane.

Each semicircular canal has an enlargement at one of its ends called the *ampulla,* and the canals are filled with a viscous fluid called *endolymph.* Flow of this fluid in the canals excites a sensory organ in the ampulla. As illustrated in Figure 16–3, located in each ampulla is a small crest called a *crista ampullaris,* and on top of the crista is a gelatinous mass similar to that in the utricle and known as the *cupula.* Into the cupula are projected cilia from hair cells located along the ampullary crest, and these hair cells in turn are connected to sensory nerve fibers that pass into the *vestibular nerve.* Bending the cupula to one side, caused by flow of fluid in

the canal, stimulates the hair cells, while bending in the opposite direction inhibits them. Thus, appropriate signals are sent through the vestibular nerve to apprise the central nervous system of fluid movement in the respective canal.

Directional Sensitivity of the Hair Cells—The Kinocilium. As illustrated in Figure 16–4, each hair cell, whether in a macula or a cupula, has an average of about 50 small cilia, called *stereocilia,* plus one very large cilium called the *kinocilium.* This kinocilium is located to one side of the hair cell, always on the same side of the cell with respect to its orientation on the ampullary crest. This is the cause of the directional sensitivity of the hair cells: namely, stimulation when the cilia are bent toward the kinocilium side and inhibition when bent in the opposite direction.

Neuronal Connections of the Vestibular Apparatus with the Central Nervous System. Figure 16–5 illustrates the central connections of the vestibular nerve. Most of the vestibular nerve fibers end in the vestibular nuclei, which are located approximately at the junction of the medulla and the pons, but some fibers pass without synapsing to the fastigial nuclei, uvula, and flocculonodular lobes of the cerebellum. The fibers that end in the vestibular nuclei synapse with second order neurons that also send fibers into these areas of the cerebellum as well as to the cortex of other portions of the cerebellum, into the vestibulospinal tract, into the medial longitudinal fasciculus, and to other areas of the brain stem, particularly the reticular formation.

Note especially the very close association between the vestibular apparatus, the vestibular nuclei, and the cerebellum. The primary pathway for the reflexes of equilibrium begins in the vestibular nerves and passes next to both the vestibular nuclei and the cerebellum. Then, along with two-way traffic of impulses between these two, signals are also sent into the reticular nuclei of the brain stem as well as down the spinal cord via the vestibulospinal and reticulospinal tracts. In turn, the signals to the cord control the interplay between facilitation and inhibition of the antigravity muscles, thus automatically controlling equilibrium.

The *flocculonodular lobes* of the cerebellum seem to be especially concerned with equilibrium functions of the

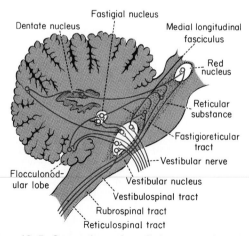

Figure 16–5. Connections of vestibular nerves in the central nervous system.

semicircular canals because destruction of these lobes gives almost exactly the same clinical symptoms as destruction of the semicircular canals themselves. That is, severe injury to either of these structures causes loss of equilibrium during *rapid changes in direction of motion* but does not seriously disturb equilibrium under static conditions, as will be discussed in subsequent sections. It is also believed that the *uvula* of the cerebellum plays an equally important role in static equilibrium.

Signals transmitted upward in the brain stem from both the vestibular nuclei and the cerebellum via the *medial longitudinal fasciculus* cause corrective movements of the eyes every time the head rotates so that the eyes can remain fixed on a specific visual object. Signals also pass upward (either through this same tract or through reticular tracts) to the cerebral cortex, probably terminating in a primary cortical center for equilibrium located in the parietal lobe deep in the Sylvian fissure, on the opposite side of the fissure from the auditory area of the superior temporal gyrus. These signals apprise the psyche of the equilibrium status of the body.

The vestibular nuclei on either side of the brain stem are divided into four separate subdivisions. These are:

1 and 2. The *superior* and *medial vestibular nuclei* that receive signals mainly from the semicircular canals and in turn send large numbers of nerve signals into the *medial longitudinal fasciculus* to cause corrective movements of the eyes as well as signals through the *medial vestibulospinal tract* to cause appropriate movements of the neck and head.

3. The *lateral vestibular nucleus* that receives its innervation primarily from the utricle and possibly saccule, and in turn transmits outflow signals to the spinal cord through the *lateral vestibulospinal tract* to control body movement.

4. The *inferior vestibular nucleus* that receives signals from both the semicircular canals and the utricle and in turn sends signals into both the cerebellum and the reticular formation of the brain stem.

FUNCTION OF THE UTRICLE (AND PROBABLY SACCULE) IN THE MAINTENANCE OF STATIC EQUILIBRIUM

It is especially important that the different hair cells are oriented in all different directions in the maculae of the utricles and saccules so that at different positions of the head, different hair cells become stimulated. The "patterns" of stimulation of the different hair cells apprise the nervous system of the position of the head with respect to the pull of gravity. In turn, the vestibular, cerebellar, and reticular motor systems reflexly excite the appropriate muscles to maintain proper equilibrium.

The maculae in the utricles function extremely effectively for maintaining equilibrium when the head is in the near-vertical position. Indeed, a person can determine as little as a half degree of mal-equilibrium when the head leans from the precise upright position. On the other hand, as the head is leaned farther and farther from the upright, the determination of head orientation by the vestibular sense becomes poorer and poorer. Obviously, extreme sensitivity in the upright position is of major importance for maintenance of precise vertical static equilibrium, which is the most essential function of the vestibular apparatus.

Detection of Linear Acceleration by the Maculae. When the body is suddenly thrust forward—that is, when the body accelerates—the statoconia, which have greater inertia than the surrounding fluids, fall backward on the hair cell cilia, and information of mal-equilibrium is sent into the nervous centers, causing the individual to feel as though he were falling backward. This automatically causes him to lean his body forward until the anterior shift of the statoconia caused by leaning exactly equals the tendency for the statoconia to fall backward. At this point, the nervous system detects a state of proper equilibrium and therefore leans the body no farther forward. Thus, the maculae operate to maintain equilibrium during linear acceleration in exactly the same manner as they operate in static equilibrium.

The maculae *do not* operate for the detection of linear *velocity*. When runners first begin to run, they must lean far forward to keep from falling over backward because of *acceleration,* but once they have achieved running speed, they would not have to lean forward at all if they were running in a vacuum. When running in air they lean forward to maintain equilibrium only because of the air resistance against their bodies, and in this instance it is not the maculae that make them lean but the pressure of the air acting on pressure end-organs in the skin, which initiate the appropriate equilibrium adjustments to prevent falling.

THE SEMICIRCULAR CANALS AND THEIR DETECTION OF HEAD ROTATION

When the head suddenly *begins* to rotate in any direction (this is called angular acceleration), the endolymph in the membranous semicircular canals, because of its inertia, tends to remain stationary while the semicircular canals themselves turn. This causes relative fluid flow in the canals in the direction opposite to the rotation of the head.

Figure 16–6 illustrates an *ampulla* of one of the semicircular canals, showing the *cupula* and its embedded hairs bending in the direction of fluid movement. And Figure 16–7 illustrates the discharge signal from a single hair cell in the crista ampullaris when an animal is rotated for 40 seconds, showing that (1) even when the cupula is in its resting position the hair cell emits a tonic discharge of approximately 200 impulses per second; (2) when the animal is rotated, the hairs bend to one side and the rate of discharge increases greatly; and (3) with continued rotation, the excess discharge of the hair cell gradually subsides back to the resting level in about 20 seconds.

The reason for this adaptation of the receptor is that within a second or more of rotation, friction in the semicircular canal causes the endolymph to

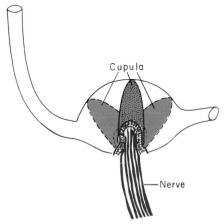

Figure 16–6. Movement of the cupula and its embedded hairs during rotation first in one direction and then in the opposite direction. (Often, the top of the cupula is attached so that it merely bulges in one direction or the other.)

rotate as rapidly as the semicircular canal itself; then in an additional 15 to 20 seconds the cupula slowly returns to its resting position in the middle of the ampulla because of its own elastic recoil.

When the rotation suddenly stops, exactly the opposite effects take place: the endolymph continues to rotate while the semicircular canal stops. This time the cupula is bent in the opposite direction, causing the hair cell to stop discharging entirely. After another few seconds, the endolymph stops moving, and the cupula returns gradually to its resting position in about 20 seconds, thus allowing the discharge of the hair cell to return to its normal tonic level as shown to the right in Figure 16–7.

Thus, the semicircular canal transmits a positive signal when the head *begins* to rotate and a negative signal when it *stops* rotating. Furthermore, at least some hair cells will always respond to rotation in any plane—horizontal, sagittal, or coronal—for fluid movement always occurs in at least one semicircular canal.

Rate of Angular Acceleration Required to Stimulate the Semicircular Canals. The angular acceleration required to stimulate the semicircular canals in the human being averages about 1 degree per second per second. In other words, when one begins to rotate, the velocity of rotation must be as much as 1 degree per second by the end of the first second, 2 degrees per second by the end of the second second, 3 degrees per second by the end of the third second, and so forth, in order for the person barely to detect that the rate of rotation is increasing.

"Predictive" Function of the Semicircular Canals in the Maintenance of Equilibrium. Since the semicircular canals do not detect that the body is off balance in the forward direction, in the side direction, or in the backward direction, one might at first ask: What is the function of the semicircular canals in the maintenance of equilibrium? All they detect is that the person's head is beginning to rotate or stopping rotation in one direction or another. Therefore, the function of the semicircular canals is not likely to be to maintain static equilib-

rium or to maintain equilibrium during linear acceleration or when the person is exposed to steady centrifugal forces. Yet loss of function of the semicircular canals causes a person to have very poor equilibrium when attempting to perform *rapid* and *intricate* body movements.

We can explain the function of the semicircular canals best by the following illustration. If a person is running forward rapidly, and then suddenly begins to turn to one side, he falls off balance a second or so later unless appropriate corrections are made *ahead of time*. But, unfortunately, the macula of the utricle cannot detect that he is off balance until *after* this has occurred. On the other hand, the semicircular canals will have already detected that the person is turning, and this information can easily apprise the central nervous system of the fact that the person *will* fall off balance within the next second or so unless some correction is made. In other words, the semicircular canal mechanism *predicts ahead of time* that mal-equilibrium is going to occur even before it does occur and thereby causes the equilibrium centers to make appropriate preventive adjustments. In this way, the person need not fall off balance before he begins to correct the situation.

Removal of the flocculonodular lobes of the cerebellum prevents normal function of the semicircular canals but does not prevent normal function of the macular receptors. It is especially interesting in this connection that the cerebellum serves as a "predictive" organ for most of the other rapid movements of the body as well as those having to do with equilibrium. These other functions of the cerebellum are discussed in the following chapter.

VESTIBULAR POSTURAL REFLEXES

Sudden changes in the orientation of an animal in space elicit reflexes that help to maintain equilibrium and posture. For instance, if an animal is suddenly pushed to the right, even before it can fall more than a few degrees

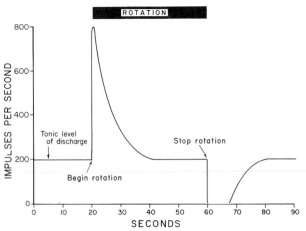

Figure 16–7. Response of a hair cell when a semicircular canal is stimulated first by rotation and then by stopping rotation.

its right legs extend instantaneously. In other words, this mechanism *anticipates* that the animal will be off balance in a few seconds and makes appropriate adjustments to prevent this.

Another type of vestibular postural reflex occurs when the animal suddenly falls forward. When this occurs, the forepaws extend forward, the extensor muscles tighten, and the muscles in the back of the neck stiffen to prevent the animal's head from striking the ground. This reflex is probably also of importance in locomotion, for, in the case of the galloping horse, the downward thrust of the head can automatically provide reflex thrust of the forelimbs to move the animal forward for the next gallop.

VESTIBULAR MECHANISM FOR STABILIZING THE EYES AND FOR NYSTAGMUS

When a person changes his direction of movement rapidly, or even leans his head sideways, forward, or backward, it would be impossible for him to maintain a stable image on the retinae of his eyes unless he had some automatic control mechanism to stabilize the direction of gaze of the eyes. In addition, the eyes would be of little use in detecting an image unless they remained "fixed" on each object long enough to gain a clear image. Fortunately, each time the head is suddenly rotated, signals from the semicircular canals cause the eyes to rotate in an equal and opposite direction to the rotation of the head. This results from reflexes transmitted from the canals through the *vestibular nuclei* and the *medial longitudinal fasciculus* to the *ocular nuclei*.

OTHER FACTORS CONCERNED WITH EQUILIBRIUM

The Neck Proprioceptors. The vestibular apparatus detects the orientation and movements *only of the head.* Therefore, it is essential that the nervous centers also receive appropriate information depicting the orientation of the head with respect to the body. This information is transmitted from the proprioceptors of the neck and body directly into the vestibular and reticular nuclei of the brain stem and also indirectly by way of the cerebellum.

By far the most important proprioceptive information needed for the maintenance of equilibrium is that derived from the *joint receptors of the neck.* When the head is leaned in one direction by bending the neck, impulses from the neck proprioceptors keep the vestibular apparatuses from giving the person a sense of mal-equilibrium. They do this by transmitting signals that exactly oppose the signals transmitted from the vestibular apparatuses. However, *when the entire body* leans in one direction, the impulses from the vestibular apparatuses *are not opposed* by the neck proprioceptors; therefore, the person in this instance does perceive a change in equilibrium status.

The Neck Reflexes. In an animal *whose vestibular apparatuses have been destroyed,* bending the neck causes immediate muscular reflexes called *neck reflexes* occurring especially in the forelimbs. For instance, bending the head forward causes both forelimbs to relax. However, when the vestibular apparatuses are *intact,* this effect does *not* occur because the vestibular reflexes function exactly oppositely to the neck reflexes. Thus, if the head

is flexed downward, the vestibular reflex tends to extend the forelimbs, while the neck reflexes tend to relax them. Since the equilibrium of the entire body and not of the head alone must be maintained, it is easy to understand that the vestibular and neck reflexes must function oppositely. Otherwise, each time the neck should bend, the animal would immediately fall off balance.

Proprioceptive and Exteroceptive Information from Other Parts of the Body. Proprioceptive information from other parts of the body besides the neck is also important in the maintenance of equilibrium. For instance, pressure sensations from the footpads can tell one whether weight is distributed equally between the two feet and whether weight is more forward or backward on the feet.

An instance in which exteroceptive information is necessary for maintenance of equilibrium occurs when a person is running. The air pressure against the front of the body signals that a force is opposing the body in a direction different from that caused by gravitational pull; as a result, the person leans forward to oppose this.

Importance of Visual Information in the Maintenance of Equilibrium. After complete destruction of the vestibular apparatuses, and even after loss of most proprioceptive information from the body, a person can still use the visual mechanisms effectively for maintaining equilibrium. Even slight linear or rotational movement of the body instantaneously shifts the visual images on the retina, and this information is relayed to the equilibrium centers. Many persons with complete destruction of the vestibular apparatuses have almost normal equilibrium as long as their eyes are open and as long as they perform all motions slowly. But, when moving rapidly or when the eyes are closed, equilibrium is immediately lost.

FUNCTIONS OF THE RETICULAR FORMATION AND SPECIFIC BRAIN STEM NUCLEI IN CONTROLLING SUBCONSCIOUS, STEREOTYPED MOVEMENTS

Rarely, a child called an *anencephalic monster* is born without brain structures above the mesencephalic region, and some of these children have been kept alive for many months. They are able to perform essentially all the functions of feeding, such as suckling, extrusion of unpleasant food from the mouth, and moving the hands to the mouth to suck the fingers. In addition, they can yawn and stretch. They can cry and follow objects with the eyes and by movements of the head. Also, placing pressure on the upper anterior parts of their legs will cause them to pull to the sitting position.

Therefore, it is obvious that many of the stereotyped motor functions of the human being are integrated in the brain stem. Unfortunately, the loci of most of the different motor control systems have not been found except for the following:

Stereotyped Body Movements. Most movements of the trunk and head can be classified into several simple movements, such as forward flexion, extension, rotation, and turning movements of the entire body. These types of movements are controlled by special nuclei located mainly in the mesencephalic and lower diencephalic region. For instance, *rotational movements* of the head and eyes are controlled by the *interstitial nucleus,* which is illustrated in Figure 16–1. This nucleus lies in close approximation to the *medial longitudinal fasciculus,* through which it transmits a major portion of its control impulses. The *raising movements* of the head and body are controlled by the *prestitial nucleus,* which is located approximately at the juncture of the diencephalon and mesencephalon. On the other hand, the *flexing movements* of the head and body are controlled by the *nucleus precommissuralis* located at the level of the posterior commissure. Finally, the *turning movements* of the entire body, which are much more complicated, involve both the pontile and mesencephalic reticular formation.

Function of the Subthalamic Areas—Forward Progression. Much less is known about function of higher brain stem centers in posture and locomotion than of the lower centers, principally because of the complexity of the neuronal connections. However, it is known that stimulation of centers in or around the subthalamic nuclei can cause rhythmic limb motions, including forward walking reflexes. This does not mean that the individual muscles of walking are controlled from this region but simply that excitation of this region sends "command" signals to activate the cord centers where *preprogrammed* neuronal circuits then cause the actual walking movements.

A cat with its brain transected beneath the thalamus but above the subthalamus can walk in an almost completely normal fashion—so much so that the observer often cannot tell the difference. However, when the animal comes to an obstruction it simply butts its head against the obstruction and tries to keep on walking. Thus, it lacks *purposefulness of locomotion.*

The function of the subthalamic region in walking is frequently described as that of controlling *forward progression.*

THE BASAL GANGLIA— THEIR MOTOR FUNCTIONS

Physiologically, the basal ganglia are considered to be comprised of the *caudate nucleus, putamen,* and *globus pallidus.* However, the *substantia nigra, subthalamus,* and important portions of both the *thalamus* and *reticular formation* operate in close association with these and therefore are actually part of the *basal ganglia system* for motor control.

The basal ganglia function in close association with the cerebral cortex for both motor control and sensory activities. However, little is known about the sensory functions of the basal ganglia despite the fact that as many nervous pathways connect the sensory areas of the cortex with the basal ganglia as with the motor areas. One of the most important recent findings has been that, when the body performs a muscle activity, action potentials appear in the basal ganglia before they appear in the cortical motor areas. And it is very probable that the basal ganglia themselves are most often set into activity not by signals from the motor cortex but instead by signals directly from the sensory and sensory association portions of the cortex, or from the thalamus and lower brain stem. Thus, there is much belief that the basal ganglia play an essential role in the initiation of most if not all motor activities of

the body besides some of the involuntary muscle contractions that originate in the brain stem or spinal cord.

Even though the basal ganglia are closely associated with the cerebral cortex in normal motor control, the basal ganglia can still provide many aspects of motor control even after the cerebral cortex has been removed. However, the motor activities are then much grosser and less determinative than when the cortex contributes its capabilities as well. We shall say more about the interrelationships between the basal ganglia and the motor cortex in the following chapter.

Physiological Anatomy of the Basal Ganglial Neuronal Connections

Figure 16–8 illustrates the complexity of the interconnections among the different basal ganglia as well as between the basal ganglia and the brain stem, the thalamus, and the cerebral cortex. However, several partially distinct neuronal pathways have been discerned among these multiple connectivities.

(1) Pathway from Cortex to Basal Ganglia and Back to Cortex. Figure 16–9 illustrates the pathway that involves the greatest number of nerve fibers in the basal ganglia system. It begins in all areas of the cerebral cortex and passes through the following four stages: (1) From the *cortex* to the *caudate nucleus* and *putamen* (which together are called the *neostriatum,* or sometimes the *striate body*). (2) From the neostriatum (caudate nucleus and putamen) to the *globus pallidus,* and eventually entering the medial segment of the globus pallidus as illustrated in the figure. (3) From the medial segment of the globus pallidus to the *ventroanterior* and *ventrolateral nuclei of the thalamus.* It is to these same thalamic nuclei that signals from the cerebellum are also transmitted. (4) From the ventroanterior and the ventrolateral nuclei of the thalamus *back to all areas of the cortex.*

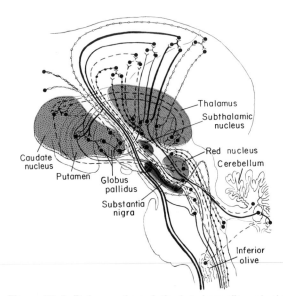

Figure 16–8. Pathways through the basal ganglia and related structures of the brain stem, thalamus, and cerebral cortex. (From Jung and Hassler: Handbook of Physiology, Sec. 1, Vol. II. Baltimore, Williams & Wilkins Company, 1960.)

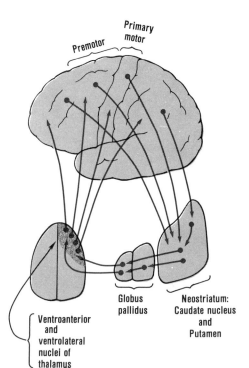

Figure 16–9. Feedback circuit from the cerebral cortex to the basal ganglia, then through the thalamus back to the cortex.

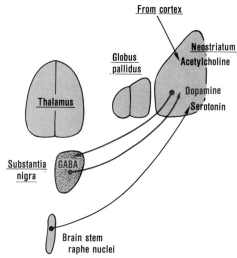

Figure 16–10. Interrelationships between the neostriatum (caudate nucleus and putamen) and the substantia nigra and raphe nuclei in the brain stem. This figure also shows several different transmitter substances involved in nerve transmission, especially secretion of GABA in the substantia nigra and dopamine in the neostriatum, both of which function as inhibitory transmitters.

Essentially all the nerve fibers from the neostriatum to the globus pallidus (stage 2 in the above circuit) are inhibitory pathways, secreting the inhibitory transmitter GABA at their nerve endings. Because of this inhibitory step, this circular pathway beginning in the cortex and returning once again to the cortex is a *negative feedback loop* that provides stability to many aspects of the motor control interactions.

(2) Mutual Inhibitory Pathways Between the Neostriatum and the Substantia Nigra. Figure 16–10 illustrates a pathway from the *caudate nucleus* and *putamen* (the neostriatum) to the *substantia nigra* that secretes the inhibitory transmitter GABA at its terminus in the substantia nigra. In turn, a group of dark-staining cells in the substantia nigra sends axons back to the caudate nucleus and putamen, secreting the inhibitory transmitter *dopamine* at their terminations. This mutual inhibitory pathway normally maintains a certain degree of inhibition of the two separate areas. Lesions of one of these pathways are the basis of a number of different clinical syndromes involving the basal ganglia, including the important syndrome Parkinson's disease that we shall discuss later.

Figure 16–10 also shows that nerve fibers from the cerebral cortex (as well as others from the thalamus) secrete *acetylcholine* in the caudate nucleus and putamen, causing excitatory effects. And still another pathway, from the brain stem raphe nuclei, secretes *serotonin*. Serotonin is an inhibitory transmitter; this pathway is believed to function primarily in relation to the sleep-producing effects of the raphe nuclei.

And not shown in this figure is still another tract that passes directly from the caudate nucleus to the substantia nigra that secretes *substance P,* an excitatory transmitter, illustrating even more the complexity of the different neurotransmitters involved in the interactions within the basal ganglia system.

(3) Interrelationships Between the Thalamic Intralam-

inar Nuclei and the Basal Ganglia. Figure 16–11 illustrates a feedback loop between the intralaminar nuclei of the thalamus and the basal ganglia that is similar to the feedback loop between the cerebral cortex and the basal ganglia. Note also in the figure the close relationship of the intralaminar nuclei with the lower brain stem. These together are older portions of the nervous system and presumably are important in the control of the more primitive aspects of motor control.

(4) Outflow Tracts from the Basal Ganglia Toward the Lower Brain Stem. Even though it is known that the basal ganglia can have important effects on the motor control functions of the brain stem, there are surprisingly few direct nerve fiber projections from the basal ganglia to the lower brain stem. Nevertheless, shown in Figure 16–12 are several pathways, all of which are relatively small, that pass from the basal ganglia to the brain stem reticular formation. Most of the signals pass from the globus pallidus through either the subthalamic nucleus or the substantia nigra before entering the reticular for-

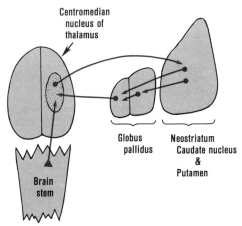

Figure 16–11. An older pathway involving the basal ganglia, showing interplay of signals among the basal ganglia, the centromedian nucleus of the thalamus, and the brain stem.

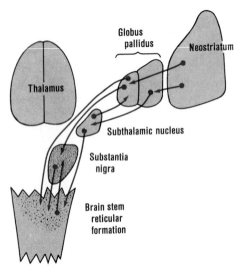

Figure 16–12. Pathway for transmission of signals from the basal ganglia to the brain stem reticular formation by way of the subthalamic nucleus and the substantia nigra.

mation. However, a few fibers pass from the medial portion of the globus pallidus directly to the brain stem.

FUNCTIONS OF THE BASAL GANGLIA

Before attempting to discuss the functions of the basal ganglia in human beings, we should speak briefly of the better known functions of these ganglia in lower animals. In birds, for instance, the cerebral cortex is poorly developed while the basal ganglia are highly developed. These ganglia perform essentially all the motor functions, even controlling the voluntary movements in much the same manner that the motor cortex of the human being controls voluntary movements. Furthermore, in the cat, and to a lesser extent in the dog, decortication removes only the discrete types of motor functions and does not interfere with the animal's ability to walk, eat, fight, develop rage, have periodic sleep and wakefulness, and even participate naturally in sexual activities. However, if a major portion of the basal ganglia is destroyed, only gross stereotyped movements remain, which were discussed earlier in relation to the mesencephalic animal.

Finally, in the human being, cortical lesions in very young individuals destroy the discrete movements of the body, particularly of the hands and distal portions of the lower limbs, but do not destroy the person's ability to walk crudely, to control equilibrium, or to perform many other subconscious types of movements. However, simultaneous destruction of a major portion of the caudate nucleus almost totally paralyzes the opposite side of the body except for a few stereotyped reflexes integrated in the cord or brain stem.

With this brief background of the overall function of the basal ganglia, we can attempt to dissect the functions of certain portions of the basal ganglia system, realizing that the system actually operates, along with the motor cortex and cerebellum, as a total unit and that individual functions cannot be ascribed to the different individual parts of the basal ganglia.

Inhibition of Motor Tone by the Basal Ganglia. Though it is wrong to ascribe a single function to all the basal ganglia, nevertheless, one of the general effects of diffuse basal ganglia excitation is to inhibit muscle tone throughout the body. This effect results from inhibitory signals transmitted from the basal ganglia to both the motor cortex and the lower brain stem. Therefore, whenever widespread destruction of the basal ganglia occurs, this causes muscle rigidity throughout the body. For instance, when the brain stem is transected at the mesencephalic level, which removes the inhibitory effects of the basal ganglia, the phenomenon of decerebrate rigidity occurs.

Yet, despite this general inhibitory effect of the basal ganglia, stimulation of certain specific areas within the basal ganglia can elicit positive muscle contractions and at times even complex patterns of movements.

Function of the Caudate Nucleus and Putamen (The Neostriatum). The caudate nucleus and putamen seem to function together to initiate and regulate gross intentional movements of the body. To perform this function they transmit impulses through two different pathways: (1) into the *globus pallidus,* thence by way of the *thalamus* to the *cerebral cortex,* and finally downward into the spinal cord through the *corticospinal pathway;* (2) downward through the *globus pallidus* and the *substantia nigra* by way of short axons into the *reticular formation* and finally into the spinal cord mainly through the *reticulospinal tracts.*

In summary, the neostriatum helps control gross intentional movements that we normally perform subconsciously. However, this control also involves the motor cortex, with which the neostriatum is closely connected.

Function of the Globus Pallidus. It is already clear that almost all the outflow of signals from the basal ganglia are channelled through the globus pallidus en route back to the cortex or on their way to lower brain centers. However, in addition to this motor relay function of the globus pallidus, the globus pallidus seems to have still another function that operates in close association with the subthalamus and brain stem to help control the axial and girdle movements of the body. These movements provide the background positioning of the body and proximal limbs so that the more discrete motor functions of the hands and feet can then be performed. That is, a person wishing to perform an exact function with a hand first positions the body, next positions the legs and arms, and finally tenses all the axial and girdle muscles to provide background positioning and stability of all the proximal portions of the body. These associated tonic contractions are supposedly initiated by circuits in the globus pallidus but operate also through the axial and girdle motor control areas of the brain stem. Lesions of the globus pallidus seriously interfere with the attitudinal movements that are necessary to position the hand and, therefore, make it difficult or impossible for one to use the hand for discrete activities.

Electrical stimulation of the globus pallidus while an animal is performing a gross body movement often will stop the movement in a static position, the animal holding that position for many seconds while the stimulation continues. This fits with the concept that the globus pallidus is involved in some type of servo feedback motor control system that is capable of locking the different parts of the body into specific positions.

CLINICAL SYNDROMES RESULTING FROM DAMAGE TO THE BASAL GANGLIA

Much of what we know about the function of the basal ganglia comes from study of patients with basal ganglia lesions whose brains have undergone pathological studies after death. Among the different clinical syndromes are:

Chorea. Chorea is a disease in which random uncontrolled "flicking-type" movements occur one after another. Normal progression of movements cannot occur; instead, the person may perform one pattern of movement for a few seconds and then suddenly another.

A particularly important type of chorea is *Huntington's chorea*, which is a hereditary disorder that begins manifesting usually in the third or fourth decade of life. It is characterized at first by flicking movements but then by progressively more severe distortional movements of the body as the disorder becomes more serious. In addition, severe dementia develops concurrently with the motor dysfunctions.

In Huntington's chorea there is diffuse and widespread degeneration of neurons in both the caudate nucleus and the putamen. The neurons most involved are those that secrete the inhibitory transmitter GABA, but some of the acetylcholine-secreting neurons also degenerate. Failure of the GABA-secreting neurons removes the inhibition of the striatonigral pathway and allows the dopamine-secreting neurons of the substantia nigra to become greatly overactive. This in turn allows excessive secretion of dopamine by the nigrostriatal fibers back in the caudate nucleus and putamen, which greatly inhibits both these nuclei. In addition, degeneration of the acetylcholine-secreting neurons adds further to the depression of these nuclei. Presumably, this depressed function interrupts some of the feedback loops from the cortex to the basal ganglia and then back to the cortex through the thalamus, thus causing the abnormal movements.

Thus, Huntington's chorea is believed to be caused by widespread depression of function in the caudate nucleus and putamen. If we also remember that at least half of all the cortical connections of the caudate nucleus and putamen are with sensory areas of the cortex rather than with motor areas, this could also explain the generalized dementia that occurs in Huntington's chorea.

Athetosis. In this disease, slow, writhing movements of a hand, the neck, the face, the tongue, or some other part of the body occur continually. The movements are likely to be wormlike, first with overextension of the hands and fingers, then flexion, then rotary twisting to the side—all these continuing in a slow, rhythmic, repetitive writhing pattern. The contracting muscles exhibit a high degree of spasm, and the movements are enhanced by emotions or by excessive signals from the sensory organs. Furthermore, voluntary movements in the affected area are greatly impaired or sometimes even impossible.

The damage in athetosis is usually found in the *lateral portion of the globus pallidus* or in this area and the *neostriatum* as well. Athetosis is usually attributed to the interruption of feedback circuits among the basal ganglia, thalamus, and cerebral cortex. The normal feedback circuits presumably allow a constant and rapid interplay between antagonistic muscle groups so that finely controlled static or progressive movements can take place. However, if the feedback circuits are blocked, it is supposed that the detouring impulses may take devious routes through the basal ganglia, thalamus, and motor cortex, causing a succession of abnormal movements.

Hemiballismus. Hemiballismus is an uncontrollable succession of violent movements of large areas of the body. These may occur once every few seconds or sometimes only once in many minutes. For instance, an entire leg might suddenly jerk uncontrollably to full flexion, or the entire trunk might go through an extreme, sudden torsion movement, or an arm might be pulled upward suddenly with great force. Hemiballismus of the legs or trunk causes the person to fall to the ground if walking, and even in bed, the person tosses violently when affected by these powerful and strong intermittent movements. Furthermore, attempts to perform voluntary movements frequently invoke ballistic movements in place of the normal movements.

Hemiballismus on one side of the body results from a *large lesion in the opposite subthalamus*. The smooth, progressive or rhythmic movements of the limbs or other parts of the body normally integrated in this area can no longer occur, but excitatory impulses attempting to evoke such movements elicit instead uncontrollable ballistic movements.

Parkinson's Disease. Parkinson's disease, which is also known as *paralysis agitans*, results almost invariably from *widespread destruction of the substantia nigra* but is often associated also with lesions of the *globus pallidus* and other related areas. It is characterized by (1) *rigidity* of the musculature either in widespread areas of the body or in isolated areas, (2) *tremor at rest* of the involved areas in most but not all instances, and (3) a serious *inability to initiate movement*, called *akinesia*.

The cause or causes of these abnormal motor activities are almost entirely unknown. However, they are almost certainly related to *loss of dopamine secretion* in the putamen and caudate nucleus by the nerve endings of the *nigrostriatal tract*. Destruction of the substantia nigra causes this tract to degenerate and the dopamine normally secreted in the putamen and caudate nucleus no longer to be present. But still present are large numbers of neurons that secrete acetylcholine, and these transmit excitatory signals throughout the basal ganglia. It is also believed that the dopamine from the nigrostriatal pathway normally acts to inhibit these acetylcholine-producing neurons or in some other way to counter their activity. But, in the absence of dopamine secretion, the acetylcholine pathways become overly active, which presumably is the basis for many of the motor symptoms in Parkinson's disease.

The rigidity in this disease is somewhat different from that which occurs in decerebrate rigidity, for decerebrate rigidity results mainly from hyperactivity of the muscle spindle system, and even slight movement of a muscle is met with rather extreme reflex resistance resulting from feedback through the stretch reflex mechanism. Parkinsonian rigidity, on the other hand, is more of a "plastic" type. That is, sudden movement usually is not met by intense resistance from the stretch reflexes, as in the decerebrate type of rigidity, but instead both protagonist and antagonist muscles remain tightly contracted throughout the movement. Therefore, it is believed that the rigidity of Parkinson's disease results to a great extent from excess impulses transmitted in the corticospinal system, thus activating the alpha motor fibers to the muscles, in addition to probably excess activation of the gamma efferent system as well.

Tremor usually, but not always, occurs in Parkinson's disease. Its frequency is normally four to six cycles per second. When the parkinsonian patient performs voluntary movements, the tremor becomes temporarily or partially blocked, presumably because other motor control signals—perhaps from the cerebral cortex and cerebellum—override the abnormal basal ganglial signals.

The mechanism of the tremor in Parkinson's disease is not known. However, a type of treatment that frequently relieves the tremor is surgical destruction of the *ventrolateral nucleus of the thalamus* which is one of the feedback pathways from the basal ganglia to the motor cortex. Therefore, it is presumed that loss of the inhibitory influence of dopamine in the basal ganglia leads to enhanced activity of the corticobasal ganglial-thalamic-cortical feedback circuit, leading to an oscillation that produces the muscle tremor.

Though the muscle rigidity and the tremor are both distressing to the parkinsonian patient, even more serious is the *akinesia* that occurs in the final stages of the disease. To perform even the simplest of movements, the person must exert the highest degree of concentration, and the mental effort, even mental anguish, that is necessary to make the movement "go" is often almost beyond the patient's willpower. Then, when the movement does occur, it is stiff and often staccato in character instead of occurring with smooth progression. For instance, when a patient begins to perform a discrete voluntary movement with the hands, the automatic "associated" adjustments of the trunk of the body and the upper arm segments do not occur. Instead, the patient must voluntarily adjust these segments before use of the hands. Furthermore, a tremendous amount of nervous effort must be made by the voluntary motor control system to overcome "motor stiffness" of the musculature. Thus, the person with Parkinson's disease has a masklike face, showing almost no automatic emotional facial expressions; he or she is usually bent forward because of the muscle rigidity; and all movements of necessity are highly deliberate rather than the many casual subconscious movements that are normally a part of our everyday life.

The cause of the akinesia in Parkinson's disease is not known, and again we must resort to theory. It is presumed that *loss of dopamine secretion in the caudate nucleus and putamen by the nigrostriatal fibers* allows excessive activity of the acetylcholine-producing neurons. But normal operation of the basal ganglia requires a balance between both excitatory and inhibitory activities, and loss of this balance, in effect, leads to a functionless basal ganglia system. We have already pointed out that the basal ganglia are responsible for many of the subconscious stereotyped movements of the body, and also responsible even for background movements of the trunk, legs, neck, and upper arms that are required preliminary to performing the more discrete movements of the hands. If the subconscious and the background movements cannot occur, then other neural mechanisms must be substituted, especially those of the motor cortex and cerebellum. Unfortunately, though, these cannot replace the movements normally controlled by the basal ganglia and certainly cannot function at a subconscious level.

Treatment with L-*Dopa and Anticholinergic Drugs.* Administration of L-dopa to patients with Parkinson's disease ameliorates many of the symptoms, especially the rigidity and the akinesia, in about two thirds of the patients. The reason for this seems to be the following: The dopamine secreted in the caudate nucleus and putamen by the nigrostriate fibers is a derivative of L-dopa. When the substantia nigra is destroyed and the person develops Parkinson's disease, the administered L-dopa is believed to substitute for the dopamine no longer secreted by the destroyed neurons. This causes more or less normal inhibition of the basal ganglia and relieves much or most of the akinesia and rigidity.

The same basal ganglia that are inhibited by dopamine are excited by acetylcholine-secreting neurons, as was discussed earlier. Therefore, as would be expected, administration of anticholinergic drugs such as scopolamine can also decrease the level of activity in the basal ganglia and therefore benefit some parkinsonian patients.

Coagulation of the Ventrolateral and Ventroanterior Nuclei of the Thalamus for Treatment of Parkinson's Disease. Neurosurgeons have treated Parkinson's disease patients, with varying success, by destroying portions of the basal ganglia, thalamus, or even motor cortex. The most prevalent treatment has been destruction of the ventrolateral and ventroanterior nuclei of the thalamus, usually by electrocoagulation. Most fiber pathways from the basal ganglia and cerebellum to the cerebral cortex pass through these nuclei so that their destruction blocks many or most of the corticobasal ganglial-thalamic-cortical feedback circuits. It is presumed that blockage of these feedbacks removes the neuronal loops that cause the tremor of Parkinson's disease.

REFERENCES

Baldessarini, R. J., and Tarsey, D.: Dopamine and the pathophysiology of dyskinesias induced by antipsychotic drugs. *Annu. Rev. Neurosci.,* 3:23, 1980.

Bird, E. D.: Chemical pathology of Huntington's disease. *Annu. Rev. Pharmacol. Toxicol.,* 20:533, 1980.

Bizzi, E.: The coordination of eye-head movements. *Sci. Am.,* 231(4):100, 1974.

Bobath, B., and Bobath, K.: Motor Development in the Different Types of Cerebral Palsy. London, W. Heinemann Medical Books, 1975.

Brodal, A. (ed.): Basic Aspects of Central Vestibular Mechanisms. New York, American Elsevier Publishing Co., 1971.

Carpenter, M. B.: Anatomy of the corpus striatum and brain stem integrating systems. *In* Brooks, V. B. (ed.): Handbook of Physiology. Sec. 1, Vol. II. Bethesda, American Physiological Society, 1981, p. 947.

Chase, T. N., *et al.* (eds.): Huntington's Disease. New York, Raven Press, 1979.

Dampney, R. A., *et al.*: Identification of cardiovascular cell groups in the brain stem. *Clin. Exp. Hypertens.*, 6:205, 1984.

DeLong, M., and Georgopoulos, A. P.: Motor functions of the basal ganglia. *In* Brooks, V. B. (ed.): Handbook of Physiology. Sec. 1, Vol. II. Bethesda, American Physiological Society, 1981, p. 1017.

Denny-Brown, D.: The Basal Ganglia: Their Relation to Disorders of Movement. New York, Oxford University Press, 1962.

Di Chiara, G. (ed.): GABA and the Basal Ganglia. New York, Raven Press, 1981.

Divac, I., and Öberg, R. G. E. (eds.): The Neostriatum. New York, Pergamon Press, 1979.

Dublin, W. B.: Fundamentals of Vestibular Pathology. St. Louis, Warren H. Green, Inc., 1985.

Duvoisin, R. C.: Parkinson's Disease. New York, Raven Press, 1978.

Elder, H. Y., and Trueman, E. R. (eds.): Aspects of Animal Movement. New York, Cambridge University Press, 1980.

Evarts, E. V.: Brain mechanisms of movement. *Sci. Am.* 241(3):164, 1979.

Fernstrom, J. D.: Role of precursor availability on control of monoamine biosynthesis in brain. *Physiol. Rev.*, 63:484, 1983.

Galanter, E.: Detection and discrimination of environmental change. *In* Darian-Smith, I. (ed.): Handbook of Physiology. Sec. 1, Vol. III. Bethesda, American Physiological Society, 1984, p. 103.

Goldberg, J. M., and Fernandez, C.: Vestibular mechanisms. *Annu. Rev. Physiol.*, 37:129, 1975.

Goldberg, J. M., and Fernandez, C.: The vestibular system. *In* Darian-Smith, I. (ed.): Handbook of Physiology. Sec. 1, Vol. III. Bethesda, American Physiological Society, 1984, p. 977.

Granit, R., and Pompeiano, O. (eds.): Reflex Control of Posture and Movement. New York, Elsevier Scientific Publishing Co., 1979.

Grillner, S.: Control of locomotion in bipeds, tetrapods, and fish. *In* Brooks, V. B. (ed.): Handbook of Physiology. Sec. 1, Vol. II. Bethesda, American Physiological Society, 1981, p. 1179.

Hobson, J. A., and Brazier, M. A. B. (eds.): The Reticular Formation Revisited: Specifying Function for a Nonspecific System. New York, Raven Press, 1980.

Hood, J. D. (ed.): Vestibular Mechanisms in Health and Disease. New York, Academic Press, 1978.

Kitai, S. T.: Electrophysiology of the corpus striatum and brain stem integrating systems. *In* Brooks, V. B. (ed.): Handbook of Physiology. Sec. 1, Vol. II. Bethesda, American Physiological Society, 1981, p. 997.

Kuypers, H. G. J. M.: Anatomy of the descending pathways. *In* Brooks, V. B. (ed.): Handbook of Physiology. Sec. 1, Vol. II. Bethesda, American Physiological Society, 1981, p. 597.

Luschei, E. S., and Goldberg, L. J.: Neural mechanisms of mandibular control: Mastication and voluntary biting. *In* Brooks, V. B. (ed.): Handbook of Physiology. Sec. 1, Vol. II. Bethesda, American Physiological Society, 1981, p. 1237.

Nauta, W. J. H., and Freitag, M.: The organization of the brain. *Sci. Am.*, 241(3):88, 1979.

Olsen, R. W.: Drug interactions at the GABA receptor-ionophore complex. *Annu. Rev. Pharmacol. Toxicol.*, 22:245, 1982.

Oosterveld, W. J. (ed.): Audio-Vestibular System and Facial Nerve. New York, S. Karger, 1977.

Orlovsky, G. N., and Shik, M. L.: Control of locomotion: A neurophysiological analysis of the cat locomotor system. *Int. Rev. Physiol.*, 10:281, 1976.

Pearson, K.: The control of walking. *Sci. Am.*, 235(6):72, 1976.

Penney, J. B., Jr., and Young, A. B.: Speculations on the functional anatomy of basal ganglia disorders. *Annu. Rev. Neurosci.*, 6:73, 1983.

Peterson, B. W.: Reticulospinal projections of spinal motor nuclei. *Annu. Rev. Physiol.*, 41:127, 1979.

Precht, W.: Vestibular mechanisms. *Annu. Rev. Neurosci.*, 2:265, 1979.

Rack, P. M. H.: Limitations of somatosensory feedback in control of posture and movement. *In* Brooks, V. B. (ed.): Handbook of Physiology. Sec. 1, Vol. II. Bethesda, American Physiological Society, 1981, p. 229.

Riklan, M.: L-Dopa and Parkinsonism. Springfield, Ill., Charles C Thomas, 1973.

Sarno, J. E., and Sarno, M. T.: Stroke; The Condition and the Patient. New York, McGraw-Hill, 1979.

Scheibel, A. B.: The brain stem reticular core and sensory function. *In* Darian-Smith, I. (ed.): Handbook of Physiology. Sec. 1, Vol. III. Bethesda, American Physiological Society, 1984, p. 213.

Sherrington, C. S.: Decerebrate rigidity and reflex coordination of movements. *J. Physiol. (Lond.)*, 22:319, 1898.

Shik, M. L., and Orlovsky, G. N.: Neurophysiology of locomotor automatism. *Physiol. Rev.*, 56:465, 1976.

Silverman, A.-J.: Magnocellular neurosecretory system. *Annu. Rev. Neurosci.*, 6:357, 1983.

Stein, P. S. G.: Motor systems with specific reference to the control of locomotion. *Annu. Rev. Neurosci.* 1:61, 1978.

Stein, R. B., and Lee, R. G.: Tremor and clonus. *In* Brooks, V. B. (ed.): Handbook of Physiology. Sec. 1, Vol. II. Bethesda, American Physiological Society, 1981, p. 325.

Talbott, R. E., and Humphrey, D. R. (eds.): Posture and Movement. New York, Raven Press, 1979.

Valentinuzzi, M.: The Organs of Equilibrium and Orientation as a Control System. New York, Harwood Academic Publishers, 1980.

Wilson, V., and Jones, G. M.: Mammalian Vestibular Physiology. New York, Plenum Press, 1979.

Wilson, V. J., and Peterson, B. W.: Peripheral and central substrates of vestibulospinal reflexes. *Physiol. Rev.*, 58:80, 1978.

Wilson, V. J., and Peterson, B. W.: Vestibulospinal and reticulospinal systems. *In* Brooks, V. B. (ed.): Handbook of Physiology. Sec. 1, Vol. II. Bethesda, American Physiological Society, 1981, p. 667.

Young, L. R.: Cross coupling between effects of linear and angular acceleration on vestibular nystagmus. *Bibl. Ophthalmol.*, 82:116, 1972.

Young, L. R.: Perception of the body in space: Mechanisms. *In* Darian-Smith, I. (ed.): Handbook of Physiology. Sec. 1, Vol. III. Bethesda, American Physiological Society, 1984. p. 1023.

17

Cortical and Cerebellar Control of Motor Functions

In preceding chapters we have been concerned with many of the subconscious motor activities integrated in the spinal cord and brain stem, especially those responsible for posture and equilibrium. In the present chapter we will discuss the control of motor function by the cerebral cortex and cerebellum as well as their relationship to the basal ganglia and the other lower centers. Much of this control is "voluntary" in contradistinction to the subconscious control effected by the lower centers. Yet we will also see that at least some motor functions of the cerebral cortex and cerebellum are not entirely "voluntary."

THE MOTOR CORTEX—THE PRIMARY AND PREMOTOR AREAS

Figure 17–1 illustrates a broad area of the cerebral cortex that is concerned either with sensation from the somatic areas of the body or with control of body movement. The posterior part of this area, the *somatic sensory cortex*, we have already discussed. Lying directly anterior to the somatic sensory area in front of the central sulcus, as illustrated in the figure, and occupying approximately the posterior one half of the frontal lobes is the *motor cortex*. Nerve signals originating from this region cause muscle contractions in different parts of the body.

The motor cortex is divided into two separate divisions, the *primary motor area* and the *premotor area*. The primary area contains very large *pyramidal motor neurons* that send their fibers all the way to the spinal cord through the *corticospinal tract* and therefore have almost direct communication with the anterior motor neurons of the cord for control of either individual muscles or small groups of muscles. Even very weak electrical stimuli in this primary motor area usually will elicit a muscle contraction somewhere in the body. The primary motor cortex is also frequently referred to as *area IV* of the cortex because this area containing the large

pyramidal cells is area IV in Brodmann's histological classification of the different cortical areas, as will be explained in Chapter 19.

The *premotor area* lies anterior to the primary motor area and is also illustrated in Figure 17–1. This area is frequently called areas VI and VIII because it occupies both these areas in the Brodmann classification of brain topology. The premotor cortex has very few neurons that project nerve fibers directly to the spinal cord. Instead, most of the nerve signals generated in this area cause more complex muscle movements, usually involving groups of muscles performing some specific task, rather than individual muscles. To achieve these results, the premotor area mainly sends its signals into the primary motor cortex to excite multiple groups of muscles. Some of these signals pass directly to the motor cortex through subcortical nerve fibers, but the premotor cortex also has extensive connections with the basal ganglia and cerebellum, both of which transmit signals back by way of the thalamus to the motor cortex. Thus the premotor cortex, the basal ganglia, the cerebellum, and the primary motor cortex constitute a complex overall system for voluntary control of muscle activity.

THE TOPOGRAPHICAL MAP OF THE PRIMARY MOTOR AREA

The neurons in each small point area of the primary motor cortex project to a single muscle or small group of muscles in a specific part of the body. Figure 17–2 illustrates four separate so-called topographical maps, two sensory and two motor, that have been discovered in the brain of a monkey. These maps show specific points in the cerebral cortex connecting with the different areas of the body. The areas labeled *Sm I* and *Sm II* are the somatic sensory areas I and II that were described in Chapter 13. The other two topographical maps, *Ms I* and *Ms II*, located more anteriorly in the brain, are topographical maps for the fiber projections from the motor cortex outward to the different body areas. The dark area, Ms I, is the *primary motor cortex*, and the lighter area, Ms II,

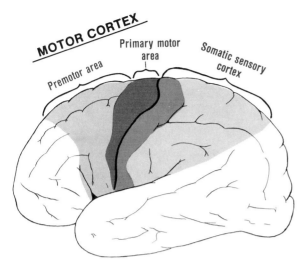

Figure 17–1. Relationship of the motor cortex to the somatic sensory cortex.

is called the *supplemental motor area*, which we shall discuss later.

Most of the primary cortex lies in the gyrus immediately anterior to the central sulcus, called the *precentral gyrus*, and, as illustrated in the figure, the head is represented most laterally in this gyrus whereas the tail end of the animal is represented most medially. In fact, the most caudal portions of the animal are represented in the portion of the precentral gyrus that curves downward into the longitudinal fissure and lies on the medial surface of the cerebral hemisphere, as illustrated in the folded-up upper portion of Figure 17–2 that shows this medial cerebral surface. Note in this figure that some parts of the body have much greater representation in the motor cortex than other parts, especially the hands, the feet, and the digits.

The Motor Topographical Map in the Human Being. The topographical map of the motor cortex in the human being is quite different from that of lower animals. The reason for this is that the human being has developed two important capabilities involving the motor cortex that are not found in lower animals. These are (1) an exceptional capability to use the hand, the fingers, and the thumb to perform highly dexterous manual tasks and (2) use of the mouth, lips, tongue, and facial muscles to talk. Therefore, there are very high degrees of representation of the hand, mouth, and facial regions in the human motor cortex.

Figure 17–3 illustrates the degrees of representation of the different muscle areas of the body in the motor cortex as mapped by Penfield and Rasmussen. This was done by stimulating the different areas of the motor cortex in human beings undergoing neurosurgical operations. Note that more than one half of the entire primary motor cortex is concerned with controlling the hands and the muscles of speech. Point stimulations in these areas of the motor cortex will cause contraction of a single muscle or even a portion of a single muscle. On the other hand, in those areas of the primary cortex with less intense degree of representation such as in the trunk area, electrical stimulation will usually contract a group of muscles instead.

The Supplemental Motor Area

Area Ms II in Figure 17–2, located on the medial surface of the frontal lobe slightly anterior to the primary motor cortex, is called the *supplemental motor area*. This area requires considerably stronger electrical stimuli to cause muscle contraction than does the primary motor area. Also, the movements involve coordinate contractions of many muscles in contradistinction to the much more discrete movements elicited from the primary area. Furthermore, many of the movements are bilateral rather than unilateral, and the contractions occur most often in the trunk or proximal portions of the limbs, causing the

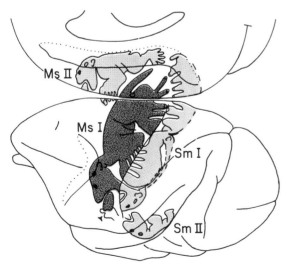

Figure 17–2. The different motor areas of the monkey cortex, illustrating especially the primary motor area (Ms I) located in the precentral gyrus. Ms II is the supplemental motor area, and Sm I and Sm II are the two somatic sensory areas. (The upper portion of the figure illustrates the medial surface of the cerebral hemisphere.) (From Woolsey, *in* Schaltenbrand and Woolsey (eds.): Cerebral Localization and Organization. Madison, University of Wisconsin Press, 1964.)

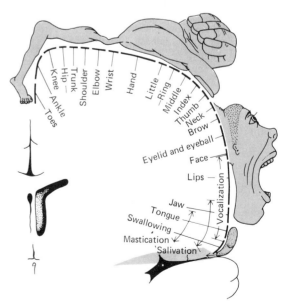

Figure 17–3. Degree of representation of the different muscles of the body in the motor cortex. (From Penfield and Rasmussen: The Cerebral Cortex of Man: A Clinical Study of Localization of Function. New York, Macmillan Company, 1968.)

animal to position itself in some special attitude. Also, there may be rotation of the head, movement of the eyes, vocalization, or yawning.

COMPLEX MOVEMENTS ELICITED BY STIMULATING THE PREMOTOR AREA

Electrical stimulation of the premotor area will often elicit complex contractions of groups of muscles. Occasionally, vocalization occurs, or rhythmic movements such as alternate thrusting of a leg forward and backward, coordinate moving of the eyes, chewing, swallowing, or contortions of parts of the body into different postural positions.

Some neurophysiologists have called this area the *motor association area* and have ascribed special capabilities to it to control coordinated movements involving many muscles simultaneously. In fact, it is peculiarly organized to perform such a function for the following reasons: (1) it has long subcortical neuronal connections with the sensory association areas of the parietal lobe; (2) it has direct subcortical connections with the primary motor cortex; (3) it connects with areas in the thalamus contiguous with the thalamic areas that connect with the primary motor cortex; and (4) most important of all, it has abundant direct connections with the basal ganglia and the cerebellum, both of which feed back to the primary motor area through the thalamus.

Broca's Area and Speech. Figure 17–4 illustrates a premotor area lying immediately anterior to the primary motor cortex and immediately above the sylvian fissure labeled "word formation." This region is called *Broca's area*. Damage to it does not prevent a person from vocalizing, but it does make it impossible for the person to speak whole words other than simple utterances such as "no" or "yes." A closely associated cortical area also causes appropriate respiratory function so that respiratory activation of vocal cords can occur simultaneously with the movements of the mouth and tongue during speech. Thus, the premotor activities that are related to Broca's area are highly complex.

The Voluntary Eye Movement Field. Immediately above Broca's area is a locus for controlling eye movements. Damage to this area prevents a person from voluntarily moving the eyes toward different objects. Instead, the eyes tend to lock on specific objects, an effect controlled by signals from the occipital region, as explained in Chapter 24. This frontal area also controls eyelid movements such as blinking.

Head Rotation Area. Still slightly higher in the motor association area, electrical stimulation will elicit head rotation. This area is closely associated with the eye movement field and is presumably related to directing the head toward different objects.

Area for Hand Skills. In the frontal area immediately anterior to the primary motor cortex for the

hands and fingers is a region neurosurgeons have called an area for hand skills. That is, when tumors or other lesions cause destruction in this area, the hand movements become incoordinate and nonpurposeful, a condition called *motor apraxia*.

FIBER PATHWAYS TO AND FROM THE MOTOR CORTEX

The functions of the motor cortex are controlled mainly by the somatic sensory system but also to a lesser extent by the other sensory systems such as hearing and vision. Once the sensory information is derived from these sources, the motor cortex operates in association with the basal ganglia and cerebellum to process the information and to determine the appropriate course of motor action. Therefore, there are many two-way fiber pathways between the motor cortex on the one hand and the sensory cortex, the basal ganglia, and the cerebellum on the other hand. In addition, the motor cortex gives rise to an especially important motor output pathway directly to the spinal cord through the pyramidal tract, as well as many other shorter pathways terminating primarily in the brain stem. Thus, the important pathways subserving all these functions are the following:

Afferent Fibers That Excite the Motor Cortex

The motor cortex is stimulated to action by signals from many different sources, including:

1. Subcortical fibers from adjacent regions of the cortex, especially from the somatic sensory areas and from the frontal areas—also subcortical fibers from the visual and auditory cortices.

2. Subcortical fibers that pass through the corpus callosum from the opposite cerebral hemisphere. These fibers connect corresponding areas of the motor cortices in the two sides of the brain.

3. Somatic sensory fibers derived directly from the ventrobasal complex of the thalamus. These transmit

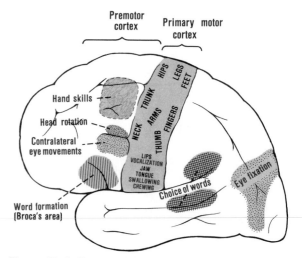

Figure 17–4. Representation of the different muscles of the body in the motor cortex and location of other cortical areas responsible for certain types of motor movements.

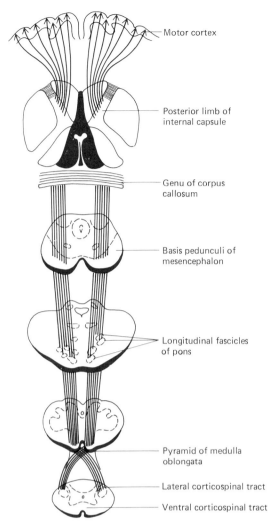

Motor cortex

Posterior limb of
internal capsule

Genu of corpus
callosum

Basis pedunculi of
mesencephalon

Longitudinal fascicles
of pons

Pyramid of medulla
oblongata

Lateral corticospinal tract

Ventral corticospinal tract

Figure 17–5. The pyramidal tract. (From Ranson and Clark: Anatomy of the Nervous System. Philadelphia, W. B. Saunders Company, 1959.)

mainly cutaneous tactile signals and joint and muscle signals.

4. Tracts from the ventrolateral and ventroanterior nuclei of the thalamus, which in turn receive tracts from the cerebellum and the basal ganglia. These tracts provide signals that are necessary for coordination between the functions of the motor cortex, the basal ganglia, and the cerebellum.

5. Fibers from the nonspecific nuclei of the thalamus. These fibers probably control the general level of excitability of the motor cortex in the same manner that they also control the general level of excitability of most other regions of the cerebral cortex.

Efferent Fibers from the Motor Cortex

The Pyramidal Tract (Corticospinal Tract). The most important output pathway from the motor cortex is the *pyramidal tract*, also called the *corticospinal tract*, which is illustrated in Figure 17–5.

The pyramidal tract originates about 60 per cent from the primary motor cortex, 20 per cent from the premotor cortex, and 20 per cent from the somatic sensory areas posterior to the central sulcus. After leaving the cortex it passes through the posterior limb of the internal capsule (between the caudate nucleus and the putamen of the basal ganglia) and then downward through the brain stem, forming the *pyramids of the medulla.* By far the majority of the pyramidal fibers then cross to the opposite side and descend in the *lateral corticospinal tracts* of the cord, finally terminating principally on the interneurons in the intermediate regions of the cord gray matter. However, some of the fibers in human beings (but not in most lower animals) terminate directly on the anterior motor neurons.

A few of the fibers do not cross to the opposite side in the medulla but pass ipsilaterally down the cord in the *ventral corticospinal tracts,* but these fibers also cross mainly to the opposite side of the cord either in the neck or the upper thoracic region.

The most impressive fibers in the pyramidal tract are a population of large myelinated fibers with mean diameter of about 16 microns. These originate from the *giant pyramidal cells,* also called *Betz cells,* that are found only in the primary motor cortex. These cells are about 60 microns in diameter, and their fibers transmit nerve impulses to the spinal cord at a velocity of about 70 meters per second, the most rapid rate of transmission of any signals from the brain to the cord. There are approximately 34,000 of these large fibers from the Betz cells in each corticospinal tract. However, the total number of fibers in each corticospinal tract is more than a million, so these large fibers represent only 3 per cent of all of them. The other 97 per cent are mainly fibers smaller than 4 microns in diameter.

Other Fiber Pathways from the Motor Cortex. The motor cortex gives rise to very large numbers of direct fibers from the cortex or collaterals from the pyramidal tract that go to the more basal regions of the cerebrum and also into the brain stem, including the following:

1. The axons from the giant Betz cells send short collaterals back to the cortex itself. It is believed that these collaterals mainly inhibit adjacent regions of the cortex when the Betz cells discharge, thereby "sharpening" the boundaries of the excitatory signal.

2. A large body of fibers passes into the *caudate nucleus* and *putamen.* From here additional pathways extend through several neurons into the brain stem, as discussed in the previous chapter.

3. A moderate number of fibers pass to the *red nuclei.* From these, additional fibers pass down the cord through the *rubrospinal tract.*

4. A moderate number of fibers deviate into the *reticular substance* of the mesencephalon; from here signals go to the cord via *reticulospinal tracts* and others go to the cerebellum via *reticulocerebellar tracts.*

5. A tremendous number of fibers synapse in the pontile nuclei, which give rise to the *pontocerebellar fibers.* Thus, whenever signals are transmitted from the motor cortex through the pyramidal tract, simultaneous signals are transmitted into the cerebellar hemispheres.

6. Collaterals also terminate in the *inferior olivary nuclei,* and from here secondary *olivocerebellar fibers* transmit signals to many areas of the cerebellum.

Thus, the basal ganglia, the brain stem, and the cerebellum all receive strong signals from the pyramidal tract every time a signal is transmitted down the spinal cord to cause a motor activity.

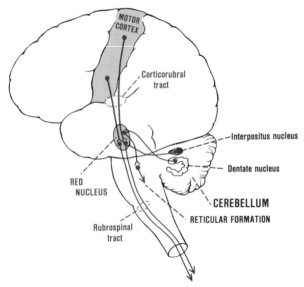

Figure 17–6. The corticorubrospinal pathway for motor control, showing also the relationship of this pathway to the cerebellum.

THE RED NUCLEUS AND THE RUBROSPINAL TRACT—THEIR RELATIONSHIP TO THE PYRAMIDAL SYSTEM

The red nucleus, illustrated in Figure 17–6, is located in the mesencephalon and functions in close association with the pyramidal tract. This nucleus has two parts, a superior portion, called the *parvocellular portion,* that is composed of small neurons, and an inferior portion, called the *magnocellular portion,* that contains many large neurons. The large neurons of the magnocellular portion give rise to the *rubrospinal tract* that crosses to the opposite side in the lower brain stem and follows a course parallel to the corticospinal tract into the lateral columns of the spinal cord. This tract partially overlaps the corticospinal tract but on the average lies slightly anterior to it. The rubrospinal fibers terminate mainly on the interneurons of the intermediate areas of the cord gray matter along with the corticospinal fibers, and a few of the rubrospinal fibers also terminate on the anterior motor neurons, along with some of the corticospinal fibers.

The red nucleus receives two major input pathways. One of these is *from the motor cortex via the corticorubral tract,* terminating mainly in the magnocellular portion of the red nucleus and thus stimulating the fibers of the rubrospinal tract. The second source of input fibers is *from the cerebellum,* which provides fibers to both the parvocellular and magnocellular portions of the red nucleus.

Function of the Corticorubrospinal System. The magnocellular portion of the red nucleus has a somatotopical representation of all the muscles of the body, as is true of the motor cortex. Therefore, stimulation of a single point in this portion of the red nucleus will cause contraction of either a single muscle or small group of muscles. However, the fineness of representation of the different muscles is far less developed than is true in the motor cortex. This is especially true in human beings who have a relatively small red nucleus.

The corticorubrospinal pathway serves as an accessory route for the transmission of relatively discrete signals from the motor cortex to the spinal cord. When the pyramidal fibers are destroyed without destroying this other pathway, discrete movements can still occur, except that the movements of the fingers and hands are considerably impaired. Wrist movements are still well developed, which is not true when the corticorubrospinal pathway is also blocked. Therefore, the pathway through the red nucleus to the spinal cord is associated far more with the pyramidal system than with the vestibuloreticulospinal system that controls mainly the axial and girdle muscles of the body. Furthermore, the rubrospinal tract lies in the lateral columns of the spinal cord, along with the corticospinal tracts, and terminates more on the interneurons and motor neurons that control the distal muscles of the limbs. Therefore, the corticospinal and rubrospinal tracts together are frequently called the *lateral motor system of the cord,* in contradistinction to the vestibuloreticulospinal system that lies mainly medially in the cord and is called the *medial motor system of the cord.*

THE EXTRAPYRAMIDAL SYSTEM

The term *extrapyramidal motor system* is widely used in clinical circles to denote all those portions of the brain and brain stem that contribute to motor control but that are not part of the direct pyramidal system. This includes the basal ganglia, the reticular formation of the brain stem, the vestibular nuclei, and often the red nuclei as well. However, this is such an all-inclusive and diverse group of motor control areas that it is difficult to ascribe specific neurophysiological functions to the extrapyramidal system as a whole. For this reason, we have discussed the functions of the separate portions of the extrapyramidal system individually.

EXCITATION OF THE SPINAL CORD BY THE PRIMARY MOTOR CORTEX AND THE RED NUCLEUS

Vertical Columnar Arrangement of the Neurons in the Motor Cortex. In Chapters 13 and 24 it is pointed out that the cells in the somatic sensory cortex and visual cortex—and perhaps in all other parts of the brain as well—are organized in vertical columns of cells. In a like manner, the cells of the motor cortex are also organized in vertical columns—columns 0.3 to 1 mm in diameter and having perhaps 50,000 to 150,000 neurons in each column.

Each column of cells functions as a unit, stimulating either a single muscle or a group of synergistic muscles. Also, each column of cells is arranged in six distinct layers, like the arrangement throughout almost all the cerebral cortex. The pyramidal cells that give rise to the corticospinal fibers all lie in the fifth layer of cells from the cortical surface, whereas the input signals to the column of cells all enter layers two through four. The sixth layer gives rise mainly to fibers that communicate with other regions of the cerebral cortex itself.

Function of Each Column of Neurons. The neurons of each column operate as an integrative processing system, utilizing information from multiple input sources to determine the output response from the column. In addition, each column can function as an amplifying system so that large numbers of pyramidal fibers to the same muscle or to synergistic muscles can be stimulated simultaneously. This is important because stimulation of a single pyramidal cell can rarely excite a muscle. Instead, as many as perhaps 50 to 100 pyramidal cells need to be excited simultaneously or in rapid succession to achieve muscle contraction.

Dynamic and Static Signals Transmitted by the Pyramidal Neurons. Characteristically, when a weak signal is transmitted to a muscle the muscle develops its force of contraction very slowly. However, if a strong signal is sent at first to cause initial rapid contraction, then a much weaker signal can maintain the contraction for long periods thereafter. This is the manner in which excitation for causing muscle contractions is usually provided. To do this, each column of cells excites two separate populations of pyramidal cell neurons, one called the *dynamic neurons* and the other the *static neurons.* The dynamic neurons are excessively excited for a short period of time at the beginning of the contraction, causing the initial development of force. Then the static neurons fire at a much slower rate, but they continue at this slow rate indefinitely to maintain the force of contraction as long as the contraction is required.

The neurons of the red nucleus have similar dynamic and static characteristics, except that more dynamic neurons are in the red nucleus and more static neurons in the primary motor cortex. This perhaps relates to the fact that the red nucleus is closely allied to the cerebellum, and we shall learn later in this chapter that the cerebellum also plays an important role in the rapid initiation of muscle contraction.

Somatic Sensory Feedback to the Motor Cortex. When nerve signals from the motor cortex cause a muscle to contract, somatic sensory signals return from the activated region of the body to the neurons in the motor cortex that are causing the action. Most of these somatic sensory signals arise in the muscle spindles or in the tactile receptors of the skin overlying the muscles. In general, the somatic signals cause a positive feedback enhancement of the muscle contraction in the following ways: In the case of the muscle spindles, if the fusimotor muscle fibers in the spindles contract more than the large skeletal muscle itself does, then the spindles become excited and the signals from these spindles stimulate the pyramidal cells in the motor cortex, which further excites the muscle, helping its contraction catch up with the contraction of the spindles. In the case of the tactile receptors, if the muscle contraction causes compression of the skin against an object, such as compression of the fingers around an object that is being grasped, the signals from these receptors cause further excitement of the muscles and therefore increase the muscle contraction—such as increasing the tightness of the grasp of the hand.

Stimulation of the Spinal Motor Neurons

Figure 17–7 shows a segment of the spinal cord, illustrating multiple motor tracts entering the cord from the brain and also showing a representative anterior motor neuron. The corticospinal tract and the rubrospinal tract lie in the dorsal portions of the lateral columns. Most of their fibers terminate on interneurons in the intermediate area of the cord gray matter; this is especially so in the trunk, leg, and arm areas of the cord. However, in the cervical enlargement of the cord where the hands and fingers are represented, the motor neurons supplying the hands and fingers lie almost entirely in the lateral portions of the anterior horns. And large numbers of both corticospinal and rubrospinal fibers terminate directly on these anterior motor neurons, thus allowing a direct route from the brain for activating muscle contraction. This is in keeping with the fact that the primary motor cortex has an extremely high degree of representation for fine control of hand, finger, and thumb actions.

Patterns of Movement Elicited by Spinal Cord Centers. From Chapter 15, recall that the spinal cord can provide specific reflex patterns of movement in response to sensory nerve stimulation.

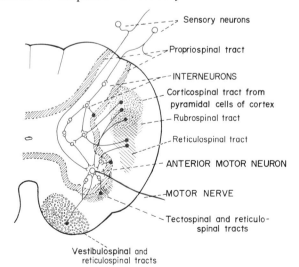

Figure 17–7. Convergence of all the different motor pathways on the anterior motor neurons.

Many of these patterns are also important when the anterior motor neurons are excited by signals from the brain. For instance, the stretch reflex is functional at all times, helping damp the motor movements initiated from the brain and probably providing at least part of the motive power required to cause the muscle contractions employing the servo-assist mechanism that was described in Chapter 15.

Also, when a brain signal excites an agonist muscle, it is not necessary to transmit an inverse signal to the antagonist at the same time; this transmission will be achieved by the reciprocal innervation circuit that is always present in the cord for coordinating the functions of antagonistic pairs of muscles.

Finally, parts of the other reflex mechanisms, such as withdrawal, stepping and walking, scratching, postural mechanisms, and so forth, can be activated by "command" signals from the brain. Thus, very simple signals from the brain can lead, at least theoretically, to many of our normal motor activities, particularly for such functions as walking and the attainment of different postural attitudes of the body.

Effect of Lesions in the Motor Cortex— The "Stroke"

The motor cortex is frequently damaged, especially by the common abnormality called a "stroke," which is caused either by a ruptured blood vessel that allows hemorrhage into the brain or by thrombosis of one of the major arteries supplying the brain, in either case causing loss of blood supply to the cortex. Also, experiments have been performed in animals to remove selectively different parts of the motor cortex.

Removal of the Primary Motor Cortex (the Area Pyramidalis). Removal of a very small portion of the primary motor cortex—the area that contains the giant Betz pyramidal cells—in a monkey causes varying degrees of paralysis of the represented muscles. If the sublying caudate nucleus and the adjacent premotor area are not damaged, gross postural and limb "fixation" movements can still be performed, but the animal *loses voluntary control of discrete movements of the distal segments of the limbs—especially of the hands and fingers.* This does not mean that the muscles themselves cannot contract but that the animal's ability to control the fine movements is gone.

From these results one can conclude that the area pyramidalis is essential for voluntary initiation of finely controlled movements, especially of the hands and fingers.

Muscle Spasticity Caused by Large Lesions of the Motor Cortex and Basal Ganglia. Ablation of the primary motor cortex alone or interruption of the pyramidal tract causes hypotonia, not spasticity, because the primary motor cortex normally exerts a continual tonic stimulatory effect on the motor neurons of the spinal cord; when they are removed, hypotonia results.

On the other hand, most lesions of the motor cortex, especially those caused by a stroke, involve both the motor cortex itself and deeper structures of the cerebrum as well, especially the basal ganglia. In these instances, muscle spasm almost invariably occurs in the afflicted muscle areas on the opposite side of the body (because all the motor pathways cross to the opposite side). Obviously, this spasm is not caused by loss of either the primary motor cortex or blockage of the pyramidal fibers to the cord. Instead, it is believed to be caused mainly by the damage in the basal ganglia. In fact, the greater the damage to the basal ganglia, the greater the degree of spasm.

It will be recalled that a major share of the output signals from the basal ganglial system are inhibitory. Much of this inhibition feeds back to the primary motor cortex to inhibit the pyramidal system itself, but still additional inhibitory signals pass into the brain stem to inhibit the reticular formation and vestibular nuclei. Therefore, release of these other motor systems from the basal ganglial inhibition allows excess excitatory motor activity, leading to the muscle spasm.

The muscle spasm that results from large lesions of the motor cortex and basal ganglia is different from the spasticity that occurs in decerebrate rigidity. In decerebrate rigidity the spasm occurs almost exclusively in the antigravity muscles, activated to a great extent by excess activity in the muscle spindle stretch reflexes; it is called *extensor spasm.* On the other hand, the spasm resulting from large cortical lesions usually involves the flexor muscles as well and is activated to a major extent by the alpha motor neurons to the muscles, in addition to activation of the muscle spindle system. This causes intense stiffening of the limbs and other parts of the body.

The Babinski Sign. Destruction of the foot region of the area pyramidalis or transection of the foot portion of the pyramidal tract causes a peculiar response of the foot called the *Babinski sign.* This response is demonstrated when a firm tactile stimulus is applied to the lateral sole of the foot: The great toe extends upward and the other toes fan outward. This is in contradistinction to the normal effect in which all the toes bend downward. The Babinski sign does not occur when damage occurs in the extrapyramidal portions of the motor control system without involving the pyramidal tract. Therefore, the sign is used clinically to detect damage specifically in the pyramidal portion of the motor control system.

The cause of the Babinski sign is believed to be the following: The pyramidal tract is a major controller of muscle activity for performance of voluntary, purposeful activity. On the other hand, the extrapyramidal system, a much older motor control system, is concerned to a great extent with protection. Therefore, when only the extrapyramidal system is functional, stimuli to the bottom of the feet cause a typical withdrawal protective type of reflex which is expressed by the upturned great toe and fanning of the other toes. But, when the pyramidal system is also fully functional, it suppresses the protective reflex and instead excites a higher order of motor function, including the normal effect of causing downward bending of the toes in response to sensory stimuli from the bottom of the feet.

THE CEREBELLUM AND ITS MOTOR FUNCTIONS

The cerebellum has long been called a *silent area* of the brain principally because electrical excitation of this structure does not cause any sensation and rarely any motor movement. However, as we shall see, removal of the cerebellum does cause the motor movements to become highly abnormal. The cerebellum is especially vital to the control of very rapid muscular activities such as running, typing, playing the piano, and even talking. Loss of this area of the brain can cause almost total incoordination of these activities even though its loss causes paralysis of no muscles.

But how is it that the cerebellum can be so important when it has no direct capability of causing muscle contraction? The answer to this is that it both *helps plan the motor activities* and also *monitors and makes corrective adjustments in the motor activities elicited by other parts of the brain.* It receives continuously updated information on the desired program of muscle contractions from the motor control areas of the other parts of the brain. And it receives continuous information from the peripheral parts of the body to determine the instantaneous status of each part of the body—its position, its rate of movement, forces acting on it, and so forth. It is believed that the cerebellum *compares* the actual instantaneous status of each part of the body as depicted by the peripheral information with the status that is intended by the motor system. If the two do not compare favorably, then appropriate corrective signals are transmitted instantaneously back into the motor system to increase or decrease the levels of activation of the specific muscles.

Since the cerebellum must make major motor corrections extremely rapidly *during the course of motor movements,* a very extensive and rapidly acting cerebellar input system is required both from the peripheral parts of the body and from the cerebral motor areas. Also, an extensive output system feeding equally as rapidly into the motor system is necessary to provide the necessary corrections of the motor signals.

THE ANATOMICAL FUNCTIONAL AREAS OF THE CEREBELLUM

Anatomically, the cerebellum is divided into three separate lobes by two deep fissures, as shown in Figure 17–8: (1) the *anterior lobe,* (2) the *posterior lobe,* and (3) the *flocculonodular lobe.* The flocculonodular lobe is the oldest of all portions of the cerebellum; it developed along with (and functions with) the vestibular system in controlling equilibrium, as was discussed in the previous chapter. Because of its ancient heritage, it is frequently called the *archicerebellum.* The anterior lobe and part of the midportion of the posterior lobe are also old; this is called the *paleocerebellum.* On the other hand, almost 90 per cent of the posterior lobe is recent in origin and is especially highly developed in primates and human beings; this is called the *neocerebellum.*

The Longitudinal Functional Divisions of the Anterior and Posterior Lobes. From a functional point of view, the anterior and posterior lobes are organized not by lobes but instead along the longitudinal axis, as illustrated in Figure 17–9, which shows the human cerebellum after

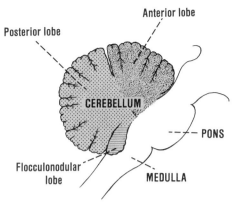

Figure 17–8. The anatomical lobes of the cerebellum as seen from the lateral side.

the lower end of the posterior cerebellum has been rolled downward from its normally hidden position. Note down the center of the cerebellum a narrow band separated from the remainder of the cerebellum by shallow grooves. This is called the *vermis.* In this area most cerebellar control functions for the muscle movements of the axial body, the neck, and the shoulders and hips are located.

To each side of the vermis is a large, laterally protruding *cerebellar hemisphere,* and each of these hemispheres is divided into an *intermediate zone* and a *lateral zone.* The intermediate zone of the hemisphere is concerned with the control of muscular contractions in the distal portions of both the upper and lower limbs, especially of the hands and fingers and feet and toes. On the other hand, the lateral zone of the hemisphere operates at a much more remote level, for this area seems to join into the overall planning of sequential motor movements. Without this lateral zone, most discrete motor activities of the body lose their appropriate timing and therefore become highly incoordinate, as we shall discuss more fully later.

Topographical Representation of the Body in the Cerebellum. In the same manner that the sensory cortex, the motor cortex, the basal ganglia, the red nuclei, and the reticular formation all have topographical representations of the different parts of the body, so also is this

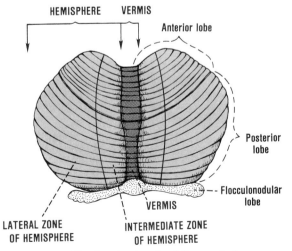

Figure 17–9. The functional parts of the cerebellum as seen from the posteroinferior view, with the inferiormost portion of the cerebellum rolled outward to flatten the surface.

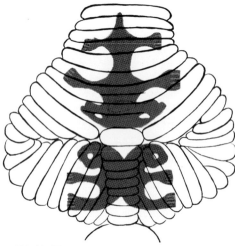

Figure 17–10. The sensory projection areas, called "homunculi," on the cortex of the cerebellum. (From Snider: *Sci. Amer., 199*:4, 1958. © 1958, by Scientific American, Inc. All rights reserved.)

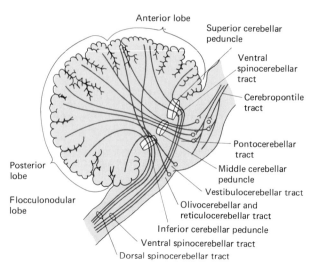

Figure 17–11. The principal afferent tracts to the cerebellum.

true for parts of the cerebellum. Figure 17–10 illustrates two separate such representations in a small monkey, showing one to be located in the anterior lobe and the other in the posterior lobe. Note that the axial portions of the body lie in the vermal part of the cerebellum whereas the limbs and facial regions lie in the intermediate zones of the two hemispheres. These topographical representations receive afferent nerve fibers from all the respective parts of the body. In turn, they send motor signals into the same respective topographical areas of the motor cortex, the basal ganglia, the red nucleus, and the reticular formation.

However, note that the large lateral portions of the cerebellar hemispheres *do not* have topographical representations of the body. These areas of the cerebellum connect mainly with the association areas of the brain, especially the premotor area of the frontal cortex and the somatic sensory and sensory association areas of the parietal cortex. Presumably this connectivity with the association areas allows the lateral portions of the cerebellar hemispheres to play important roles in planning and coordinating the sequential patterns of muscular activities.

The Input Pathways to the Cerebellum

Afferent Pathways from the Brain. The basic input pathways to the cerebellum are illustrated in Figure 17–11. An extensive and important afferent pathway is the *corticopontocerebellar pathway,* which originates mainly in the *motor cortex* but to a lesser extent in the sensory cortex as well and then passes by way of the *pontile nuclei* and *pontocerebellar tracts* to the contralateral hemisphere of the cerebellum. In addition, important afferent tracts originate in the brain stem; they include (1) an extensive *olivocerebellar* tract, which passes from the *inferior olive* to all parts of the cerebellum; this tract is excited by fibers from the *motor cortex,* the *basal ganglia,* widespread areas of the *reticular formation,* and the *spinal cord;* (2) *vestibulocerebellar fibers,* some of which originate in the vestibular apparatus itself and others from the vestibular nuclei; most of these terminate in the *flocculonodular lobe* and *fastigial nucleus* of the cerebellum; and (3) *reticulocerebellar*

fibers, which originate in different portions of the reticular formation and terminate mainly in the midline cerebellar areas (the vermis).

Afferent Pathways from the Periphery. The cerebellum also receives important sensory signals directly from the peripheral parts of the body through four separate tracts, two of which are located dorsally in the cord and two ventrally. The two most important of these tracts are illustrated in Figure 17–12: the *dorsal spinocerebellar tract* and the *ventral spinocerebellar tract.* These two tracts originate in the sacral, lumbar, and thoracic segments of the cord. Similar tracts, not shown in Figure 17–12, originate in the neck segments of the cord and course roughly along with the dorsal and ventral spinocerebellar tracts in their passage to the cerebellum. These are the *cuneocerebellar tract* that joins the dorsal spinocerebellar tract and the *rostral spinocerebellar tract* that joins the ventral

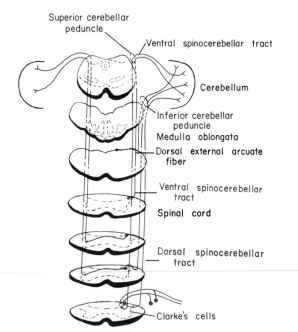

Figure 17–12. The spinocerebellar tracts.

spinocerebellar tract. The dorsal tracts enter the cerebellum through the inferior cerebellar peduncle and terminate in the cerebellum on the same side as their origin. The two ventral tracts enter the cerebellum through the superior cerebellar peduncle, but they terminate in both sides of the cerebellum.

The signals transmitted in the dorsal spinocerebellar tracts come mainly from the muscle spindles and to a lesser extent from other somatic receptors throughout the body, such as from the Golgi tendon organs, the large tactile receptors of the skin, and the joint receptors. All these signals apprise the cerebellum of the momentary status of muscle contraction, degree of tension on the muscle tendons, positions and rates of movement of the parts of the body, and forces acting on the surfaces of the body.

On the other hand, the ventral spinocerebellar tracts receive less information from the peripheral receptors. Instead, they are excited mainly by the motor signals arriving in the spinal cord from the brain through the corticospinal and rubrospinal tracts. Thus, this ventral fiber pathway tells the cerebellum that the motor signals have indeed arrived at the cord, and it also apprises the cerebellum of the intensity of the signals.

The spinocerebellar pathways can transmit impulses at velocities as great as 100 meters per second, which is the most rapid conduction of any pathway in the entire central nervous system. This extremely rapid conduction is important for the instantaneous apprisal of the cerebellum of changes that take place in the status of the body.

In addition to the signals in the spinocerebellar tracts, other signals are transmitted through the dorsal and dorsolateral columns to the medulla and then relayed from there to the cerebellum. Likewise, signals are transmitted through the *spinoreticular pathway* to the reticular formation of the brain stem and through the *spino-olivary pathway* to the inferior olivary nucleus and then relayed from both these areas to the cerebellum. Thus, the cerebellum continually collects information about all parts of the body even though it is operating at a subconscious level.

Output Signals from the Cerebellum

The Deep Cerebellar Nuclei and the Efferent Pathways. Located deep in the cerebellar mass are three *deep cerebellar nuclei*—the *dentate, interpositus,* and *fastigial nuclei.* The *vestibular nuclei* in the medulla also function in some respects as if they were deep cerebellar nuclei because of their direct connections with the cortex of the flocculonodular lobe. All the deep cerebellar nuclei receive signals from two different sources: the cerebellar cortex and the sensory afferent tracts to the cerebellum. Each time an input signal arrives in the cerebellum, it divides and goes in two directions: (1) directly to one of the deep nuclei and (2) to a corresponding area of the cerebellar cortex overlying the deep nucleus; then, a short time later, the cerebellar cortex relays its output signals also to the same deep nucleus. Thus, all the input signals that enter the cerebellum eventually end in the deep nuclei. We shall discuss this circuit in greater detail later.

Three major efferent pathways lead out of the cerebellum, as illustrated in Figure 17–13:

1. A pathway that begins in the *cortex of the lateral zone of the cerebellar hemisphere,* then passes to the *dentate nucleus,* next to the *ventrolateral and ventroanterior nuclei of*

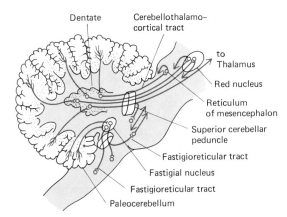

Figure 17–13. Principal efferent tracts from the cerebellum.

the thalamus, and finally to the *cerebral cortex.* This pathway plays an important role in helping coordinate "voluntary" motor activities initiated by the cerebral cortex.

2. A pathway that originates in the *midline structures of the cerebellum* (the *vermis*) and then passes through the *fastigial nuclei* into the *medullary* and *pontile regions of the brain stem.* This circuit functions in close association with the equilibrium apparatus to help control equilibrium and also, in association with the reticular formation of the brain stem, helps control the postural attitudes of the body. It was discussed in detail in the previous chapter in relation to equilibrium.

3. A pathway that originates in the *intermediate zone of the cerebellar hemisphere,* between the vermis and the lateral zone of the cerebellar hemisphere, then passes (1) through the *nucleus interpositus* to the *ventrolateral and ventroanterior nuclei of the thalamus,* and thence to the *cerebral cortex,* (2) to several *midline structures* of the *thalamus* and thence to the *basal ganglia,* and (3) to the *red nucleus* and *reticular formation* of the upper portion of the brain stem. This circuit is believed to coordinate mainly the reciprocal contractions of agonist and antagonist muscles in the peripheral portions of the limbs—especially in the hands, fingers, and thumbs.

THE NEURONAL CIRCUIT OF THE CEREBELLUM

The human cerebellar cortex is actually a large folded sheet, approximately 17 cm wide by 120 cm long, with the folds lying crosswise, as illustrated in Figures 17–9 and 17–10. Each fold is called a *folium.* And lying deep in the folded mass of cortex are the deep nuclei.

The Functional Unit of the Cerebellar Cortex—the Purkinje Cell. The cerebellum has approximately 30 million nearly identical functional units, one of which is illustrated to the left in Figure 17–14, shown mainly in red color. This functional unit centers on the *deep nuclear cell* and on the *Purkinje cell,* of which there are also 30 million in the cerebellar cortex.

Note to the right in Figure 17–14 the three major layers of the cerebellar cortex: the *molecular layer,* the *Purkinje cell layer,* and the *granular cell layer.*

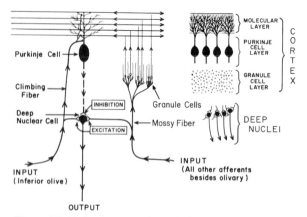

Figure 17–14. Basic neuronal circuit of the cerebellum, showing excitatory pathways in color. At right are the three major layers of the cerebellar cortex and also the deep nuclei.

Then, beneath these layers, the *deep nuclei* are located far within the center of the cerebellar mass.

The Neuronal Circuit of the Functional Unit. As illustrated in Figure 17–14, the output from the functional unit is from a deep nuclear cell. However, this cell is continually under the influence of both excitatory and inhibitory influences. The excitatory influences arise from direct connections with the afferent fibers that enter the cerebellum. The inhibitory influences arise entirely from the Purkinje cells in the cortex of the cerebellum.

The afferent inputs to the cerebellum are mainly of two types, one called the *climbing fiber type* and the other called the *mossy fiber type.* There is one climbing fiber for about ten Purkinje cells. After sending collaterals to several deep nuclear cells, the climbing fiber projects all the way to the molecular layer of the cerebellar cortex where it makes about 300 synapses with the soma and dendrites of each Purkinje cell. This climbing fiber is distinguished by the fact that a single impulse in it will always cause a single, very prolonged, and peculiar oscillatory type of action potential in each Purkinje cell with which it connects. Another distinguishing feature of the climbing fibers is that *they all originate in the inferior olive of the medulla,* whereas the cerebellar afferent fibers from all other sources are almost entirely of the mossy type.

The mossy fibers also send collaterals to excite deep nuclear cells. Then these fibers proceed to the granular layer of the cortex where they synapse with hundreds of *granule cells.* These in turn send very small axons, less than 1 micron in diameter, up to the outer surface of the cerebellar cortex to enter the molecular layer. Here the axons divide into two branches that extend 1 to 2 millimeters in each direction parallel to the folia. There are literally millions of these *parallel nerve fibers* in each small segment of the cerebellar cortex (there are about 1000 granule cells for every Purkinje cell). It is into this molecular layer that the dendrites of the Purkinje cells project, and 80,000 to 200,000 of these parallel fibers synapse with each Purkinje cell; as

these fibers pass along their 1 to 2 mm course, each of them contacts about 50 Purkinje cells. Yet, the mossy fiber input to the Purkinje cell is quite different from the climbing fiber input because stimulation of a single mossy fiber will never elicit an action potential in the Purkinje cell; instead, large numbers of mossy fibers must be stimulated simultaneously to activate the Purkinje cell. Furthermore, this activation usually takes the form of prolonged facilitation or excitation that, when it reaches threshold for stimulation, causes repetitive Purkinje cell firing of normal, short-duration action potentials rather than the single prolonged action potential occurring in response to the climbing fiber input.

Thus, the Purkinje cells are stimulated by two types of input circuits—one that causes a highly specific output in response to the incoming signal and the other that causes a less specific but tonic type of response. It should be noted that by far the greater proportion of the afferent input to the cerebellum is of the mossy fiber type, because this represents the afferent input from almost all the cerebellar afferent tracts besides those from the inferior olive.

Balance Between Excitation and Inhibition in the Deep Cerebellar Nuclei. The output signals from the Purkinje cells to the deep nuclei are entirely inhibitory. Therefore, referring again to the circuit of Figure 17–14, *one should note that direct stimulation of the deep nuclear cells by both the climbing and the mossy fibers excites them, whereas the signals arriving from the Purkinje cells inhibit them.* Normally, there is a continual balance between these two effects so that the degree of output from the deep nuclear cell remains relatively constant at a moderate level of continuous stimulation. On the other hand, in the execution of rapid motor movements, the *timing* of the two effects on the deep nuclei is such that the excitation appears before the inhibition. Then a few milliseconds later inhibition occurs. In this way, there is first a very rapid excitatory signal fed back into the motor pathway to modify the motor movement, but this is followed within a few milliseconds by an inhibitory signal. This inhibitory signal resembles a "delay-line" negative feedback signal of the type that is very effective in providing *damping.* That is, when the motor system is excited, a negative feedback signal presumably occurs after a short delay to stop the muscle movement from overshooting its mark, which is the usual cause of oscillation.

Other Inhibitory Cells in the Cerebellar Cortex. In addition to the granule cells and Purkinje cells, three other types of neurons are also located in the cerebellar cortex: *basket cells, stellate cells,* and *Golgi cells.* All these are inhibitory cells with very short axons. Both the basket cells and the stellate cells are located in the molecular layer of the cortex, lying among and stimulated by the parallel fibers. These cells in turn send their axons at right angles across the parallel fibers and cause *lateral inhibition* of the adjacent Purkinje cells, thus sharpening the signal in the same manner that lateral inhibition sharpens the contrast of signals in many other areas of the nervous system. The Golgi cells lie in the Purkinje cell layer of the cortex, and their dendrites are also stimulated by the parallel fibers of the molecular layer, but the axons from these cells feed back to and inhibit the granule cells instead of the Purkinje cells. The function of this feedback is to limit the duration of the signal transmitted into the cerebellar cortex from the granule cells. That is, within a short fraction of a second after the granule cells are stimulated, they are then inhibited by the feedback. Therefore, a short, transient, pulselike signal, not a prolonged signal, is transmitted into the parallel fibers and thence to the Purkinje cells.

Special Features of the Cerebellar Neuronal Circuit. A special feature of the cerebellum is that there are no reverberatory pathways in the cerebellar neuronal circuits, so that the input-output signals of the cerebellum are very rapid transients that never persist for long periods of time.

Another special feature is that many of the cells of the cerebellum are constantly active. This is especially true of the deep nuclear cells; they continually send output signals to the other areas of the motor system. The importance of this is that *decrease* of the nuclear cell firing rate can provide an *inhibitory output signal* from the cerebellum, while an *increase* in firing rate can provide an *excitatory output signal.*

FUNCTION OF THE CEREBELLUM IN CONTROLLING MOVEMENTS

The cerebellum functions in motor control only in association with motor activities initiated elsewhere in the nervous system. These activities may originate in the spinal cord, in the reticular formation, in the basal ganglia, or in areas of the cerebral cortex. We will discuss, first, the operation of the cerebellum in association with the spinal cord and lower brain stem for control of postural movements and equilibrium and then discuss its function in association with the motor cortex for control of voluntary movements.

FUNCTION OF THE CEREBELLUM WITH THE SPINAL CORD AND BRAIN STEM TO CONTROL POSTURAL AND EQUILIBRIUM MOVEMENTS

The cerebellum originated phylogenetically at about the same time that the vestibular apparatus developed. Furthermore, as was discussed in the previous chapter, loss of the flocculonodular lobes of the cerebellum causes extreme disturbance of equilibrium. Yet, we still must ask the question, what role does the cerebellum play in equilibrium that cannot be provided by the other neuronal machinery of the brain stem? A clue is the fact that in persons with cerebellar dysfunction equilibrium is far more disturbed during performance of rapid motions than during stasis. This suggests that the cerebellum is especially important in controlling the balance between agonist and antagonist muscle

contractions during rapid changes in body positions as dictated by the vestibular apparatuses. One of the major problems in controlling this balance is the time required to transmit position signals and kinesthetic signals from the different parts of the body to the brain. Even when utilizing the most rapidly conducting sensory pathways at 100 meters per second, as used by the spinocerebellar system, the delay for transmission from the feet to the brain is still 15 to 20 milliseconds. The feet of a person running rapidly can move as much as 10 inches during this time. Therefore, it is impossible for the brain to know at any given instant during rapid motion the exact position of the different parts of the body.

On the other hand, with appropriate neuronal circuitry, it would be possible for the cerebellum or some other portion of the brain to know how rapidly and in what direction a part of the body was moving 15 to 20 milliseconds earlier and then to predict from this information where the parts of the body should be at the present time. And this seems to be one of the major functions of the cerebellum.

As we have already discussed in relation to the neuronal circuitry of the cerebellum, there are abundant sensory pathways from the somatic areas of the body, especially from the muscles, joints, and skin surface, that feed both into the brain stem and into the older areas of the cerebellum—into the flocculonodular lobes through the vestibular nuclei and into the vermis and intermediate areas of the cerebellum through the dorsal and ventral spinocerebellar tracts and reticulocerebellar tracts. Also, the vestibular apparatus is located within a few centimeters of the flocculonodular lobes, allowing no more than a millisecond or so delay in transmission of the vestibular information.

Therefore, during the control of equilibrium, it is presumed that the extremely rapidly conducted vestibular apparatus information is used in a typical feedback control circuit to provide almost instantaneous correction of postural motor signals as necessary for maintaining equilibrium even during extremely rapid motion, including rapidly changing directions of motion. The feedback signals from the peripheral areas of the body help in this process, but their help is presumably contingent upon some function of the cerebellum to compute positions of the respective parts of the body at any given time, despite the long delay time from the periphery to the cerebellum.

Relationship of Cerebellar Function to the Spinal Cord Stretch Reflex

One major component of cerebellar control of posture and equilibrium is an extreme amount of information transmitted from the muscle spindles to the cerebellum through the dorsal spinocerebellar tracts. In turn, signals are transmitted into the brain stem through the cerebellar fastigial nuclei to stimulate the gamma efferent fibers that innervate the muscle spindles themselves. Therefore, a cerebellar stretch reflex occurs that is similar to but more complex than the spinal cord stretch reflex. It utilizes signals that pass all the way to the cerebellum and back again to the muscles. In general, this reflex adds additional support to the cord stretch reflex, but its feedback time is considerably longer, thus prolonging the effect. Through this feedback pathway many of the postural adjustments of the body are believed to occur.

FUNCTION OF THE CEREBELLUM IN VOLUNTARY MUSCLE CONTROL

In addition to the feedback circuitry between the body periphery and the cerebellum, an almost entirely independent feedback circuitry exists between the motor cortex and the cerebellum. This is illustrated in its simplest form in Figure 17–15 and in a much more complex form, involving the basal ganglia also in the control circuit, in Figure 17–16. Most of the signals of this circuit pass from the motor cortex and adjacent cortical areas to the cerebellar hemispheres and then back to the cortex again, successively, through the dentate and interpositus cerebellar nuclei and the ventrolateral and ventroanterior nuclei of the thalamus. These circuits are not involved in the control of the axial and girdle muscles of the body. Instead, they serve two other motor control functions involving respectively the intermediate zone of the cerebellar hemisphere, and the large lateral zone of this hemisphere. Let us discuss each of these separately.

CEREBELLAR FEEDBACK CONTROL OF THE DISTAL LIMBS THROUGH THE INTERMEDIATE CEREBELLAR ZONE AND INTERPOSITUS NUCLEUS

The intermediate zone of each cerebellar hemisphere receives information from two sources: direct information from the motor cortex and feedback information from the peripheral parts of the body, especially from the distal portions of the limbs. After the cerebellum has integrated this information, output signals are then transmitted mainly to the cerebral cortex through relays in the interpositus nucleus and the thalamus. In addition, signals pass directly from the interpositus nucleus to the magnocellular portion (the lower portion) of the red nucleus that gives rise to the rubrospinal tract. The rubrospinal tract in turn innervates especially those portions of the spinal cord gray matter that control the distal parts of the limbs, particularly the hands and fingers.

It is believed that this part of the cerebellar motor control system provides smooth, coordinate movements of the agonist and antagonist muscles of the distal limbs for the performance of acute purposeful

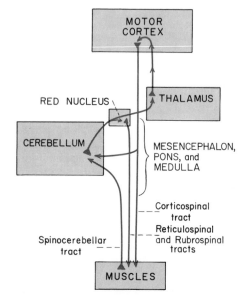

Figure 17–15. Pathways for cerebellar control of voluntary movements.

intricate movements. The cerebellum seems to compare the "intentions" of the higher levels of the motor control system, as transmitted to the intermediate cerebellar hemisphere through the corticopontocerebellar tract, with the "performance" by the respective parts of the body as transmitted back to the cerebellum from the periphery. In fact, the ventral spinothalamic tract even transmits back to

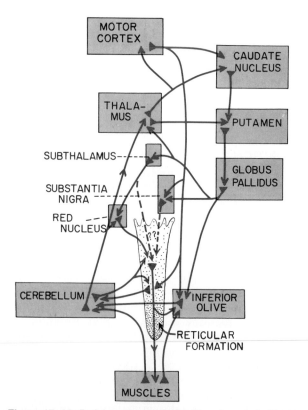

Figure 17–16. Pathways for cerebellar "error" control of involuntary movements.

the cerebellum a "copy" of the actual motor control signals that reach the anterior motor neurons, and this too is integrated with the signals arriving from the muscle spindles and other proprioceptor sensory organs.

Ordinarily, during rapid movements, the motor cortex transmits far more impulses than are needed to perform each intended movement, and the cerebellum therefore must act to inhibit the motor cortex at the appropriate time after the muscle has begun to move. The cerebellum is believed to assess the rate of movement and calculate the length of time that will be required to reach the point of intention. Then appropriate inhibitory impulses are transmitted to the motor cortex to inhibit the agonist muscle and to excite the antagonist muscle. In this way, appropriate "brakes" are applied to stop the movement at the precise point of intention.

Thus, when a rapid movement is made toward a point of intention, the agonist muscle contracts strongly throughout the early course of movement. Then, suddenly, shortly before the point of intention is reached, the agonist muscle becomes completely inhibited while the antagonist muscle becomes strongly excited. Furthermore, the point at which this reversal of excitation occurs depends on the rate of movement and on the previously learned knowledge of the inertia of the system. The faster the movement and the greater the inertia, the earlier the reversal point appears in the course of movement.

Since all these events transpire much too rapidly for the motor cortex to reverse the excitation "voluntarily," it is evident that the excitation of the antagonist muscle toward the end of a movement is an entirely automatic and subconscious function and is not a "willed" contraction of the same nature as the original contraction of the agonist muscle. We shall see later that in patients with serious cerebellar damage, excitation of the antagonist muscles does not occur at the appropriate time but instead always too late. Therefore, it is almost certain that one of the major functions of the cerebellum is automatic excitation of antagonist muscles at the end of a movement while at the same time inhibiting agonist muscles that have started the movement.

The "Damping" Function of the Cerebellum. One of the byproducts of the cerebellar feedback mechanism is its ability to "damp" muscular movements. To explain the meaning of "damping" we must first point out that essentially all movements of the body are "pendular." For instance, when an arm is moved, momentum develops, and the momentum must be overcome before the movement can be stopped. And, because of the momentum, all pendular movements have a tendency to overshoot. If overshooting does occur in a person whose cerebellum has been destroyed, the conscious centers of the cerebrum eventually recognize this and initiate a movement in the opposite direction to bring the arm to its intended position. But again

the arm, by virtue of its momentum, overshoots, and appropriate corrective signals must again be instituted. Thus, the arm oscillates back and forth past its intended point for several cycles before it finally fixes on its mark. This effect is called an *action tremor*, or *intention tremor*.

However, if the cerebellum is intact, appropriate subconscious signals stop the movement precisely at the intended point, thereby preventing the overshoot and also the tremor. This is the basic characteristic of a damping system. All servo control systems regulating pendular elements that have inertia must have damping circuits built into the servo mechanisms. In the motor control system of our central nervous system, the cerebellum seems to provide much of this damping function.

Cerebellar Control of Ballistic Movements. Many rapid movements of the body, such as the movements of the fingers in typing, occur so rapidly that it is not possible to receive feedback information either from the periphery to the cerebellum or from the cerebellum back to the motor cortex before the movements are over. These movements are called *ballistic movements*, meaning that the entire movement is preplanned and is set into motion to go a specific distance and then to stop. Another important example is the saccadic movements of the eyes, in which the eyes jump from one position to the next when reading or when looking at successive points along a road when a person is moving in a car.

Much can be understood about the function of the cerebellum by studying the changes that occur in the ballistic movements when the cerebellum is removed. Three major changes occur: (1) the movements are slow to begin, (2) the force development is weak, and (3) the movements are slow to turn off. Therefore, it becomes very difficult to perform the very rapid ballistic movements. Furthermore, it is almost impossible to control how far the movement will go because of the difficulty of turning the movement off once it is begun. Thus, in the absence of the cerebellar circuit, the motor cortex has to think very hard to turn ballistic movements on and again has to think hard and take extra time to turn the movement off. Thus, the automatism of ballistic movements is lost.

But, how does the cerebellum function in the control of ballistic movements? We do not know the answer to this. The supposition is that when the motor cortex first initiates the movement, it immediately sends signals to the cerebellum at the same time. The first effect of the signals is to excite the deep cerebellar nuclei, and these immediately send an excitatory signal back to the motor cortex, red nucleus, or other motor nuclei to reinforce strongly the onset of the ballistic movement. A few milliseconds later, the signal entering the cerebellum will have had time to go through the delay circuits of the cerebellar cortex and to return by way of the Purkinje cells to the deep cerebellar nuclei, but this time inhibiting these rather than exciting them. Therefore, after this given delay time, this automatic delayed inhibitory signal presumably stops the ballistic movement by turning off the agonist muscle and, because of reciprocal innervation, turning on the antagonist at the same time.

If the student will consider once again the circuitry of the cerebellum as described earlier in the chapter, she or he will see that it is beautifully organized to perform this biphasic, first excitatory and then delayed inhibitory, function that is required for ballistic movements. The student will also see that the time delay circuits of the cerebellar cortex almost undoubtedly are fundamental to this particular ability of the cerebellum.

FUNCTION OF THE LARGE LATERAL ZONE OF THE CEREBELLAR HEMISPHERE—THE "PLANNING" AND "TIMING" FUNCTIONS

In human beings, the lateral zones of the two cerebellar hemispheres have become very highly developed and greatly enlarged, along with the human capability to perform intricate movements with the hands and fingers and along with the ability to speak. Yet, strangely enough, these large lateral portions of the cerebellar hemispheres have no direct input of information from the peripheral parts of the body. Also, almost all the communication between these lateral cerebellar areas and the cortex is not with the primary motor cortex itself but instead with the premotor area and primary and association somatic sensory areas. Even so, destruction of the lateral portions of the cerebellar hemispheres along with their deep nuclei, the dentate nuclei, can lead to extreme incoordination of the purposeful movements of the hands, fingers, feet, and speech apparatus. This has been hard to understand because of lack of direct communication between this part of the cerebellum and the primary motor cortex. However, recent experimental studies suggest that these portions of the cerebellum are concerned with two important aspects of motor control: the "planning" of sequential movements and the "timing" of the sequential movements.

The Planning Function. The planning of sequential movements seems to be related to the fact that the lateral hemispheres communicate with the premotor and sensory portions of the cerebral cortex and that there is in turn two-way communication between these areas and corresponding areas of the basal ganglia. It seems that the "plan" of the sequential movements is transmitted from the sensory and premotor areas of the cortex to the lateral zones of the cerebellar hemispheres, and two-way traffic between the cerebellum and the cortex is necessary to provide appropriate transition from one movement to the next. An exceedingly interesting observation that supports this view is that many of the neurons in the dentate nuclei display the activity pattern of the next movement at the same time that the present movement is occurring. Thus, the lateral hemispheres appear to be involved not with what is happening at a given moment but instead with *what will be happening during the next sequential movement.*

To summarize, one of the most important features of normal motor function is one's ability to progress smoothly from one movement to the next in orderly succession. In the absence of the cerebellar hemispheres this capability is seriously disturbed, especially for rapid movements.

The Timing Function. Another important function of the lateral cerebellar hemispheres is to provide appropriate timing for each movement. In the absence of these lateral areas, one loses the subconscious ability to predict ahead of time how far the different parts of the body will move in a given time. And without this timing capability, the person becomes unable to control the beginning of the next movement. As a result, the succeeding movement may begin much too early or much too late. Therefore, cerebellar lesions cause complex movements, such as those required for writing, running, or even talking, to become completely incoordinate, lacking completely in the ability to progress in an orderly sequence from one movement to the next. Such cerebellar lesions are said to cause *failure of smooth progression of movements.*

Extramotor Predictive Functions of the Cerebellum. The cerebellum also plays a role in predicting other events besides movements of the body. For instance, the rates of progression of both auditory and visual phenomena can be predicted. As an example, a person can predict from the changing visual scene how rapidly he or she is approaching an object. A striking experiment that demonstrates the importance of the cerebellum in this ability is the effect of removing the "head" portion of the cerebellum in monkeys. Such a monkey occasionally charges the wall of a corridor and literally bashes its brains out because it is unable to predict when it will reach the wall.

Unfortunately, we are only now beginning to learn about these extramotor predictive functions of the cerebellum. It is quite possible that the cerebellum provides a "time base," perhaps utilizing time-delay circuits, against which signals from other parts of the central nervous system can be compared. It is often stated that the cerebellum is especially important in interpreting *spatiotemporal relationships* in sensory information.

CLINICAL ABNORMALITIES OF THE CEREBELLUM

Essentially all lesions or malfunctions of the cerebellum cause abnormal motor movements on the *same side*—the *ipsilateral side*—of the body as the side of the malfunction in the cerebellum. The reason for this is that almost all tracts feeding sensory information into the cerebellum, especially the dorsal spinocerebellar tract, are uncrossed, whereas all tracts in both directions between the cerebral cortex and the cerebellum cross to the opposite side in the same manner that the pyramidal tract crosses to the opposite side of the peripheral body.

A second important feature of clinical cerebellar abnormalities is that destruction of small portions of the cerebellar cortex rarely causes a detectable abnormality in motor function. In fact, several months after as much as half the cerebellar cortex has been removed, if the deep cerebellar nuclei are not removed along with the cortex the motor functions of an animal appear to be almost entirely normal as long as the animal performs all movements slowly. Thus, the remaining portions of the motor control system are capable of compensating tremendously for loss of parts of the cerebellum.

To cause serious and continuous dysfunction of the cerebellum, the cerebellar lesion must usually involve the deep cerebellar nuclei—the *dentate, interpositus,* and *fastigial nuclei*—as well as the cerebellar cortex.

Dysmetria and Ataxia. Two of the most important symptoms of cerebellar disease are dysmetria and ataxia. It was pointed out earlier that in the absence of the cerebellum the subconscious motor control system cannot predict ahead of time how far movements will go. Therefore, the movements ordinarily overshoot their intended mark, though sometimes they are short of the mark. This effect is called *dysmetria,* and it results in incoordinate movements that are called *ataxia.*

Dysmetria and ataxia can also result from lesions in the spinocerebellar tracts, for the feedback information from the moving parts of the body is essential for accurate control of the movements.

Past Pointing. Past pointing means that in the absence of the cerebellum a person ordinarily moves the hand or some other moving part of the body considerably beyond the point of intention. This probably results from the following effect: The motor cortex normally transmits more impulses to the muscles to perform a given motor function than are actually needed. The cerebellum automatically corrects this by inhibiting the movement after it has begun. However, if the cerebellum is not available to cause this inhibition, the movement ordinarily goes beyond the intended point. Therefore, past pointing is actually a manifestation of dysmetria.

Failure of Progression. *Dysdiadochokinesia.* When the motor control system fails to predict ahead of time where the different parts of the body will be at a given time, it temporarily "loses" the parts during rapid motor movements. As a result, the succeeding movement may begin much too early or much too late so that no orderly "progression of movement" can occur. One can demonstrate this readily by having a patient with cerebellar damage turn one hand upward and downward at a rapid rate. The patient rapidly "loses" the hand and does not know its position during any portion of the movement. As a result, a series of jumbled movements occurs instead of the normal coordinate upward and downward motions. This is called *dysdiadochokinesia.*

Dysarthria. Another instance in which failure of progression occurs is in talking, for the formation of words depends on rapid and orderly succession of individual muscular movements in the larynx, mouth, and respiratory system. Lack of coordination between these and inability to predict either the intensity of the sound or the duration of each successive sound cause jumbled vocalization, with some syllables loud, some weak, some held long, some held for short intervals, and resultant speech that is almost completely unintelligible. This is called *dysarthria.*

Intention Tremor. When a person who has lost the cerebellum performs a voluntary act, the muscular movements are jerky; this reaction is called an *intention tremor* or an *action tremor,* and it results from failure of the cerebellar system to damp the motor movements.

Cerebellar Nystagmus. Cerebellar nystagmus is a tremor of the eyeballs that occurs usually when one attempts to fixate the eyes on a scene to one side of the head. This off-center type of fixation results in rapid, tremulous movements of the eyes rather than a steady fixation, and it is probably another manifestation of the failure of damping by the cerebellum. It occurs especially when the flocculonodular lobes are damaged; in this instance it is associated with loss of equilibrium, presumably because of dysfunction of the pathways through the cerebellum from the semicircular canals.

Rebound. If a person with cerebellar disease is asked to pull upward strongly on an arm while the physician holds it back at first and then lets go, the arm will fly back until it strikes the face instead of being automatically stopped. This is called *rebound,* and it results from *loss of the cerebellar component of the stretch reflex.* That is, the normal cerebellum ordinarily instantaneously and powerfully sensitizes this spinal cord reflex mechanism whenever a portion of the body begins to move unexpectedly in an unwilled direction. But, without the cerebellum, strong activation of the antagonist muscles fails to occur, thus allowing overmovement of the limb.

Hypotonia. Loss of the deep cerebellar nuclei, particularly the dentate and interpositus nuclei, causes decreased tone of the peripheral musculature on the side of the lesion, though after several months the motor cortex usually compensates for this by an increase in its intrinsic activity. The hypotonia results from loss of facilitation of the motor cortex and brain stem nuclei by the tonic discharge of the deep nuclei.

SENSORY FEEDBACK CONTROL OF MOTOR FUNCTIONS

THE "SENSORY ENGRAM" FOR MOTOR CONTROL

When large portions of the somatic sensory cortex are removed or damaged, a person or an animal loses the ability to perform many complex motor activities previously learned. The reason for this is believed to be that, when a person learns to perform a motor function, he or she experiences in the somatic sensory areas the effects of the motor movement each time it is performed, and "memories" of the different patterns of movements are recorded. These are called *sensory engrams of the motor movements.* Once a sensory engram has been established in the sensory cortex—that is, once the movement has been learned—the person then uses this sensory engram as a guide for the motor system of the brain to follow in reproducing the same pattern of movement. For instance, as a person learns to cut out a paper doll with scissors, the movements involved in this process cause a particular sequential pattern of sensory signals to pass to the somatic sensory area. Once this pattern has been "learned" by the sensory cortex, the memory engram of the pattern can be used to activate the motor system to perform the same sequential pattern whenever it is required—even when the person is blindfolded.

To do this, the sensory signals from the fingers, hands, and arms are compared with the engram, and if the two do not match each other, the difference, called the "error," supposedly initiates additional motor signals that automatically activate appropriate muscles to bring the fingers, hands, and arms into the necessary sequential attitudes for performance of the task. Each successive portion of the engram presumably is projected according to a time sequence, and the motor control system automatically follows from one point to the next so that the fingers go through the precise motions necessary to duplicate the sensory engram.

Thus, one can see that the motor system in this case acts as a *servo mechanism*, for it is not the motor cortex itself that controls the pattern of activity to be accomplished. Instead, the pattern is located in the sensory part of the brain, and the motor system merely "follows" the pattern, which is the definition of a servo mechanism. If ever the motor system fails to follow the pattern, sensory signals are fed back to the sensory cortex to apprise the sensorium of this failure, and appropriate corrective signals are transmitted to the muscles.

Other sensory signals besides somesthetic signals are also involved in motor control, particularly visual signals. However, these other sensory systems are often slower to recognize error than is the somatic system. Therefore, when the sensory engram depends on visual feedback for control purposes, the movements are usually considerably slowed in comparison with those that depend on somatic feedback.

An extremely interesting experiment that demonstrates the importance of the sensory engram for control of motor movements is one in which a monkey has been trained to perform some complex but slow-moving activity, and then various portions of its cortex are removed. Removal of small portions of the motor cortex that control the muscles normally used for the activity does not prevent the monkey from performing the activity. Instead it automatically uses other muscles in place of the paralyzed ones to perform the same activity. On the other hand, if the corresponding somatic sensory cortex is removed while the motor cortex is left intact, the monkey loses all ability to perform the activity. Thus, this experiment demonstrates that the motor system acts automatically as a servo mechanism to use whatever muscles are available to follow the pattern of the sensory engram, and if some muscles are missing, other muscles are substituted automatically. The experiment also demonstrates forcefully that the somatic sensory cortex is essential for performance of most complex types of "learned" motor activities.

ESTABLISHMENT OF RAPID MOTOR PATTERNS

Many motor activities are performed so rapidly that there is insufficient time for sensory feedback signals to control these activities. For instance, the movements of the fingers during typing occur much too rapidly for somatic sensory signals to be transmitted either to the somatic sensory cortex or even directly to the motor cortex and for these then to control each discrete movement. It is believed that the patterns for control of these rapid, coordinate muscular movements are established in the motor system itself, probably involving complex circuitry in the primary motor cortex, in the premotor cortex, the basal ganglia, and even the cerebellum. Indeed, lesions in any of these areas can destroy one's ability to perform rapid coordinated muscular contractions, such as those required during the acts of typing, talking, or writing by hand.

Role of Sensory Feedback During Establishment of the Rapid Motor Patterns. Even a highly skilled motor activity can be performed the very first time if it is performed extremely slowly—slowly enough for sensory feedback to guide the movements through each step. However, to be really useful, many skilled motor activities must be performed rapidly. This probably is achieved by successive performance of the same skilled activity until finally an engram for the skilled activity is laid down in the motor control areas of the cortex as well as in the sensory system. This *motor engram* causes a precise set of muscles to go through a specific sequence of movements required to perform the skilled activity. Therefore, such an engram is called a *pattern of skilled motor function,* and the motor areas are primarily concerned with this.

After a person has performed a skilled activity many times, the motor pattern of this activity can thereafter cause the hand or arm or other part of the body to go through the same pattern of activity again and again, now entirely *without* sensory feedback control. However, even though sensory feedback control is no longer present, the sensory system still determines whether or not the act has been performed correctly. This determination is made in retrospect rather than while the act is being performed. If the pattern has not been performed correctly, information from the sensory system can help correct the pattern the next time it is performed.

Thus, eventually, hundreds of patterns of different coordinate movements are believed to be laid down in the motor system, and these can be called upon one at a time in different sequential orders to perform literally thousands of complex motor activities.

An interesting experiment that demonstrates the applicability of these theoretical methods of muscular control is one in which the eyes are made to "follow" an object that moves around and around in a circle. At first, the eyes can follow the object only when it moves around the circle slowly, and even then the movements of the eyes are extremely jerky. Thus, sensory feedback is being utilized to control the eye movements for following the object. However, after a few seconds, the eyes begin to follow the moving object rather faithfully, and the rapidity of movement around the circle can be increased to many times per second, and still, the eyes continue to follow the object. Sensory feedback control of each stage of the eye movements at these rapid rates would be completely impossible. Therefore, by this time, the eyes have developed a pattern of movement that is not dependent upon step-by-step sensory feedback. Nevertheless, if the eyes should fail to follow the object around the circle, the sensory system would immediately become aware of this and presumably could make corrections in the pattern of movement.

INITIATION OF VOLUNTARY MOTOR ACTIVITY

Because of the spectacular properties of the primary motor cortex (the area pyramidalis) and of the instantaneous muscle contractions that can be achieved by stimulating this area, it has become customary to think that the initial brain signals that elicit voluntary muscle contractions begin in the primary motor cortex. However, this almost certainly is far from the truth. Indeed, experiments have shown that the cerebellum and the basal ganglia are activated at almost exactly the same time as or even before the motor cortex is activated. Furthermore, there is no known mechanism by which the motor cortex can conceive the entire sequential pattern that is to be achieved by the motor movements.

Therefore, we are left with an unanswered question: What is the locus of the initiation of voluntary motor activity? A partial answer to this comes from the fact that neuronal activity occurs in sensory areas of the brain as long as a second before a voluntary motor activity occurs. Also, neuronal activity begins in the premotor areas of the cortex and in some areas of the basal ganglia many milliseconds before motor activity occurs in the motor cortex. Therefore, it is beginning to be believed that *cerebration* occurring in these "integrative" portions of the brain, operating in association with the cerebellum, conceives and plans the complex sequence of movements that is to be executed. Only after the "plan" has been established is the primary motor system involving the primary motor cortex set into action to cause the sequential events. In the following chapter, we shall discuss the planning and execution of speech, which is an excellent illustration of these principles of voluntary motor control.

REFERENCES

Allen, G. I., and Tsukahara, N.: Cerebrocerebellar communication systems. *Physiol. Rev.*, 54:957, 1974.

Armstrong, D. M.: The mammalian cerebellum and its contribution to movement control. *In* Porter, R. (ed.): International Review of Physiology: Neurophysiology III. Vol. 17. Baltimore, University Park Press, 1978, p. 239.

Asanuma, H.: Cerebral cortical control of movement. *Physiologist*, 16:143, 1973.

Asanuma, H.: Recent developments in the study of the columnar arrangement of neurons within the motor cortex. *Physiol. Rev.*, 55:143, 1975.

Asanuma, H.: The pyramidal tract. *In* Brooks, V. B. (ed.): Handbook of Physiology. Sec. 1, Vol. II. Bethesda, American Physiological Society, 1981, p. 703.

Bloedel, J. R., and Courville, J.: Cerebellar afferent systems. *In* Brooks, V. B. (ed.): Handbook of Physiology. Sec. 1, Vol. II. Bethesda, American Physiological Society, 1981, p. 735.

Brooks, V. B., and Stoney, S. D., Jr.: Motor mechanisms: The role of the pyramidal system in motor control. *Annu. Rev. Physiol.*, 33:337, 1971.

Brooks, V. B., and Thach, W. T.: Cerebellar control of posture and movement. *In* Brooks, V. B. (ed.): Handbook of Physiology. Sec. 1, Vol. II. Bethesda, American Physiological Society, 1981, p. 877.

Cooper, I. S., *et al.* (eds.): The Cerebellum, Epilepsy, and Behavior. New York, Plenum Press, 1974.

Crowley, W. J.: Neural control of skeletal muscle. *In* Frohlich, E. D. (ed.): Pathophysiology, 2nd Ed. Philadelphia, J. B. Lippincott Co., 1976, p. 735.

Desmedt, J. E. (ed.): Cerebral Motor Control in Man: Long Loop Mechanisms. New York, S. Karger, 1978.

Eccles, J. C.: The Understanding of the Brain. New York, McGraw-Hill, 1973.

Evarts, E. V.: Brain mechanisms in movement. *Sci. Am.*, 229:96, 1973.

Evarts, E. V.: Brain mechanisms of movement. *Sci. Am.*, 241(3):164, 1979.

Evarts, E. V.: Role of motor cortex in voluntary movements in primates. *In* Brooks, V. B. (ed.): Handbook of Physiology. Sec. 1, Vol. II. Bethesda, American Physiological Society, 1981, p. 1083.

Evarts, E. V., and Thach, W. T.: Motor mechanisms of the CNS: Cerebrocerebellar interrelations. *Annu. Rev. Physiol.*, 31:451, 1969.

Fuster, J. M.: Prefrontal cortex in motor control. *In* Brooks, V. B. (ed.): Handbook of Physiology. Sec. 1, Vol. II. Bethesda, American Physiological Society, 1981, p. 1149.

Gallistel, C. R.: The Organization of Action: A New Synthesis. New York, Halsted Press, 1979.

Granit, R.: The Basis of Motor Control. New York, Academic Press, 1970.

Grillner, S.: Locomotion in vertebrates: Central mechanisms and reflex interaction. *Physiol. Rev.*, 55:247, 1975.

Keele, S. W.: Behavioral analysis of movement. *In* Brooks, V. B. (ed.): Handbook of Physiology. Sec. 1, Vol. II. Bethesda, American Physiological Society, 1981, p. 1391.

Kuypers, H. G. J. M.: Anatomy of the descending pathways. *In* Brooks, V. B. (ed.): Handbook of Physiology. Sec. 1, Vol. II. Bethesda, American Physiological Society, 1981, p. 597.

Llinas, R.: Eighteenth Bowditch lecture. Motor aspects of cerebellar control. *Physiologist*, 17:19, 1974.

Llinas, R.: Electrophysiology of the cerebellar networks. *In* Brooks, V. B. (ed.): Handbook of Physiology. Sec. 1, Vol. II. Bethesda, American Physiological Society, 1981, p. 831.

Massion, J., and Sasaki, K. (eds.): Cerebro-Cerebellar Interactions. New York, Elsevier/North-Holland, 1979.

McCloskey, D. I.: Corollary discharges: Motor commands and perception. *In* Brooks, V. B. (ed.): Handbook of Physiology. Sec. 1, Vol. II. Bethesda, American Physiological Society, 1981, p. 1415.

McHenry, L. C., Jr.: Cerebral Circulation and Stroke. St. Louis, W. H. Green, 1978.

O'Connell, A. L., and Gardner, E. B.: Understanding the Scientific Bases of Human Movement. Baltimore, Williams & Wilkins, 1972.

Orlovsky, G. N., and Shik, M. L.: Control of locomotion: A neurophysiological analysis of the cat locomotor system. *Int. Rev. Physiol.*, 10:281, 1976.

Paillard, J.: The patterning of skilled movements. *In* Magoun, H. W. (ed.): Handbook of Physiology. Sec. 1, Vol. 3. Baltimore, Williams & Wilkins, 1960, p. 1679.

Pearson, K.: The control of walking. *Sci. Am.*, 235(6):72, 1976.

Penfield, W., and Rasmussen, T.: The Cerebral Cortex of Man. New York, The Macmillan Co., 1950.

Porter, R.: Functions of the mammalian cerebral cortex in movement. *Prog. Neurobiol.*, 1:3, 1973.

Porter, R.: The neurophysiology of movement performance. *In* MTP International Review of Science: Physiology. Vol. 3. Baltimore, University Park Press, 1974, p. 151.

Porter, R.: Influences of movement detectors on pyramidal tract neurons in primates. *Annu. Rev. Physiol.*, 38:121, 1976.

Porter, R.: Internal organization of the motor cortex for input-output arrangements. *In* Brooks, V. B. (ed.): Handbook of Physiology. Sec. 1, Vol. II. Bethesda, American Physiological Society, 1981, p. 1063.

Poulton, E. C.: Human manual control. *In* Brooks, V. B. (ed.): Handbook of Physiology. Sec. 1, Vol. II. Bethesda, American Physiological Society, 1981, p. 1337.

Shik, M. L., and Orlovsky, G. N.: Neurophysiology of locomotor automatism. *Physiol. Rev.*, 56:465, 1976.

Stein, P. S. G.: Motor systems with specific reference to the control of locomotion. *Annu. Rev. Neurosci.*, 1:61, 1978.

Wiesendanger, M.: Organization of secondary motor areas of cerebral cortex. *In* Brooks, V. B. (ed.): Handbook of Physiology. Sec. 1, Vol. II. Bethesda, American Physiological Society, 1981, p. 1121.

Wiesendanger, M., and Miles, T. S.: Ascending pathway of low-threshold muscle afferents to the cerebral cortex and its possible role in motor control. *Physiol. Rev.*, 62:1234, 1982.

Wilson, D. M.: The flight-control system of the locust. *Sci. Am.*, 218:(5):83, 1968.

18

The Cerebral Cortex and Intellectual Functions of the Brain

It is ironic that we know least about the mechanisms of the cerebral cortex of almost all parts of the brain, even though it is by far the largest portion of the nervous system. Yet, we do know the effects of destruction or of specific stimulation of various portions of the cortex, and still more is known from electrical recordings from the cortex or from the surface of the scalp. In the early part of the present chapter the facts known about cortical functions are discussed and then some basic theories of the neuronal mechanisms involved in thought processes, memory, analysis of sensory information, and so forth are presented briefly.

PHYSIOLOGICAL ANATOMY OF THE CEREBRAL CORTEX

The functional part of the cerebral cortex is composed mainly of a thin layer of neurons 2 to 5 millimeters in thickness, covering the surface of all the convolutions of the cerebrum and having a total area of about one quarter square meter. The total cerebral cortex probably contains 50 to 100 billion neurons.

Figure 18–1 illustrates the typical structure of the cerebral cortex, showing successive layers of different types of cells. Most of the cells are of three types: *granular* (also called *stellate), fusiform,* and *pyramidal,* the latter named for their characteristic pyramidal shape. To the right in Figure 18–1 is illustrated the typical organization of nerve fibers within the different layers of the cortex. Note particularly the large number of *horizontal fibers* extending between adjacent areas of the cortex, but note also the *vertical fibers* that extend to and from the cortex to lower areas of the brain and to the spinal cord or to distant regions of the cerebral cortex through long association bundles of fibers.

Neurohistologists have divided the cerebral cortex into almost 100 different areas, which have slightly different architectural characteristics. Yet in all these different areas except the hippocampal region there still persist representations of all the six major layers of the cortex. To the untrained histologist, only five major architectural types of cortex can be distinguished as follows: type 1 contains large numbers of pyramidal cells with few granular cells and, therefore, is often called the *agranular cortex.* At the other extreme, type 5 contains almost no pyramidal cells but is filled with closely packed granular cells and is called the *granular cortex.* Types 2, 3, and 4 have intermediate characteristics containing graded proportions of pyramidal and granular cells.

The agranular cortex, which contains large numbers of pyramidal cells, is characteristic of the motor areas of the cerebral cortex, whereas the granular cortex, containing almost no pyramidal cells, is characteristic of the primary sensory areas. The other three intermediate types of cortex are characteristic of the association areas between the primary sensory and motor regions. The pyramidal cells give rise to the long axons that transmit motor signals to the basal ganglia, the brain stem and cerebellum, and the spinal cord. The granular cells have short axons that transmit multiple signals from neuron to neuron within the neural network of the cortex itself.

Figure 18–2 shows a map of cortical areas classified on the basis of histological studies by Brodmann. This classification provides a basis for discussion of functional areas of the brain, even though different architectural types of cortex often have similar functions.

Anatomical Relationship of the Cerebral Cortex to the Thalamus and Other Lower Centers. All areas of the cerebral cortex have direct afferent and efferent connections with the thalamus. Figure 18–3 shows the areas of the cerebral cortex connected with specific parts of the thalamus. These connections are in *two* directions, both from the thalamus to the cortex and then from the cortex back to essentially the same area of the thalamus. Furthermore, when the thalamic connections are cut, the functions of the corresponding cortical area become entirely or almost entirely abrogated. Therefore, the cortex operates in close association with the thalamus and can almost be considered both anatomically and functionally to be a large outgrowth of the thalamus; for this reason the thalamus and the cortex together are often called the *thalamocortical system,* as we shall discuss further in the following chapter. Also, all pathways from the sensory organs to the cortex pass through the thalamus, with the single exception of the sensory pathways of the olfactory tract.

FUNCTIONS OF CERTAIN SPECIFIC CORTICAL AREAS

Studies in human beings by neurosurgeons have shown that some specific functions are localized to

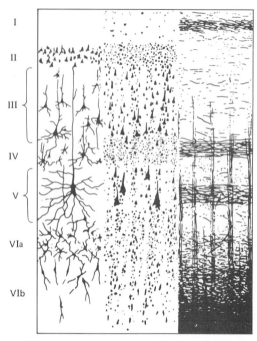

Figure 18–1. Structure of the cerebral cortex, illustrating *I*, molecular layer; *II*, external granular layer; *III*, layer of pyramidal cells; *IV*, internal granular layer; *V*, large pyramidal cell layer; *VI*, layer of fusiform or polymorphic cells. (From Ranson and Clark (after Brodmann): Anatomy of the Nervous System. Philadelphia, W. B. Saunders Company, 1959.)

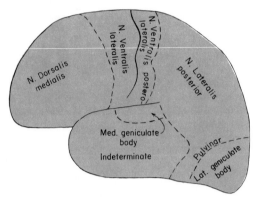

Figure 18–3. Areas of the cerebral cortex that connect with specific portions of the thalamus. (Modified from Elliott: Textbook of the Nervous System. Philadelphia, J. B. Lippincott Co.)

more general functions that we call association or cerebration.

SPECIFIC FUNCTIONS OF THE PRIMARY SENSORY AREAS

The primary sensory areas all have certain functions in common. For instance, the somatic sensory areas, visual sensory areas, and auditory sensory areas all have spatial localizations of signals from the peripheral receptors (which are discussed in detail in Chapters 13, 24, and 25).

Electrical stimulation of the *primary somatic sensory area* in the parietal lobe in awake patients elicits relatively uncomplicated sensations. For instance, in the somatic sensory area the patient expresses feelings of tingling in the skin, numbness, mild "electric" feeling, or, rarely, mild degrees of temperature sensations. And these sensations are localized to discrete areas of the body in accord with the spatial representation in the somatic sensory cortex, as described in Chapter 13. Therefore, it is believed that the primary somatic sensory cortex analyzes only the simple aspects of sensations and that analysis of intricate patterns of sensory experience requires also adjacent parts of the parietal lobes called the *somatic sensory association area*.

Electrical stimulation of the *primary visual cortex* in the occipital lobe causes the person to see flashes of light, bright lines, colors, or other simple visions. Here again, the visual images are localized to specific regions of the visual fields in accord with the portion of the primary visual cortex stimulated, as described in Chapter 24. But the visual cortex alone is not capable of complete analysis of complicated visual patterns; for this, the visual cortex must operate in association with adjacent regions of the occipital, temporal, and parietal cortex, the *visual association areas*.

Electrical stimulation of the *primary auditory cortex* in the temporal lobe causes a person to hear a simple sound which may be weak or loud, have low or high frequency, or have other uncomplicated

certain general areas of the cerebral cortex. Figure 18–4 gives a map of some of these areas as determined by Penfield and Rasmussen from direct electrical stimulation of the cortex or by neurological examination of patients after portions of the cortex had been removed. The lightly shaded areas are *primary sensory areas*, while the darkly shaded area is the *primary motor area* (also called *voluntary motor area*) from which muscular movements can be elicited with relatively weak electrical stimuli. These primary sensory and motor areas have highly specific functions as we have discussed in previous chapters, whereas other areas of the cortex perform

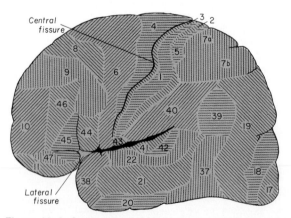

Figure 18–2. Structurally distinct areas of the human cerebral cortex. (From Everett: Functional Neuroanatomy. 5th ed. Philadelphia, Lea & Febiger, 1965. Modified from Brodmann.)

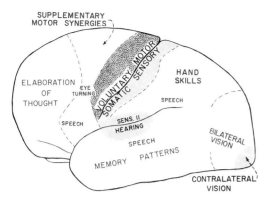

Figure 18–4. Functional areas of the human cerebral cortex as determined by electrical stimulation of the cortex during neurosurgical operations and by neurological examinations of patients with destroyed cortical regions. (From Penfield and Rasmussen: The Cerebral Cortex of Man: A Clinical Study of Localization of Function. New York, Macmillan Company, 1968.)

characteristics, such as a squeak or even an undulation. But never are words or any other fully intelligible sound heard. Thus, the primary auditory cortex, like the other primary sensory areas, can detect the individual elements of auditory experience but cannot analyze complicated sounds. Therefore, the primary auditory cortex alone is not sufficient to give one even the usual auditory experiences; these can be achieved, however, when the primary area operates together with the *auditory association areas* in adjacent regions of the temporal lobes.

Despite the inability of the primary sensory areas to analyze the incoming sensations fully, when these primary areas are destroyed the ability of the person to utilize the respective sensations usually suffers drastically. For instance, loss of the primary visual cortex in one occipital lobe causes a person to become blind in the ipsilateral halves of both retinae, and loss of the primary visual cortices in both hemispheres causes total blindness. Likewise, loss of both primary auditory cortices causes almost total deafness. Loss of the primary somatic sensory areas in the postcentral gyri causes *depression* of somatic sensory sensations—though not total loss—presumably because of additional thalamic and cortical representation of these sensations in other cortical areas: somatic sensory area II and the motor cortex, for example. (In animals far down the phylogenetic scale, loss of the visual and auditory cortices may have little effect on vision and hearing, and even an anencephalic human infant having no brain above the mesencephalon detects some visual cues in the absence of the visual cortex, for such a child can observe a moving object and even follow it by movement of the eyes and head.)

Therefore, we can summarize the functions of the primary sensory areas of the human cerebral cortex in the following way: The lower centers of the brain relay a large part of the sensory signals to the cerebral cortex for analysis. In turn, the primary sensory areas transmit the results of their analyses,

albeit still simple analyses, back to the lower centers and to other regions of the cerebral cortex, as is discussed later in the chapter.

THE SENSORY ASSOCIATION AREAS

Around the borders of the primary sensory areas are regions called *sensory association areas* or *secondary sensory areas*. In general, these areas extend 1 to 5 centimeters in one or more directions from the primary sensory areas; each time a primary area receives a sensory signal, secondary signals spread, after a delay of a few milliseconds, into the respective association area as well. Part of this spread occurs directly from the primary area through subcortical fiber tracts, but part also occurs in the thalamus, beginning in the sensory relay nuclei, passing next to corresponding *thalamic association areas*, and then traveling to the association cortex.

The general function of the sensory association areas is to provide a higher level of interpretation of the sensory experiences. The general areas for the interpretative functions for somatic, visual, and auditory experiences are illustrated in Figure 18–5.

Destruction of the *sensory association area* greatly reduces the capability of the brain to analyze different characteristics of sensory experiences. For instance, damage in the temporal lobe below and behind the primary auditory area in the "dominant hemisphere" of the brain often causes a person to lose the ability to understand words or other auditory experiences even though they are heard.

Likewise, destruction of the *visual association area* in Brodmann's areas 18 and 19 of the occipital lobe in the dominant hemisphere (see Figure 18–2), or the presence of a brain tumor or other lesion in these areas, does not cause blindness or prevent normal activation of the primary visual cortex but does greatly reduce the person's ability to interpret what is seen. Such a person often loses the ability

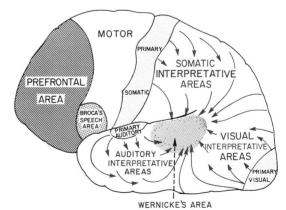

Figure 18–5. Organization of the somatic, auditory, and visual association areas into a general mechanism for interpretation of sensory experience. All these feed also into *Wernicke's area* located in the posterosuperior portion of the temporal lobe. Note also the prefrontal area and Broca's speech area.

to recognize the meanings of words, a condition that is called *word blindness* or *dyslexia.*

Finally, destruction of the *somatic sensory association area* in the parietal cortex posterior to primary somatic area I causes the person to lose spatial perception for location of the different parts of the body. In the case of the hand that has been "lost," the skills of the hand are greatly reduced. Thus, this area of the cortex seems to be necessary for interpretation of somatic sensory experiences.

The functions of the association areas are described in more detail in Chapter 13 for somatic, in Chapter 24 for visual, and in Chapter 25 for auditory experiences.

INTERPRETATIVE FUNCTION OF THE POSTERIOR SUPERIOR TEMPORAL LOBE—"WERNICKE'S AREA" (A GENERAL INTERPRETATIVE AREA)

The somatic, visual, and auditory association areas, which can actually be called "interpretative areas," all meet one another in the posterior part of the superior temporal lobe where the temporal, parietal, and occipital lobes all come together. This area of confluence of the different sensory interpretative areas is especially highly developed in the dominant side of the brain—the *left side* in right-handed persons—and it plays the greatest single role of any part of the cerebral cortex in the higher levels of brain function that we call *cerebration.* Therefore, this region has frequently been called by different names suggestive of the area having almost global importance: the *general interpretative area,* the *gnostic area,* the *knowing area,* the *tertiary association area,* and so forth. However, it is best known as *Wernicke's area* in honor of the neurologist who first described its special significance in intellectual processes.

Following severe damage in Wernicke's area, a person might hear perfectly well and even recognize different words but still might be unable to arrange these words into a coherent thought. Likewise, the person may be able to read words from the printed page but be unable to recognize the thought that is conveyed.

Electrical stimulation in Wernicke's area of the conscious patient occasionally causes a highly complex thought. This is particularly true when the stimulatory electrode is passed deep enough into the brain to approach the corresponding connecting areas of the thalamus. The types of thoughts that might be experienced include memories of complicated visual scenes that one might remember from childhood, auditory hallucinations such as a specific musical piece, or even a discourse by a specific person. For this reason it is believed that complicated memory patterns involving more than one sensory modality are stored at least partially in this area, or that activation of Wernicke's area can call

forth the memories even if they may be stored elsewhere. This belief is in accord with the importance of Wernicke's area in interpretation of the complicated meanings of different sensory experiences.

The Angular Gyrus—Interpretation of Visual Information. The angular gyrus is the most inferior portion of the posterior parietal lobe, lying immediately behind Wernicke's area and fusing posteriorly into the visual areas of the occipital lobe as well. If this region is destroyed while Wernicke's area in the temporal lobe is still intact, the person can still interpret auditory experiences as usual, but the stream of visual experiences passing into Wernicke's area from the visual cortex is mainly blocked. Therefore, the person may be able to see words and even know they are words but, nevertheless, not be able to interpret their meanings. As mentioned previously, this is the condition called dyslexia, or word blindness.

Let us again emphasize the global importance of Wernicke's area for most intellectual functions of the brain. Loss of this area in an adult usually leads thereafter to a lifetime of almost demented existence.

The Concept of the Dominant Hemisphere

The general interpretative functions of Wernicke's area and of the angular gyrus, and also the functions of the speech and motor control areas, are usually much more highly developed in one cerebral hemisphere than in the other. Therefore, this hemisphere is called the *dominant hemisphere.* In about 95 per cent of all persons the left hemisphere is the dominant one. Wernicke's area of the brain is as much as 50 per cent larger in the left hemisphere than in the right in more than one half of newborn babies. Therefore, it is easy to understand why the left side of the brain might become dominant over the right side. However, if for some reason the dominant Wernicke's area is removed in early childhood, the opposite side of the brain can develop full dominant characteristics.

A theory that can explain the capability of one hemisphere to dominate the other hemisphere is the following:

The attention of the "mind" seems to be directed to one portion of the brain at a time. Presumably, because its size is usually larger at birth, the left temporal lobe normally begins to be used to a greater extent than the right, and, thenceforth, because of the tendency to direct one's attention to the better developed region, the rate of learning in the cerebral hemisphere that gains the first start increases rapidly while that in the opposite side remains slight. Therefore, in the normal human being, one side becomes dominant over the other.

In about 95 per cent of all persons the left temporal lobe and angular gyrus become dominant, and in the remaining 5 per cent of the population either both sides develop simultaneously to have dual dominance, or, more rarely, the right side alone becomes highly developed.

Usually associated with the dominant temporal lobe and angular gyrus is dominance of certain portions of the somatic sensory cortex and motor cortex for control of voluntary motor functions. For instance, as is discussed later in the chapter, the premotor speech area (Broca's area), located far laterally in the intermediate frontal lobe, is almost always dominant also on the left side of the brain. This speech area causes the formation of words by exciting simultaneously the laryngeal muscles, the respiratory muscles, and the muscles of the mouth. The motor areas for controlling the hands are dominant on the left side of the brain in about nine of ten persons, thus causing "right-handedness" in most people.

Though the interpretative areas of the temporal lobe and angular gyrus, as well as many of the motor areas, are highly developed in only a single hemisphere, they are capable of receiving sensory information from both hemispheres and are also capable of controlling motor activities in both hemispheres, utilizing mainly fiber pathways in the *corpus callosum* for communication between the two hemispheres. This unitary cross-feeding organization prevents interference between the functions of the two sides of the brain; such interference, obviously, could create havoc with both thoughts and motor responses.

Role of Language in Function of Wernicke's Area and in Intellectual Functions

A major share of our sensory experience is converted into its language equivalent before being stored in the memory areas of the brain and before being processed for other intellectual purposes. For instance, when we read a book, we do not store the visual images of the printed words but, instead, store the words themselves in language form. Also, the information conveyed by the words is usually converted to language form before its meaning is discerned.

The sensory area of the dominant hemisphere for interpretation of language is Wernicke's area, and this is very closely associated with both the primary hearing area and the auditory association areas of the temporal lobe. This very close relationship probably results from the fact that the first introduction to language is by way of hearing. Later in life, when visual perception of language through the medium of reading develops, the visual information is then presumably channeled into the already developed language regions of the dominant temporal lobe.

Wernicke's Area in the Nondominant Hemisphere. When Wernicke's area in the dominant hemisphere is destroyed, the person normally loses almost all intellec-

tual functions associated with language or verbal symbolism, such as ability to read, ability to perform mathematical operations, and even the ability to think through logical problems. However, many other types of interpretative capabilities, some of which utilize the temporal lobe and angular gyrus regions of the opposite hemisphere, are retained. Psychological studies in patients with damage to their nondominant hemispheres have suggested that this hemisphere may be especially important for understanding and interpreting music, nonverbal visual experiences (especially visual patterns), spatial relationships between the person and the surroundings, and probably also interpreting many somatic experiences related to use of the limbs and hands. Thus, even though we speak of the "dominant" hemisphere, this dominance is primarily for language- or verbal symbolism-related intellectual functions; the opposite hemisphere is actually dominant for some other types of intelligence.

An Area for Recognition of Faces

An interesting type of brain abnormality called *prosopagnosia* is the inability to recognize faces. This occurs in persons who have extensive damage on the medial undersides of both occipital lobes and along the medioventral surfaces of the temporal lobes, as illustrated in Figure 18–6. Loss of these face recognition areas, strangely enough, results in very little other abnormality of brain function.

One wonders why so much of the cerebral cortex should be reserved for the simple task of face recognition. However, when it is remembered that most of our daily tasks involve associations with other people, one can see the importance of this intellectual function.

The occipital portion of this area is contiguous with the primary visual cortex, and the temporal portion is closely associated with the limbic system that has to do with emotions, brain activation, and control of one's behavioral response to the environment, as we shall discuss in Chapter 20.

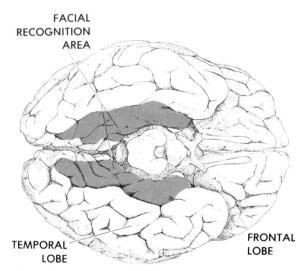

FACIAL RECOGNITION AREA

TEMPORAL LOBE

FRONTAL LOBE

Figure 18–6. Facial recognition areas located on the underside of the brain in the medial occipital and temporal lobes. (From Geschwind: *Sci. Am.*, 241:180, 1979. © 1979 by Scientific American, Inc. All rights reserved.)

THE PREFRONTAL AREAS

The prefrontal areas are those portions of the frontal lobes that lie anterior to the motor regions, as shown in Figure 18–5. For years, this part of the cortex has been considered to be the locus of the higher intellect of the human being, principally because the main difference between the brain of monkeys and that of human beings is the great prominence of the human prefrontal areas. Yet efforts to show that the prefrontal cortex is more important in higher intellectual functions than other portions of the cortex have not been successful. Indeed, destruction of the posterior temporal lobe (Wernicke's area) and the angular gyrus region in the dominant hemisphere causes infinitely more harm to the intellect than does destruction of both prefrontal areas.

Yet, the prefrontal areas do have some specific functions that are all their own. One of these has to do with control of some types of behavior, especially choice of behavioral options for each social or physical situation. For this purpose, the prefrontal areas transmit signals into the limbic areas of the brain, as will be described in Chapter 20. Some of the other possible functions of the prefrontal lobes include:

Prevention of Distractibility—Importance for Sequencing Thoughts. One of the outstanding characteristics of a person who has lost the prefrontal areas is the ease with which he or she can be *distracted* from a sequence of thoughts. Likewise, in lower animals whose prefrontal areas have been removed, the ability to concentrate on psychological tests is almost completely lost. The human being without prefrontal areas is still capable of performing many intellectual tasks, such as answering short questions and performing simple arithmetic computations (such as $9 \times 6 = 54$), thus illustrating that the basic intellectual activities of the cerebral cortex are still intact without the prefrontal areas. Yet if concerted *sequences* of cerebral functions are required of the person, he becomes completely disorganized. Therefore, the prefrontal areas seem to be important in keeping the mental functions directed toward goals.

Elaboration of Thought, Prognostication, and Performance of Higher Intellectual Functions by the Prefrontal Areas. Another function that has been ascribed to the prefrontal areas by psychologists and neurologists is *elaboration of thought*. This means simply an increase in depth and abstractness of the different thoughts. Psychological tests have shown that prefrontal lobectomized lower animals presented with successive bits of sensory information fail to store these bits even in temporary memory—probably because they are distracted so easily that they cannot hold thoughts long enough for storage to take place. This ability of the prefrontal areas to cause storage—even though it be temporary—of many bits of information simultaneously, and then to cause recall of this information bit by bit as it is needed for subsequent thoughts, could well explain the many functions of the brain that we associate with higher intelligence, such as the abilities to (1) prognosticate, (2) plan for the future, (3) delay action in response to incoming sensory signals so that the sensory information can be weighed until the best course of response is decided, (4) consider the consequences of motor actions even before these are performed, (5) solve complicated mathematical, legal, or philosophical problems, (6) correlate all avenues of information in diagnosing rare diseases, and (7) control one's activities in accord with moral laws.

Effects of Destruction of the Prefrontal Areas

Human beings without prefrontal areas ordinarily act precipitously in response to incoming sensory signals, such as reacting angrily to slight provocations but also forgetting the event equally as rapidly. In addition, they are likely to lose many or most of their morals; they have little embarrassment in relation to excretory, sexual, and social activities; and they are prone to quickly changing moods of sweetness, hate, joy, sadness, exhilaration, and rage. And they lose both ambition and drive toward goals. In short, they are highly *distractible* persons with lack of ability to pursue long and complicated thoughts.

THOUGHTS, CONSCIOUSNESS, AND MEMORY

Our most difficult problem in discussing consciousness, thoughts, memory, and learning is that we do not know the neural mechanism of a thought. We know that destruction of large portions of the cerebral cortex does not prevent a person from having thoughts, but it usually does reduce the *degree* of awareness of the surroundings.

Each thought almost certainly involves simultaneous signals in many portions of the cerebral cortex, thalamus, limbic system, and reticular formation of the brain stem. Some crude thoughts probably depend almost entirely on lower centers; the thought of pain is probably a good example, for electrical stimulation of the human cortex rarely elicits anything more than the mildest degrees of pain, whereas stimulation of certain areas of the hypothalamus and mesencephalon in animals appears to cause excruciating pain. On the other hand, a type of thought pattern that requires mainly the cerebral cortex is that involving vision, because loss of the visual cortex causes complete inability to perceive visual form or color.

Therefore, we might formulate a definition of a thought in terms of neural activity as follows: a thought probably results from the momentary "pattern" of stimulation of many different parts of the nervous system at the same time, probably involving most importantly the cerebral cortex, the thalamus, the limbic system, and the upper reticular formation of the brain stem. This is called the *holistic theory* of thoughts. The stimulated areas of the limbic system, thalamus, and reticular formation perhaps determine the general nature of the thought, giving it such qualities as pleasure, displeasure, pain, comfort, crude modalities of sensation, localization to gross areas of the body, and other general characteristics. On the other hand, the stimulated areas of the cerebral cortex probably determine the discrete characteristics of the thought such as specific localization of sensations on the body and of objects in the fields of vision, discrete patterns of sensation such as the rectangular pattern of a concrete block wall or the texture of a rug, and other individual characteristics that enter into the overall awareness of a particular instant.

And consciousness can perhaps be described as our continuing stream of awareness of either our surroundings or our sequential thoughts.

MEMORY AND TYPES OF MEMORY

If we accept the above approximation of what constitutes a thought, we can see immediately that the mechanism of memory must be equally as complex as the mechanism of a thought, for, to provide memory, the nervous system must recreate the same spatial and temporal pattern (the "holistic" pattern) of stimulation in the central nervous system at some future date. Though we cannot explain in detail what a memory is, we do know some of the basic psychological and neuronal processes that probably lead to the process of memory.

All of us know that all degrees of memory occur, some memories lasting a few seconds and others lasting hours, days, months, or years. Possibly all these types of memory are caused by the same mechanism operating to different degrees of fulfillment. Yet, it is also possible that different mechanisms of memory do exist. Indeed, most physiologists classify memory into from two to four different types. For the purpose of the present discussion, we will use the following classification: 1. *Sensory memory*; 2. *Primary memory*; 3. *Secondary memory*.

The basic characteristics of these types of memory are the following:

Sensory Memory. Sensory memory means the ability to retain sensory signals in the sensory areas of the brain for a very short interval of time following the actual sensory experience. Usually these signals remain available for analysis for several hundred milliseconds but are replaced by new sensory signals in less than one second. Nevertheless, during the short interval of time that the instantaneous sensory information remains in the brain it can continue to be used for further processing; most important, it can be "scanned" to pick out the important points. Thus, this is the initial stage of the memory process.

Primary Memory. Primary memory is the memory of facts, words, numbers, letters, or other information for a few seconds to a few minutes at a time. This is typified by a person's memory of the digits in a telephone number for a short period of time after he has looked up the number in the telephone directory. It is also typified by the ability of a person to look at a visual scene, then to turn the head away and still be able to recall for seconds or a minute or more many features of the scene.

One of the most important characteristics of primary memory is that the information in this memory store is instantaneously available so that the person does not have to search through his or her mind for it as one does for information that has been put away in the secondary memory stores. However, still another feature of primary memory is that when new bits of information are put into the primary store, old information is displaced. Thus, if a person looks up a second telephone number, the first is usually lost. Also, if one sees a rapid succession of visual scenes, it is usually the last of these that remains most prominently in the primary memory store.

Secondary Memory. Secondary memory is the storage in the brain of information that can be recalled at some later time—hours, days, months, or years later. This type of memory has been called *long-term memory*, *fixed memory*, *permanent memory*, and several other names. One of its characteristics is that, except when the memory is very deeply engrained, one must "search" through the memory stores for seconds to minutes before it is possible to recall the memory.

"Short-term" and "Long-term" Memory. Memory is also frequently divided into either "short-term" or "long-term." However, use of these terms is extremely loose. Psychologists frequently classify short-term memory to be the same as primary memory and long-term memory the same as secondary memory. However, many physiologists and clinicians include in short-term memory the early stages of secondary memory lasting for as long as several days to a week or more, and reserve the term long-term memory for memories that can be recalled weeks, months, or years after the initial experience.

PHYSIOLOGICAL BASIS OF MEMORY

Despite the many advances in neurophysiology during the past half century, we still cannot explain what is perhaps the most important function of the brain: its capability for memory. Yet, physiological experiments are beginning to generate conceptual theories of the means by which memory could occur. Some of these are discussed in the following few sections.

Possible Mechanisms for Primary Memory. Primary memory requires a neuronal mechanism that can hold specific information signals for a few seconds to at most a minute or more. Several such mechanisms are the following:

Reverberating Circuit Theory of Primary Memory. When an appropriate tetanizing electrical stimulus is applied directly to the surface of the cerebral cortex and then is removed after a second or more, the local area excited by this stimulus often continues to emit rhythmic action potentials for short periods of time. This effect is believed to result from local reverberating circuits, the signals passing through a multistage circuit of neurons in the local area of the cortex itself or perhaps even back and forth between the cortex and the thalamus or other subcortical areas.

It is postulated that sensory signals reaching the cerebral cortex can set up similar reverberating oscillations and that these could be the basis for primary memory. Then, as the reverberating circuit fatigues, or as new signals interfere with the reverberations, the primary memory fades away.

One of the principal observations in support of this theory is that any factor that suddenly blocks brain function, such as a blow on the head that causes temporary coma or such as anesthesia, erases the primary memory. The memory cannot be recalled when the disturbance is over unless a portion of this memory had already been placed into the secondary memory store, as will be discussed in subsequent sections.

Post-Tetanic Potentiation Theory of Primary Memory. In most parts of the nervous system, including even the anterior motor neurons of the spinal cord, tetanic stimulation of a synapse for a few seconds causes a short period of synaptic fatigue for the next few seconds but then increased excitability of the synapse for another few seconds to a few hours. If during this time of increased excitability the synapse is stimulated again, the neuron responds much more vigorously than normally, a phenomenon called *post-tetanic potentiation.* This is obviously a type of memory that depends on change in the excitability of the synapse, and it could be the basis for primary memory. Recent experiments have shown that post-tetanic potentiation is caused by excessive accumulation of calcium ions in the presynaptic terminals, these ions in turn increasing the release of transmitter substance by the terminals, as was explained in Chapter 10.

Presynaptic Facilitation and Inhibition as Possible Causes of Primary Memory. Many presynaptic terminals of the central nervous system lie on the surfaces of other presynaptic terminals or even on terminal nerve fibrils. When such terminals are stimulated, they can cause either inhibition or facilitation of the secondary terminals depending on the type of transmitter released. Furthermore, this inhibition or facilitation can last at times for many minutes and perhaps even for an hour or more. Such events are a type of memory, though it still is not known whether this is one of the mechanisms of primary memory.

Mechanism of Secondary Memory— Enhancement of Synaptic Transmission Facility

Secondary memory is the ability of the nervous system to recall thoughts long after initial elicitation of the thoughts is over. We know that secondary memory does not depend on continued activity of the nervous system, because the brain can be totally inactivated by cooling, by general anesthesia, by hypoxia, by ischemia, or by any other method and yet secondary memories that have been previously stored are still retained when the brain becomes active once again. Therefore, secondary memory must result from some actual alterations of the synapses, either physical or chemical.

Many different theories have been offered to explain the synaptic changes that cause long-term memory. Among the most important of these are:

1. Anatomical Changes in the Synapses. Cajal, almost a century ago, discovered that the number of terminal fibrils ending on neuronal cells and dendrites in the cerebral cortex increases with age. Conversely, physiologists have shown that inactivity of regions of the cortex causes thinning of the cortex: for instance, thinning of the primary visual cortex in animals that have lost their eyesight. Also, intense activity of a particular part of the cortex can cause excessive thickening of the cortical shell in that area alone. This has been demonstrated especially in the visual cortex of animals subjected to repeated visual experiences. Finally, some neuroanatomists have observed electron micrographic changes in presynaptic terminals that have been subjected to intense and prolonged activity.

All these observations have led to a widely held belief that fixation of memories in the brain results from anatomical changes in the synapses themselves: perhaps changes in numbers of presynaptic terminals, perhaps in sizes of the terminals, or perhaps in the sizes and conductivities of the dendrites. Such anatomical changes could cause permanent or semipermanent increase in the degree of facilitation of specific neuronal circuits, thus allowing signals to pass through the circuits with more ease the more often the memory trace is used. This obviously would explain the tendency for memories to become more and more deeply fixed in the nervous system the more often they are recalled or the more often the person repeats the sensory experience that leads to the memory trace.

Another variant of the anatomical theory is based on the experimental observation that in early life an excess of synaptic connections is made, and those synapses that are active continue to remain functional whereas the others eventually degenerate. Thus, the pattern of synaptic transmission could be established by destroying unused synapses rather than by enhancing the used ones. This theory fits the finding that unused synapses and even unused neurons often disappear completely.

2. Physical or Chemical Changes in the Presynaptic Terminal or the Postsynaptic Membrane. Recent studies by Kandel and others in the large snail *Aplysia* have uncovered several mechanisms of memory that result from either physical or chemical changes in the presynaptic terminal or possibly even in the entire presynaptic neuron. One such

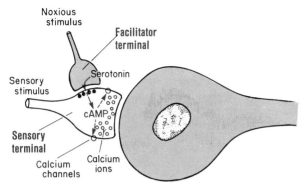

Figure 18–7. A memory system that has been discovered in the snail *Aplysia.*

mechanism, illustrated in Figure 18–7, functions in the following way. In this figure there are two separate presynaptic terminals, one of which is from a primary input sensory neuron and terminates on the surface of a secondary neuron that is to be stimulated; this is called the *sensory terminal.* The other presynaptic terminal lies on the surface of the sensory terminal and is called the *facilitator terminal.* When the sensory terminal is stimulated repeatedly but without stimulating the facilitator terminal, signal transmission at first is very great, but this becomes less and less intense with repeated stimulation until transmission almost ceases. This phenomenon is called *habituation.* It is a type of memory that causes the neuronal circuit to lose its response to repeated events that are insignificant.

On the other hand, if a noxious stimulus excites the facilitator terminal at the same time that the sensory terminal is stimulated, then, instead of the transmitted signal becoming progressively weaker, the ease of transmission becomes much stronger and will remain strong for hours, days, or perhaps weeks even without further stimulation of the facilitator terminal. Thus, the noxious stimulus causes the memory pathway to become facilitated for days or weeks thereafter. It is especially interesting that only a few repeated action potentials are required to cause either habituation or facilitation. However, once habituation has occurred, the synapses can become facilitated very rapidly with only a few noxious stimuli.

At the molecular level, the habituation effect in the sensory terminal results from progressive closure of calcium channels of the terminal membrane, though the cause of this is not fully known. As a result, much smaller than normal amounts of calcium diffuse into this terminal when action potentials occur, and much less transmitter is therefore released because calcium entry is the stimulus for transmitter release (as was discussed in Chapter 10).

In the case of facilitation, the molecular mechanism is believed to be the following:

1. Stimulation of the facilitator neuron at the same time that the sensory neuron is stimulated causes serotonin release at the facilitator synapse on the sensory presynaptic terminal.

2. The serotonin acts on *serotonin receptors* in the sensory terminal membrane, and these activate the enzyme *adenylate cyclase* inside the membrane. This causes the formation of *cyclic AMP* inside the sensory presynaptic terminal.

3. The cyclic AMP activates a *protein kinase* that is believed to cause phosphorylation of the channel surfaces of the potassium channels in the sensory terminal membrane. This blocks these channels for potassium conductance. This blockage of the potassium channels can last for days and maybe even weeks or longer.

4. Lack of potassium conductance causes a greatly prolonged action potential in the presynaptic terminal because the flow of potassium ions out of the terminal is the usual mechanism for recovery from the action potential.

5. The prolonged action potential causes prolonged activation of the calcium pores, allowing tremendous quantities of calcium ions to enter the sensory terminal. These calcium ions then cause greatly increased transmitter release, thereby greatly facilitating synaptic transmission.

Thus, in a very indirect way the associative effect of stimulating the facilitator neuron at the same time that the sensory neuron is stimulated causes a prolonged change in the sensory terminal that produces a long-term memory trace.

Recent studies by Byrne in the snail *Aplysia* have suggested still another mechanism of cellular memory; his studies have shown that stimuli from two separate sources acting on a single sensory neuron can, under appropriate conditions, cause long-term changes in the membrane properties of the entire sensory neuron, and these changes can increase the excitability of the neuron for many minutes thereafter. Thus, this is another possible mechanism of memory, either primary memory or secondary memory.

Summary. The theory that at present seems most likely for explaining secondary memory is that some actual anatomical, physical, or chemical change occurs in the presynaptic terminals or perhaps in whole neurons that permanently facilitates the transmission of impulses at the synapses. If all the synapses are thus facilitated in a thought circuit, this circuit can be re-excited by any one of many diverse signals at later dates, thereby causing memory. The overall facilitated circuit is called a *memory engram* or a *memory trace.*

Consolidation of Memory

For a primary memory to be converted into a secondary memory that can be recalled days later, it must become "consolidated"—that is, the synapses must become permanently facilitated. This process requires 5 to 10 minutes for minimal consolidation and an hour or more for maximal consolidation. For instance, if a strong sensory impression is made on the brain but is then followed within a minute or so by an electrically induced brain convulsion, the sensory experience will not be remembered at all. Likewise, brain concussion, sudden application of deep general anesthesia, and other effects that temporarily block the dynamic function of the brain can prevent consolidation.

However, if the same sensory stimulus is impressed on the brain and the strong electrical shock is delayed for more than 5 to 10 minutes, at least part of the memory trace will have become established. If the shock is delayed for an hour, the memory will have become fully consolidated.

The process of consolidation and the time required for consolidation can probably be explained by the phenomenon of *rehearsal* of the primary memory as follows:

Role of Rehearsal in Transference of Primary Memory into Secondary Memory. Psychological studies have shown that rehearsal of the same information again and again accelerates and potentiates the degree of transfer of primary memory into secondary memory, and therefore also accelerates and potentiates the process of consolidation. The brain has a natural tendency to rehearse newfound information, and especially to rehearse newfound information that catches the mind's attention. Therefore, over a period of time the important features of sensory experiences become progressively more and more fixed in the secondary memory stores. This explains why a person can remember large amounts of information studied in depth far better than small amounts of information studied only superficially. And it also explains why a person who is wide-awake will consolidate memories far better than will a person who is in a state of mental fatigue.

Codifying of Memories During the Process of Consolidation. One of the most important features of the process of consolidation is that memories to be placed permanently into the secondary memory storehouse are first codified into different classes of information. During this process similar information is recalled from the secondary storage bins and is used to help process the new information. The new and old are compared for similarities and for differences, and part of the storage process is to store the information about these similarities and differences rather than simply to store the information unprocessed. Thus, during the process of consolidation, the new memories are not stored randomly in the brain but instead are stored in direct association with other memories of the same type. This is obviously necessary if one is to be able to "search" the memory store at a later date to find the required information.

Role of Specific Parts of the Brain in the Memory Process

Role of the Hippocampus for Rehearsal, Codification, and Consolidation of Memories—Anterograde Amnesia Following Hippocampal Lesions.

The hippocampus is the most medial portion of the temporal lobe cortex where it folds underneath the brain and then upward into the lower surface of the lateral ventricle. The two hippocampi have been removed for the treatment of epilepsy in a number of patients. This procedure hardly affects the person's memory for information stored in the brain prior to removal of the hippocampi. However, after removal, these persons have very little capability for transferring *verbal and symbolic types* of primary memories into secondary memories. That is, they do not have the ability to separate out the important information; to codify it, to rehearse it, and to consolidate it in the long-term memory store. Therefore, these persons are unable to establish new long-term memories of those types of information that are the basis of intelligence. This is called *anterograde amnesia.*

Lesions in other parts of the temporal lobes besides the hippocampi are also frequently associated with reduced ability to store new memories. This probably results from two factors: (1) the possible association of the other parts of the temporal lobes with the hippocampi and therefore failure of the usual consolidation process for memories, and (2) the fact that Wernicke's area, which is the major locus of intellectual operations of the brain, is located in the temporal lobe; the reason that lesions affecting Wernicke's area might diminish memory storage is probably that consolidation of memories requires analysis of the memory so that it can be stored in association with other memories of like kind.

Retrograde Amnesia. *Retrograde amnesia* means inability to recall memories from the past—that is, from the long-term memory storage bins—even though the memories are known to be still there. When retrograde amnesia occurs, the degree of amnesia for recent events is likely to be much greater than for events of the distant past. The reason for this difference is probably that the distant memories have been rehearsed so many times that elements of these memories are stored in widespread areas of the brain.

In some persons who have hippocampal lesions, some degree of retrograde amnesia usually occurs along with the anterograde amnesia just discussed, which suggests that these two types of amnesia are at least partially related and that hippocampal lesions can cause both. However, it has also been claimed that damage in some thalamic areas can lead specifically to retrograde amnesia without causing significant anterograde amnesia. This perhaps can be explained by the possibility that the thalamus might normally play a role in helping the person "search" the memory storehouses and thus be able to "read out" the memories. That is, the memory process not only requires the storing of memories but also the ability to search and find the memory at a later date. The possible function of the thalamus in this process will be discussed in the following chapter.

It should be noted, however, that persons with either temporal lobe or hippocampal lesions usually do not have difficulty in learning physical skills that do not involve verbalization or symbolic types of intelligence. For instance, these persons can still learn hand skills such as those required in carpentry.

ANALYTICAL OPERATIONS OF THE BRAIN

Thus far, we have considered the approximate nature of thoughts and possible mechanisms by which memory and learning can occur. Now we need to consider the mechanisms by which the brain performs complex intellectual operations, such as the analysis of sensory information and the establishment of abstract thoughts. About these mechanisms we know almost nothing, but experiments along these lines have established the following important facts: First, the brain can focus its attention on specific types of information (which will be discussed in the following chapter). Second, separate qualities of each set of information signals are split away from the central signal and are transmitted to multiple areas of the brain. Third, the brain compares new information with old information in its memory loci. And, fourth, the brain determines patterns of stimulation.

Analysis of Information by Splitting Its Qualities. When sensory information enters the nervous system, one of the first steps in its analysis is to transmit the signal to separate parts of the brain that are selectively adapted for detecting specific qualities. For instance, if the hand is placed on a hot stove, (1) pain information is sent through the spinoreticular and spinothalamic tracts into the reticular formation of the brain stem and into certain thalamic and hypothalamic nuclei, (2) tactile information is sent through the dorsal column system to the somatic sensory cortex, giving the cortex a detailed description of the part of the hand that is touching the hot stove, and (3) position sense information from the muscles and joints is sent to the cerebellum, the reticular formation, and to higher centers of the brain to give momentary information on the position of the hand. Thus, the different qualities of the overall information are dissected and transmitted to different parts of the brain. On the basis of analyses in all these parts of the brain, motor responses to the incoming sensory information are formulated.

One can see that different centers of the brain react to specific qualities of information—the reticular formation and certain regions of the thalamus and hypothalamus to pain, regions of the mesencephalon and hypothalamus to the affective nature of the sensation (that is, whether it is pleasant or unpleasant), the somatic sensory cortex to the localization of sensation, other areas to kinesthetic activities, and others to visual, auditory, gustatory, olfactory, and vestibular information.

Analysis of New Information by Comparison with Memories. We all know that new sensory experiences are immediately compared with previous experiences of the same or similar types. For instance, this is the way we recognize a person whom we know. Yet, it still remains a mystery how we can make these comparisons. One theory suggests that if the new pattern of stimulation matches a memory engram, some interaction between the two gives the person a sense of recognition.

Analysis of Patterns. In analyzing information, the brain depends to a great extent on "patterns" of stimulation. For instance, a square is detected as a square regardless of its position or angle of rotation in the visual field. Likewise, a series of parallel bars is detected as parallel bars regardless of their orientation, or a fly is detected as a fly whether it is seen in the peripheral or central field of vision. We can extend the same logic to the somatic sensory areas, for a person can detect a cube simply by feeling, whether it be in an upright, horizontal, or angulated position. Also, it can be detected even by one's feet even though one's feet may have never felt a cube before.

Processing of Information so That Patterns Can Be Determined. Beautiful examples of the ability of the brain to process information for determination of patterns have been discovered in relation to the visual system. In Chapter 24 we shall point out that the retina itself processes visual information to a great extent even before it is transmitted into the brain. For instance, the neuronal circuits in the retina are organized to detect lines or boundaries between light and dark areas. That is, the visual neural mechanisms bring out strongly the contrast boundaries of the scene but de-emphasize the flat areas. This explains why a few lines drawn on a paper can give one the impression of seeing the image of a person. Certainly the lines do not represent the actual picture of the person, but they do give the visual cortex the same pattern of contrasts that one's own visual system would give.

One can see, therefore, that the visual cortex utilizes transformed types of information to point up the most striking characteristics of the visual scene while neglecting unimportant information. Then, the patterns of the visual scene can be extracted from this "preselected" information.

FUNCTION OF THE BRAIN IN COMMUNICATION

One of the most important differences between the human being and lower animals is the facility with which human beings can communicate with one another. Furthermore, because neurological tests can easily assess the ability of a person to communicate with others, we know perhaps more about the sensory and motor systems related to communication than about any other segment of cortical function. Therefore, we will review rapidly the function of the cortex in communication, and from this one can see immediately how the principles of sensory analysis and motor control apply to this art.

There are two aspects to communication: first, the *sensory aspect*, involving the ears and eyes, and, second, the *motor aspect*, involving vocalization and its control.

Sensory Aspects of Communication. We noted earlier in the chapter that destruction of portions of the *auditory* and *visual association areas* of the cortex can result in inability to understand the spoken word or the written word. These effects are called, respectively, *auditory receptive aphasia* and *visual receptive aphasia* or, more commonly, *word deafness* and *word blindness* (also called *dyslexia*).

Wernicke's Aphasia (Sensory Aphasia). Some persons are perfectly capable of understanding either the spoken word or the written word but are *unable to interpret the thought* that is expressed. This results most frequently when *Wernicke's area* in the *posterior portion of the dominant hemisphere superior temporal gyrus* is damaged or destroyed. Therefore, this type of aphasia is generally called *Wernicke's aphasia*: also, it is frequently called simply "sensory aphasia."

When the lesion in Wernicke's area is widespread and extends (1) backward into the angular gyrus region, (2) inferiorly into the lower areas of the temporal lobe, and (3) superiorly into the superior border of the sylvian fissure, the person is likely to be almost totally demented and therefore is said to have *global aphasia*.

Motor Aspects of Communication. The process of speech involves two principal stages of mentation: (1) formation in the mind of thoughts to be expressed and choice of words to be used, then (2) motor control of vocalization and the actual act of vocalization itself. The formation of thoughts and choice of words is the function of the sensory areas of the brain. Again, it is Wernicke's area in the posterior part of the superior temporal gyrus that is most important for this ability. Therefore, persons with either Wernicke's aphasia or global aphasia are unable to formulate the thoughts that are to be communicated. Or, if the lesion is less severe, the person may be able to formulate thoughts but yet be unable to put together the appropriate words to express the thought. Often, a person may be very fluent in words but the words may present a jumbled mass of confusion.

Motor Aphasia. Often a person is perfectly capable of deciding what he wishes to say, and he is capable of vocalizing, but he simply cannot make his vocal system emit words instead of noises. This effect, called *motor aphasia*, results from damage to *Broca's speech area*, which lies in the *premotor* facial region of the cortex—about 95 per cent of the time in the left hemisphere, as illustrated in Figures 18–5 and 18–8. Therefore, we assume that the *skilled motor patterns* for control of the larynx, lips, mouth, respiratory system, and other accessory muscles of articulation are all controlled in this area.

Articulation. Finally, we have the act of articulation itself, which means the muscular movements of the mouth, tongue, larynx, and so forth, that are responsible for the actual emission of sound. The *facial and laryngeal regions of the motor cortex* activate these muscles, and the *cerebellum, basal ganglia,* and *sensory cortex* all help control the muscle contractions by feedback mechanisms described in Chapter 17. Destruction of these regions can cause either total or partial inability to speak distinctly.

Summary. Figure 18–8 illustrates two principal pathways for communication. The upper half of the figure shows the pathway involved in hearing and speaking a word. This sequence is the following: (1) reception in the primary auditory area of the sound signals that encode the word; (2) interpretation of the word in Wernicke's area; (3) determination also in Wernicke's area that the word is to be spoken; (4) transmission of signals from Wernicke's area to Broca's area via the *arcuate fasciculus*; (5) activation of the skilled motor programs in Broca's area for control of word formation; and (6) transmission of appropriate signals into the motor cortex to control the speech muscles.

The lower figure illustrates the comparable steps in reading a word and then speaking it. The initial receptive area for the word is in the primary visual area rather than in the primary auditory area. Then the word information passes through early stages of interpretation in the *angular gyrus region* and finally reaches its full level of recognition in Wernicke's area. From here, the sequence is the same as for speaking a heard word.

FUNCTION OF THE CORPUS CALLOSUM AND ANTERIOR COMMISSURE TO TRANSFER THOUGHTS, MEMORIES, AND OTHER INFORMATION TO THE OPPOSITE HEMISPHERE

Fibers in the *corpus callosum* connect the respective cortical areas of the two hemispheres with each other except for the anterior portions of the temporal lobes; these temporal areas, including especially the *amygdala*, are interconnected by fibers that pass through the *anterior commissure*. Because of the tremendous number of fibers in the corpus callosum, it was assumed from the beginning that this massive structure must have some important function to correlate activities of the two cerebral hemispheres. However, after cutting the corpus callosum in experimental animals, it was difficult to discern changes in brain function. Therefore, for a long time the function of the corpus callosum was a mystery.

Yet, properly designed psychological experiments have now demonstrated the extremely important functions of the corpus callosum and anterior commissure. These can be explained best by recounting one of the experiments. A monkey is first prepared by cutting the corpus callosum and splitting the optic chiasm longitudinally. Then it is taught to recognize different types of objects with its right eye while its left eye is covered. Next, the right eye is covered and the monkey is tested to determine whether or not its left eye can recognize the same object. The answer to this is that the left eye *cannot* recognize the object. Yet, on repeating the same experiment in another monkey with the optic chiasm split but the corpus callosum intact, it is found invariably that recognition in one hemisphere of the brain creates recognition also in the opposite hemisphere.

Thus, one of the functions of the corpus callosum and the anterior commissure is to make information stored in the cortex of one hemisphere available to the corresponding cortical area of the opposite hemisphere. Three important examples of such cooperation between the two hemispheres are:

1. Cutting of the corpus callosum blocks transfer of information from Wernicke's area of the dominant hemisphere to the motor cortex on the opposite side of the brain. Therefore, the intellectual functions of the brain, located primarily in the dominant hemisphere, lose their control over the right motor cortex and therefore also of the voluntary motor functions of the left hand and arm even though the usual subconscious movements of the left hand and arm are completely normal.

2. Cutting of the corpus callosum prevents transfer of somatic and visual information from the right hemisphere into Wernicke's area of the dominant hemisphere. Therefore, somatic and visual information from the left side of the body frequently fails to reach this general interpretative area of the brain and, therefore, cannot be used for decision making.

3. Finally, a teen-aged boy whose corpus callosum had been completely sectioned but whose anterior commissure was not sectioned recently was found to have two entirely separate conscious portions to his brain. Only the left half of his brain could understand the spoken word, because it was the dominant hemisphere. On the other hand, the right side of the brain could understand the written word and could elicit a motor response to it

SPEAKING A HEARD WORD

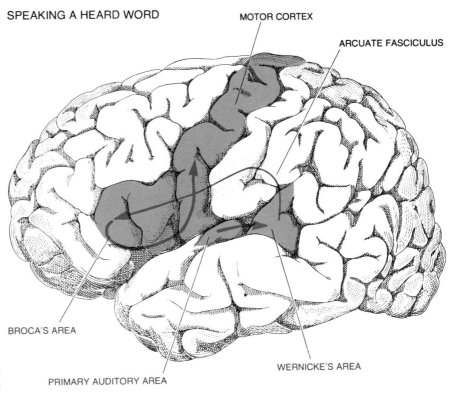

SPEAKING A WRITTEN WORD

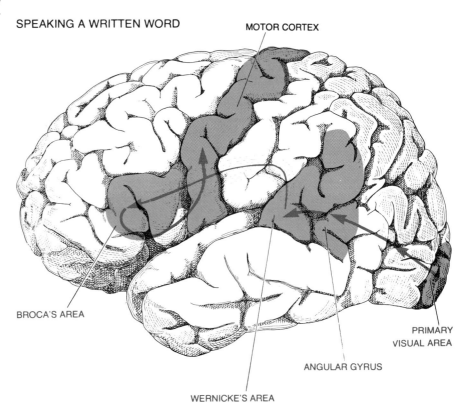

Figure 18–8. Brain pathways for (*top*) perception of the heard word and then speaking the same word, and (*bottom*) perception of the written word and then speaking the same word. (From Geschwind: *Sci. Am.,* *241*:180, 1979 © 1979 by Scientific American, Inc. All rights reserved.)

without the left side of the brain ever knowing why the response was performed. Yet, the effect was somewhat different when an emotional response was evoked in the right side of the brain: in this case a subconscious emotional response occurred in the left side of the brain as well. This undoubtedly occurred because the temporal lobe areas and other basal brain areas of the two sides of the brain were still communicating with each other through the anterior commissure that was not sectioned. For instance, when the command "kiss" was written for the right half of his brain to see, the boy immediately and with full emotion, said "No way!" This response obviously required function of Wernicke's area and the motor areas for speech in the left hemisphere. But, when questioned why he said this, the boy could not explain. Thus, the two halves of the brain have independent capabilities for consciousness, memory storage, communication, and control of motor activities. The corpus callosum is required for the two sides to operate cooperatively, and the anterior commissure plays an important role in unifying the emotional responses of the two brain sides.

REFERENCES

Bannister, R. (rev.): Brain's Clinical Neurology. New York, Oxford University Press, 1978.

Bekhtereva, N. P.: The Neurophysiological Aspects of Human Mental Activity. New York, Oxford University Press, 1978.

Benson, D. F.: Aphasia, Alexia, and Agraphia. New York, Churchill Livingstone, 1979.

Bindman, L.: The Neurophysiology of the Cerebral Cortex. Austin, University of Texas Press, 1981.

Buchtel, H. A.: The Conceptual Nervous System. New York, Pergamon Press, 1982.

Buser, P.: Higher functions of the nervous system. *Annu. Rev. Physiol., 38*:217, 1978.

Damasio, A. R., and Geschwind, N.: The neural basis of language. *Annu. Rev. Neurosci., 7*:127, 1984.

Daniloff, R., *et al.*: The Physiological Bases of Verbal Communication. Englewood Cliffs, N.J., Prentice-Hall, 1980.

De Silva, F. H. L., and Arnolds, D.E.A.T.: Physiology of the hippocampus and related structures. *Annu. Rev. Physiol., 40*:185, 1978.

Dimond, S. J.: Neuropsychology: A Textbook of Systems and Psychological Functions of the Human Brain. Boston, Butterworths, 1979.

Edelman, G. M., and Mountcastle, V. B.: The Mindful Brain: Cortical Organization and the Group-Selective Theory of Higher Brain Function. Cambridge, Mass., MIT Press, 1978.

Geschwind, N.: Specializations of the human brain. *Sci. Am., 241*(3):180, 1979.

Hixon, T. J., *et al.* (eds.): Introduction to Communicative Disorders. Englewood Cliffs, N.J., Prentice-Hall, 1980.

Hubel, D. H.: The brain. *Sci. Am., 241*(3):44, 1979.

Hyvarinen, J.: Posterior parietal lobe of the primate brain. *Physiol. Rev., 62*:1060, 1982.

Kandel, E. R.: Neuronal plasticity and the modification of behavior. *In* Brookhart, J. M., and Mountcastle, V. B. (eds.): Handbook of Physiology. Sec. 1, Vol. I, Baltimore. Williams & Wilkins, 1977, p. 1137.

Kandel, E. R.: A Cell-Biological Approach to Learning. Bethesda, Md., Society for Neuroscience, 1978.

Klopf, A. H.: The Hedonistic Neuron. A Theory of Memory, Learning, and Intelligence. Washington, D.C., Hemisphere Publishers, 1982.

Laduron, P. M.: Presynaptic heteroreceptors in regulation of neuronal transmission. *Biochem. Pharmacol., 34*:467, 1985.

McCloskey, D. I.: Corollary discharges: Motor commands and perception. *In* Brooks, V. B. (ed.): Handbook of Physiology. Sec. 1, Vol. II. Bethesda, American Physiological Society, 1981, p. 1415.

McNeil, M. R. (ed.): The Dysarthrias. Physiology, Acoustics, and Perception Management. San Diego, College-Hill Press, 1984.

Mitzdorf, U.: Current source-density method and application in cat cerebral cortex: Investigation of evoked potentials and EEG phenomena. *Physiol. Rev., 65*:37, 1985.

Moskowitz, B. A.: The acquisition of language. *Sci. Am., 239*(5):92, 1978.

Quinn, W. G., and Greenspan, R. J.: Learning and courtship in Drosophila: Two stories with mutants. *Annu. Rev. Neurosci., 7*:67, 1984.

Rosenbek, J. C. (ed.): Apraxia of Speech. Physiology, Acoustics, Linguistics, Management. San Diego, College-Hill Press, 1984.

Sperry, R. W.: Changing concepts of consciousness and free will. *Perspect. Biol. Med., 20*:9, 1976.

Thompson, R. F., *et al.*: Cellular processes of learning and memory in the mammalian CNS. *Annu. Rev. Neurosci., 6*:447, 1983.

Trevarthen, C.: Hemispheric specialization. *In* Darian-Smith, I. (ed.): Handbook of Physiology. Sec. 1, Vol. III. Bethesda, American Physiological Society, 1984, p. 1129.

Truman, J. W.: Cell death in invertebrate nervous systems. *Annu. Rev. Neurosci., 7*:171, 1984.

Uttal, W. R.: The Physiology of Mind. New York, Halsted Press, 1978.

Vellutino, F. R.: Dyslexia: Theory and Research. Cambridge, Mass., MIT Press, 1979.

Walters, E. T., and Byrne, J. H.: Associative conditioning of single sensory neurons suggests a cellular mechanism for learning. Science, *219*:405, 1983.

Wong, R. K., *et al.*: Local circuit interactions in synchronization of cortical neurones. *J. Exp. Biol., 112*:169, 1984.

19

Activation of the Brain— the Reticular Activating System and Wakefulness; Attention and Searching of Memory; Brain Waves; Sleep; Epilepsy

One of the remaining great mysteries of the brain is how the brain itself controls itself. For instance, what sets the overall level of activity? Also, why do we go to sleep or wake up? And perhaps even more mysterious is the mechanism by which we can focus our attention on certain functions of the brain while ignoring others.

Though the answers to these questions are mainly unknown, glimmers of information are beginning to appear that will at least let us construct plausible, even though questionable, theories about activation of the brain, wakefulness, sleep, and so forth.

THE RETICULAR ACTIVATING SYSTEM AND ITS ROLE IN WAKEFULNESS

Diffuse electrical stimulation in the *mesencephalic and pontile portions of the reticular formation*—an area discussed in Chapter 16 in relation to the motor functions of the nervous system—causes immediate and marked activation of the cerebral cortex and will even cause a sleeping animal to awaken instantaneously. This area is represented in Figure 19–1 by the bold arrow directed upward through the brain stem. Extending upward into the cerebrum from the mesencephalic reticular formation are multiple diffuse pathways that terminate in almost all areas of both the diencephalon and the cerebrum. This entire system is called the *reticular activating system*.

When the reticular activating system was first discovered almost 40 years ago, it was believed that this entire system was represented by a diffuse matrix of neurons that operated mainly as a single unit to provide generalized and uniform activation

of all regions of the diencephalon and cerebrum at the same time. We now know, however, that certain regions of the reticular formation as well as portions of the upward radiating distribution system have discrete anatomical organizations, discrete distribution pathways, and different effects on different parts of the brain—at some times causing increased activity and at other times decreased activity—and even utilize different transmitter substances to perform these different functions. We shall discuss these more specific systems later, but for now let us address the more general functions.

Two Different Pathways into the Cerebrum from the Reticular Formation. Signals are transmitted from the mesencephalic portion of the reticular activating system to the cortex mainly through two different general pathways. One pathway passes upward to the intralaminar, midline, and reticular nuclei of the thalamus and thence through relay pathways to essentially all parts of the cerebral cortex and basal ganglia.

The second pathway, probably a less important pathway, passes through the subthalamus, hypothalamus, and adjacent areas.

Function of the Mesencephalic Portion of the Reticular Activating System. To understand the function of the mesencephalic portion of the reticular activating system it is instructive to consider two different experiments performed by cutting the brain stem at two different levels, as follows:

1. Cutting the brain stem at the upper end of the mesencephalon causes the cerebrum to become inactive—that is, to go into coma.

2. Cutting the brain stem in the midpontile region causes the cerebrum to become active and to remain active indefinitely as if it remains continuously awake.

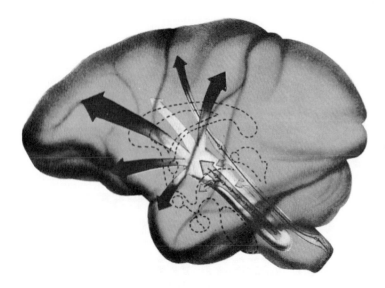

Figure 19–1. The reticular activating system schematically projected on a monkey brain. (From Lindsley: Reticular Formation of the Brain. Boston, Little, Brown and Co.)

Therefore, the reticular formation of the mesencephalon and upper pons seems to provide intrinsic activation of the brain. On the other hand, areas in the brain stem below the midlevel of the pons can inhibit this activating system and cause sleep.

Function of the Thalamic Portion of the Activating System. Electrical stimulation in different areas of the thalamic portion of the activating system activates specific regions of the cerebral cortex more than others. This is distinctly different from stimulation in the mesencephalic portion, which activates large areas of the brain at the same time. Therefore, it is postulated that selective stimulation of portions of the thalamus by the internal signals of the brain might be the cause of specific activation of certain areas of the cerebral cortex in distinction to other areas.

Stimulation of the Reticular Activating System by Nerve Signals from Elsewhere

The reticular activating system itself is subject to stimulation and therefore subject to increased levels of activation. Also, it is subject to inhibition, which can lead to sleep, as we shall discuss in detail later in the chapter.

Two basic types of stimuli are especially likely to increase the activity of the activating system. These are (1) sensory stimuli from almost any part of the body and (2) retrograde stimuli from the cerebrum, feeding mainly into the mesencephalic portion of the reticular formation.

Almost any sensory signal entering the nervous system will cause at least some degree of activation of the reticular activating system. However, some signals are much more stimulatory than others, especially pain and proprioceptive somatic impulses, both of which are likely to require some immediate action by the brain. It will be recalled that the reticular formation receives tremendous numbers of signals either directly or through collaterals from the *spinoreticular tracts*, the *spinothalamic tracts*,

and the *spinotectal tracts*. When an animal is asleep and appropriate sensory signals suddenly enter the reticular activating system, this can cause the animal to awaken immediately. This is called the *arousal reaction*.

Stimulation of the reticular activating system by the cerebrum, especially by the cerebral cortex, is mediated through direct fiber pathways into the reticular formation from almost all parts of the cerebrum, including (1) the somatic sensory cortex, (2) the motor cortex, (3) the frontal cortex, (4) the basal ganglia, (5) the hippocampus and other limbic structures, and (6) the hypothalamus. An especially large number of nerve fibers pass from the motor regions of the cerebral cortex to the reticular formation; therefore, motor activity in particular is associated with a high degree of reticular activation, which partially explains the importance of moving around when one wishes to remain awake.

Wakefulness—Its Relationship to Activation of the Brain

We shall see later that the brain is exceedingly active in the course of generalized epileptic seizures, and yet the person is not awake. Likewise, the brain remains active to varying degrees during sleep and at some stages of sleep is perhaps equally as active as during wakefulness.

On the other hand, wakefulness does not occur in the absence of a reasonable degree of activation of the brain.

Therefore, wakefulness can be defined as activity in the brain directed into appropriate channels to give the person a sense of conscious awareness.

Coma

Coma is the opposite of brain activation. It can result from any factor that diminishes or stops activity in the mesencephalic portion of the reticular activating system. This can include such factors as:

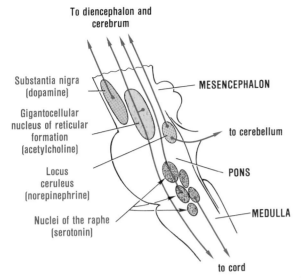

Substantia nigra (dopamine)

Gigantocellular nucleus of reticular formation (acetylcholine)

Locus ceruleus (norepinephrine)

Nuclei of the raphe (serotonin)

To diencephalon and cerebrum

MESENCEPHALON

to cerebellum

PONS

MEDULLA

to cord

Figure 19–2. Multiple centers in the brain stem, the neurons of which secrete different transmitter substances. These neurons send control signals upward into the diencephalon and cerebrum and downward into the spinal cord.

(1) Brain tumors pressing on the brain stem, such as tumors of the pineal gland or the pituitary gland. (2) Vascular lesions that interrupt the blood supply to the midbrain. (3) Prolonged hypoxia that causes death of brain neurons. (4) Infectious processes in the brain stem, such as the encephalitis that causes sleeping sickness. (5) Poisons that destroy brain tissue.

Coma is distinct from sleep in that a person cannot be aroused from coma. In some coma patients all parts of the brain are inactivated, not just the reticular activating system. In this case all electrical activity of the brain ceases—that is, the brain waves are said to be "flat." This is the condition called *brain death*, and the person can then remain alive only by being sustained on artificial respiration, administration of nutrition by stomach tube or intravenously, and use of various supportive drugs and fluids to maintain appropriate blood circulation.

SPECIFIC NEURONAL SYSTEMS ASSOCIATED WITH THE RETICULAR FORMATION

We noted earlier that as more has been learned about the reticular formation, specific anatomically distinct neuronal systems have been discovered. Four of these have special importance in controlling specific activities of the diencephalon and cerebrum. Illustrated in Figure 19–2, these are:

1. *The gigantocellular nucleus of the reticular formation.* This area lies in the medial portions of the reticular formation in the mesencephalon and upper pons. The neurons of this nucleus are very large and their fibers divide immediately into two branches, one passing upward into the higher levels of the brain and the other passing downward

through the reticulospinal tracts into the spinal cord. This is a principal activator portion of the reticular activating system.

The neurons of this nucleus release *acetylcholine* at their terminals, and this normally functions as an excitatory transmitter.

2. *The substantia nigra.* This nucleus was discussed in Chapter 16 in relation to the basal ganglia. It lies in the anterior portion of the mesencephalon and contains neuronal cell bodies that secrete *dopamine* at their nerve endings. Additional neurons that secrete dopamine are also found in adjacent regions of the ventral tegmentum of the mesencephalon. In addition to the basal ganglia, fibers from these areas pass to the hypothalamus, the cerebral cortex, and the limbic system. The dopamine released at the nerve endings functions in the basal ganglia as an inhibitory transmitter, which is perhaps also true in other areas of the brain, but not necessarily so because some dopamine receptors are excitatory.

It will be recalled from Chapter 16 that destruction of the dopaminergic neurons in the substantia nigra eliminates their normal inhibitory effect on the basal ganglia, and that is the basic cause of Parkinson's disease.

3. *The locus ceruleus.* This is a small area located bilaterally and posteriorly at the junction point between the mesencephalon and the pons. Nerve fibers from this area secrete norepinephrine. They spread very widely through the diencephalon and the cerebrum, as well as into the cerebellum and lower regions of the brain stem. The norepinephrine released by the endings of these neurons may have either excitatory or inhibitory effects on different structures, depending on the character of the receptors in the postsynaptic neurons. Later in the chapter we shall see that the locus ceruleus probably plays a role in one type of sleep called REM sleep.

4. *The raphe nuclei.* In the midline of the lower pons and medulla are several very thin nuclei called the raphe nuclei. Many of the neurons in these nuclei secrete serotonin, and they send fibers to widespread areas in the diencephalon and also to the cord. The cord fibers have the capability of suppressing pain, which was discussed in Chapter 14. The serotonin released in the diencephalon and cerebrum almost certainly plays an essential role in causing normal sleep, as we shall discuss later in the chapter.

THE GENERALIZED THALAMOCORTICAL SYSTEM— ITS POSSIBLE FUNCTION IN ATTENTION AND SEARCHING THE MEMORY STORE

The thalamus is the entryway for all sensory nervous signals to the cerebral cortex, with the single exception of signals from the olfactory sys-

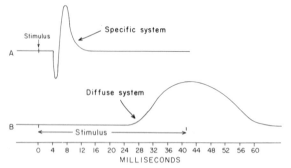

Figure 19–3. Comparison of the response of the visual cortex following stimulation of the lateral geniculate body (record A), which is part of the specific thalamocortical system, with the response of the visual cortex following stimulation of the visual portion of the generalized thalamocortical system (record B). Note in record B the long latent period before appearance of the diffuse response and also the prolonged duration of the response.

tem. Those thalamic nuclei that relay these sensory signals to the cerebral cortex are called the *specific thalamic nuclei*, and this sensory input system to the cerebral cortex is known as the *specific thalamocortical system*.

In addition to the *specific* thalamocortical system, another thalamocortical system separate from the specific system is called the *generalized thalamocortical system*. This is composed principally of the nerve pathway discussed earlier feeding upward from the mesencephalic portion of the reticular formation by way of the thalamus to the cortex. The signals of this pathway are relayed in the thalamus by multiple small diffuse neurons that lie mainly between the specific thalamic nuclei or on the outer surface of the thalamus. Many of these neurons make multiple connections with the specific thalamic nuclei, but especially they project very small fibers to all parts of the cerebral cortex.

Mechanism of Cortical Activation by the Generalized Thalamocortical System. The way in which the generalized thalamocortical system activates the cerebral cortex is entirely different from activation by the specific sensory systems. Some of the differences are the following:

1. Stimulation of a specific thalamic nucleus—such as the ventrobasal complex that transmits somatic signals to the somatic sensory cortex—activates the cortex within 1 to 2 milliseconds, whereas stimulation of the generalized system causes no activation for approximately the first 25 milliseconds. The activation level builds up over a period of many milliseconds. These differences are illustrated in Figure 19–3.

2. At the end of stimulation, the activation of the cortex by the specific nuclei dies away within another few milliseconds, whereas the activation by the generalized system sometimes continues as an "after-discharge" for as long as 30 seconds.

3. Signals from the specific nuclei to the cortex activate mainly layer IV of the cortex, as was explained in Chapter 13, whereas activation of the generalized thalamic system activates mainly layers I and II of the cortex. Since this latter activation is prolonged and because layers I and II are the loci of many of the dendrites of the deeper cortical neurons, it is supposed that the stimulation by the generalized thalamic system mainly causes partial depolarization of large numbers of dendrites near the surface of the cortex; this in turn causes a generalized increase in the degree of facilitation of the cortex. When the cortex is thus facilitated, specific signals that enter the cortex from other sources are exuberantly received.

4. Stimulation in the generalized thalamic system *facilitates* an *area* of several square centimeters in the cortex, while stimulation at a point in a specific thalamic nucleus *excites* a specific point in the cortex.

In summary, the generalized thalamocortical system controls the overall degree of activity of the cortex. It can at times facilitate activity in regional areas of the cortex distinct from the remainder of the cortex. Collateral signals from this system also control the level of activity in the specific nuclei of the thalamus, the basal ganglia, the hypothalamus, and other structures of the cerebrum and diencephalon as well.

Possible Mechanisms for Attention and for Searching the Memory Store

We are all aware that we can direct our attention toward certain of our mental activities individually and can also search through our memory store for specific memories. Because of the capability of the generalized thalamocortical system to activate small areas of the cerebral cortex at a time, it is tempting to believe that specific activation of regional portions of the cortex might be the way in which we do indeed direct our attention, and might also be the basis for searching through memory stores.

One other bit of information also suggests that the generalized thalamocortical system might be important in searching for memories: It has been reported that specific lesions in the thalamus are sometimes associated with retrograde amnesia—that is, inability to recall memories that are known to be stored within the brain.

BRAIN WAVES

Electrical recordings from the surface of the brain or from the outer surface of the head demonstrate continuous electrical activity in the brain. Both the intensity and patterns of this electrical activity are determined to a great extent by the overall level of excitation of the brain resulting from functions in the reticular activating system. The undulations in the recorded electrical potentials, shown in Figure 19–4, are called *brain waves*, and the entire record is called an *electroencephalogram* (EEG).

The intensities of the brain waves on the surface of the scalp range from 0 to 300 microvolts, and their frequencies range from once every few seconds to 50 or more per second. The character of the waves is highly dependent on the degree of activity of the cerebral cortex, and the

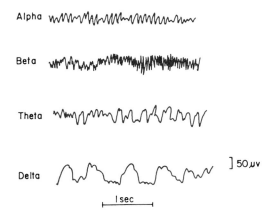

Figure 19–4. Different types of normal electroencephalographic waves.

waves change markedly between the states of wakefulness and sleep and coma.

Much of the time, the brain waves are irregular, and no general pattern can be discerned in the EEG. However, at other times, distinct patterns do appear. Some of these are characteristic of specific abnormalities of the brain, such as epilepsy, which is discussed later. Others occur even in normal persons and can be classified as *alpha, beta, theta,* and *delta waves,* which are all illustrated in Figure 19–4.

Alpha waves are rhythmic waves occurring at a frequency of between 8 and 13 per second and are found in the EEGs of almost all normal adult persons when they are awake in a quiet, resting state of cerebration. These waves occur most intensely in the occipital region but can also be recorded at times from the parietal and frontal regions of the scalp. Their voltage usually is about 50 microvolts. During sleep the alpha waves disappear entirely, and when the awake person's attention is directed to some specific type of mental activity, the alpha waves are replaced by asynchronous, higher frequency but lower voltage beta waves. Figure 19–5 illustrates the effect on the alpha waves of simply opening the eyes in bright light and then closing the eyes again. Note that the visual sensations cause immediate cessation of the alpha waves and that these are replaced by low voltage, asynchronous beta waves.

Beta waves occur at frequencies of more than 14 cycles per second and as high as 25 and rarely 50 cycles per second. These are most frequently recorded from the parietal and frontal regions of the scalp. Most beta waves appear during activation of the central nervous system or during tension.

Theta waves have frequencies of between 4 and 7 cycles per second. These occur mainly in the parietal and temporal regions in children, but they also occur during emotional stress in some adults, particularly during disappointment and frustration. They can often be brought out in the EEG of a frustrated person by allowing enjoyment of some pleasant experience and then suddenly removing this element of pleasure; this causes approximately 20 seconds of theta waves. These same waves also occur in many brain disorders.

Delta waves include all the waves of the EEG below 3.5 cycles per second and sometimes as low as 1 cycle every 2 to 3 seconds. These occur in deep sleep, in infancy, and in serious organic brain disease. And they occur in the cortex of animals that have had subcortical transec-

tions separating the cerebral cortex from the thalamus. Therefore, delta waves can occur strictly in the cortex independently of activities in lower regions of the brain.

ORIGIN OF THE DIFFERENT TYPES OF BRAIN WAVES

The discharge of a single neuron or single nerve fiber in the brain cannot be recorded from the surface of the head. Instead, for an electrical potential to be recorded all the way through the skull, large portions of nervous tissue must emit electrical current simultaneously. There are two ways in which this can occur. First, tremendous numbers of nerve fibers can discharge in synchrony with each other, thereby generating very strong electrical currents. Second, large numbers of neurons can partially discharge, though not emit action potentials; furthermore, these partially discharged neurons can cause electrical potentials that undulate with changing degrees of excitability of the neurons. Simultaneous electrical measurements within the brain while recording brain waves from the scalp indicate that it is the second of these that causes the usual brain waves.

To be more specific, the surface of the cerebral cortex is composed almost entirely of a mat of dendrites extending to the surface from neuronal cells in the lower layers of the cortex. When signals impinge on these dendrites, the dendrites become partially discharged. This makes the neurons of the cortex highly excitable—that is, facilitates them, and the negative potential is simultaneously recorded from the surface of the scalp, indicating this high degree of excitability.

One of the principal sources of signals to excite the outer dendritic layer of the cerebral cortex is the generalized thalamocortical fibers of the reticular activating system. Therefore, brain wave intensity is closely related to the degree of activity in either the brain stem or the thalamic portions of the reticular activating system.

Origin of Delta Waves. Transection of the fiber tracts from the thalamus to the cortex, which blocks the reticular activating system fibers, causes delta waves in the cortex. This indicates that some synchronizing mechanism can occur in the cortical neurons themselves—entirely independently of lower structures in the brain—to cause the delta waves.

Delta waves also occur in very deep "slow wave" sleep, and this suggests that the cortex then might be released from the activating influences of the reticular activating system.

Origin of Alpha Waves. Alpha waves will *not* occur in the cortex without connections with the thalamus. Also, stimulation in the generalized thalamic nuclei often sets up waves in the generalized thalamocortical system at a frequency of between 8 and 13 per second, the natural frequency of the alpha waves. Therefore, it is assumed that the alpha waves result from spontaneous activity in the generalized thalamocortical system, which causes both the periodicity of the alpha waves and the synchronous activation of literally millions of cortical neurons during each wave.

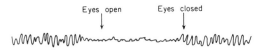

Figure 19–5. Replacement of the alpha rhythm by an asynchronous discharge of opening the eyes.

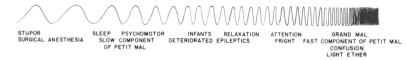

STUPOR   SLEEP   PSYCHOMOTOR   INFANTS   RELAXATION   ATTENTION   GRAND MAL
SURGICAL ANESTHESIA   SLOW COMPONENT DETERIORATED EPILEPTICS   FRIGHT FAST COMPONENT OF PETIT MAL
               OF PETIT MAL   CONFUSION
                                                                LIGHT ETHER

|⊢——— I SECOND ———⊣|

Figure 19–6. Effect of varying degrees of cerebral activity on the basic rhythm of the EEG. (From Gibbs and Gibbs: Atlas of Electroencephalography, 2nd Ed. Vol. I. Addison-Wesley, 1974. Reprinted by permission.)

EFFECT OF VARYING DEGREES OF CEREBRAL ACTIVITY ON THE BASIC RHYTHM OF THE ELECTROENCEPHALOGRAM

There is a general relationship between the degree of cerebral activity and the average frequency of the electroencephalographic rhythm, the average frequency increasing progressively with higher and higher degrees of activity. This is illustrated in Figure 19–6, which shows the existence of delta waves in stupor, surgical anesthesia, and sleep; theta waves in psychomotor states and in infants; alpha waves during relaxed states; and beta waves during periods of intense mental activity. However, during periods of mental activity the waves usually become asynchronous rather than synchronous so that the voltage falls considerably, despite increased cortical activity, as illustrated in Figure 19–5.

CLINICAL USE OF THE ELECTROENCEPHALOGRAM

One of the most important uses of the EEG is to diagnose different types of epilepsy and to find the focus in the brain causing the epilepsy. This is discussed further later. But, in addition, the EEG can be used to localize brain tumors or other space-occupying lesions of the brain and to diagnose certain types of psychopathic disturbances.

Localization of Brain Tumors. There are two means by which brain tumors can be localized. Some brain tumors are so large that they block electrical activity from a given portion of the cerebral cortex, and when this occurs the voltage of the brain waves is considerably reduced in the region of the tumor. However, more frequently a brain tumor compresses the surrounding neuronal tissue and causes abnormal electrical excitation of these surrounding areas; this in turn leads to synchronous discharges of very high voltage waves in the EEG, as shown in the middle two records of Figure 19–7. Localization of the origin of these spikes on the surface of the scalp is a valuable means for locating the brain tumor; this is achieved in the following way:

The upper part of Figure 19–7 shows the placement of 16 different electrodes on the scalp, and the lower part of the figure shows the brain waves from 4 of these electrodes marked in the figure by Xs. Note that in two of these, intense brain waves are recorded and, furthermore, that the two waves are essentially of reverse polarity to each other. This reverse polarity means that the origin of the spikes is somewhere in the area *between* the two respective electrodes. Thus, the excessively excitable area of the brain has been located, and this is a lead to the location of the brain tumor.

Diagnosing Psychopathic Disturbances. Use of brain waves in diagnosing psychopathic abnormalities is generally not very satisfactory because only a few of these cause distinct brain wave patterns. Yet by observing

combinations of different types of basic rhythms, reactions of the rhythms to attention, changes of the rhythms during alkalosis caused by forced breathing, the appearance of particular characteristics in the brain waves (such as "spindles" of alpha waves), and so forth, an experienced electroencephalographer can detect at least certain types of psychopathic disturbances. Also, theta waves are frequently found in persons with brain abnormalities.

SLEEP

Sleep is defined as a state of unconsciousness from which a person can be aroused by appropriate sensory or other stimuli.

Two Different Types of Sleep—(1) Slow Wave Sleep and (2) REM Sleep. During each night a person goes through stages of two different types of sleep that alternate with each other. These are called *slow wave sleep,* because in this type of sleep the brain waves are very slow, and *REM sleep,* which stands for *rapid eye movement* sleep, because in this type of sleep the eyes undergo rapid movements despite the fact that the person is still asleep.

Most of the sleep during each night is of the slow wave variety; this is the deep, restful type of sleep that the person experiences during the first hour of sleep after having been kept awake for many hours. Episodes of REM sleep occur periodically during sleep and occupy about 25 per cent of the sleep time of the young adult; they normally recur about every 90 minutes. This type of sleep is not so restful,

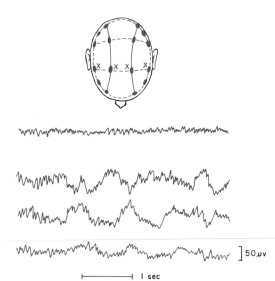

Figure 19–7. Localization of a brain tumor by means of the EEG, illustrating (*above*) the placement of electrodes and (*below*) the records from the four electrodes designated by Xs.

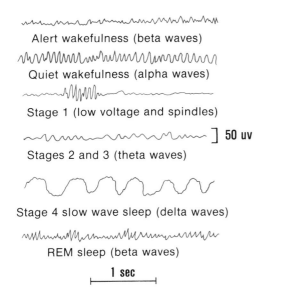

Alert wakefulness (beta waves)

Quiet wakefulness (alpha waves)

Stage 1 (low voltage and spindles)

] 50 uv

Stages 2 and 3 (theta waves)

Stage 4 slow wave sleep (delta waves)

REM sleep (beta waves)

⊢ 1 sec ⊣

Figure 19–8. Progressive change in the characteristics of the brain waves during different stages of sleep.

and it is usually associated with dreaming, as we shall discuss later.

Electroencephalographic Changes in the Different Stages of Wakefulness and Sleep

Figure 19–8 illustrates the electroencephalogram from a typical person in different stages of wakefulness and sleep. Alert wakefulness is characterized by high frequency *beta waves*, whereas quiet wakefulness is usually associated with *alpha waves*, as illustrated by the first two electroencephalograms of the figure.

Slow wave sleep is generally divided into four stages. In the first stage, a stage of very light sleep, the voltage of the electroencephalographic waves becomes very low but this is broken by *"sleep spindles,"* that is, short spindle-shaped bursts of alpha waves that occur periodically. In stages 2, 3, and 4 of slow wave sleep the frequency of the electroencephalogram becomes progressively slower until it reaches a frequency of only two to three waves per second; these are typical *delta waves.*

In REM sleep, the electroencephalogram suddenly changes back to the characteristics of the early stages of wakefulness, indicating a high level of activity in the brain during this period of sleep.

SLOW WAVE SLEEP

Most of us can understand the characteristics of deep slow wave sleep by remembering the last time that we were kept awake for more than 24 hours and the deep sleep that occurred within 30 minutes to an hour after going to sleep. This sleep is exceedingly restful and is associated with a decrease in both peripheral vascular tone and many other vegetative functions of the body as well. In addi-

tion, there is a 10 to 30 per cent decrease in blood pressure, respiratory rate, and basal metabolic rate.

Though slow wave sleep is frequently called "dreamless sleep," dreams actually occur very often during slow wave sleep, and nightmares even occur during this type of sleep. However, the difference between the dreams occurring in slow wave sleep and those in REM sleep is that those of REM sleep are remembered whereas those of slow wave sleep usually are not. That is, during slow wave sleep the process of consolidation of the dreams in memory does not occur.

Origin of the Delta Waves in Sleep. In experimental animals in which the fiber tracts between the thalamus and the cortex have been transected, delta waves are generated in the isolated cortex, indicating that this type of wave probably occurs intrinsically in the cortex when the cortex is not driven from below by the reticular activating system. Therefore, it is assumed that the degree of activity in the activating system has fallen to a level during deep slow wave sleep that is too low to maintain normal excitability of the cortex.

REM SLEEP (PARADOXICAL SLEEP, DESYNCHRONIZED SLEEP)

In a normal night of sleep, bouts of REM sleep lasting 5 to 30 minutes usually appear on the average every 90 minutes, the first such period occurring 80 to 100 minutes after the person falls asleep. When the person is extremely tired, the duration of each bout of REM sleep is very short, and it may even be absent. On the other hand, as the person becomes more rested through the night, the duration of the REM bouts greatly increases.

There are several very important characteristics of REM sleep:

1. It is usually associated with active dreaming.

2. The person is even more difficult to arouse by sensory stimuli than during deep slow wave sleep, and yet persons usually awaken in the morning during an episode of REM sleep, not from slow wave sleep.

3. The muscle tone throughout the body is exceedingly depressed, indicating strong inhibition of the spinal projections from the reticular formation of the brain stem.

4. The heart rate and respiration usually become irregular, which is characteristic of the dream state.

5. Despite the extreme inhibition of the peripheral muscles, a few irregular muscle movements occur. These include, in particular, rapid movements of the eyes; this is the origin of the name acronym REM, for "rapid eye movements."

6. The electroencephalogram shows a desynchronized pattern of beta waves similar to those that occur during wakefulness. Therefore, this type of sleep is also frequently called *desynchronized sleep,* meaning desynchronized brain waves; or, it is also

called *paradoxical sleep* because it is a paradox that a person can still be asleep despite marked activity in the brain.

In summary, REM sleep is a type of sleep in which the brain is quite active. However, the brain activity is not channeled in the proper direction for persons to be aware of their surroundings and therefore to be awake.

BASIC THEORIES OF SLEEP

The Active Theory of Sleep. An earlier theory of sleep was that the reticular activating system and other parts of the brain simply fatigued over the period of a waking day and therefore became inactive as a result. This was called the *passive theory of sleep.* However, an important experiment quoted earlier in this chapter changed this view to the current belief that sleep most likely is caused by an active inhibitory process. This was the experiment in which it was discovered that transecting the brain stem in the midpontile region leads to a brain that never goes to sleep. In other words, there seems to be some center or centers located below the midpontile level of the brain stem that actively cause sleep by inhibiting other parts of the brain. This is called the *active theory* of sleep.

Neuronal Centers, Transmitters, and Mechanisms That Can Cause Sleep

Stimulation of several specific areas of the brain can produce sleep with characteristics very near those of natural sleep. Some of these are the following:

1. The most conspicuous stimulation area for causing almost natural sleep is the raphe nuclei in the lower half of the pons and in the medulla. These are a thin sheet of nuclei located in the midline. Nerve fibers from these nuclei spread widely in the reticular formation and also upward into the thalamus and neocortex, hypothalamus, and most areas of the limbic cortex. In addition, they extend downward into the spinal cord, terminating in the posterior horns where they can inhibit incoming pain signals, as was discussed in Chapter 14. It is also known that the endings of fibers from these raphe neurons secrete *serotonin.* Therefore, it is assumed that serotonin is the major transmitter substance associated with production of sleep.

2. Stimulation of some areas in the *nucleus of the tractus solitarius,* which is the sensory region of the medulla and pons for the visceral sensory signals entering the brain via the vagi and glossopharyngeal nerves, will also promote sleep. However, this will not occur if the raphe nuclei have been destroyed. Therefore, these regions probably act by exciting the raphe nuclei.

3. Stimulation of several other regions in the lower brain stem and diencephalon can also help promote sleep, including the rostral part of the hypothalamus, mainly in the suprachiasmal area, and an occasional area in the diffuse nuclei of the thalamus.

Effect of Lesions in the Sleep-Promoting Centers. Discrete lesions in the raphe nuclei lead to a high state of wakefulness. This is also true of bilateral lesions in the mediorostral suprachiasmal portion of the anterior hypothalamus. In both instances, the reticular activating system seems to become released from inhibition. Indeed, the lesions of the anterior hypothalamus can sometimes cause such intense wakefulness that the animal actually dies of exhaustion.

Other Possible Transmitter Substances Related to Sleep. Experiments have shown that the cerebrospinal fluid and also the blood of animals that have been kept awake for several days contain a substance or substances that cause sleep when injected into the ventricular system of an animal. One of these substances is a small polypeptide with a molecular weight of less than 500. When cerebrospinal fluid containing this sleep-producing substance or substances is injected into the third ventricle, almost natural sleep occurs within a few minutes, and the animal may then stay asleep for several hours. Another substance that has similar effects in causing sleep is a nonapeptide isolated from the blood of sleeping animals. And still a third and different sleep factor has been isolated from the neuronal tissues of the brain stem of animals kept awake for days. Therefore, it is possible that prolonged wakefulness causes progressive accumulation of a sleep factor in the brain stem or in the cerebrospinal fluid that leads to sleep.

Possible Causes of REM Sleep

Why slow wave sleep is broken periodically by REM sleep is not understood. However, a lesion in the *locus ceruleus* on each side of the brain stem can reduce REM sleep, and if the lesion includes other contiguous areas of the brain stem, REM sleep can be prevented altogether. Therefore, it has been postulated that when stimulated, the norepinephrine-secreting nerve fibers that originate in the locus ceruleus can activate many portions of the brain. This theoretically causes the excess activity that occurs in certain regions of the brain in REM sleep, but the signals are not channeled appropriately in the brain to cause normal conscious awareness that is characteristic of the wakefulness state.

The Cycle Between Sleep and Wakefulness

The preceding discussions have merely identified neuronal areas, transmitters, and mechanisms that are related to sleep. However, they have not explained the cyclic, reciprocal operation of the sleep-wakefulness cycle. It is quite possible that this is caused by a free-running intrinsic oscillator within the brain stem that cycles back and forth between the sleep centers and areas in the reticular activating system that cause wakefulness.

However, there is much reason to believe that feedback signals from the cerebral cortex and also from the peripheral nerve receptors might also play an important role in helping control the sleep-wakefulness rhythm. One reason for believing this is that sensory signals feeding into the reticular activating system will often arouse a person from deep sleep. Also, as explained earlier, stimulation of the cerebral cortex will cause powerful activation of the reticular activating system.

Therefore, a very likely mechanism for causing the rhythmicity of the sleep-wakefulness cycle is the following:

When the sleep centers are not activated, the reticular activating system then presumably begins spontaneous activity. This in turn excites both the cerebral cortex and the peripheral nervous system. Next, positive feedback signals come from both these areas back to the reticular activating system to activate it still further. Thus, once the wakefulness state begins, it has a natural tendency to sustain itself.

However, after the brain remains activated for many hours, even the neurons within the activating system presumably will fatigue to some extent, and other factors presumably activate the sleep centers. Consequently, the positive feedback cycle between the reticular activating system and the cortex, and also that between the reticular activating system and the periphery, will fade, and the inhibitory effects of the sleep centers as well as inhibition by possible sleep-producing chemical transmitter substances will take over, leading to rapid transition from the wakefulness state to the sleep state.

Then, one could postulate that during sleep the excitatory neurons of the reticular activating system gradually become more and more excitable because of the prolonged rest, while the inhibitory neurons of the sleep centers become less excitable, thus leading to a new cycle of wakefulness.

This theory obviously can explain the rapid transitions from sleep to wakefulness and from wakefulness to sleep. It can also explain arousal, the insomnia that occurs when a person's mind becomes preoccupied with a thought, the wakefulness that is produced by bodily activity, and many other conditions that affect the person's state of sleep or wakefulness.

PHYSIOLOGICAL EFFECTS OF SLEEP

Sleep causes two major types of physiological effects: first, effects on the nervous system itself and, second, effects on other structures of the body. The first of these seems to be by far the more important, for any person who has a transected

spinal cord in the neck shows no physiological effects in the body beneath the level of transection that can be attributed to a sleep and wakefulness cycle; that is, lack of sleep and wakefulness causes neither significant harm to the bodily organs nor even any deranged function. On the other hand, lack of sleep certainly does affect the functions of the central nervous system.

Prolonged wakefulness is often associated with progressive malfunction of the mind and also causes abnormal behavioral activities of the nervous system. We are all familiar with the increased sluggishness of thought that occurs toward the end of a prolonged wakeful period, but in addition, a person can become irritable or even psychotic following forced wakefulness for prolonged periods of time. Therefore, one can assume that sleep in some way not presently understood restores both normal sensitivities of and normal "balance" among the different parts of the central nervous system. This might be likened to the "rezeroing" of electronic analog computers after prolonged use, for all computers of this type gradually lose their "base line" of operation; it is reasonable to assume that the same effect occurs in the central nervous system, because overuse of some neurons during wakefulness could easily throw all these out of balance with the remainder of the nervous system. Therefore, in the absence of any definitely demonstrated functional value of sleep, we might postulate that the principal value of sleep is to restore the natural balance among the neuronal centers.

Even though, as pointed out earlier, wakefulness and sleep have not been shown to be necessary for somatic functions of the body, the cycle of enhanced and depressed nervous excitability that follows the cycle of wakefulness and sleep does have moderate effects on the peripheral body. For instance, there is enhanced sympathetic activity during wakefulness and also enhanced numbers of impulses to the skeletal musculature to increase muscle tone. Conversely, during sleep, sympathetic activity decreases while parasympathetic activity occasionally increases. Therefore, arterial blood pressure falls, pulse rate decreases, skin vessels dilate, activity of the gastrointestinal tract sometimes increases, muscles fall into a mainly relaxed state, and the overall basal metabolic rate of the body falls by 10 to 30 per cent.

EPILEPSY

Epilepsy is characterized by uncontrolled excessive activity of either a part or all of the central nervous system. A person who is predisposed to epilepsy has attacks when the basal level of excitability of the nervous system (or of the part that is susceptible to the epileptic state) rises above a certain critical threshold. But, as long as the degree of excitability is held below this threshold, no attack occurs.

Basically, epilepsy can be classified into three major

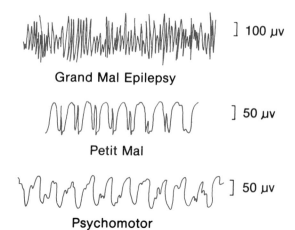

Figure 19–9. Electroencephalograms in different types of epilepsy.

types: *grand mal epilepsy*, *petit mal epilepsy*, and *focal epilepsy*.

GRAND MAL EPILEPSY

Grand mal epilepsy is characterized by extreme neuronal discharges in all areas of the brain—in the cortex, in the deeper parts of the cerebrum, and even in all areas of the reticular activating system. Also, discharges are transmitted from the reticular formation into the spinal cord to cause generalized *tonic convulsions* of the entire body, followed toward the end of the attack by alternating muscular contractions called *tonic-clonic convulsions*. Often the person bites or "swallows" the tongue and usually has difficulty in breathing, sometimes to the extent of developing cyanosis. Also, signals to the viscera frequently cause urination and defecation.

The grand mal seizure lasts from a few seconds to as long as three to four minutes and is characterized by postseizure depression of the entire nervous system; the person remains in stupor for one to many minutes after the attack is over and then often remains severely fatigued for many hours thereafter.

The top recording of Figure 19–9 illustrates a typical electroencephalogram from almost any region of the cortex during the tonic phase of a grand mal attack. This illustrates that high voltage, synchronous discharges occur over the entire cortex. Furthermore, the same type of discharge occurs on both sides of the brain at the same time, illustrating that the abnormal neuronal circuitry responsible for the attack strongly involves the basal regions of the brain that drive the cortex.

In experimental animals or even in human beings, grand mal attacks can be initiated by administering neuronal stimulants, such as the well-known drug Metrazol, or they can be caused by insulin hypoglycemia or by the passage of alternating electrical current directly through the brain. Electrical recordings from the thalamus and also from the reticular formation of the brain stem during the grand mal attack show typical high voltage activity in both of these areas similar to that recorded from the cerebral cortex.

Presumably, therefore, a grand mal attack is caused by abnormal activation in the lower portions of the brain activating system itself.

What Initiates a Grand Mal Attack? Most persons who have grand mal attacks have a hereditary predisposition to epilepsy, a predisposition that occurs in about 1 of every 50 to 100 people. In such persons, some of the factors that can increase the excitability of the abnormal "epileptogenic" circuitry enough to precipitate attacks are (1) strong emotional stimuli, (2) alkalosis caused by hyperventilation, (3) drugs, (4) fever, or (5) loud noises or flashing lights. Also, even in persons not genetically predisposed, traumatic lesions in almost any part of the brain can cause excess excitability of local brain areas as we shall discuss shortly, and these too can transmit signals into the reticular activating system to elicit grand mal seizures.

What Stops the Grand Mal Attack? The cause of the extreme neuronal overactivity during a grand mal attack is presumed to be massive activation of many reverberating pathways throughout the brain. It is presumed that the major factor, or at least one of the major factors, that stops the attack after a few minutes is the phenomenon of neuronal *fatigue*. However, a second factor is probably *active inhibition* by certain structures of the brain. The stupor and total body fatigue that occur after a grand mal seizure is over are believed to result from the intense fatigue of the neurons following their intensive activity during the grand mal attack.

PETIT MAL EPILEPSY

Petit mal epilepsy is closely allied to grand mal epilepsy in that it too almost certainly involves the reticular activating system. It is usually characterized by 3 to 30 seconds of unconsciousness during which the person has several twitchlike contractions of the muscles, usually in the head region—especially blinking of the eyes; this is followed by return of consciousness and resumption of previous activities. The patient may have one such attack in many months or in rare instances may have a rapid series of attacks, one following the other. However, the usual course is for the petit mal attacks to appear in late childhood and then to disappear entirely by the age of 30. On occasion, a petit mal epileptic attack will initiate a grand mal attack.

The brain wave pattern in petit mal epilepsy is illustrated by the middle record of Figure 19–9, which is typified by a *spike and dome pattern*. The spike portion of this recording is almost identical to the spikes that occur in grand mal epilepsy, but the dome portion is distinctly different. The spike and dome can be recorded over most or all of the cerebral cortex, illustrating that the seizure involves the activating system of the brain.

FOCAL EPILEPSY

Focal epilepsy can involve almost any part of the brain, either localized regions of the cerebral cortex or deeper structures of both the cerebrum and brain stem. And almost always, focal epilepsy results from some localized organic lesion or functional abnormality, such as a scar that pulls on the neuronal tissue, a tumor that compresses an area of the brain, a destroyed area of brain tissue, or congenitally deranged local circuitry. Lesions such as these can promote extremely rapid discharges in the local neurons, and when the discharge rate rises above approximately 1000 per second, synchronous waves begin to spread over the adjacent cortical regions. These waves presumably result from *localized reverberating circuits* that gradually recruit adjacent areas of the cortex into the discharge zone. The process spreads to adjacent areas at a rate as slow as a few millimeters a minute to as fast as several centimeters per second. When such a wave of excitation spreads over the motor cortex, it causes a progressive "march" of muscular contractions throughout the opposite side of the body, beginning most characteristically in the mouth region and marching progressively downward to the legs, but at other times marching in the opposite direction. This is called *jacksonian epilepsy.*

A focal epileptic attack may remain confined to a single area of the brain, but in many instances the strong signals from the convulsing cortex or other part of the brain excite the mesencephalic portion of the brain activating system so greatly that a grand mal epileptic attack ensues as well.

Another type of focal epilepsy is the so-called *psychomotor seizure,* which may cause (1) a short period of amnesia, (2) an attack of abnormal rage, (3) sudden anxiety, discomfort, or fear, (4) a moment of incoherent speech or mumbling of some trite phrase, or (5) a motor act to attack someone, to rub the face with the hand, or so forth. Sometimes the person cannot remember his activities during the attack, but at other times he will have been conscious of everything that he had been doing but unable to control it. Attacks of this type characteristically involve part of the limbic portion of the brain, such as the hippocampus, the amygdala, the septum, or the temporal cortex.

The lower tracing of Figure 19–9 illustrates a typical electroencephalogram during a psychomotor attack, showing a low frequency rectangular wave with a frequency of between 2 and 4 per second and with superimposed 14 per second waves.

The electroencephalogram can often be used to localize abnormal spiking waves originating in areas of organic brain disease that might predispose to focal epileptic attacks. Once such a focal point is found, surgical excision of the focus frequently prevents future attacks.

REFERENCES

Arkin, J. S., *et al.* (eds.): The Mind in Sleep. New York, Halsted Press, 1978.

Bindman, L.: The Neurophysiology of the Cerebral Cortex. Austin, University of Texas Press, 1981.

Block, G. D., and Page, T. L.: Circadian pacemakers in the nervous system. *Annu. Rev. Neurosci.,* 1:19, 1978.

Buser, P.: Higher functions of the nervous system. *Annu. Rev. Physiol., 38*:217, 1978.

Enright, J. T.: The Timing of Sleep and Wakefulness: On the Substructure and Dynamics of the Circadian Pacemakers Underlying the Wake-Sleep Cycle. New York, Springer-Verlag, 1979.

Fuller, R. W.: Pharmacology of central serotonin neurons. *Annu. Rev. Pharmacol. Toxicol.,* 20:111, 1980.

Glaser, G. H., *et al.* (eds.): Antiepileptic Drugs. New York, Raven Press, 1980.

Hobson, J. A., and Brazier, M. A. B. (eds.): The Reticular Formation Revisited: Specifying Function for a Nonspecific System. New York, Raven Press, 1980.

Hyvarinen, J.: Posterior parietal lobe of the primate brain. *Physiol. Rev., 62*:1060, 1982.

Ito, M., *et al.* (eds.): Integrative Control Functions of the Brain. New York, Elsevier/North-Holland, 1978.

Jones, E. G.: Organization of the thalamocortical complex and its relation to sensory processes. *In* Darian-Smith, I. (ed.): Handbook of Physiology. Sec. 1, Vol. III. Bethesda, American Physiological Society, 1984, p. 149.

Klee, M. (ed.): Physiology and Pharmacology of Epileptogenic Phenomena. New York, Raven Press, 1982.

Livingston, R. B.: Sensory Processing, Perception, and Behavior. New York, Raven Press, 1978.

Mitzdorf, U.: Current source-density method and application in cat cerebral cortex: Investigation of evoked potentials and EEG phenomena. *Physiol. Rev.,* 65:37, 1985.

Newmark, M. E., and Penry, J. K.: Genetics of Epilepsy: A Review. New York, Churchill Livingstone, 1980.

O'Keefe, J., and Nadel, L.: The Hippocampus as a Cognitive Map. New York, Oxford University Press, 1978.

Pappenheimer, J. R.: The sleep factor. *Sci. Am., 235*(2):24, 1976.

Passouant, P., and Oswald, I. (eds.): Pharmacology of the States of Alertness. New York, Pergamon Press, 1979.

Plum, F., and Posner, J. B.: The Diagnosis of Stupor and Coma, 3rd Ed. Philadelphia, F. A. Davis, 1980.

Pollack, M. H., *et al.*: Propranolol and depression revisited: Three cases and a review. *J. Nerv. Ment. Dis., 173*:118, 1985.

Regan, D.: Electrical responses evoked from the human brain. *Sci. Am., 241*(6):134, 1979.

Schneider, A. M., and Tarshis, B.: An Introduction to Physiological Psychology. New York, Random House, 1979.

Stern, R. M., *et al.*: Psychophysiological Recording. New York, Oxford University Press, 1980.

Tucek, S.: Regulation of acetylcholine synthesis in the brain. *J. Neurochem.,* 44:11, 1985.

20

Behavioral Functions of the Brain: The Limbic System, Role of the Hypothalamus, and Control of Vegetative Functions of the Body

Behavior is a function of the entire nervous system, not of any particular portion. Even the discrete cord reflexes are an element of behavior, and the wakefulness and sleep cycle discussed in Chapter 19 is certainly one of the most important of our behavioral patterns. However, in this chapter we will deal with those special types of behavior associated with emotions, subconscious motor and sensory drives, and the intrinsic feelings of punishment and pleasure. These functions of the nervous system are performed mainly by subcortical structures located in the basal regions of the brain.

The word "limbic" means "border," and the original usage of the term *limbic system* was to describe the brain structures that lie in the border region between the hypothalamus and its related structures, on the one hand, and the cerebral cortex. However, as we have learned more about the functions of the hypothalamus and the limbic system, it has become clear that they mainly function together as a total system. Therefore, the term limbic system has now been expanded in common usage to mean this entire basal system of the brain that mainly controls the person's emotional behavior and drive.

The hypothalamus and its related structures also control many internal conditions of the body as well as aspects of behavior—such conditions as body temperature, osmolality of the body fluids, the drives to eat and drink, body weight, and so forth. These internal functions are collectively called *vegetative functions* of the body, and their control is obviously closely related to behavior.

FUNCTIONAL ANATOMY OF THE LIMBIC SYSTEM; ITS RELATION TO THE HYPOTHALAMUS

Figure 20–1 illustrates the anatomical structures of the limbic system and its relationship to the hypothalamus, showing these to be an interconnected complex of basal brain elements. Located in the midst of all these is the hypothalamus, which is considered by many anatomists to be a separate structure from the remainder of the limbic system but which, from a physiological point of view, is one of the central elements of the system. Therefore, Figure 20–2 illustrates schematically this key position of the hypothalamus in the limbic system and shows that surrounding it are the other subcortical structures of the limbic system, including the *septum*, the *paraolfactory area*, the *epithalamus*, the *anterior nuclei of the thalamus*, portions of the *basal ganglia*, the *hippocampus*, and the *amygdala*.

Surrounding the subcortical limbic areas is the *limbic cortex* composed of a ring of cerebral cortex (1) beginning in the *orbitofrontal area* on the ventral surface of the frontal lobes, (2) extending upward in the *subcallosal gyrus* beneath the anterior limb of the corpus callosum, (3) over the top of the corpus callosum onto the medial aspect of the cerebral hemisphere in the *cingulate gyrus*, and finally (4) passing behind the corpus callosum and downward onto the ventromedial surface of the temporal lobe to the *parahippocampal gyrus* and *uncus*. Thus, on the medial and ventral surfaces of each cerebral hemisphere is a ring of mostly *paleocortex* that surrounds a group of deep structures intimately associated with overall behavior and with emotions. In turn, this ring of limbic cortex functions as a two-way communication and association linkage between the *neocortex* and the lower limbic structures.

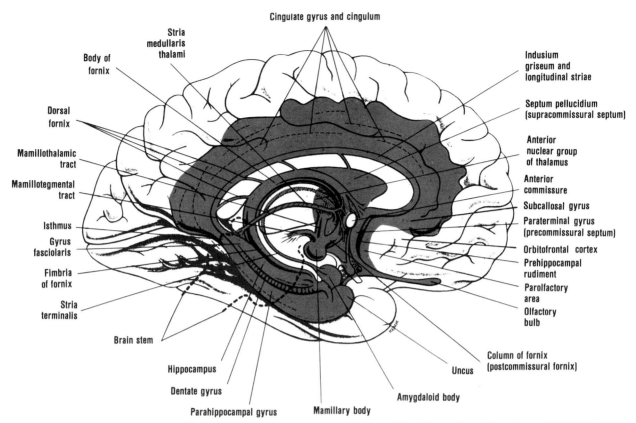

Figure 20–1. Anatomy of the limbic system illustrated by the shaded areas of the figure. (From Warwick and Williams: Gray's Anatomy. 35th Br. ed. London, Longman Group, Ltd., 1973.)

It is also important to recognize that many of the behavioral functions elicited from the hypothalamus and from other limbic structures are mediated through the reticular formation of the brain stem. It was pointed out in Chapters 16 and 19 that stimulation of the excitatory portion of the reticular formation can cause high degrees of somatic excitability; in Chapter 21 we will see that most of the signals for control of the autonomic nervous system also are transmitted through nuclei located in the brain stem.

Therefore, from a physiological point of view the reticular formation and allied regions of the brain stem are a very important part of the limbic system even though anatomically they are considered to be a separate entity. A very important route of communication between the limbic system and the brain stem is the *medial forebrain bundle* that extends from the septal and orbitofrontal cortical regions downward through the hypothalamus to the reticular formation. This bundle carries fibers in both directions, forming a trunk-line communication system. A second route of communication is through short pathways among the reticular formation, the thalamus, the hypothalamus, and most of the other contiguous areas of the basal brain.

THE HYPOTHALAMUS, A MAJOR OUTPUT PATHWAY OF THE LIMBIC SYSTEM

Note in Figure 20–2 that the hypothalamus lies in the very middle of the limbic system. It also has communicating pathways with all levels of this system. In turn, it and its closely allied structures send output signals in three directions: (1) downward through the brain stem mainly into the reticular formation of the mesencephalon, pons, and medulla, (2) upward toward many higher areas of the diencephalon and cerebrum, especially the anterior thalamus and the limbic cortex, and (3) into the infundibulum to control most of the secretory functions of both the posterior and anterior pituitary glands.

In summary, the hypothalamus, which represents less than 1 per cent of the brain mass, nevertheless is the most important of all the motor output pathways of the limbic system. It controls most of the vegetative and endocrine functions of the body as well as many aspects of emotional behavior. Let us discuss first the vegetative and endocrine control functions of the hypothalamus and then return to its behavioral functions to see how all these operate together.

VEGETATIVE AND ENDOCRINE CONTROL FUNCTIONS OF THE HYPOTHALAMUS

The different hypothalamic mechanisms for controlling the vegetative and endocrine functions of the body along with the functions that they control are discussed in many different chapters through-

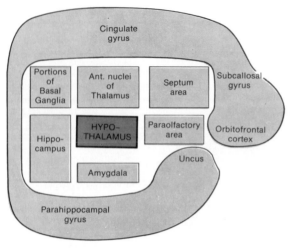

Figure 20–2. The limbic system.

out this text. For instance, the role of the hypothalamus in arterial pressure regulation and in thirst and water conservation in Chapter 27, temperature regulation in Chapter 28, and endocrine control in Chapter 29. However, to illustrate the organization of the hypothalamus as a functional unit, let us summarize the more important of its vegetative and endocrine functions here as well.

Figure 20–3 shows an enlargement of the hypothalamus, which represented only a small area in Figure 20–1. Please take a few minutes to study this diagram, especially to read the multiple activities that are excited or inhibited when respective hypothalamic nuclei are stimulated. In addition to those centers that are illustrated, a large *lateral hypothalamic* area overlies the illustrated areas on each side of the hypothalamus. The lateral areas are especially important in controlling thirst, hunger, and many of the emotional drives.

A word of caution must be issued for studying this diagram, however, for the areas that cause specific activities are not nearly so discrete nor so accurately localized as suggested in the figure. Also, it is not known whether the effects noted in the figure result from stimulation of specific control nuclei or whether they result merely from activation of fiber tracts leading from control nuclei located elsewhere. For instance, stimulation of either the lateral hypothalamus or the posterior hypothalamus, through which many fiber pathways pass, can at times elicit many functions believed to be controlled primarily by other hypothalamic nuclei or even by nuclei outside the hypothalamus. With this caution in mind, we can give the following general description of the vegetative and control functions of the hypothalamus.

Cardiovascular Regulation. Stimulation of different areas throughout the hypothalamus can cause every known type of neurogenic effect on the cardiovascular system, including increased arterial pressure, decreased arterial pressure, increased heart rate, and decreased heart rate. In general, stimulation in the *posterior* and *lateral hypothalamus* increases the arterial pressure and heart rate, while stimulation in the *preoptic area* often has opposite effects, causing a decrease in both heart rate and arterial pressure. These effects are transmitted mainly through the cardiovascular control centers in the reticular substance of the medulla and pons.

Regulation of Body Temperature. Large areas in the anterior portion of the hypothalamus, especially in the *preoptic area*, are concerned with regulation of body temperature. An increase in the temperature of the blood

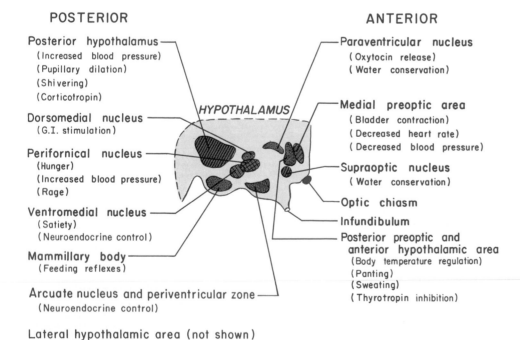

Figure 20–3. Control centers of the hypothalamus.

flowing through these areas increases the activity of temperature-sensitive neurons, whereas a decrease in temperature decreases their activity. In turn, these neurons control the mechanisms for increasing or decreasing body temperature, as discussed in Chapter 28.

Regulation of Body Water. The hypothalamus regulates body water in two separate ways: by creating the sensation of thirst, which makes an animal drink water and by controlling the excretion of water into the urine. An area called the *thirst center* is located in the lateral hypothalamus. When the electrolytes inside the neurons either of this center or allied areas of the hypothalamus become too concentrated, the animal develops an intense desire to drink water; it will search out the nearest source of water and drink enough to return the electrolyte concentration of the thirst center neurons to normal.

Control of renal excretion of water is vested mainly in the *supraoptic* nucleus. When the body fluids become too concentrated, the neurons of this area become stimulated. The nerve fibers from these neurons project downward through the infundibulum into the posterior pituitary gland where they secrete a hormone called *antidiuretic hormone* (also called *vasopressin*). This hormone is then absorbed into the blood and acts on the collecting ducts of the kidneys to cause massive reabsorption of water, thereby decreasing the loss of water into the urine. These functions will be presented in Chapter 27.

Regulation of Uterine Contractility and of Milk Ejection by the Breasts. Stimulation of the *paraventricular nuclei* causes its neuronal cells to secrete the hormone *oxytocin.* This in turn causes increased contractility of the uterus and also contraction of the myoepithelial cells that surround the alveoli of the breasts, which then causes the alveoli to empty the milk through the nipples. At the end of pregnancy, especially large quantities of oxytocin are secreted, and this secretion helps to promote labor contractions that expel the baby. Also, when a baby suckles the mother's breast, a reflex signal from the nipple to the hypothalamus causes oxytocin release, and the oxytocin then performs the necessary function of expelling the milk through the nipples so that the baby can nourish itself. These functions are discussed in Chapter 29.

Gastrointestinal and Feeding Regulation. Stimulation of several areas of the hypothalamus causes an animal to experience extreme hunger, a voracious appetite, and an intense desire to search for food. The area most associated with hunger is the *lateral hypothalamic area.* On the other hand, damage to this causes the animal to lose desire for food, sometimes causing starvation that results in death.

A center that opposes the desire for food, called the *satiety center,* is located in the *ventromedial nucleus.* When this center is stimulated, an animal that is eating food suddenly stops eating and shows complete indifference to the food. On the other hand, if this area is destroyed, the animal cannot be satiated, but instead, its hypothalamic hunger centers become overactive so that it has a voracious appetite, resulting in tremendous obesity.

Another area of the hypothalamus that enters into the overall control of gastrointestinal activity is the *mammillary bodies* that activate many feeding reflexes, such as licking the lips and swallowing.

Hypothalamic Control of the Anterior Pituitary Gland

Stimulation of certain areas of the hypothalamus also causes the anterior pituitary gland to secrete its hormones. This subject will be discussed in detail in Chapter 29 in relation to the neural control of the endocrine glands, but, briefly, the basic mechanism of the control of the anterior pituitary is the following.

The anterior pituitary gland receives its blood supply mainly from veins that flow into the anterior pituitary sinuses from the lower part of the hypothalamus. As the blood courses through the hypothalamus before reaching the anterior pituitary, *releasing hormones* and *inhibitory hormones* are secreted into the blood by various hypothalamic nuclei. They are then transported in the blood to the anterior pituitary where they act on the glandular cells to control the release of the anterior pituitary hormones.

The cell bodies of the neurons that secrete these releasing hormones and inhibitory hormones are located mainly in the medial basal nuclei of the hypothalamus, especially in the *paraventricular zone,* the *arcuate nucleus,* and part of the *ventromedial nucleus.* However, the axons from these nuclei then project to the *median eminence,* which is an enlarged area of the infundibulum where it arises from the inferior border of the hypothalamus. It is here that the nerve terminals actually secrete their releasing and inhibitory hormones. These hormones are then absorbed into the blood capillaries in the median eminence and carried in the venous blood down along the infundibulum to the anterior pituitary gland.

Summary. A number of discrete areas of the hypothalamus have now been found that control specific vegetative functions. However, these areas are still poorly delimited, so much so that the above separation of different areas for different hypothalamic functions is partially artificial.

BEHAVIORAL FUNCTIONS OF THE HYPOTHALAMUS AND ASSOCIATED LIMBIC STRUCTURES

Aside from the vegetative and endocrine functions of the hypothalamus, experiments have shown that stimulation of or lesions in the hypothalamus often have profound effects on emotional behavior of animals or human beings.

In animals, some of the behavioral effects of stimulation are the following:

1. Stimulation in the *lateral hypothalamus* not only causes thirst and hunger as discussed above in relation to the vegetative functions but also increases the general level of activity of the animal, sometimes leading to overt rage and fighting as will be discussed subsequently.

2. Stimulation in the *ventromedial nuclei* and surrounding areas mainly causes effects opposite to those caused by lateral hypothalamic stimulation— that is, a sense of *satiety, decreased eating,* and *tranquility.*

3. Stimulation of a *thin zone of periventricular nuclei,* located immediately adjacent to the third ventricle (or also stimulation of the central gray area of the mesencephalon that is continuous with this portion of the hypothalamus) often leads to *fear* and *punishment reactions.*

4. *Sexual drive* can be stimulated from several areas of the hypothalamus, especially the most

anterior and most posterior portions of the hypothalamus.

Lesions in the hypothalamus, in general, cause the opposite effects. For instance:

1. Bilateral lesions in the lateral hypothalamus will decrease drinking and eating almost to zero, often leading to lethal starvation, as was discussed above in relation to the vegetative functions of the lateral hypothalamus. But these lesions cause extreme *passivity* of the animal as well, with loss of most of its overt activities.

2. Bilateral lesions of the ventromedial areas of the hypothalamus cause exactly opposite effects: excessive drinking and eating, as well as hyperactivity and often continuous savagery along with frequent bouts of extreme rage on the slightest provocation.

Lesions or stimulation in other regions of the limbic system, especially the amygdala, the septal area, and areas in the mesencephalon, often also cause effects similar to those elicited directly from the hypothalamus. We will discuss some of these in more detail later.

The Reward and Punishment Function of the Limbic System

From the preceding discussion it is already clear that the hypothalamus and other limbic structures are particularly concerned with the affective nature of sensory sensations—that is, whether the sensations are *pleasant* or *unpleasant*. These affective qualities are also called *reward* and *punishment* or *satisfaction* and *aversion*. Electrical stimulation of certain regions pleases or satisfies the animal, whereas electrical stimulation of other regions causes terror, pain, fear, defense, escape reactions, and all the other elements of punishment. Obviously, these two oppositely responding systems greatly affect the behavior of the animal.

Reward Centers. Figure 20–4 illustrates a technique that has been used for localizing the specific reward and punishment areas of the brain. In this figure a lever is placed at the side of the cage and is arranged so that depressing the lever makes electrical contact with a stimulator. Electrodes are placed successively at different areas in the brain so that the animal can stimulate the area by pressing the lever. If stimulating the particular area gives the animal a sense of reward, then it will press the lever again and again, sometimes as much as 10,000 times per hour. Furthermore, when offered the choice of eating some delectable food as opposed to the opportunity to stimulate the reward center, it often chooses the electrical stimulation.

By using this procedure, the major reward centers have been found to be located *along the course of the medial forebrain bundle*, especially in the *lateral* and *ventromedial nuclei of the hypothalamus*. It is strange that the lateral nuclei should be included among the reward areas—indeed it is one of the most

potent reward areas of all—because even stronger stimuli in this area can cause rage. But this is true in many areas, with weaker stimuli giving a sense of reward and stronger ones a sense of punishment.

Less potent reward centers, which are perhaps secondary to the major ones in the hypothalamus, are found in the septum, the amygdala, certain areas of the thalamus and basal ganglia, and finally extending downward into the basal tegmentum of the mesencephalon.

Punishment Centers. The apparatus illustrated in Figure 20–4 can also be connected so that pressing the lever turns off rather than turns on an electrical stimulus. In this case, the animal will not turn the stimulus off when the electrode is in one of the reward areas, but when it is in certain other areas it immediately learns to turn it off. Stimulation in these areas causes the animal to show all the signs of displeasure, fear, terror, and punishment. Furthermore, prolonged stimulation for 24 hours or more can cause the animal to become severely sick and actually lead to death.

By means of this technique, the most potent areas for punishment and escape tendencies have been found in the *central gray area surrounding the aqueduct of Sylvius in the mesencephalon* and extending upward into the *periventricular zones of the hypothalamus and thalamus*. Also, less potent punishment areas are found in the *amygdala* and the *hippocampus*.

It is particularly interesting that stimulation in the punishment centers can frequently inhibit the reward and pleasure centers completely, illustrating that punishment and fear can take precedence over pleasure and reward.

Importance of Reward and Punishment in Behavior. Almost everything that we do is related in some way to reward and punishment. If we are

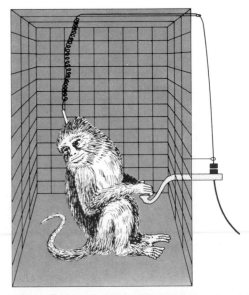

Figure 20–4. Technique for localizing reward and punishment centers in the brain of a monkey.

doing something that is rewarding, we continue to do it; if it is punishing, we cease to do it. Therefore, the reward and punishment centers undoubtedly constitute one of the most important of all the controllers of our bodily activities, our drives, and so forth.

Importance of Reward and Punishment in Learning and Memory—Habituation or Reinforcement. Animal experiments have shown that a sensory experience causing neither reward nor punishment is remembered hardly at all. Electrical recordings show that new and novel sensory stimuli always excite the cerebral cortex. But repetition of the stimulus over and over leads to almost complete extinction of the cortical response if the sensory experience does not elicit either a sense of reward or punishment. Thus, the animal becomes *habituated* to the sensory stimulus, and thereafter ignores it.

However, if the stimulus causes either reward or punishment rather than indifference, the cortical response becomes progressively more and more intense with repeated stimulation instead of fading away, and the response is said to be *reinforced*. Thus, an animal builds up strong memory traces for sensations that are either rewarding or punishing but, on the other hand, develops complete habituation to indifferent sensory stimuli. Therefore, it is evident that the reward and punishment centers of the limbic system have much to do with selecting the information that we learn.

Effect of Tranquilizers on the Reward and Punishment Centers. Administration of a tranquilizer, such as chlorpromazine, inhibits both the reward and punishment centers, thereby greatly decreasing the affective reactivity of the animal. Therefore, it is presumed that tranquilizers function in psychotic states by suppressing many of the important behavioral areas of the hypothalamus and its associated regions of the brain, a subject that we will discuss more fully later.

Rage

An emotional pattern that involves the hypothalamus and has been well characterized is the *rage pattern*. This can be described as follows:

Strong stimulation of the punishment centers of the brain, especially the *periventricular zone of the hypothalamus* or in the *lateral hypothalamus*, causes the animal to (1) develop a defense posture, (2) extend its claws, (3) lift its tail, (4) hiss, (5) spit, (6) growl, and (7) develop piloerection, wide-open eyes, and dilated pupils. Furthermore, even the slightest provocation causes an immediate savage attack. This is approximately the behavior that one would expect from an animal being severely punished, and it is a pattern of behavior that is called *rage*.

Stimulation of the more rostral areas of the punishment areas—in the midline preoptic areas—causes mainly fear and anxiety, associated with a tendency for the animal to run away.

In the normal animal the rage phenomenon is held in check mainly by counterbalancing activity of the ventromedial nuclei of the hypothalamus. In addition, the hippocampus, the amygdala, and the anterior portions of the limbic cortex, especially the limbic cortex of the anterior cingulate gyrus and the subcallosal gyrus, help suppress the rage phenomenon. Conversely, if these portions of the limbic system are damaged or destroyed, the animal (also the human being) becomes far more susceptible to bouts of rage.

Placidity and Tameness. Exactly the opposite emotional behavioral patterns occur when the reward centers are stimulated: placidity and tameness.

Function of the Hypothalamus and Other Limbic Areas in Sleep, Wakefulness, Alertness, and Excitement

Stimulation of regions of the hypothalamus dorsal to the mammillary bodies greatly excites the reticular activating system and therefore causes wakefulness, alertness, and excitement. In addition, the sympathetic nervous system becomes excited in general, increasing the arterial pressure, causing pupillary dilatation, and enhancing other activities associated with sympathetic activity.

On the other hand, stimulation of some areas in the septum, in the anterior hypothalamus, or in isolated points of the thalamic portions of the reticular activating system often inhibits the mesencephalic portion of the reticular activating system, causing somnolence and sometimes actual sleep. Thus, the hypothalamus and other limbic structures indirectly contribute much to the control of the degree of excitement and alertness.

SPECIFIC FUNCTIONS OF OTHER PARTS OF THE LIMBIC SYSTEM

FUNCTIONS OF THE AMYGDALA

The amygdala is a complex of nuclei located immediately beneath the medial surface of the cerebral cortex in the anterior pole of each temporal lobe, and it has abundant bidirectional connections with the hypothalamus. In lower animals, this complex is concerned to a great extent with association of olfactory stimuli with stimuli from other parts of the brain. Indeed, it is pointed out in Chapter 26 that one of the major divisions of the olfactory tract leads directly to a portion of the amygdala called the *corticomedial nuclei* that lie immediately beneath the cortex in the pyriform area of the temporal lobe. However, in the human being, another portion of the amygdala, the *basolateral nuclei*, has become much more highly developed than the olfactory portion and plays important roles in many behavioral activities not generally associated with olfactory stimuli.

The amygdala receives impulses from all portions of the limbic cortex, from the orbital surfaces of the frontal lobes, from the cingulate gyrus, from the parahippocampal gyrus, and from the neocortex of the temporal, parietal, and occipital lobes, especially from the auditory and visual association areas. Because of these multiple connections, the amygdala has been called the "window" through which the limbic system sees the place of the person in the world. In turn, the amygdala transmits signals (1) back into these same cortical areas, (2) into the hippocampus, (3) into the septum, (4) into the thalamus, and (5) especially into the hypothalamus.

Effects of Stimulating the Amygdala. In general, stimulation in the amygdala can cause almost all the same effects as those elicited by stimulation of the hypothalamus, plus still other effects. The effects that are mediated through the hypothalamus include (1) increases or decreases in arterial pressure, (2) increases or decreases in heart rate, (3) increases or decreases in gastrointestinal motility and secretion, (4) defecation and micturition, (5) pupillary dilatation or, rarely, constriction, (6) piloerection, (7) secretion of the various anterior pituitary hormones, including especially the gonadotropins and ACTH.

Aside from these effects mediated through the hypothalamus, amygdala stimulation can also cause different types of involuntary movement. These include (1) tonic movements, such as raising the head or bending the body, (2) circling movements, (3) occasionally clonic, rhythmic movements, and (4) different types of movements associated with olfaction and eating, such as licking, chewing, and swallowing.

In addition, stimulation of certain amygdaloid nuclei can, rarely, cause a pattern of rage, escape, punishment, and fear similar to the rage pattern elicited from the hypothalamus as described earlier. And stimulation of other nuclei can give reactions of reward and pleasure.

Finally, excitation of still other portions of the amygdala can cause sexual activities that include erection, copulatory movements, ejaculation, ovulation, uterine activity, and premature labor.

Effects of Bilateral Ablation of the Amygdala—The Klüver-Bucy Syndrome. When the anterior portions of both temporal lobes are destroyed in a monkey, this not only removes the temporal cortex but also the amygdalas that lie deep in these parts of the temporal lobes. This causes a combination of changes in behavior called the Klüver-Bucy syndrome, which includes (1) excessive tendency to examine objects orally, (2) loss of fear, (3) decreased aggressiveness, (4) tameness, (5) changes in dietary habits, even to the extent that a herbivorous animal frequently becomes carnivorous, (6) sometimes psychic blindness, and (7) often excessive sex drive. The characteristic picture is of an animal that is not afraid of anything, has extreme curiosity about everything, forgets very rapidly, has a tendency to place everything in its mouth and sometimes even tries to eat solid objects, and, finally, often has a sex drive so strong that it attempts to copulate with immature animals, animals of the wrong sex, or animals of a different species.

Though similar lesions in human beings are rare, afflicted persons respond in a manner not too different from that of the monkey.

Overall Function of the Amygdala. The amygdala seems to be a behavioral awareness area that operates at a semiconscious level. It also seems to project into the limbic system one's present status in relation both to surroundings and thoughts. Based on this information, the amygdala is believed to help pattern the person's behavioral response so that it is appropriate for each occasion.

FUNCTIONS OF THE HIPPOCAMPUS

The hippocampus is an elongated structure composed of a modified type of cerebral cortex. In fact it is that portion of the temporal lobe cortex that folds inward to form the ventral surface of the inferior horn of the lateral ventricle. One end of the hippocampus abuts the amygdaloid nuclei, and it also fuses along one of its borders with the parahippocampal gyrus, which is the cortex of the ventromedial surface of the temporal lobe.

The hippocampus has numerous connections with most portions of the cerebral cortex as well as with the basic structures of the limbic system—the amygdala, the hypothalamus, the septum, and the mammillary bodies. Almost any type of sensory experience causes instantaneous activation of different parts of the hippocampus, and the hippocampus in turn distributes many outgoing signals to the hypothalamus and other parts of the limbic system, especially through the *fornix*, one of its major output pathways. Thus, the hippocampus, like the amygdala, is an additional channel through which incoming sensory signals can lead to appropriate limbic reactions, but perhaps for different purposes as we shall see later.

As in other limbic structures, stimulation of different areas in the hippocampus can cause almost any one of different behavioral patterns, such as rage, passivity, excess sex drive, or so forth.

Another feature of the hippocampus is that very weak electrical stimuli can cause local epileptic seizures that persist for many seconds after the stimulation is over, suggesting that the hippocampus can perhaps give off prolonged output signals even under normal functioning conditions. During the hippocampal seizures, the person experiences various psychomotor effects, including olfactory, visual, auditory, tactile, and other types of hallucinations that cannot be suppressed even though the person has not lost consciousness and knows these hallucinations to be unreal. Probably one of the reasons for this hyperexcitability of the hippocampus is that it is composed of a different type of cortex from that elsewhere in the cerebrum, having only three neuronal layers instead of the six layers found elsewhere.

Effect of Bilateral Removal of the Hippocampi—Inability to Learn. The hippocampi have been surgically removed bilaterally in a few human beings for the treatment of epilepsy. These persons can perform most previously learned activities satisfactorily. However, they can learn essentially nothing new. In fact, they cannot even learn the names or the faces of persons with whom they come in contact every day. Yet, they can remember for a moment or so what transpires during the course of their activities. Thus, they do have a type of short-term primary memory even though their ability to establish new long-term secondary memories is either completely or almost completely abolished, which is the phenomenon called *anterograde amnesia* that was discussed in Chapter 18.

Destruction of the hippocampi also causes some deficit in previously learned memories (retrograde amnesia), a little more so for recent memories than for memories of the distant past.

Theoretical Function of the Hippocampus in Learning. The hippocampus originated as part of the olfactory cortex. In the very lowest animals it plays essential roles in determining whether the animal will eat a particular food, whether the smell of a particular object suggests danger, whether the odor is sexually inviting, and in making other decisions that are of life and death importance. Thus, very early in the development of the brain, the hippocampus presumably became a critical decision-making neuronal mechanism, determining the importance and type of importance of the incoming sensory signals. Presumably, as the remainder of the brain developed, the connections from the other sensory areas into the hippocampus have continued to utilize this decision-making capability.

Earlier in this chapter (and also in the previous chapter), it was pointed out that reward and punishment play a major role in determining the importance of information and especially whether or not the information will be stored in memory. A person rapidly becomes habituated to indifferent stimuli but learns assiduously any sensory experience that causes either pleasure or punishment. Yet, what is the mechanism by which this occurs? It has been suggested that the hippocampus provides the drive that causes translation of primary memory into secondary memory—that is, it transmits some type of signal to the long-term memory storage area directing that permanent storage shall take place.

Whatever the mechanism, without the hippocampi *consolidation* of long-term memories does not take place. This is especially true for verbal information, perhaps because the temporal lobes, in which the hippocampi are located, are particularly concerned with verbal information.

FUNCTION OF THE LIMBIC CORTEX

Probably the most poorly understood portion of the entire limbic system is the ring of cerebral cortex called the *limbic cortex* that surrounds the subcortical limbic structures. This cortex functions as a transitional zone through which signals are transmitted from the remainder of the cortex into the limbic system. Therefore, it is presumed that the limbic cortex functions as a cerebral *association area for control of behavior.*

Stimulation of the different regions of the limbic cortex has failed to give any real idea of their functions. However, as is true of so many other portions of the limbic system, essentially all the behavioral patterns that have already been described can also be elicited by stimulation in different portions of the limbic cortex. Likewise, ablation of a few limbic cortical areas can cause persistent changes in an animal's behavior, though ablation in most areas has little effect. Some of the areas that have been noted to cause specific changes include:

Ablation of the Temporal Cortex. When the anterior temporal cortex is ablated bilaterally, the amygdala is almost invariably damaged as well. This was discussed earlier, and it was pointed out that the Klüver-Bucy syndrome occurs. The animal develops consummatory behavior especially, investigates any and all objects, has intense sex drives toward inappropriate animals or even inanimate objects, and loses all fear—thus develops tameness as well.

Ablation of the Posterior Orbital Frontal Cortex. Bilateral removal of the posterior portion of the orbital frontal cortex often causes an animal to develop insomnia and an intense degree of motor restlessness, becoming unable to sit still but moving about continually.

Ablation of the Anterior Cingulate Gyri and Subcallosal Gyri. The anterior cingulate gyri and the subcallosal gyri are the portions of the limbic cortex that communicate between the prefrontal cerebral cortex and the subcortical limbic structures. Destruction of these gyri bilaterally releases the rage centers of the septum and hypothalamus from an inhibitory influence. Therefore, the animal can become vicious and much more subject to fits of rage than normally.

Summary. Until further information is available, it is perhaps best to state that the cortical regions of the limbic system occupy intermediate associative positions between the functions of the remainder of the cerebral cortex and the functions of the subcortical limbic structures for control of behavioral patterns. Thus, in the anterior temporal cortex one especially finds gustatory and olfactory associations. In the parahippocampal gyri there is a tendency for complex auditory associations and also complex thought associations derived from Wernicke's area of the posterior temporal lobe. In the cingulate cortex, there is reason to believe that sensorimotor associations occur.

FUNCTION OF SPECIFIC CHEMICAL TRANSMITTER SYSTEMS FOR BEHAVIOR CONTROL

In previous chapters it has already been pointed out that several special collections of neurons in the brain stem radiate to multiple areas of the forebrain, each releasing a specific chemical transmitter substance. Three of these special chemical transmitter systems have received particular attention as behavior modifiers; these are the norepinephrine system, the serotonin system, and the dopamine system.

The Norepinephrine and Serotonin Systems and Their Relationship to Depression and Manic-Depressive Psychoses. In the previous chapter it was pointed out that large numbers of *norepinephrine-secreting neurons* are located in the reticular formation, especially in the *locus ceruleus,* and that these send fibers upward to most parts of the limbic system, the thalamus, and cerebral cortex. Also, many *serotonin-producing neurons* are located in the *midline raphe nuclei* of the lower pons and medulla and also project fibers to many areas of the limbic system and to some other areas of the brain as well.

In the past few years much evidence has accumulated to show that the *mental depression psychosis,* which afflicts about 8 million people in the United States at any one time, might be caused by diminished formation of either norepinephrine or serotonin or both. These patients experience symptoms of grief, unhappiness, despair, and misery. In addition, they lose their appetite and sex drive and also have severe insomnia. And associated with all these is a state of psychomotor agitation despite the depression.

A principal reason for believing that depression is caused by diminished activity of the norepinephrine and serotonin systems is that drugs that block the secretion of norepinephrine and serotonin, such as the drug reserpine, frequently cause depression. Conversely, about 70 per cent of depressive patients can be treated very effectively with one of two types of drugs that increase norepinephrine and serotonin at the nerve endings: *monoamine oxidase inhibitors* that block destruction of norepinephrine and serotonin once they are formed and *tricyclic antidepressants* that block reuptake of norepinephrine and serotonin by the nerve endings so that these transmitters remain active for longer periods of time after secretion.

(Mental depression can also be treated effectively by electroconvulsive therapy—commonly called "shock therapy." In this therapy an electric shock is used to cause a generalized seizure similar to that of an epileptic attack. This causes considerable retrograde memory loss that recovers in about two to three weeks. Mental depression is one of the very few mental illnesses in which such shock therapy is of real value. However, the reason for its value is still to be determined.)

Some patients with mental depression alternate between depression and mania, which is called the *manic-depressive psychosis*, and a few persons exhibit only mania without the depressive episodes. Drugs that block the formation or action of norepinephrine and serotonin, such as lithium compounds, can be effective in treating the manic condition.

Therefore, it is presumed that the norepinephrine and serotonin systems normally function to provide motor drive to the limbic system to increase a person's sense of well being, to create happiness, contentment, good appetite, appropriate sex drive, and psychomotor balance, though too much of a good thing can cause mania.

The Dopamine System and Its Relationship to Schizophrenia. There are many reasons to believe that schizophrenia might be caused by excess secretion of dopamine in the brain. In Chapter 16 we discussed the dopaminergic neurons that project from the substantia nigra to the basal ganglia and exert an important inhibitory restraint on basal ganglial activity. In addition to the dopaminergic neurons in the substantia nigra, still other dopaminergic neurons are located in the ventral tegmentum of the mesencephalon medial and superior to the substantia nigra. These neurons give rise to the so-called *mesolimbic dopaminergic system* that projects nerve fibers mainly into the medial and anterior portions of the limbic system, especially into the amygdala, the anterior caudate nucleus, and the anterior cingulate gyrus of the cortex, all of which are powerful behavioral control centers.

Some of the reasons for believing the mesolimbic dopaminergic system to be related to schizophrenia are the following: When Parkinson's disease patients are treated with L-dopa, which releases dopamine in the brain, the parkinsonian patient sometimes develops schizophrenic symptoms, indicating that excess dopaminergic activity can cause dissociation of a person's drives and thought patterns. However, an even more compelling reason for believing that schizophrenia might be caused by excess production of dopamine is that those drugs that are effective in treating schizophrenia, such as chlorpromazine and haloperidol, all decrease the secretion of dopamine by the dopaminergic nerve endings or decrease the effect of dopamine on the subsequent neurons.

Almost certainly there are other factors in schizophrenia besides excess secretion of dopamine, but, nevertheless, the symptoms of schizophrenia are believed to be similar to the behavioral effects of excessive dopamine as follows: (1) a sense of persecution from outside sources, (2) hearing of voices, (3) incoherent speech, (4) dissociation of ideas and abnormal sequences of thought, and (5) sometimes abnormal postures or rigidities.

The Enkephalin-Endorphin System. Very little is yet known about the behavioral functions of the enkephalin-endorphin system. However, the probable role of this system for suppression of pain was discussed in Chapter 14. It presumably has many other activities as well,

because it is secreted in many areas of the brain stem and thalamus.

Effects of the General Hormones on Behavior. Several of the general hormones have specific effects on behavior. Some of these are:

Thyroid hormone increases the overall *metabolism of the body* and increases overall activity of the nervous system as well.

Both *testosterone* in the male and *estrogen* in the female increase *libido*. Also, injection of a minute quantity of estrogen into the anterior hypothalamus of some lower animals will cause estrous behavior (heat). The sex drive of the human female seems to be increased near the time of ovulation when estrogen secretion is high.

A small, 6 or 7 amino acid *fragment of ACTH*, when injected into the brain of an animal, can cause *intense fear*.

Injection of *norepinephrine*, or excess secretion of norepinephrine or epinephrine by the adrenal medullae, increases the overall activity of the brain, which is essentially the same effect as produced by stimulating the reticular activating system.

Thus, it is becoming clear that various chemical and transmitter systems play important roles in determining an animal's behavior. Furthermore, abnormalities of some of the brain's chemical transmitter systems seem to be the bases of some of the common psychoses.

PSYCHOSOMATIC EFFECTS OF THE BEHAVIORAL SYSTEM

We are all familiar with the fact that abnormal function in the central nervous system can frequently lead to serious dysfunction of the different somatic organs of the body. This is also true in experimental animals. Indeed, prolonged electrical stimulation in the punishment regions of the brain can actually lead to severe sickness of the animal, culminating in death within 24 to 48 hours. We need, therefore, to discuss briefly the mechanisms by which stimulatory effects in the brain can affect the peripheral organs. Ordinarily, this occurs through three routes: (1) through the motor nerves to the skeletal muscles throughout the body, (2) through the autonomic nerves to the different internal organs of the body, and (3) through the hormones secreted by the pituitary gland in response to nervous activity in the hypothalamus, as will be explained in Chapter 29.

Psychosomatic Disorders Transmitted Through the Skeletal Nervous System. In neurotic and psychotic states such as anxiety, tension, and mania, generalized overactivity of both the muscles and sympathetic system often occurs throughout the body. This in turn results in intense feedback from the muscle proprioceptors to the reticular activating system, and the norepinephrine and epinephrine circulating in the blood as a result of the sympathetic activity also excite the reticular activating system, all of which undoubtedly help maintain an extreme degree of wakefulness and alertness that characterizes these emotional states. Unfortunately, though, the wakefulness prevents adequate sleep and also leads to progressive bodily fatigue and mental dissociations.

Transmission of Psychosomatic Effects Through the Autonomic Nervous System. Many psychosomatic abnormalities result from hyperactivity of either the sympathetic or parasympathetic system. In general, hyperactivity of the sympathetic system occurs in many areas of the body at the same time rather than in focal areas, and the usual effects are (1) increased heart rate—sometimes with palpitation of the heart, (2) increased arterial pressure, (3) constipation, and (4) increased metabolic rate. On the other hand, parasympathetic signals are likely to be much more focal. For instance, stimulation or inhibition of specific areas in the dorsal motor nuclei of the vagus nerves can cause more or less specifically (1) increased or decreased heart rate or palpitation of the heart, (2) esophageal spasm, (3) increased peristalsis in the upper gastrointestinal tract, or (4) increased hyperacidity of the stomach with resultant development of peptic ulcer. Stimulation of the sacral region of the parasympathetic system, on the other hand, is likely to cause extreme colonic glandular secretion and peristalsis with resulting diarrhea.

One can readily see, then, that emotional patterns controlling the sympathetic and parasympathetic centers of the hypothalamus and lower brain stem can cause wide varieties of peripheral psychosomatic effects.

Psychosomatic Effects Transmitted Through the Anterior Pituitary Gland. Electrical stimulation of the midbasal hypothalamus increases the secretion of corticotropin (ACTH) by the anterior pituitary gland (as explained earlier in the chapter) and therefore indirectly increases the output of adrenocortical hormones. One of the effects of this is a gradual increase in stomach hyperacidity because of the effect of glucocorticoids on stomach secretion. Over a prolonged period of time this obviously could lead to peptic ulcer, which is a well-known effect of hypersecretion by the adrenal cortex. Likewise, activity in the preoptic area of the hypothalamus increases the pituitary secretion of thyrotropin, which in turn increases the output of thyroxine and leads to an elevated basal metabolic rate. It is well known that different types of emotional disturbances can lead to thyrotoxicosis (as will be explained in Chapter 76), this presumably resulting from overactivity in the hypothalamus.

From these examples, therefore, it is evident that many types of psychosomatic diseases of the body can be caused by abnormal control of anterior pituitary secretion.

REFERENCES

Baldessarini, R. J., and Tarsy, D.: Dopamine and the pathophysiology of dyskinesias induced by antipsychotic drugs. *Annu. Rev. Neurosci.*, 3:23, 1980.

Berger, P. A., *et al.*: Behavioral pharmacology of the endorphins. *Annu. Rev. Med.*, 33:397, 1982.

Burchfield, S. R. (ed.): Stress. Physiological and Psychological Interactions. Washington, D.C., Hemisphere Publishing Corp., 1985.

Buzsaki, G.: Feed-forward inhibition in the hippocampal formation. *Prog. Neurobiol.*, 22:131, 1984.

Cohen, D. H., and Randall, D. C.: Classical conditioning of cardiovascular responses. *Annu. Rev. Physiol.*, 46:187, 1984.

Cotman, C. W., and McGaugh, J. L.: Behavioral Neuroscience. New York, Academic Press, 1979.

de Wied, D., and Jolles, J.: Neuropeptides derived from pro-opiocortin: Behavioral, physiological, and neurochemical effects. *Physiol. Rev.*, 62:976, 1982.

Doris, P. A.: Vasopressin and central integrative processes. *Neuroendocrinology*, 38:75, 1984.

Engel, B. T., and Schneiderman, N.: Operant conditioning and the modulation of cardiovascular function. *Annu. Rev. Physiol.*, 46:199, 1984.

Fink, M.: Convulsive and drug therapies of depression. *Annu. Rev. Med.*, 32:405, 1981.

Foote, S. L., *et al.*: Nucleus locus ceruleus: New evidence of anatomical and physiological specificity. *Physiol. Rev.*, 63:844, 1983.

Fuller, R. W.: Pharmacology of brain epinephrine neurons. *Annu. Rev. Pharmacol. Toxicol.*, 22:31, 1982.

Ganong, W. F.: The brain renin-angiotensin system. *Annu. Rev. Physiol.*, 46:17, 1984.

Givens, J. R.: The Hypothalamus in Health and Disease. Chicago, Year Book Medical Publishers, 1984.

Guillemin, R.: Neuroendocrine interrelations. *In* Bondy, P. K., and Rosenberg, L. E. (eds.): Metabolic Control and Disease, 8th Ed. Philadelphia, W. B. Saunders Co., 1980, p. 1155.

Iversen, L. L.: Nonopioid neuropeptides in mammalian CNS. *Annu. Rev. Pharmacol. Toxicol.*, 23:1, 1983.

Kelly, D.: Anxiety and Emotions: Physiological Basis and Treatment. Springfield, Ill., Charles C Thomas, 1979.

Klimov, P. K.: Behavior of the organs of the digestive system. *Neurosci. Behav. Physiol.*, 14:333, 1984.

Lechtenberg, R.: Psychiatrist's Guide to Diseases of the Nervous System. New York, John Wiley & Sons, 1982.

Malick, J. B. (ed.): Anxiolytics. Neurochemical, Behavioral, and Clinical Perspectives. New York, Raven Press, 1983.

McFadden, D. (ed.): Neural Mechanisms in Behavior. New York, Springer-Verlag, 1980.

Russell, R. W.: Cholinergic system in behavior: The search for mechanisms of action. *Annu. Rev. Pharmacol. Toxicol.*, 22:435, 1982.

Siddle, D.: Orienting and Habituation. Perspectives in Human Research. New York, John Wiley & Sons, 1982.

Skodol, A. E., and Spitzer, R. L.: The development of reliable diagnostic criteria in psychiatry. *Annu. Rev. Med.*, 33:317, 1982.

Smith, O. A., and DeVito, J. L.: Central neural integration for the control of autonomic responses associated with emotion. *Annu. Rev. Neurosci.*, 7:43, 1984.

Snyder, S.: Biological Aspects of Mental Disorders. New York, Oxford University Press, 1980.

Stephenson, R. B.: Modification of reflex regulation of blood pressure by behavior. *Annu. Rev. Physiol.*, 46:133, 1984.

Swanson, L. W., and Sawchenko, P. E.: Hypothalamic integration: Organization of the paraventricular and supraoptic nuclei. *Annu. Rev. Neurosci.*, 6:269, 1983.

Tucek, S.: Regulation of acetylcholine synthesis in the brain. *J. Neurochem.*, 44:11, 1985.

Usdin, E.: Stress. The Role of Catecholamines and Other Neurotransmitters. New York, Gordon Press Publishers, 1984.

Verrier, R. L., and Lown, B.: Behavioral stress and cardiac arrhythmias. *Annu. Rev. Physiol.*, 46:155, 1984.

21

The Autonomic Nervous System; The Adrenal Medulla

The portion of the nervous system that controls the visceral functions of the body is called the *autonomic nervous system*. This system helps control arterial pressure, gastrointestinal motility and secretion, urinary bladder emptying, sweating, body temperature, and many other activities, some of which are controlled almost entirely and some only partially by the autonomic nervous system.

One of the most striking characteristics of the autonomic nervous system is the rapidity and intensity with which it can change visceral functions. For instance, within 3 to 5 seconds it can increase the heart rate to two times normal, and the arterial pressure can be doubled within as little as 10 to 15 seconds; or, at the other extreme, the arterial pressure can be decreased low enough within 4 to 5 seconds to cause a faint. Sweating can begin within seconds, and the bladder may empty involuntarily, also within seconds. Thus, the nervous system, acting through the autonomic nerve fibers, can exert rapid and effective control of many if not most of the internal functions of the body. It is these extremely rapid changes that are measured by the lie detector polygraph, reflecting the innermost feelings of a person.

GENERAL ORGANIZATION OF THE AUTONOMIC NERVOUS SYSTEM

The autonomic nervous system is activated mainly by centers located in the *spinal cord, brain stem*, and *hypothalamus*. Also, portions of the cerebral cortex and especially of the limbic system can transmit impulses to the lower centers and in this way influence autonomic control. Often the autonomic nervous system also operates by means of *visceral reflexes*. That is, sensory signals enter the centers of the autonomic ganglia, cord, brain stem, or hypothalamus, and these in turn transmit appropriate reflex responses back to the visceral organs to control their activities.

The autonomic signals are transmitted to the body through two major subdivisions called the *sympa-thetic* and *parasympathetic systems*, the characteristics and functions of which follow.

PHYSIOLOGICAL ANATOMY OF THE SYMPATHETIC NERVOUS SYSTEM

Figure 21–1 illustrates the general organization of the sympathetic nervous system, showing one of the two *paravertebral sympathetic chains* to the side of the spinal column and nerves extending to the different internal organs. The sympathetic nerves originate in the spinal cord between the segments T-1 and L-2 and pass from here first into the sympathetic chain, thence to the tissues and organs that are stimulated by the sympathetic nerves.

Preganglionic and Postganglionic Sympathetic Neurons. The sympathetic nerves are different from skeletal motor nerves in the following way: Each motor pathway from the cord to a skeletal muscle is comprised of a single fiber. Each sympathetic pathway, on the other hand, is comprised of two fibers, a *preganglionic neuron* and a *postganglionic neuron*. The cell body of a preganglionic neuron lies in the *intermediolateral horn* of the spinal cord, and its fiber passes, as illustrated in Figure 21–2, through an *anterior root* of the cord into a *spinal nerve*.

Immediately after the spinal nerve leaves the spinal column, the preganglionic sympathetic fibers leave the nerve and pass through the *white ramus* into one of the *ganglia* of the *sympathetic chain*. Then the course of the fibers can be one of the following three: (1) It can synapse with postganglionic neurons in the ganglion that it enters. (2) It can pass upward or downward in the chain and synapse in one of the other ganglia of the chain. Or (3) it can pass for variable distances through the chain and then through one of the nerves radiating outward from the chain, finally terminating in an *outlying sympathetic ganglion*.

The postganglionic neuron, therefore, can originate either in one of the sympathetic chain ganglia or in one of the outlying ganglia. From either of these two sources, the postganglionic fibers then travel to their destinations in the various organs.

Sympathetic Nerve Fibers in the Skeletal Nerves. Many of the postganglionic fibers pass back from the sympathetic chain into the spinal nerves through *gray rami* (see Fig. 21–2) at all levels of the cord. These pathways are made up of type C fibers that extend to all parts of the body in the skeletal nerves. They control the

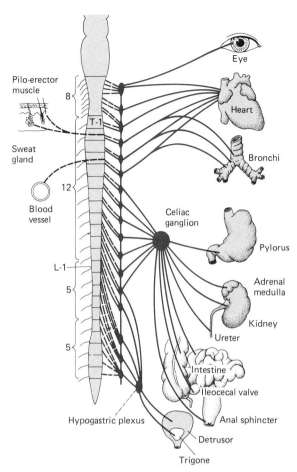

Figure 21–1. The sympathetic nervous system. Dashed lines represent postganglionic fibers in the gray rami leading into the spinal nerves for distribution to blood vessels, sweat glands, and piloerector muscles.

blood vessels, sweat glands, and piloerector muscles of the hairs. Approximately 8 per cent of the fibers in the average skeletal nerve are sympathetic fibers, a fact that indicates their importance.

Segmental Distribution of Sympathetic Nerves. The sympathetic pathways originating in the different segments of the spinal cord are not necessarily distributed to the same part of the body as the spinal nerve fibers from the same segments. Instead, the *sympathetic fibers from T-1 generally pass up the sympathetic chain into the head; from T-2 into the neck; T-3, T-4, T-5, and T-6 into the thorax; T-7, T-8, T-9, T-10, and T-11 into the abdomen; and T-12, L-1, and L-2 into the legs.* This distribution is only approximate and overlaps greatly.

The distribution of sympathetic nerves to each organ is determined partly by the position in the embryo at which the organ originates. For instance, the heart receives many sympathetic nerves from the neck portion of the sympathetic chain because the heart originates in the neck of the embryo. Likewise, the abdominal organs receive their sympathetic innervation from the lower thoracic segments because the primitive gut originates in this area.

Special Nature of the Sympathetic Nerve Endings in the Adrenal Medullae. Preganglionic sympathetic nerve fibers pass, without synapsing, all the way from the intermediolateral horn cells of the spinal cord, through the sympathetic chains, through the splanchnic nerves, and finally into the adrenal medullae. There they end directly on special cells that secrete epinephrine and norepinephrine directly into the circulatory blood. These secretory cells embryologically are derived from nervous tissue and are analogous to postganglionic neurons; indeed, they even have rudimentary nerve fibers, and it is these fibers that secrete the hormones.

PHYSIOLOGICAL ANATOMY OF THE PARASYMPATHETIC NERVOUS SYSTEM

The parasympathetic nervous system is illustrated in Figure 21–3, showing that parasympathetic fibers leave the central nervous system through several of the cranial nerves, the second and third sacral spinal nerves, and occasionally the first and fourth sacral nerves. About 75 per cent of all parasympathetic nerve fibers are in the vagus nerves, passing to the entire thoracic and abdominal regions of the body. Therefore, a physiologist speaking of the parasympathetic nervous system often thinks mainly of the two vagus nerves. The vagus nerves supply parasympathetic nerves to the heart, the lungs, the esophagus, the stomach, the small intestine, the proximal half of the colon, the liver, the gallbladder, the pancreas, and the upper portions of the ureters.

Parasympathetic fibers in the *third nerve* flow to the pupillary sphincters and ciliary muscles of the eye. Fibers from the *seventh nerve* pass to the lacrimal, nasal, and submandibular glands, and fibers from the *ninth nerve* pass to the parotid gland.

The sacral parasympathetic fibers congregate in the form of the *nervi erigentes*, also called the *pelvic nerves*, which leave the sacral plexus on each side of the cord and distribute their peripheral fibers to the descending colon, rectum, bladder, and lower portions of the ureters. Also, this sacral group of parasympathetics supplies fibers to the external genitalia to cause various sexual reactions.

Preganglionic and Postganglionic Parasympathetic Neurons. The parasympathetic system, like the sympathetic, has both preganglionic and postganglionic neurons, but, except in the case of a few cranial parasym-

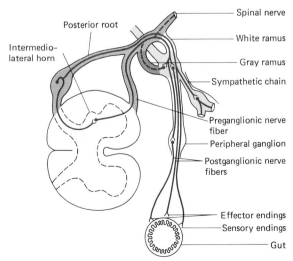

Figure 21–2. Nerve connections between the spinal cord, sympathetic chain, spinal nerves, and peripheral sympathetic nerves.

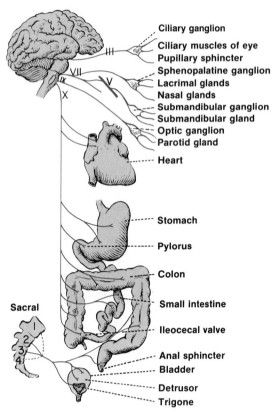

Figure 21–3. The parasympathetic nervous system.

pathetic nerves, the *preganglionic fibers* pass uninterrupted to the organ that is to be controlled. In the wall of the organ are located the *postganglionic neurons* of the parasympathetic system. The preganglionic fibers synapse with these; then short postganglionic fibers, 1 millimeter to several centimeters in length, leave the neurons to spread in the substance of the organ. This location of the parasympathetic postganglionic neurons in the visceral organ itself is quite different from the arrangement of the sympathetic ganglia, for the cell bodies of the sympathetic postganglionic neurons are almost always located in ganglia of the sympathetic chain or in various other discrete ganglia in the abdomen rather than in the excited organ itself.

BASIC CHARACTERISTICS OF SYMPATHETIC AND PARASYMPATHETIC FUNCTION

CHOLINERGIC AND ADRENERGIC FIBERS—SECRETION OF ACETYLCHOLINE OR NOREPINEPHRINE BY THE POSTGANGLIONIC NEURONS

The sympathetic and parasympathetic nerve endings secrete one of the two synaptic transmitter substances, *acetylcholine* or *norepinephrine*. Those fibers that secrete acetylcholine are said to be *cholinergic*. Those that secrete norepinephrine are said to be *adrenergic*, a term derived from *adrenalin*, which is the British name for epinephrine.

All *preganglionic neurons* are *cholinergic* in both the sympathetic and parasympathetic nervous systems. Therefore, acetylcholine or acetylcholine-like substances, when applied to the ganglia, will excite both sympathetic and parasympathetic postganglionic neurons.

The *postganglionic neurons of the parasympathetic system are* also *all cholinergic*. On the other hand, *most of the postganglionic sympathetic neurons are adrenergic*, though this is not entirely so because the sympathetic nerve fibers to the sweat glands, to the piloerector muscles, and to a few blood vessels are cholinergic.

Thus, in general, the terminal nerve endings of the parasympathetic system secrete acetylcholine, and most of the sympathetic nerve endings secrete norepinephrine. These hormones, in turn, act on the different organs to cause the respective parasympathetic and sympathetic effects. Therefore, these substances are often called respectively *parasympathetic* and *sympathetic transmitters*. These are the molecular structures of acetylcholine and norepinephrine:

$$CH_3-\underset{\underset{O}{\|}}{C}-O-CH_2-CH_2-\underset{\underset{CH_3}{|}}{\overset{+}{N}}\diagup\overset{\diagup CH_3}{\diagdown CH_3}$$

Acetylcholine

Norepinephrine

Mechanism of Secretion of Acetylcholine and Norepinephrine by Autonomic Nerve Endings. Some of the autonomic nerve endings, especially those of the parasympathetic nerves, are similar to but much smaller in size than those of the skeletal neuromuscular junction. However, most of the sympathetic nerve fibers merely touch the effector cells of the organs that they innervate as they pass by; in some instances they terminate in connective tissue located adjacent to the cells that are to be stimulated. Where these filaments pass over or near the effector cells, they usually have bulbous enlargements called *varicosities*, and it is in these varicosities that the transmitter vesicles of acetylcholine and norepinephrine are found. Also in the varicosities are large numbers of mitochondria to supply the ATP required to energize acetylcholine or norepinephrine synthesis.

When an action potential spreads over the terminal fibers, the depolarization process increases the permeability of the fiber membrane to calcium ions, thus allowing these to diffuse in moderate numbers into the nerve terminals. There they interact with the vesicles adjacent to the membrane, causing them to fuse with the membrane and to empty their contents to the exterior. Thus, the transmitter substance is secreted.

Synthesis of Acetylcholine, Its Destruction After Secretion, and Duration of Action. Acetylcholine is synthesized in the terminal endings of cholinergic nerve fibers. Most of this synthesis occurs in the axoplasm, and most of the acetylcholine is then transported to the interior of the vesicles. The basic chemical reaction of this synthesis is the following:

$$\text{Acetyl-CoA} + \text{Choline} \xrightarrow{\text{choline acetyl-transferase}} \text{Acetylcholine}$$

Once the acetylcholine has been secreted by the cholinergic nerve ending, most of it is split into acetate ion and choline by the enzyme *acetylcholinesterase* that is present in the synaptic area bound with the local collagen and glycosaminoglycans. Thus, this is the same mechanism of acetylcholine destruction that occurs at the neuromuscular junctions of skeletal nerve fibers. The choline that is formed is in turn transported back into the terminal nerve ending where it is used again for synthesis of new acetylcholine. Though most of the acetylcholine is usually destroyed within a fraction of a second after its secretion, it sometimes persists for as long as several seconds, and a small amount also diffuses into the surrounding fluids. These fluids contain a different type of cholinesterase called *serum cholinesterase* that destroys the remaining acetylcholine within another few seconds. Therefore, the action of acetylcholine released by cholinergic nerve fibers usually lasts for a few seconds at most.

Synthesis of Norepinephrine, Its Removal, and Duration of Action. Synthesis of norepinephrine begins in the axoplasm of the terminal nerve endings of adrenergic nerve fibers but is completed inside the vesicles. The basic steps are the following:

1. $\text{Tyrosine} \xrightarrow{\text{hydroxylation}} \text{DOPA}$

2. $\text{DOPA} \xrightarrow{\text{decarboxylation}} \text{Dopamine}$

3. Transport of dopamine into the vesicles

4. $\text{Dopamine} \xrightarrow{\text{hydroxylation}} \text{Norepinephrine}$

In the adrenal medulla this reaction goes still one step further to form epinephrine, as follows:

5. $\text{Norepinephrine} \xrightarrow{\text{methylation}} \text{Epinephrine}$

Following secretion of norepinephrine by the terminal nerve endings, it is removed from the secretory site in three different ways: (1) re-uptake into the adrenergic nerve endings themselves by an active transport process—accounting for removal of 50 to 80 per cent of the secreted norepinephrine; (2) diffusion away from the nerve endings into the surrounding body fluids and thence into the blood—accounting for removal of most of the remainder of the norepinephrine; and (3) destruction by enzymes to a slight extent (one of these enzymes is *monoamine oxidase*, which is found in the nerve endings themselves, and another is *catechol-O-methyl transferase*, which is present diffusely in all tissues).

Ordinarily, the norepinephrine secreted directly in a tissue by adrenergic nerve endings remains active for only a few seconds, illustrating that its re-uptake and diffusion away from the tissue are rapid. However, the norepinephrine and epinephrine secreted into the blood by the adrenal medullae remain active until they diffuse into tissue where they are destroyed by catechol-O-methyl transferase; this occurs mainly in the liver. Therefore, when secreted into the blood, both norepinephrine and epinephrine remain very active for 10 to 30 seconds, followed by decreasing activity thereafter for 1 to several minutes.

RECEPTORS OF THE EFFECTOR ORGANS

The acetylcholine, norepinephrine, and epinephrine transmitters secreted by the autonomic nervous system all stimulate the effector organs by first binding with *receptors* of the effector cells. The receptor in most instances is in the cell membrane and is a protein molecule. The usual mechanism for function of the receptor is that the transmitter first binds with the receptor and this causes a basic change in the structure of the protein molecule in the manner described in Chapters 5 and 6. Because the receptor is an integral part of the cell membrane, this structural change often opens or closes *ion channels*, thus altering the permeability of the cell membrane to various ions—for instance, to allow rapid influx or to diminish influx of sodium, chloride, or calcium ions into the cell or to alter the efflux of potassium ions out of the cell. These ionic changes then usually alter the membrane potential, sometimes causing increased negativity (hyperpolarization) or at other times causing decreased negativity (depolarization) to elicit action potentials (as occurs in some smooth muscle cells) and at other times causing electrotonic effects on the cells (as occurs in glandular cells) to produce the responses. The ions themselves have direct effects within the receptor cells, such as the effect of calcium ions to promote smooth muscle contraction.

Another way that the receptor can function, besides changing the membrane permeability, is to activate an enzyme in the cell membrane; this enzyme in turn promotes chemical reactions within the cell. For instance, epinephrine increases the activity of *adenyl cyclase* in some cell membranes, and this then causes the formation of cyclic AMP at the inner surfaces of the membranes; the cyclic AMP then initiates many intracellular activities.

The effect that occurs in each instance is determined by the nature of the receptors, as we shall see in the following paragraphs.

The Acetylcholine Receptors—"Muscarinic" and "Nicotinic" Receptors. Acetylcholine activates two different types of receptors. These are called *muscarinic* and *nicotinic* receptors. The reason for these names is that muscarine, a poison from toadstools, also activates the muscarinic receptors but will not activate the nicotinic receptors, whereas nicotine will activate only the other receptors; acetylcholine activates both of them.

The muscarinic receptors are found in all the effector cells stimulated by the postganglionic neurons of the parasympathetic nervous system, as well as those stimulated by the postganglionic cholinergic neurons of the sympathetic system.

The nicotinic receptors are found in the synapses between the pre- and postganglionic neurons of both the sympathetic and parasympathetic systems and also in the membranes of skeletal muscle fibers at the neuromuscular junction (discussed in Chapter 8).

An understanding of the two different types of receptors is especially important because specific drugs are frequently used in the practice of medicine to stimulate or to block one or the other of the two types of receptors.

The Adrenergic Receptors—"Alpha" and "Beta" Receptors. Research experiments using different drugs (called *sympathomimetic drugs*) that mimic the action of norepinephrine on sympathetic effector organs have shown that there are two major types of adrenergic receptors, called *alpha receptors* and *beta receptors*. (The beta receptors in turn are divided into *beta₁* and *beta₂* receptors because certain drugs affect some beta receptors but not all.)

Norepinephrine and epinephrine, both of which are secreted by the adrenal medulla, have somewhat different effects in exciting the alpha and beta receptors. Norepinephrine excites mainly alpha receptors but excites the beta receptors to a very slight extent as well. On the other hand, epinephrine excites both types of receptors approximately equally. Therefore, the relative effects of norepinephrine and epinephrine on different effector organs is determined by the types of receptors in the organs. Obviously, if they are all beta receptors, epinephrine will be the more effective excitant.

Table 21–1 gives the distribution of alpha and beta receptors in some of the organs and systems controlled by the sympathetics. Note that certain alpha functions are excitatory while others are inhibitory. Likewise, certain beta functions are excitatory and others are inhibitory. Therefore, alpha and beta receptors are not necessarily associated with excitation or inhibition but simply with the affinity of the hormone for the receptors in a given effector organ.

A synthetic hormone chemically similar to epinephrine and norepinephrine, *isopropyl norepinephrine*, has an extremely strong action on beta receptors but essentially no action on alpha receptors. Later in the chapter we will discuss various drugs that can mimic the adrenergic actions of epinephrine and norepinephrine or that will block specifically the alpha or beta receptors.

EXCITATORY AND INHIBITORY ACTIONS OF SYMPATHETIC AND PARASYMPATHETIC STIMULATION

Table 21–2 lists the effects on different visceral functions of the body caused by stimulating the parasympathetic and sympathetic nerves. From this

Table 21–1. ADRENERGIC RECEPTORS AND FUNCTION

Alpha Receptor	Beta Receptor
Vasoconstriction	Vasodilatation (β_2)
Iris dilatation	Cardioacceleration (β_1)
Intestinal relaxation	Increased myocardial strength (β_1)
Intestinal sphincter contraction	Intestinal relaxation (β_2)
Pilomotor contraction	Bronchodilatation (β_2)
Bladder sphincter contraction	Calorigenesis (β_2)
	Glycogenolysis (β_2)
	Lipolysis (β_1)
	Bladder relaxation (β_2)

table it can be seen that *sympathetic stimulation causes excitatory effects in some organs but inhibitory effects in others. Likewise, parasympathetic stimulation causes excitation in some organs but inhibition in others.* Also, when sympathetic stimulation excites a particular organ, parasympathetic stimulation sometimes inhibits it, illustrating that the two systems occasionally act reciprocally to each other. However, most organs are dominantly controlled by one or the other of the two systems.

There is no generalization one can use to explain whether sympathetic or parasympathetic stimulation will cause excitation or inhibition of a particular organ. Therefore, to understand sympathetic and parasympathetic function, one must learn the functions of these two nervous systems as listed in Table 21–2. Some of these functions need to be clarified in still greater detail as follows.

EFFECTS OF SYMPATHETIC AND PARASYMPATHETIC STIMULATION ON SPECIFIC ORGANS

The Eye. Two functions of the eye are controlled by the autonomic nervous system. These are the pupillary opening and the focus of the lens. Sympathetic stimulation contracts the meridional *fibers of the iris* and, therefore, dilates the pupil, while parasympathetic stimulation contracts the *circular muscle of the iris* to constrict the pupil. The parasympathetics that control the pupil are reflexly stimulated when excess light enters the eyes; this reflex reduces the pupillary opening and decreases the amount of light that strikes the retina. On the other hand, the sympathetics become stimulated during periods of excitement and, therefore, increase the pupillary opening at these times.

Focusing of the lens is controlled almost entirely by the parasympathetic nervous system. The lens is normally held in a flattened state by tension of its radial ligaments. Parasympathetic excitation contracts the *ciliary muscle*, which releases this tension and allows the lens to become more convex. This causes the eye to focus on objects near at hand. The focusing mechanism is discussed in Chapters 22 and 24 in relation to function of the eyes.

The Glands of the Body. The *nasal, lacrimal, salivary,* and many *gastrointestinal glands* are all strongly stimulated by the parasympathetic nervous system, resulting in copious quantities of secretion. The glands of the alimentary tract most strongly stimulated by the parasympathetics are those of the upper tract, especially those of

Table 21–2. AUTONOMIC EFFECTS ON VARIOUS ORGANS OF THE BODY

Organ	Effect of Sympathetic Stimulation	Effect of Parasympathetic Stimulation
Eye: Pupil	Dilated	Constricted
Ciliary muscle	Slight relaxation	Constricted
Glands: Nasal	Vasoconstriction and slight secretion	Stimulation of copious (except pancreas) secretion (containing many enzymes for enzyme-secreting glands)
Lacrimal		
Parotid		
Submandibular		
Gastric		
Pancreatic		
Sweat glands	Copious sweating (cholinergic)	None
Apocrine glands	Thick, odoriferous secretion	None
Heart: Muscle	Increased rate	Slowed rate
	Increased force of contraction	Decreased force of contraction (especially of atrium)
Coronaries	Dilated (β_2); constricted (α)	Dilated
Lungs: Bronchi	Dilated	Constricted
Blood vessels	Mildly constricted	? Dilated
Gut: Lumen	Decreased peristalsis and tone	Increased peristalsis and tone
Sphincter	Increased tone (most times)	Relaxed (most times)
Liver	Glucose released	Slight glycogen synthesis
Gallbladder and bile ducts	Relaxed	Contracted
Kidney	Decreased output and renin secretion	None
Bladder: Detrusor	Relaxed (slight)	Excited
Trigone	Excited	Relaxed
Penis	Ejaculation	Erection
Systemic arterioles:		
Abdominal	Constricted	None
Muscle	Constricted (adrenergic α)	None
	Dilated (adrenergic β_2)	
	Dilated (cholinergic)	
Skin	Constricted	None
Blood: Coagulation	Increased	None
Glucose	Increased	None
Basal metabolism	Increased up to 100%	None
Adrenal medullary secretion	Increased	None
Mental activity	Increased	None
Piloerector muscles	Excited	None
Skeletal muscle	Increased glycogenolysis	None
	Increased strength	

the mouth and stomach. The glands of the small and large intestines are controlled principally by local factors in the intestinal tract itself and not by the autonomic nerves.

Sympathetic stimulation has a slight direct effect on glandular cells in causing formation of a concentrated secretion. However, it also causes vasoconstriction of the blood vessels supplying the glands and in this way often reduces their rates of secretion.

The *sweat glands* secrete large quantities of sweat when the sympathetic nerves are stimulated, but no effect is caused by stimulating the parasympathetic nerves. However, the sympathetic fibers to most sweat glands are *cholinergic* (except for a few adrenergic fibers to palms of the hand and the soles of the feet), in contrast to most other sympathetic fibers, which are adrenergic. Furthermore, the sweat glands are stimulated primarily by centers in the hypothalamus that are usually considered to be parasympathetic centers. Therefore, sweating could be called a parasympathetic function.

The *apocrine glands* secrete a thick, odoriferous secretion as a result of sympathetic stimulation, but they do not react to parasympathetic stimulation. Furthermore, the apocrine glands, despite their close embryological relationship to sweat glands, are controlled by adrenergic

fibers rather than by cholinergic fibers and are controlled by the sympathetic centers of the central nervous system rather than by the parasympathetic centers.

The Gastrointestinal System. The gastrointestinal system has its own intrinsic set of nerves known as the *intramural plexus.* However, both parasympathetic and sympathetic stimulation can affect gastrointestinal activity—parasympathetic especially. Parasympathetic stimulation, in general, increases the overall degree of activity of the gastrointestinal tract by promoting peristalsis and relaxing the sphincters, thus allowing rapid propulsion of contents along the tract. This propulsive effect is associated with simultaneous increases in rates of secretion by many of the gastrointestinal glands, which was described earlier.

Normal function of the gastrointestinal tract is not very dependent on sympathetic stimulation. However, strong sympathetic stimulation inhibits peristalsis and increases the tone of the sphincters. The net result is greatly slowed propulsion of food through the tract.

The Heart. In general, sympathetic stimulation increases the overall activity of the heart. This is accomplished by increasing both the rate and force of the heartbeat. Parasympathetic stimulation causes mainly the opposite effects, decreasing the overall activity of the heart. To express these effects in another way, sympathetic stimulation increases the effectiveness of the heart as a pump, whereas parasympathetic stimulation decreases its pumping capability.

Systemic Blood Vessels. Most blood vessels, especially those of the abdominal viscera and the skin of the limbs, are constricted by sympathetic stimulation. Parasympathetic stimulation generally has almost no effects on blood vessels but does dilate vessels in certain restricted areas such as in the blush area of the face. Under some conditions, the beta stimulatory function of the sympathetics causes vascular dilatation, especially when drugs have paralyzed the sympathetic alpha effects.

Effect of Sympathetic and Parasympathetic Stimulation on Arterial Pressure. The arterial pressure is caused by propulsion of blood by the heart and by resistance to flow of this blood through the blood vessels. In general, sympathetic stimulation increases both propulsion by the heart and resistance to flow, which can cause the pressure to increase greatly.

On the other hand, parasympathetic stimulation decreases the pumping by the heart, which lowers the pressure a moderate amount, though usually not nearly so much as the sympathetics can increase the pressure.

Effects of Sympathetic and Parasympathetic Stimulation on Other Functions of the Body. In general, most of the entodermal structures, such as the ducts of the liver, the gallbladder, the ureter, the bladder, and the bronchi, are inhibited by sympathetic stimulation but excited by parasympathetic stimulation. Sympathetic stimulation also has metabolic effects, causing release of glucose from the liver, increase in blood glucose concentration, increase in glycogenolysis in muscle, increase in muscle strength, increase in basal metabolic rate, and increase in mental activity. Finally, the sympathetics and parasympathetics are involved in the execution of the male and female sexual acts, as will be explained in Chapter 29.

FUNCTION OF THE ADRENAL MEDULLAE

Stimulation of the sympathetic nerves to the adrenal medullae causes large quantities of epinephrine and norepinephrine to be released into the circulating blood, and these two hormones in turn are carried in the blood to all tissues of the body. On the average, approximately 80 per cent of the secretion is epinephrine and 20 per cent is norepinephrine, though the relative proportions of these change considerably under different physiological conditions.

The circulating epinephrine and norepinephrine have almost the same effects on the different organs as those caused by direct sympathetic stimulation, except that *the effects last 5 to 10 times as long* because these hormones are removed from the blood slowly.

The circulating norepinephrine causes constriction of essentially all the blood vessels of the body; it causes increased activity of the heart, inhibition of the gastrointestinal tract, dilation of the pupils of the eyes, and so forth.

Epinephrine causes almost the same effects as those caused by norepinephrine, but the effects differ in the following respects: First, epinephrine, because of its greater effect in stimulating the beta receptors, has a greater effect on cardiac activity than norepinephrine. Second, epinephrine causes only weak constriction of the blood vessels of the muscles in comparison with a much stronger constriction that results from norepinephrine. Since the muscle vessels represent a major segment of all vessels of the body, this difference is of special importance because norepinephrine greatly increases the total peripheral resistance and thereby greatly elevates arterial pressure, whereas epinephrine raises the arterial pressure to a lesser extent but increases the cardiac output considerably more because of its effect on the heart and veins.

A third difference between the action of epinephrine and norepinephrine relates to their effects on tissue metabolism. Epinephrine has several times as great a metabolic effect as norepinephrine. Indeed, the epinephrine secreted by the adrenal medullae can increase the metabolic rate of the body often to as much as 100 per cent above normal, in this way increasing the activity and excitability of the whole body. It also increases the rate of other metabolic activities, such as glycogenolysis in the liver and muscle and glucose release into the blood.

In summary, stimulation of the adrenal medullae causes the release of hormones that have almost the same effects throughout the body as direct sympathetic stimulation, except that the effects are greatly prolonged, up to a minute or two after the stimulation is over. The only significant differences are caused by the beta effects of the epinephrine in the secretion, which increase the rate of metabolism and cardiac output to a greater extent than is caused by direct sympathetic stimulation.

Value of the Adrenal Medullae to the Function of the Sympathetic Nervous System. Epinephrine and norepinephrine are almost always released by the adrenal medullae at the same time that the different organs are stimulated directly by the sympathetic nerves. Therefore, the organs are actually stimulated in two different ways simultaneously, directly by the sympathetic nerves and indirectly by the medullary hormones. The two means of stimulation support each other, and either can usually substitute for the other. For instance, destruction of the direct sympathetic pathways to the organs does not abrogate excitation of the organs because norepinephrine and epinephrine are still released into the circulating fluids and indirectly cause stimulation. Likewise, total loss of the two adrenal medullae usually has little significant effect on the operation of the sympathetic nervous system because the direct pathways can still perform almost all the necessary duties. Thus, the dual mechanism of sympathetic stimulation provides a safety factor, one mechanism substituting for the other when the second is missing.

Another important value of the adrenal medullae is the capability of epinephrine and norepinephrine to stimulate structures of the body that are not innervated by direct sympathetic fibers. For instance, the metabolic rate of every cell of the body is increased by these hormones, especially by epinephrine, even though only a small proportion of all the cells in the body are innervated directly by sympathetic fibers.

RELATIONSHIP OF STIMULUS RATE TO DEGREE OF SYMPATHETIC AND PARASYMPATHETIC EFFECT

A special difference between the autonomic nervous system and the skeletal nervous system is the low frequency of stimulation required for full activation of autonomic effectors. In general, only one impulse every second or so suffices to maintain normal sympathetic or parasympathetic effect, and full activation occurs when the nerve fibers discharge 10 to 20 times per second. This compares with full activation in the skeletal nervous system at about 50 to 200 impulses per second.

SYMPATHETIC AND PARASYMPATHETIC "TONE"

The sympathetic and parasympathetic systems are continually active, and the basal rates of activity are known, respectively, as *sympathetic tone* or *parasympathetic tone.*

The value of tone is that it allows a single nervous system to increase or to decrease the activity of a stimulated organ. For instance, sympathetic tone normally keeps almost all the blood vessels of the body constricted to approximately half their maximum diameter. By increasing the degree of sympathetic stimulation, the vessels can be constricted even more; but, on the other hand, by inhibiting the normal tone, the vessels can be dilated. If it were not for the continual sympathetic tone, the sympathetic system could cause only vasoconstriction, never vasodilatation.

Another interesting example of tone is that of the parasympathetics in the gastrointestinal tract. Surgical removal of the parasympathetic supply to the gut by cutting the vagi can cause serious and prolonged gastric and intestinal "atony," thus illustrating that in normal function the parasympathetic tone to the gut is strong. This tone can be decreased by the brain, thereby inhibiting gastrointestinal motility, or it can be increased, thereby promoting increased gastrointestinal activity.

Tone Caused by Basal Secretion of Epinephrine and Norepinephrine by the Adrenal Medullae. The normal resting rate of secretion by the adrenal medullae is about 0.2 μgm/kg/min of epinephrine and about 0.05 μgm/kg/min of norepinephrine. These quantities are considerable—indeed, enough to maintain the blood pressure almost up to the normal value even if all direct sympathetic pathways to the cardiovascular system are removed. Therefore, it is obvious that much of the overall tone of the sympathetic nervous system results from basal secretion of epinephrine and norepinephrine in addition to the tone resulting from direct sympathetic stimulation.

Effect of Loss of Sympathetic or Parasympathetic Tone Following Denervation. Immediately after a sympathetic or parasympathetic nerve is cut, the innervated organ loses its sympathetic or parasympathetic tone. In the case of the blood vessels, for instance, cutting the sympathetic nerves results immediately in almost maximal vasodilatation. However, over minutes, hours, days, or weeks, the *intrinsic tone* in the smooth muscle of the vessels increases, usually restoring almost normal vasoconstriction.

Essentially the same events occur in most effector organs whenever sympathetic or parasympathetic tone is lost. That is, intrinsic compensation soon develops to return the function of the organ almost to its normal basal level. However, in the parasympathetic system, the compensation sometimes requires many months. For instance, loss of parasympathetic tone to the heart increases the heart rate to 160 beats per minute in a dog, and this will still be about 120 beats six months later.

DENERVATION SUPERSENSITIVITY OF SYMPATHETIC AND PARASYMPATHETIC ORGANS FOLLOWING DENERVATION

During the first week or so after a sympathetic or parasympathetic nerve is destroyed, the innervated organ becomes more and more sensitive to injected norepinephrine or acetylcholine, respectively. This effect is illustrated in Figure 21–4; the blood flow in the forearm before removal of the sympathetics is about 200 ml per minute, and a test dose of norepinephrine causes only a slight depression in flow. Then the stellate ganglion is removed, and normal sympathetic tone is lost. At first, the blood flow rises markedly because of the lost vascular tone, but over a period of days to weeks the blood flow returns almost to normal because of progressive increase in intrinsic tone of the vascular musculature itself, thus compensating for the loss of sympathetic tone. Another test dose of norepinephrine is then administered and the blood flow decreases much more than before, illustrating that the blood vessels become about two to four times as responsive to norepinephrine as previously. This phenomenon is called *denervation supersensitivity.* It occurs in both sympathetic and parasympathetic organs and to a far greater extent in some organs than in others, often increasing the response as much as tenfold or more.

Mechanism of Denervation Supersensitivity. The cause of denervation supersensitivity is only partially known. Part of the answer is that the number of receptors in the postsynaptic membranes of the effector cells in-

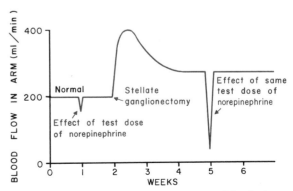

Figure 21–4. Effect of sympathectomy on blood flow in the arm, and the effect of a test dose of norepinephrine before and after sympathectomy, showing sensitization of the vasculature to norepinephrine.

creases—sometimes manyfold—when norepinephrine or acetylcholine are no longer released at the synapses, a process called "up-regulation" of the receptors. Therefore, when these hormones appear in the circulating blood, the effector reaction is vastly enhanced.

THE AUTONOMIC REFLEXES

Many of the visceral functions of the body are regulated by *autonomic reflexes*. Throughout this text the functions of these reflexes are discussed in relation to individual organ systems, but, to illustrate their importance, a few are presented here briefly.

Cardiovascular Autonomic Reflexes. Several reflexes in the cardiovascular system help to control the arterial blood pressure, cardiac output, and heart rate. One of these is the *baroreceptor reflex*, which was described in Chapter 27 along with other cardiovascular reflexes. Briefly, stretch receptors called *baroreceptors* are located in the walls of the major arteries, including the carotid arteries and the aorta. When these become stretched by high pressure, signals are transmitted to the brain stem, where they inhibit the sympathetic impulses to the heart and blood vessels, which allows the arterial pressure to fall back toward normal.

The Gastrointestinal Autonomic Reflexes. The uppermost part of the gastrointestinal tract and also the rectum are controlled principally by autonomic reflexes. For instance, the smell of appetizing food initiates signals from the nose to the vagal, glossopharyngeal, and salivary nuclei of the brain stem. These in turn transmit signals through the parasympathetic nerves to the secretory glands of the mouth and stomach, causing secretion of digestive juices even before food enters the mouth. And when fecal matter fills the rectum at the other end of the alimentary canal, sensory impulses initiated by stretching the rectum are sent to the sacral portion of the spinal cord, and a reflex signal is retransmitted through the parasympathetics to the distal parts of the colon; these result in strong peristaltic contractions that empty the bowel.

Other Autonomic Reflexes. Emptying of the bladder is controlled in the same way as emptying the rectum; stretching of the bladder sends impulses to the sacral cord, and this in turn causes contraction of the bladder as well as relaxation of the urinary sphincters, thereby promoting micturition.

Also important are the sexual reflexes, which are initiated both by psychic stimuli from the brain and stimuli from the sexual organs. Impulses from these sources converge on the sacral cord and, in the male, result, first, in erection, mainly a parasympathetic function, and then in ejaculation, a sympathetic function.

Other autonomic reflexes include reflex contributions to the regulation of pancreatic secretion, gallbladder emptying, renal excretion of urine, sweating, blood glucose concentration, and many other visceral functions.

STIMULATION OF DISCRETE ORGANS IN SOME INSTANCES, MASS STIMULATION IN OTHER INSTANCES, BY THE SYMPATHETIC AND PARASYMPATHETIC SYSTEMS

The Sympathetic System. In many instances, the sympathetic nervous system discharges almost as a complete unit, a phenomenon called *mass discharge*. This frequently occurs when the hypothalamus becomes activated by fright or fear or severe pain. The result is a widespread reaction throughout the body called the *alarm* or *stress response*, which we shall discuss shortly.

However, at other times sympathetic activation occurs in isolated portions of the system. The most important of these are: (1) In the process of heat regulation, the sympathetics control sweating and blood flow in the skin without affecting other organs innervated by the sympathetics. (2) During muscular activity in some animals, cholinergic vasodilator fibers of the skeletal muscles are stimulated independently of all the remainder of the sympathetic system. (3) Many "local reflexes" involving the spinal cord but usually not the higher nervous centers affect local areas. For instance, heating a local skin area causes local vasodilatation and enhanced local sweating, while cooling causes the opposite effects. (4) Many of the sympathetic reflexes that control gastrointestinal functions are very discrete, operating sometimes by way of nerve pathways that do not even enter the spinal cord, merely passing from the gut to the sympathetic ganglia and then back to the gut through the sympathetic nerves to control motor or secretory activity.

The Parasympathetic System. In contrast to the sympathetic system, most control functions of the parasympathetic system are very specific. For instance, parasympathetic cardiovascular reflexes usually act only on the heart to increase or decrease its rate of beating. Likewise, parasympathetic reflexes frequently cause secretion mainly in the mouth or, in other instances, secretion mainly in the stomach glands. Finally, the rectal emptying reflex does not affect other parts of the bowel to a major extent.

Yet there is often association between closely allied parasympathetic functions. For instance, though salivary secretion can occur independently of gastric secretion, these two often also occur together, and pancreatic secretion frequently occurs at the same time. Also, the rectal emptying reflex often initiates a bladder emptying reflex, resulting in simultaneous emptying of both the bladder and rectum. Conversely, the bladder emptying reflex can help initiate rectal emptying.

"ALARM" OR "STRESS" RESPONSE OF THE SYMPATHETIC NERVOUS SYSTEM

When large portions of the sympathetic nervous system discharge at the same time—that is, a mass discharge—this increases in many different ways the capability of the body to perform vigorous muscle activity. Let us quickly summarize these ways:

1. increased arterial pressure
2. increased blood flow to active muscles concurrent with decreased blood flow to organs that are not needed for rapid activity
3. increased rates of cellular metabolism throughout the body
4. increased blood glucose concentration
5. increased glycolysis in muscle
6. increased muscle strength
7. increased mental activity
8. increased rate of blood coagulation

The sum of these effects permits the person to perform far more strenuous physical activity than would otherwise be possible. Since it is physical *stress* that usually excites the sympathetic system, it is frequently said that the purpose of the sympathetic system is to provide extra activation of the body in states of stress: this is often called the sympathetic *stress response*.

The sympathetic system is also strongly activated in many emotional states. For instance, in the state of *rage*, which is elicited mainly by stimulating the hypothalamus, signals are transmitted downward through the reticular formation and spinal cord to cause massive sympathetic discharge, and all of the sympathetic events listed above ensue immediately. This is called the sympathetic *alarm reaction*. It is also frequently called the *fight or flight reaction* because an animal in this state decides almost instantly whether to stand and fight or to run. In either event, the sympathetic alarm reaction makes the animal's subsequent activities extremely vigorous.

MEDULLARY, PONTINE, AND MESENCEPHALIC CONTROL OF THE AUTONOMIC NERVOUS SYSTEM

Many areas in the reticular substance of the medulla, pons, and mesencephalon, as well as many special nuclei (Fig. 21–5), control different autonomic functions such as arterial pressure, heart rate, glandular secretion in the upper part of the gastrointestinal tract, gastrointestinal peristalsis, the degree of contraction of the urinary bladder, and many others. The most important factors controlled in the lower brain stem are arterial pressure, heart rate, and respiration. Indeed, transection of the brain stem at the midpontine level allows normal

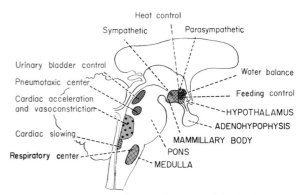

Figure 21–5. Autonomic control centers of the brain stem.

basal control of arterial pressure to continue as before but prevents its modulation by higher nervous centers, particularly the hypothalamus. On the other hand, transection immediately below the medulla causes the arterial pressure to fall to about one-half normal for several hours or several days after the transection.

Closely associated with the cardiovascular regulatory centers in the medulla are the medullary and pontine centers for regulation of respiration discussed in detail in Chapter 27. Though this is not considered to be an autonomic function, it is one of the *involuntary* functions of the body.

Control of Lower Brain Stem Autonomic Centers by Higher Areas. Signals from the hypothalamus and even from the cerebrum can affect the activities of almost all the lower brain stem autonomic control centers. For instance, stimulation in appropriate areas of the hypothalamus can activate the medullary cardiovascular control centers strongly enough to increase the arterial pressure to more than double normal. Likewise, other hypothalamic centers can control body temperature, increase or decrease salivation and gastrointestinal activity, or cause bladder emptying. To some extent, therefore, the autonomic centers in the lower brain stem act as relay stations for control activities initiated at higher levels of the brain.

In the previous chapter it was also pointed out that many of the behavioral responses of an animal are mediated through the hypothalamus, reticular formation, and the autonomic nervous system. Indeed, the higher areas of the brain can alter the function of the whole autonomic nervous system or of portions of it strongly enough to cause severe autonomic-induced disease, such as peptic ulcer, constipation, heart palpitation, and even heart attacks.

PHARMACOLOGY OF THE AUTONOMIC NERVOUS SYSTEM

DRUGS THAT ACT ON ADRENERGIC EFFECTOR ORGANS—THE SYMPATHOMIMETIC DRUGS

From the foregoing discussion, it is obvious that intravenous injection of norepinephrine causes essentially the same effects throughout the body as sympathetic stimulation. Therefore, norepinephrine is called a *sympathomimetic*, or *adrenergic*, *drug*. Epinephrine and *methoxamine* are sympathomimetic drugs, and there are many others. These differ from each other in the degree to which they stimulate different sympathetic effector organs and in their duration of action. Norepinephrine and epinephrine have actions as short as 1 to 2 minutes, whereas the actions of most other commonly used sympathomimetic drugs last 30 minutes to 2 hours.

Important drugs that stimulate specific adrenergic receptors but not the others are *phenylephrine*—α receptors; *isoproterenol*—β receptors; and *salbutamol*—only β_2 receptors.

Drugs That Cause Release of Norepinephrine from Nerve Endings. Certain drugs have a sympathomimetic action in an indirect manner rather than by directly exciting adrenergic effector organs. These drugs include *ephedrine, tyramine,* and *amphetamine.* Their effect is to cause release of norepinephrine from its storage vesicles in the sympathetic nerve endings. The norepinephrine in turn causes the sympathetic effects.

Drugs That Block Adrenergic Activity. Adrenergic activity can be blocked at several different points in the stimulatory process as follows:

1. The synthesis and storage of norepinephrine in the sympathetic nerve endings can be prevented. The best known drug that causes this effect is *reserpine.*

2. Release of norepinephrine from the sympathetic endings can be blocked. This is caused by *guanethidine.*

3. The *alpha* receptors can be blocked. Two drugs that cause this effect are *phenoxybenzamine* and *phentolamine.*

4. The beta receptors can be blocked. A drug that blocks all beta receptors is *propranolol.* One that blocks only beta₁ receptors is *practolol.*

5. Sympathetic activity can be blocked by drugs that block transmission of nerve impulses through the autonomic ganglia. These are discussed in the following section, but the most important drug for blockade of both sympathetic and parasympathetic transmission through the ganglia is *hexamethonium.*

DRUGS THAT ACT ON CHOLINERGIC EFFECTOR ORGANS

Parasympathomimetic Drugs (Muscarinic Drugs). Acetylcholine injected intravenously usually does not cause exactly the same effects throughout the body as parasympathetic stimulation because the acetylcholine is destroyed by cholinesterase in the blood and body fluids before it can reach all the effector organs. Yet a number of other drugs that are not so rapidly destroyed can produce typical parasympathetic effects, and these are called *parasympathomimetic drugs.*

Two commonly used parasympathomimetic drugs are *pilocarpine* and *methacholine.* These act directly on the muscarinic type of cholinergic receptors.

Parasympathomimetic drugs act on the effector organs of cholinergic *sympathetic* fibers also. For instance, these drugs cause profuse sweating. Also, they cause vascular dilatation in some organs, this effect occurring even in vessels not innervated by cholinergic fibers.

Drugs That Have a Parasympathetic Potentiating Effect. Some drugs do not have a direct effect on parasympathetic effector organs but do potentiate the effects of the naturally secreted acetylcholine at the parasympathetic endings. These are the same drugs as those listed in Chapter 8 that potentiate the effect of acetylcholine at the neuromuscular junction—that is, *neostigmine, physostigmine,* and *diisopropyl fluorophosphate.* These inhibit acetylcholinesterase, thus preventing rapid destruction of the acetylcholine liberated by the parasympathetic nerve endings. As a consequence, the quantity of acetylcholine acting on the effector organs progressively increases with successive stimuli, and the degree of action also increases.

Drugs That Block Cholinergic Activity at Effector Organs. *Atropine* and similar drugs, such as *homatropine* and *scopolamine,* block the action of acetylcholine on the muscarinic type of cholinergic effector organs. However, these drugs do not affect the nicotinic action of acetylcholine on the postganglionic neurons or on skeletal muscle.

DRUGS THAT STIMULATE THE POSTGANGLIONIC NEURONS— "NICOTINIC DRUGS"

The preganglionic neurons of both the parasympathetic and sympathetic nervous systems secrete acetylcholine at their endings, and the acetylcholine in turn stimulates the postganglionic neurons. Therefore, injected acetylcholine can also stimulate the postganglionic neurons of both systems, thereby causing both sympathetic and parasympathetic effects in the body. *Nicotine* is a drug that can also stimulate postganglionic neurons in the same manner as acetylcholine because the neuronal membranes contain *nicotinic receptors.* However, nicotine cannot directly stimulate the autonomic effector organs, which have muscarinic receptors as explained earlier in the chapter. Therefore, drugs that cause autonomic effects by stimulating the postganglionic neurons are frequently called *nicotinic drugs.* Some drugs, such as *acetylcholine* itself and *methacholine,* have both nicotinic and muscarinic actions, whereas pilocarpine has only muscarinic actions.

Nicotine excites both the sympathetic and parasympathetic postganglionic neurons at the same time, resulting in strong sympathetic vasoconstriction in the abdominal organs and limbs, but at the same time resulting in parasympathetic effects, such as increased gastrointestinal activity and, sometimes, slowing of the heart.

Ganglionic Blocking Drugs. Many important drugs block impulse transmission from the preganglionic neurons to the postganglionic neurons, including *tetraethyl ammonium ion, hexamethonium ion,* and *pentolinium.* These inhibit impulse transmission in both the sympathetic and parasympathetic systems simultaneously. They are often used for blocking sympathetic activity but rarely for blocking parasympathetic activity, because the sympathetic blockade usually far overshadows the effects of parasympathetic blockade. The ganglionic blocking drugs can especially reduce the arterial pressure in patients with hypertension, but these drugs are not very useful for this purpose because they are hard to control.

REFERENCES

Abboud, F. M. (ed.): Disturbances in Neurogenic Control of the Circulation. Baltimore, Williams and Wilkins, 1981.

Aviado, D. M., *et al.* (eds.): Pharmacology of Ganglionic Transmission. New York, Springer-Verlag, 1979.

Axelrod, J.: Neurotransmitters. *Sci. Am.*, 230(6):58, 1974.

Bhagat, B. D.: Mode of Action of Autonomic Drugs. Flushing, N.Y., Graceway Publishing Company, 1979.

Black, I. B.: Regulation of autonomic development. *Annu. Rev. Neurosci.*, 1:183, 1978.

Brooks, C. M., *et al.* (eds.): Integrative Functions of the Autonomic Nervous System. Tokyo, University of Tokyo Press, 1979.

Burattini, R., and Borgdorff, P.: Closed-loop baroreflex control of total peripheral resistance in the cat: Identification of gains by aid of a model. *Cardiovasc. Res.*, 18:715, 1984.

Burchfield, S. R. (ed.): Stress. Physiological and Psychological Interactions. Washington, D.C., Hemisphere Publishing Corp., 1985.

Carrier, O., Jr.: Pharmacology of the Peripheral Autonomic Nervous System. Chicago, Year Book Medical Publishers, 1972.

Christensen, N. J., and Galbo, H.: Sympathetic nervous activity during exercise. *Annu. Rev. Physiol.*, 45:139, 1983.

Davies, A. O., and Lefkowitz, R. J.: Regulation of β-adrenergic receptors by steroid hormones. *Annu. Rev. Physiol.*, 46:119, 1984.

DeQuattro, V., *et al.*: Anatomy and biochemistry of the sympathetic nervous system. *In* DeGroot, L. J., *et al.* (eds.): *Endocrinology*. Vol. 2. New York, Grune & Stratton, 1979, p. 1241.

Donald, D. E., and Shepherd, J. T.: Autonomic regulation of the peripheral circulation. *Annu. Rev. Physiol.*, 42:429, 1980.

Geffen, L. B., and Jarrott, B.: Cellular aspects of catecholaminergic neurons. *In* Brookhart, J. M., and Mountcastle, V. B. (eds.): Handbook of Physiology. Sec. 1, Vol. 1. Baltimore, Williams & Wilkins, 1977, p. 521.

Gillis, C. N., and Pitt, B. R.: The fate of circulating amines within the pulmonary circulation. *Annu. Rev. Physiol.*, 44:269, 1982.

Givens, J. R.: The Hypothalamus in Health and Disease. Chicago, Year Book Medical Publishers, 1984.

Guyton, A. C., and Gillespie, W. M., Jr.: Constant infusion of epinephrine: Rate of epinephrine secretion and destruction in the body. *Am. J. Physiol.*, 165:319, 1951.

Guyton, A. C., and Reeder, R. C.: Quantitative studies on the autonomic actions of curare. *J. Pharmacol. Exp. Ther.*, 98:188, 1950.

Haber, E., and Wrenn, S.: Problems in identification of the beta-adrenergic receptor. *Physiol. Rev.*, 56:317, 1976.

Hayward, J. N.: Functional and morphological aspects of hypothalamic neurons. *Physiol. Rev.*, 57:574, 1977.

Hoffman, B. B., and Lefkowitz, R. J.: Radioligand binding studies of adrenergic receptors: New insights into molecular and physiological regulation. *Annu. Rev. Pharmacol. Toxicol.*, 20:581, 1980.

Kalsner, S. (ed.): Trends in Autonomic Pharmacology. Baltimore, Urban & Schwarzenberg, 1979.

Kunos, G.: Adrenoceptors. *Annu. Rev. Pharmacol. Toxicol.*, 18:291, 1978.

Landsberg, L., and Young, J. B.: Catecholamines and the adrenal medulla. *In* Bondy, P. K., and Rosenberg, L. E. (eds.): Metabolic Control and Disease, 8th Ed. Philadelphia, W. B. Saunders Co., 1980, p. 1621.

Levitzki, A.: Catecholamine receptors. *In* Adrian, R. H., *et al.* (eds.): Reviews of Physiology, Biochemistry, and Pharmacology. New York, Springer-Verlag, 1978, p. 1.

Livett, B. G.: Adrenal medullary chromaffin cells in vitro. *Physiol. Rev.*, 64:1103, 1984.

Mason, C. A., and Bern, H. A.: Cellular biology of the neurosecretory neuron. *In* Brookhart, J. M., and Mountcastle, V. B. (eds.): Handbook of Physiology. Sec. 1, Vol. 1. Baltimore, Williams & Wilkins, 1977, p. 651.

Moore, R. Y., and Bloom, F. E.: Central catecholamine neuron systems: Anatomy and physiology of the dopamine system. *Annu. Rev. Neurosci.*, 1:129, 1978.

Morgane, P. J., and Panksepp, J. (eds.): Handbook of the hypothalamus. New York, Marcel Dekker, 1979.

Paton, D. M. (ed.): The Release of Catecholamines from Adrenergic Neurons. New York, Pergamon Press, 1979.

Patterson, P. H.: Environmental determination of autonomic neurotransmitter functions. *Annu. Rev. Neurosci.*, 1:1, 1978.

Rémond, A., and Izard, C. (eds.): Electrophysiological Effects of Nicotine. New York, Elsevier/North Holland, 1979.

Robinson, R.: Tumours That Secrete Catecholamines: A Study of Their Natural History and Their Diagnosis. New York, John Wiley & Sons, 1980.

Rowell, L. B.: Reflex control of regional circulations in humans. *J. Auton. Nerv. Syst.*, 11:101, 1984.

Simon, P. (ed.): Neurotransmitters. New York, Pergamon Press, 1979.

Stiles, G. L., *et al.*: β-Adrenergic receptors: Biochemical mechanisms of physiological regulation. *Physiol. Rev.*, 64:661, 1984.

Szabadi, E., *et al.*: Recent Advances in the Pharmacology of Adrenoceptors. New York, Elsevier/North-Holland, 1978.

Tauc, L.: Nonvesicular release of neurotransmitter. *Physiol. Rev.*, 62:857, 1982.

Torretti, J.: Sympathetic control of renin release. *Annu. Rev. Pharmacol. Toxicol.*, 22:167, 1982.

Tŭcek, S. (ed.): The Cholinergic Synapse. New York, Elsevier/North-Holland, 1979.

Ungar, A., and Phillips, J. H.: Regulation of the adrenal medulla. *Physiol. Rev.*, 63:787, 1983.

Usdin, E.: Stress. The Role of Catecholamines and Other Neurotransmitters. New York, Gordon Press Publishers, 1984.

Usdin, E., *et al.* (eds.): Catecholamines: Basic and Clinical Frontiers. New York, Pergamon Press, 1979.

von Euler, U. S.: Noradrenaline. Springfield, Ill., Charles C Thomas, 1956.

Westfall, T. C.: Local regulations of adrenergic neurotransmission. *Physiol. Rev.*, 57:659, 1977.

V

THE SPECIAL SENSES

22

The Eye: I. Optics of Vision

PHYSICAL PRINCIPLES OF OPTICS

Before it is possible to understand the optical system of the eye, the student must be thoroughly familiar with the basic physical principles of optics, including the physics of refraction, a knowledge of focusing, depth of focus, and so forth. Therefore, in the present study of the optics of the eye, a brief review of these physical principles is first presented, and then the optics of the eye is discussed.

REFRACTION OF LIGHT

The Refractive Index of a Transparent Substance. Light rays travel through air at a velocity of approximately 300,000 kilometers per second but much slower through transparent solids and liquids. The refractive index of a transparent substance is the *ratio* of the velocity of light in air to that in the substance. Obviously, the refractive index of air itself is 1.00.

If light travels through a particular type of glass at a velocity of 200,000 kilometers per second, the refractive index of this glass is 300,000 divided by 200,000, or 1.50.

Refraction of Light Rays at an Interface Between Two Media with Different Refractive Indices. When light waves traveling forward in a beam, as shown in the upper part of Figure 22–1, strike an interface that is perpendicular to the beam, the waves enter the second refractive medium without deviating in their course. The only effect that occurs is decreased velocity of transmission and shorter wavelength. On the other hand, as illustrated in the lower part of Figure 22–1, if the light waves strike an angulated interface, the light waves bend if the refractive indices of the two media are different from each other. In this particular figure the light waves are leaving air, which has a refractive index of 1.00, and are entering a block of glass having a refractive index of 1.50. When the beam first strikes the angulated interface, the lower edge of the beam enters the glass ahead of the upper edge. The wave front in the upper portion of the beam continues to travel at a velocity of 300,000 kilometers per second while that which has entered the glass travels at a velocity of 200,000 kilometers per second. This causes the upper portion of the wave front to move ahead of the lower portion so that the wave front is no longer vertical but is angulated to the right. Because the *direction in which light travels is always perpendicular to the*

plane of the wave front, the direction of travel of the light beam now bends downward.

The bending of light rays at an angulated interface is known as *refraction*. Note particularly that the degree of refraction increases as a function of (1) the ratio of the two refractive indices of the two transparent media and (2) the degree of angulation between the interface and the entering wave front.

APPLICATION OF REFRACTIVE PRINCIPLES TO LENSES

The Convex Lens—Focusing of Light Rays. Figure 22–2 shows parallel light rays entering a convex lens. The light rays passing through the center of the lens strike the lens exactly perpendicular to the lens surface and therefore pass through the lens without being refracted at all. Toward either edge of the lens, however, the light rays strike a progressively more angulated interface. Therefore, the outer rays bend more and more toward the center. Half the bending occurs when the rays enter the lens and half as they exit from the opposite side. (At this time the student should pause and analyze why the rays still bend toward the center upon leaving the lens.)

Finally, if the lens is ground with exactly the proper curvature, parallel light rays passing through each part of the lens will be bent exactly enough so that all the rays will pass through a single point, which is called the *focal point*.

The Concave Lens. Figure 22–3 shows the effect of a concave lens on parallel light rays. The rays that enter the very center of the lens strike an interface that is absolutely perpendicular to the beam and, therefore, do not refract at all. The rays at the edge of the lens enter the lens ahead of the rays toward the center. This is opposite to the effect in the convex lens, and it causes the peripheral light rays to *diverge* away from the light rays that pass through the center of the lens.

Thus, the concave lens *diverges* light rays, whereas the convex lens *converges* light rays.

Spherical Versus Cylindrical Lenses. Figure 22–4 illustrates both a convex *spherical* lens and a convex *cylindrical* lens. Note that the cylindrical lens bends light rays from the two sides of the lens but not from either the top or the bottom. Therefore, parallel light rays are bent to a focal *line*. On the other hand, light rays that pass through the spherical lens are refracted at all edges of the lens toward the central ray, and all the rays come to a *focal point*.

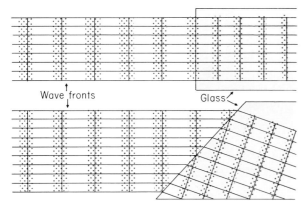

Figure 22–1. Wave fronts entering (*top*) a glass surface perpendicular to the light rays and (*bottom*) a glass surface angulated to the light rays. This figure illustrates that the distance between waves after they enter the glass is shortened to approximately two thirds that in air. It also illustrates that light rays striking an angulated glass surface are refracted.

The cylindrical lens is well illustrated by a test tube full of water. If the test tube is placed in a beam of sunlight and a piece of paper is brought progressively closer to the tube, a certain distance will be found at which the light rays come to a *focal line*. On the other hand, the spherical lens is illustrated by an ordinary magnifying glass. If such a lens is placed in a beam of sunlight and a piece of paper is brought progressively closer to the lens, the light rays will impinge on a common focal point at an appropriate distance.

Concave cylindrical lenses *diverge* light rays in only one plane in the same manner that *convex* cylindrical lenses *converge* light rays in one plane.

Figure 22–5 shows two convex cylindrical lenses at right angles to each other. The vertical cylindrical lens causes convergence of the light rays that pass through the two sides of the lens. The horizontal lens converges the top and bottom rays. Thus, all the light rays come to a single point focus. In other words, *two cylindrical lenses crossed at right angles to each other perform the same function as one spherical lens of the same refractive power.*

FOCAL LENGTH OF A LENS

The distance from a convex lens at which parallel rays converge to a common focal point is the *focal length* of the lens. The diagram at the top of Figure 22–6 illustrates this focusing of parallel light rays. In the middle diagram, the light rays that enter the convex lens are not parallel but are diverging because the origin of the light is a point

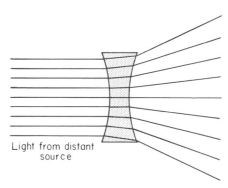

Figure 36–3. Bending of light rays at each surface of a concave spherical lens, illustrating that parallel light rays are diverged by a concave lens.

source not far away from the lens itself. The rays striking the center of the lens pass through the lens without any refraction as pointed out above. And the rays striking the edges are refracted toward the center. However, because these rays are diverging outward from the point source, it can be seen from the diagram that they do not come to a point focus at the same distance away from the lens as do parallel rays. In other words, when rays of light that are already diverging enter a convex lens, the distance of focus on the other side of the lens is farther from the lens than is the case when the entering rays are parallel to each other.

In the lower diagram of Figure 22–6 are shown light rays that are diverging toward a convex lens with far

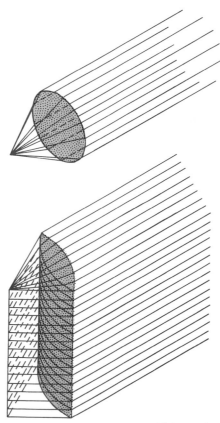

Figure 22–4. *Top*: Point focus of parallel light rays by a spherical convex lens. *Bottom*: Line focus of parallel light rays by a cylindrical convex lens.

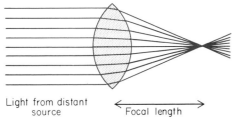

Figure 36–2. Bending of light rays at each surface of a convex spherical lens, showing that parallel light rays are focused to a point focus.

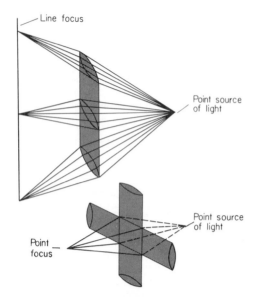

Figure 22–5. Two cylindrical convex lenses at right angles to each other, illustrating that one lens converges light rays in one plane and the other lens converges light rays in the plane at right angles. The two lenses combined give the same point focus as that obtained with a spherical convex lens.

greater curvature than that of the upper two lenses of the figure. In this diagram the distance from the lens at which the light rays come to a focus is exactly the same as that from the lens in the first diagram, in which the lens was less convex but the rays entering it were parallel. This illustrates that both parallel rays and diverging rays can be focused at the same distance behind a lens provided the lens changes its convexity.

The relationship of focal length of the lens, distance of

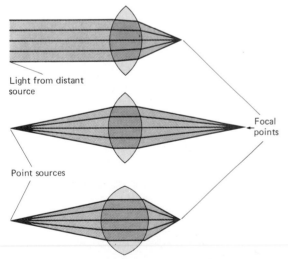

Figure 22–6. The upper two lenses of this figure have the same strength, but the light rays entering the top lens are parallel whereas those entering the second lens are diverging; the effect of parallel versus diverging rays on the focal distance is illustrated. The bottom lens has far more refractive power than either of the other two lenses, illustrating that the stronger the lens the nearer to the lens is the point focus.

the point source of light, and distance of focus is expressed by the following formula:

$$\frac{1}{f} = \frac{1}{a} + \frac{1}{b}$$

in which *f* is the focal length of the lens, *a* the distance of the point source of light from the lens, and *b* the distance of focus from the lens.

FORMATION OF AN IMAGE BY A CONVEX LENS

The upper drawing of Figure 22–7 illustrates a convex lens with two point sources of light to the left. Because light rays pass through the center of a convex lens without being refracted in either direction, the light rays from each point source of light are shown to come to a point focus on the opposite side of the lens *directly in line with the point source and the center of the lens.*

Any object in front of the lens is in reality a mosaic of point sources of light. Some of these points are very bright, some are very weak, and they vary in color. The light rays from each point entering the very center of the lens pass directly through without any of the rays bending. Furthermore, the light rays that enter the edges of the lens come to focal points behind the lens in line with the rays that pass through the center. Therefore, every point source of light on the object comes to a separate point focus on the opposite side of the lens. If all portions of the object are the same distance in front of the lens, all the focal points behind the lens will fall in a common plane a certain distance behind the lens. If a white piece of paper is placed at this distance, one can see an image of the object, as is illustrated in the lower portion of Figure 22–7. However, this image is upside down with respect to the original object, and the two lateral sides of the image are reversed with respect to the original. This is the method by which the lens of a camera focuses light rays on the camera film.

MEASUREMENT OF THE REFRACTIVE POWER OF A LENS—THE DIOPTER

The more a lens bends light rays, the greater is its "refractive power." This refractive power is measured in terms of *diopters.* The refractive power of a convex lens is equal to 1 meter divided by its focal length. Thus a spherical lens has a refractive power of +1 diopter if it converges parallel light rays to a focal point 1 meter beyond the lens, as illustrated in Figure 22–8. If the lens is capable of bending parallel light rays twice as much as a lens with a power of +1 diopter, it is said to have a strength of +2 diopters, and, obviously, the light rays come to a focal point 0.5 meter beyond the lens. A lens capable of converging parallel light rays to a focal point only 10 cm (0.10 meter) beyond the lens has a refractive power of +10 diopters.

The refractive power of concave lenses cannot be stated in terms of the focal distance beyond the lens because the light rays diverge rather than focusing to a point. Therefore, the power of a concave lens is stated in terms of its ability to diverge light rays in comparison with the ability of convex lenses to converge light rays. That is, if a concave lens diverges light rays the same amount that

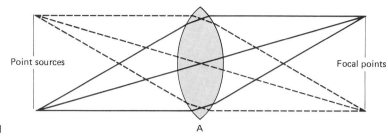

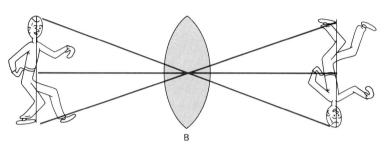

Figure 22–7. *A*, Two point sources of light focused at two separate points on the opposite side of the lens. *B*, Formation of an image by a convex spherical lens.

a 1 diopter convex lens converges them, the concave lens is said to have a dioptric strength of −1. Likewise, if the concave lens diverges the light rays as much as a +10 diopter lens converges them, it is said to have a strength of −10 diopters.

Note particularly that concave lenses can "neutralize" the refractive power of convex lenses. Thus, placing a 1 diopter concave lens immediately in front of a 1 diopter convex lens results in a lens system with zero refractive power.

The strengths of cylindrical lenses are computed in the same manner as the strengths of spherical lenses. If a cylindrical lens focuses parallel light rays to a line focus 1 meter beyond the lens, it has a strength of +1 diopter. On the other hand, if a cylindrical lens of a concave type *diverges* light rays as much as a +1 diopter cylindrical lens *converges* them, it has a strength of −1 diopter.

THE OPTICS OF THE EYE

THE EYE AS A CAMERA

The eye, as illustrated in Figure 22–9, is optically equivalent to the usual photographic camera, for it has a lens system, a variable aperture system (the

pupil), and a retina that corresponds to the film. The lens system of the eye is composed of four refractive interfaces: (1) the interface between air and the anterior surface of the cornea, (2) the interface between the posterior surface of the cornea and the aqueous humor, (3) the interface between the aqueous humor and the anterior surface of the crystalline lens of the eye, and (4) the interface between the posterior surface of the lens and the vitreous humor. The refractive index of air is 1; the cornea, 1.38; the aqueous humor, 1.33; the crystalline lens (on the average), 1.40; and the vitreous humor, 1.34.

The Reduced Eye. If all the refractive surfaces of the eye are algebraically added together and then considered to be one single lens, the optics of the normal eye may be simplified and represented schematically as a "reduced eye." This is useful in simple calculations. In the reduced eye, a single lens is considered to exist with its central point 17 mm in front of the retina and to have a total refractive power of approximately 59 diopters when the lens is accommodated for distant vision.

Most of the refractive power of the eye is provided not by the crystalline lens but instead by the anterior surface of the cornea. The principal reason for this is that the refractive index of the cornea is markedly different from that of air.

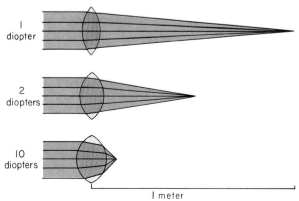

Figure 22–8. Effect of lens strength on the focal distance.

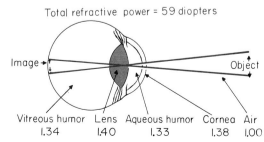

Figure 22–9. The eye as a camera. The numbers are the refractive indices.

On the other hand, the total refractive power of the crystalline lens of the eye, as it normally lies in the eye surrounded by fluid on each side, is only 15 diopters, about one fourth the total refractive power of the eye's lens system. If this lens were removed from the eye and then surrounded by air, its refractive power would be about six times as great. The reason for this difference is that the fluids surrounding the lens have refractive indices not greatly different from the refractive index of the lens itself, and the smallness of the differences greatly decreases the amount of light refraction at the lens interfaces. But the importance of the crystalline lens is that its curvature can be increased markedly to provide "accommodation," which will be discussed later in the chapter.

Formation of an Image on the Retina. In exactly the same manner that a glass lens can focus an image on a sheet of paper, the lens system of the eye can focus an image on the retina. The image is inverted and reversed with respect to the object. However, the mind perceives objects in the upright position despite the upside-down orientation on the retina because the brain is trained to consider an inverted image as the normal.

THE MECHANISM OF ACCOMMODATION

The refractive power of the crystalline lens of the eye can be voluntarily increased from 15 diopters to approximately 29 diopters in young children; this is a total "accommodation" of 14 diopters. To do this, the shape of the lens is changed from that of a moderately convex lens to that of a very convex lens. The mechanism of this is the following:

In the young person, the lens is composed of a strong elastic capsule filled with viscous, proteinaceous, but transparent fibers. When the lens is in a relaxed state, with no tension on its capsule, it assumes a spherical shape, owing entirely to the elasticity of the lens capsule. However, as illustrated in Figure 22–10, approximately 70 ligaments attach radially around the lens, pulling the lens edges toward the edge of the choroid. These ligaments are constantly tensed by the elastic pull of their attachments to the choroid, and the tension on the ligaments causes the lens to remain relatively flat under normal resting conditions of the eye. At the insertions of the ligaments in the choroid is the ciliary muscle, which has two sets of smooth muscle fibers, the *meridional fibers* and the *circular fibers*. The meridional fibers extend from the corneoscleral junction to the insertions of the lens ligaments in the choroid approximately 2 to 3 mm behind the corneoscleral junction. When these muscle fibers contract, the insertions of the ligaments are pulled forward, thereby releasing a certain amount of tension on the crystalline lens. The circular fibers are arranged circularly all the way around the eye so that when they contract a sphincter-like action occurs, decreasing the diameter of the circle of liga-

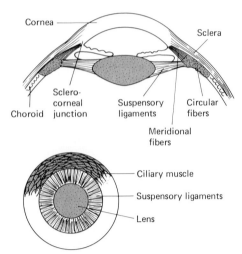

Figure 22–10. Mechanism of accommodation (focusing).

ment attachments and allowing the ligaments to pull less on the lens capsule.

Thus, contraction of both sets of smooth muscle fibers in the ciliary muscle relaxes the ligaments to the lens capsule, and the lens assumes a more spherical shape, like that of a balloon, because of the natural elasticity of its capsule. When the ciliary muscle is completely relaxed, the dioptric strength of the lens is as weak as it can become. On the other hand, when the ciliary muscle contracts as strongly as possible, the dioptric strength of the lens becomes maximal.

Autonomic Control of Accommodation. The ciliary muscle is controlled almost entirely by the parasympathetic nervous system. Stimulation of the parasympathetic nerves to the eye contracts the ciliary muscle, which in turn relaxes the lens ligaments and increases the refractive power. With an increased refractive power, the eye is capable of focusing on objects nearer at hand than when the eye has less refractive power. Consequently, as a distant object moves toward the eye, the number of parasympathetic impulses impinging on the ciliary muscle must be progressively increased for the eye to keep the object constantly in focus. (Sympathetic stimulation has a weak effect in relaxing the ciliary muscle but this plays almost no role in the normal accommodation mechanism, the neurology of which will be discussed in Chapter 24.)

Presbyopia. As a person grows older, the lens loses its elastic nature and becomes a relatively solid mass, partly because of progressive denaturation of the lens proteins. Therefore, the ability of the lens to assume a spherical shape progressively decreases, and the power of accommodation decreases from approximately 14 diopters in the young child to less than 2 diopters at the age of 45 to 50. Thereafter, the lens may be considered to be almost totally nonaccommodating, a condition known as "presbyopia."

Once a person has reached the state of presbyopia, each eye remains focused permanently at an almost constant distance; this distance depends on the physical characteristics of each individual's eyes. Obviously, the eyes can no longer accommodate for both near and far vision. Therefore, to see clearly both in the distance and nearby, an older person must wear bifocal glasses with the upper segment normally focused for far-seeing and the lower segment focused for near-seeing.

THE PUPILLARY APERTURE

A major function of the iris is to increase the amount of light that enters the eye during darkness and to decrease the light in bright light. The reflexes for controlling this mechanism will be considered in the discussion of the neurology of the eye in Chapter 24. The amount of light that enters the eye through the pupil is proportional to the *area* of the pupil or to the *square of the diameter* of the pupil. The pupil of the human eye can become as small as approximately 1.5 mm and as large as 8 mm in diameter. Therefore, the quantity of light entering the eye may vary approximately 30 times as a result of changes in pupillary aperture.

Depth of Focus of the Lens System of the Eye. Figure 22–11 illustrates two separate eyes that are exactly alike except for the diameters of the pupillary apertures. In the upper eye the pupillary aperture is small, and in the lower eye the aperture is large. In front of each of these two eyes are two small point sources of light, and light from each passes through the pupillary aperture and focuses on the retina. Consequently, in both eyes the retina sees two spots of light in perfect focus. It is evident from the diagrams, however, that if the retina is moved forward or backward to an out-of-focus position, the size of each spot will not change much in the upper eye, but in the lower eye the size of each spot will increase greatly, becoming a "blur circle." In other words, the upper lens system has far greater *depth of focus* than the bottom lens system. When a lens system has great depth of focus, the retina can be considerably displaced from the

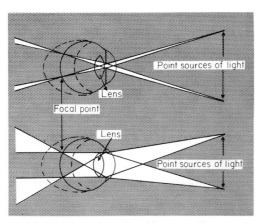

Figure 22–11. Effect of small and large pupillary apertures on the depth of focus.

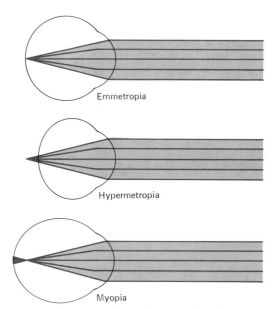

Figure 22–12. Parallel light rays focus on the retina in emmetropia, behind the retina in hypermetropia, and in front of the retina in myopia.

focal plane and still the image remains in sharp focus; whereas, when a lens system has a shallow depth of focus, moving the retina only slightly away from the focal plane causes extreme blurring.

The greatest possible depth of focus occurs when the pupil is extremely small. The reason for this is that with a very small aperture all light rays must pass through the center of the lens, and the centralmost rays are always in focus, as was explained earlier.

ERRORS OF REFRACTION

Emmetropia. As shown in Figure 22–12, the eye is considered to be normal, or "emmetropic," if parallel light rays from distant objects are in sharp focus on the retina when the ciliary muscle is completely relaxed. This means that the emmetropic eye can see all distant objects clearly, with its ciliary muscle completely relaxed, but to focus objects at close range it must contract its ciliary muscle and thereby provide various degrees of accommodation.

Hypermetropia (Hyperopia). Hypermetropia, which is also known as "far-sightedness," is usually due either to an eyeball that is too short or occasionally to a lens system that is too weak when the ciliary muscle is relaxed. In this condition, as seen in the middle panel of Figure 22–12, parallel light rays are not bent sufficiently by the lens system to come to a focus by the time they reach the retina. To overcome this abnormality, the ciliary muscle may contract to increase the strength of the lens. Therefore, the far-sighted person is capable, by using his mechanism of accommodation, of focusing distant objects on the retina. If he has used only a small amount of strength in his ciliary muscle to accommodate for the distant objects, then he still has much accommodative power left, and objects closer and closer to the eye can also be focused sharply until the ciliary muscle has contracted to its limit. The distance of the object away from the eye at this point is known as the "near point" of vision.

In old age, when the lens becomes presbyopic, the far-sighted person often is not able to accommodate his or her lens sufficiently to focus even distant objects, much less to focus near objects.

Myopia. In myopia, or "near-sightedness," when the ciliary muscle is completely relaxed, the light rays coming from distant objects are focused in front of the retina, as shown in the lower panel of Figure 22–12. This is usually due to too long an eyeball but it can occasionally result from too much refractive power of the lens system of the eye.

No mechanism exists by which the eye can decrease the strength of its lens to less than that which exists when the ciliary muscle is completely relaxed. Therefore, the myopic person has no mechanism by which he can ever focus distant objects sharply on his retina. However, as an object comes nearer to his eye it finally comes near enough that its image will focus on the retina. Then, when the object comes still closer to the eye, the person can use his mechanism of accommodation to keep the image focused clearly. Therefore, a myopic person has a definite limiting "far point" for clear vision as well as a "near point."

Correction of Myopia and Hypermetropia by Use of Lenses. It will be recalled that light rays passing through a concave lens diverge. Therefore, if the refractive surfaces of the eye have too much refractive power, as in myopia, some of this excessive refractive power can be neutralized by placing in front of the eye a concave spherical lens, which will diverge rays. On the other hand, in a person who has hypermetropia—that is, someone who has too weak a lens system—the abnormal vision can be corrected by adding refractive power with a convex lens in front of the eye. These corrections are illustrated in Figure 22–13. One usually determines the strength of the concave or convex lens needed for clear vision by "trial and error"—that is, by trying first a strong lens and then a stronger or weaker lens until the one that gives the best visual acuity is found.

Astigmatism

Astigmatism is a refractive error of the lens system, caused usually by an oblong shape of the cornea or, rarely, an oblong shape of the lens. A lens surface like the side of an egg lying edgewise to the incoming light would be an example of an astigmatic lens. The degree of curvature in the plane through the long axis of the egg is not nearly so great as the degree of curvature in the plane through the short axis. Because the curvature of the astigmatic lens along one plane is less than the curvature along the other plane, light rays striking the peripheral portions of the lens in one plane are not bent nearly so much as are rays striking the peripheral portions of the other plane.

This is illustrated in Figure 22–14, which shows rays of light emanating from a point source and passing through an oblong, astigmatic lens. The light rays in the vertical plane, indicated by plane *BD*, are refracted greatly by the astigmatic lens because of the greater curvature in the vertical direction than in the horizontal direction. However, the light rays in the horizontal plane, indicated by plane *AC*, are bent not nearly so much as the light rays in the vertical plane. It is obvious, therefore, that the light rays passing through an astigmatic lens do not all

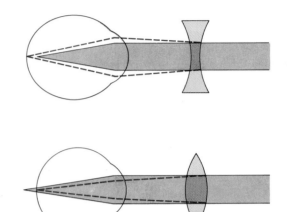

Figure 22–13. Correction of myopia with a concave lens, and correction of hypermetropia with a convex lens.

come to a common focal point because the light rays passing through one plane of the lens focus far in front of those passing through the other plane.

The accommodative powers of the eyes can never compensate for astigmatism because, during accommodation, the curvature of the eye lens changes equally in both planes. Therefore, when the accommodation corrects the refractive error in one plane, the error in the other plane is not corrected. That is, each of the two planes requires a different degree of accommodation to be corrected, so that the two planes are never corrected at the same time. Thus, vision never occurs with a sharp focus.

Correction of Astigmatism with a Cylindrical Lens. One may consider an astigmatic eye as having a lens system made up of two cylindrical lenses of different strengths and placed at right angles to each other. Therefore, to correct for astigmatism the usual procedure is to find a spherical lens by "trial and error" that corrects the focus in one of the two planes of the astigmatic lens. Then an additional cylindrical lens is used to correct the error in the remaining plane. To do this, both the *axis* and the *strength* of the required cylindrical lens must be determined.

There are several methods for determining the axis of the abnormal cylindrical component of the lens system of an eye. One of these methods is based on the use of

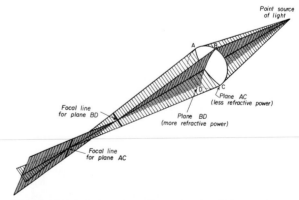

Figure 22–14. Astigmatism, illustrating that light rays focus at one focal distance in one focal plane and at another focal distance in the plane at right angles.

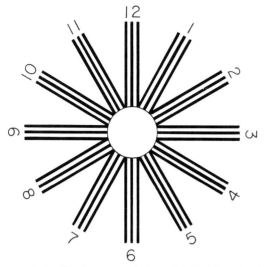

Figure 22–15. Chart composed of parallel black bars for determining the axis of astigmatism.

parallel black bars as shown in Figure 22–15. Some of these parallel bars are vertical, some horizontal, and some at various angles to the vertical and horizontal axes. After placing various spherical lenses in front of the astigmatic eye by trial and error, a strength of lens usually will be found that will cause sharp focus of one set of these parallel bars on the retina of the astigmatic eye but will cause fuzziness of the set of bars at right angles to the sharp bars.

It can be shown from the physical principles of optics discussed earlier in this chapter that the axis of the *out-of-focus* cylindrical component of the optical system is parallel to the bars that are fuzzy. Once this axis is found, the examiner tries progressively stronger and weaker positive or negative cylindrical lenses, the axes of which are placed parallel to the out-of-focus bars, until the patient sees all the crossed bars with equal clarity. When this has been accomplished, the examiner directs the optician to grind a special lens having the spherical correction as well as the cylindrical correction at the appropriate axis.

Correction of Optical Abnormalities by Use of Contact Lenses

In recent years, either glass or plastic contact lenses have been fitted snugly against the anterior surface of the cornea. These lenses are held in place by a thin layer of tears that fill the space between the contact lens and the anterior eye surface.

A special feature of the contact lens is that it nullifies almost entirely the refraction that normally occurs at the anterior surface of the cornea. The reason for this is that the tears between the contact lens and the cornea have a refractive index almost equal to that of the cornea so that no longer does the anterior surface of the cornea play a significant role in the eye's optical system. Instead, the anterior surface of the contact lens now plays the major role and its posterior surface a minor role. Thus, the refraction of this lens now substitutes for the cornea's usual refraction. This is especially important in persons whose eye refractive errors are caused by an abnormally shaped cornea, such as persons who have an odd-shaped, bulging cornea—a condition called *keratoconus*. Without

the contact lens the bulging cornea causes such severe abnormality of vision that almost no glasses can correct the vision satisfactorily; when a contact lens is used, however, the corneal refraction is neutralized, and normal refraction by the anterior surface of the contact lens is substituted in its place.

The contact lens has several other advantages as well, including (1) the lens turns with the eye and gives a broader field of clear vision than do usual glasses, and (2) the contact lens has little effect on the size of the object that the person sees through the lens; on the other hand, lenses placed several centimeters in front of the eye do affect the size of the image in addition to correcting the focus.

Cataracts

Cataracts are an especially common eye abnormality that occurs in older people. A cataract is a cloudy or opaque area in the lens. In the early stage of cataract formation the proteins in the lens fibers immediately beneath the capsule become denatured. Later, these same proteins coagulate to form opaque areas in place of the normal transparent protein fibers of the lens. Finally, in still later stages, calcium is often deposited in the coagulated proteins, thus further increasing the opacity.

When a cataract has obscured light transmission so greatly that it seriously impairs vision, the condition can be corrected by surgical removal of the entire lens. When this is done, however, the eye loses a large portion of its refractive power, which must be replaced by a powerful convex lens (about +15 diopters) in front of the eye, or an artificial lens may be implanted inside the eye in place of the removed lens.

VISUAL ACUITY

Theoretically, light from a distant point source, when focused on the retina, should be infinitely small. However, since the lens system of the eye is not perfect, such a retinal spot ordinarily has a total diameter of about 11 microns even with maximal resolution of the optical system. However, it is brightest in its very center and shades off gradually toward the edges, as illustrated by the two point images in Figure 22–16.

The average diameter of cones *in the fovea* of the retina, the central part of the retina where vision is most highly developed, is approximately 1.5 microns, which is one seventh the diameter of the spot of light. Nevertheless, since the spot of light has a bright center point and shaded edges, a person can distinguish two separate points if their centers lie approximately 2 microns apart on the retina, which is slightly greater than the width of a foveal cone. This discrimination between points is illustrated in Figure 22–16.

The maximum visual acuity of the human eye for discriminating between point sources of light is 26 seconds. That is, when light rays from two separate points strike the eye with an angle of at least 26 seconds between them, they can usually be recognized as two points instead of one. This means that a person with maximal acuity looking at two bright

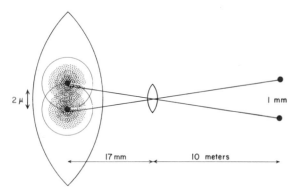

Figure 22–16. Maximum visual acuity for two point sources of light.

pinpoint spots of light 10 meters away can barely distinguish the spots as separate entities when they are 1 millimeter apart.

The fovea is less than one half a millimeter in diameter, which means that maximum visual acuity occurs in only 3 degrees of the visual field. Outside this foveal area the visual acuity is reduced five- to tenfold, and it becomes progressively poorer as the periphery is approached. This is caused by the connection of many rods and cones to the same nerve fiber, as will be discussed in Chapter 24.

Clinical Method for Stating Visual Acuity. Usually the test chart for testing eyes is placed 20 feet away from the tested person, and if the person can see the letters of the size that he should be able to see at 20 feet, he is said to have 20/20 vision: that is, normal vision. If he can see only letters that he should be able to see at 200 feet, he is said to have 20/200 vision. In other words, the clinical method for expressing visual acuity is to use a mathematical fraction that expresses the ratio of two distances, which is also the ratio of one's visual acuity to that of the normal person.

DETERMINATION OF DISTANCE OF AN OBJECT FROM THE EYE— DEPTH PERCEPTION

The visual apparatus normally perceives distance by three major means. This phenomenon is known as *depth perception*. These means are (1) size of the image of known objects on the retina, (2) the phenomenon of moving parallax, and (3) the phenomenon of stereopsis.

Determination of Distance by Sizes of Retinal Images of Known Objects. If one knows that a man whom he is viewing is 6 feet tall, he can determine how far away the man is simply by the size of the man's image on his retina. He does not consciously think about the size, but his brain has learned to calculate automatically from image sizes the distances of objects when the dimensions are known.

Determination of Distance by Moving Parallax. Another important means by which the eyes deter-

mine distance is that of moving parallax. If a person looks off into the distance with his eyes completely still, he perceives no moving parallax, but, when he moves his head to one side or the other, the images of objects close to him move rapidly across his retinae while the images of distant objects remain rather stationary. For instance, if he moves his head 1 inch and an object is only 1 inch in front of his eye, the image moves almost all the way across his retinae, whereas the image of an object 200 feet away from his eyes does not move perceptibly. Thus, by this mechanism of moving parallax, one can tell the *relative distances* of different objects even though only one eye is used.

Determination of Distance by Stereopsis—Binocular Vision. Another method by which one perceives parallax is that of binocular vision. Because one eye is a little more than 2 inches to one side of the other eye, the images on the two retinae are different one from the other—that is, an object that is 1 inch in front of the bridge of the nose forms an image on the temporal portion of the retina of each eye, whereas a small object 20 feet in front of the nose has its image at closely corresponding points in the middle of each retina. This type of parallax is illustrated in Figure 22–17, which shows the images of a black spot and a square actually reversed on the two retinas because they are at different distances in front of the eyes. This gives a type of parallax that is present all the time when both eyes are being used. It is almost entirely this binocular parallax (or stereopsis) that gives a person with two eyes far greater ability to judge relative distances *when objects are nearby* than a person who has only one eye. However, stereopsis is virtually useless for depth perception at distances beyond 200 feet.

OPTICAL INSTRUMENTS

THE OPHTHALMOSCOPE

The ophthalmoscope is an instrument through which an observer can look into another person's eye and see the retina with clarity. Though the ophthalmoscope appears to be a relatively complicated instrument, its prin-

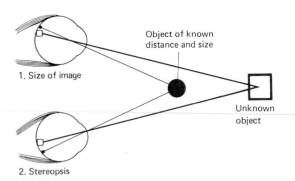

Figure 22–17. Perception of distance (1) by the size of the image on the retina, and (2) as a result of stereopsis.

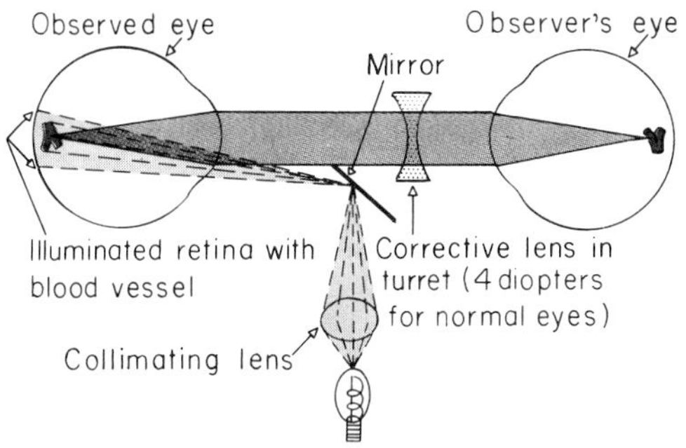

Observed eye   Observer's eye
              Mirror

Illuminated retina with   Corrective lens in
blood vessel   turret (4 diopters
                           for normal eyes)

Collimating lens

Figure 22–18. The optical system of the ophthalmoscope.

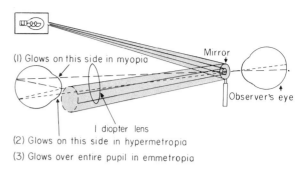

(1) Glows on this side in myopia

Mirror

1 diopter lens

Observer's eye

(2) Glows on this side in hypermetropia

(3) Glows over entire pupil in emmetropia

Figure 22–19. The retinoscope.

ciples are simple. The basic components are illustrated in Figure 22–18 and may be explained as follows.

If a bright spot of light is on the retina of an *emmetropic eye*, light rays from this spot diverge toward the lens system of the eye, and, after passing through the lens system, they are parallel with each other because the retina is located exactly one focal length distance behind the lens. Then, when these parallel rays pass into an emmetropic eye of another person, they focus back again to a point focus on the retina of the second person because his retina is also one focal length distance behind the lens. Therefore, any spot of light on the retina of the observed eye comes to a focal spot on the retina of the observing eye. Likewise, when the bright spot of light is moved to different points on the observed retina, the focal spot on the retina of the observer also moves an equal amount. Thus, if the retina of one person is made to emit light, the image of his retina will be focused on the retina of the observer provided the two eyes are simply looking into each other. These principles, of course, apply only to completely emmetropic eyes.

To make an ophthalmoscope, one need only devise a means for illuminating the retina to be examined. Then, the reflected light from that retina can be seen by the observer simply by putting the two eyes close to each other. To illuminate the retina of the observed eye, an angulated mirror or a segment of a prism is placed in front of the observed eye in such a manner, as illustrated in Figure 22–18, that light from a bulb is reflected into the observed eye. Thus, the retina is illuminated through the pupil, and the observer sees into the subject's pupil by looking over the edge of the mirror or prism, or *through* an appropriately designed prism so that the light will not have to enter the pupil at an angle.

It was noted above that these principles apply only to persons with completely emmetropic eyes. If the refractive power of either eye is abnormal, it is necessary to correct this refractive power in order for the observer to see a sharp image of the observed retina. Therefore, the usual ophthalmoscope has a series of about 20 lenses mounted on a turret so that the turret can be rotated from one lens to another, and the correction for abnormal refractive power of either or both eyes can be made by selecting a lens of appropriate strength. In normal young adults, when the two eyes come close together a natural accommodative reflex occurs that causes an approximate +2 diopters increase in the strength of the lens of each eye. To correct for this, it is necessary that the lens turret be rotated to approximately −4 diopters correction.

THE RETINOSCOPE

The retinoscope, illustrated in Figure 22–19, is an instrument that can be used to determine the refractive power of an eye even though the subject cannot converse with the observer. Such a procedure is valuable for fitting glasses to an infant.

To use the retinoscope, one places a bright spot of light behind and to one side of the observed eye, and the observer stands 1 meter away, looking through a hole in the middle of a small round mirror. The observer then rotates this mirror from side to side, making a reflected beam of light travel across the pupil of the observed eye while the subject keeps his gaze intently on the observer's eye. If the observed eye is exactly focused on the observer's eye, when the edge of this beam of light first enters the pupil the entire pupil suddenly glows red. If the eye has abnormal refractive power, the red glow appears either on the side of the pupil into which the light edge first shines or on the opposite side of the pupil—one or the other. *In hypermetropia the first glow appears on the side of the pupil from which the light beam is being moved. In myopia the first glow appears on the opposite side of the pupil.* The cause of this difference is that the lens of the hyperopic eye is too weak and that of the myopic eye too strong to focus the light from the edge of the pupil on the retina exactly in line with the observer's eye. For a fuller understanding of this effect, however, the student is referred to texts on physiological optics.

One can fit glasses to a patient by placing selected lenses in front of the observed eye one at a time until the glow suddenly covers the pupil over its entire extent rather than spreading from one side of the pupil to the other. However, it should be noted that in retinoscopy one tests an eye that is focused on the observer's eye at 1 meter's distance. This must be taken into consideration in prescribing glasses; 1 diopter strength must be subtracted for far vision.

REFERENCES

Allen, E. W.: Essentials of Ophthalmic Optics. New York, Oxford University Press, 1979.

Campbell, C. J., *et al.*: Physiological Optics. Hagerstown, Md., Harper & Row, 1974.

Collins, R., and Van der Werff, T. J.: Mathematical Models of the Dynamics of the Human Eye. New York, Springer-Verlag, 1980.

Davson, H.: The Physiology of the Eye, 3rd Ed. New York, Academic Press, 1972.

Davson, H., and Graham, L. T., Jr.: The Eye. Vols. 1–6. New York, Academic Press, 1969–1974.

Dick, G. L.: Studies in Ocular Anatomy and Physiology. Kensington, N. S. W., New South Wales University Press, 1976.

Duncan, G., and Jacob, T. J.: Calcium and the physiology of cataract. *Ciba Found. Symp.*, 106:132, 1984.

Fischbarg, J., and Lim, J. J.: Fluid and electrolyte transports across corneal endothelium. *Curr. Top. Eye Res.*, 4:201, 1984.

Hartstein, J.: Basics of Contact Lenses, 3rd Ed. San Francisco, American Academy of Ophthalmology, 1979.

Jaffe, N. S.: Cataract Surgery and Its Complications. St. Louis, C. V. Mosby, 1981.

Kavner, R. S., and Dusky, L.: Total Vision. New York, A & W Publishers, 1980.

Kolder, H. E. J. W. (ed.): Cataracts. Boston, Little, Brown, 1978.

Kuszak, J. R., et al.: Sutures of the crystalline lens: A review. *Scan. Electron Microsc.*, *(Pt. 3)*:1369, 1984.

Lerman, S.: Radiant Energy and the Eye. New York, The Macmillan Co., 1979.

Lesperace: Ophthalmic Lasers. Photocoagulation, Photoradiation and Surgery. St. Louis, C. V. Mosby, 1983.

Miller, D.: Ophthalmology; The Essentials. Boston, Houghton Mifflin, 1979.

Morgan, M. W.: The Optics of Ophthalmic Lenses. Chicago, Professional Press, 1978.

Moses, R. A.: Adler's Physiology of the Eye; Clinical Application. 7th Ed. St. Louis, C. V. Mosby, 1981.

Polyak, S.: The Vertebrate Visual System. Chicago, University of Chicago Press, 1957.

Records, R. E.: Physiology of the Human Eye and Visual System. Hagerstown, Md., Harper & Row, 1979.

Regan, D., et al.: The visual perception of motion in depth. *Sci. Am.*, 241(1):136, 1979.

Roth, H. W., and Roth-Wittig, M.: Contact Lenses. Hagerstown, Md., Harper & Row, 1980.

Ruben, M.: Understanding Contact Lenses (and the Correction of the Abnormal Eye). London, Heinemann Health Books, 1975.

Safir, A. (ed.): Refraction and Clinical Optics. Hagerstown, Md., Harper & Row, 1980.

Sloane, A. E. (ed.): Manual of Refraction. Boston, Little, Brown, 1979.

Toates, F. M.: Accommodation function of the human eye. *Physiol. Rev.*, 52:828, 1972.

Van Heyningen, R.: What happens to the human lens in cataract. *Sci. Am.*, 233(6):70, 1975.

Whitnall, S. E.: The Anatomy of the Human Orbit and Accessory Organs of Vision. Huntington, N.Y., R. E. Kreiger Publishing Co., 1979.

Whitteridge, D.: Binocular vision and cortical function. *Proc. R. Soc. Med.*, 65:947, 1972.

Witkovsky, P.: Peripheral mechanisms of vision. *Annu. Rev. Physiol.*, 33:257, 1971.

Yellott, J. I., Jr., et al.: The beginnings of visual perception: The retinal image and its initial encoding. *In* Darian-Smith, I. (ed.): Handbook of Physiology. Sec. 1, Vol. III. Bethesda, American Physiological Society, 1984, p. 257.

23

The Eye: II. Receptor and Neural Function of the Retina

The retina is the light-sensitive portion of the eye, containing the cones which are responsible for color vision and the rods which are mainly responsible for vision in the dark. When the rods and cones are excited, signals are transmitted through successive neurons in the retina itself and finally into the optic nerve fibers and cerebral cortex. The purpose of the present chapter is to explain specifically the mechanisms by which the rods and cones detect both white and colored light.

ANATOMY AND FUNCTION OF THE STRUCTURAL ELEMENTS OF THE RETINA

The Layers of the Retina. Figure 23–1 shows the functional components of the retina arranged in layers from the outside to the inside as follows: (1) pigment layer, (2) layer of rods and cones projecting into the pigment, (3) outer lining membrane, (4) outer nuclear layer, (5) outer plexiform layer, (6) inner nuclear layer, (7) inner plexiform layer, (8) ganglionic layer, (9) layer of optic nerve fibers, and (10) inner limiting membrane.

After light passes through the lens system of the eye and then through the vitreous humor, it enters the retina from the inside (see Figure 23–1); that is, it passes through the ganglion cells, the plexiform layer, the nuclear layer, and the limiting membranes before it finally reaches the layer of rods and cones located all the way on the outer side of the retina. This distance is a thickness of several hundred microns; visual acuity is obviously decreased by this passage through such non-homogeneous tissue. However, in the central region of the retina, as will be discussed below, the initial layers are pulled aside to prevent this loss of acuity.

The Foveal Region of the Retina and Its Importance in Acute Vision. A minute area in the center of the retina, illustrated in Figure 23–2, called the *macula* and occupying a total area of less than 1 square millimeter, is especially capable of acute and detailed vision. The central portion of the macula, only 0.4 millimeter in diameter, is called the *fovea*; this area is composed entirely of cones, and the cones have a special structure that aids their detection of detail in the visual image, especially a long slender body in contradiction to much larger cones located further

peripherally in the retina. Also, in this region the blood vessels, the ganglion cells, the inner nuclear layer of cells, and the plexiform layers are all displaced to one side rather than resting directly on top of the cones. This allows light to pass unimpeded to the cones rather than through several layers of retina, which aids immensely in the acuity of visual perception.

The Rods and Cones. Figure 23–3 is a diagrammatic representation of a photoreceptor (either a rod or a cone) though the cones are distinguished by having a conical upper end (the outer segment), as shown in Figure 23–4. In general, the rods are narrower and longer than the cones, but this is not always the case. In the peripheral portions of the retina the rods are 2 to 5 microns in diameter whereas the cones are 5 to 8 microns in diameter; in the central part of the retina, in the fovea, the cones have a diameter of only 1.5 microns.

To the right in Figure 23–3 are labeled the four major functional segments of either a rod or a cone: (1) the *outer segment*, (2) the *inner segment*, (3) the *nucleus*, and (4) the *synaptic body*. In the outer segment the light-sensitive photochemical is found. In the case of the rods, this is *rhodopsin*, and in the cones it is one of several photochemicals collectively called *iodopsin*, which are almost exactly the same as rhodopsin except for differences in spectral sensitivity.

Note in Figures 23–3 and 23–4 the large numbers of discs in both the rods and the cones. In the cones, each of the discs is actually an infolded shelf of cell membrane; in the rods this is also true near the base of the rod. However, toward the tip of the rod the discs separate from the membrane and are flat sacs lying totally inside the cell. There are as many as 1000 discs in each rod or cone. At the tips of the rods the discs are continually degenerating, but new ones are also being formed at a rate of about 50 to 100 per day at the base of the outer segment. In the cones, similar degeneration and replacement occurs, but it occurs along the entire extent of the outer segment.

Both rhodopsin and iodopsin are conjugated proteins. These are incorporated into the membranes of the discs in the form of transmembrane proteins. The concentrations of these photosensitive pigments in the disc are so great that they constitute approximately 40 per cent of the entire mass of the outer segment.

The inner segment contains the usual cytoplasm of the cell with the usual cytoplasmic organelles. Particularly important are the mitochondria, for we shall see later

OUTSIDE

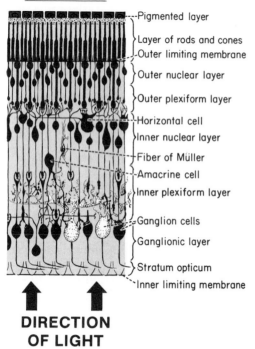

Pigmented layer

Layer of rods and cones

Outer limiting membrane

Outer nuclear layer

Outer plexiform layer

Horizontal cell

Inner nuclear layer

Fiber of Müller

Amacrine cell

Inner plexiform layer

Ganglion cells

Ganglionic layer

Stratum opticum

Inner limiting membrane

DIRECTION OF LIGHT

Figure 23–1. Plan of the retinal neurons. (Modified from Polyak: The Retina. Chicago, University of Chicago Press.)

that the mitochondria in this segment play an important role in providing most of the energy for function of the photoreceptors.

The synaptic body is the portion of the rod and cone that connects with the subsequent neuronal cells, the horizontal and bipolar cells, that represent the next stages in the vision chain.

The Pigment Layer of the Retina. The black pigment *melanin* in the pigment layer, and still more melanin in the choroid, prevent light reflection throughout the globe of the eyeball; this is extremely important for clear vision. This pigment performs the same function in the eye as does the black coloring inside the bellows of a camera.

Without it, light rays would be reflected in all directions within the eyeball and would cause diffuse lighting of the retina rather than the contrast between dark and light spots required for formation of precise images.

The importance of melanin in the pigment layer and choroid is well illustrated by its absence in *albinos*, persons hereditarily lacking in melanin pigment in all parts of their bodies. When an albino enters a bright area, light that impinges on the retina is reflected in all directions by the white surface of the unpigmented choroid so that a single discrete spot of light that would normally excite only a few rods or cones is reflected everywhere and excites many of the receptors. Therefore, the visual acuity of albinos, even with the best of optical correction, is rarely better than 20/100 to 20/200.

The pigment layer also stores large quantities of *vitamin A*. This vitamin A is exchanged back and forth through the membranes of the outer segments of the rods and cones, which themselves are embedded in the pigment layer. We shall see later that vitamin A is an important precursor of the photosensitive pigments and that this interchange of vitamin A is very important for adjustment of the light sensitivity of the receptors.

The Blood Supply of the Retina—The Retinal Arterial System and the Choroid. The nutrient blood supply for the inner layers of the retina is derived from the central retinal artery, which enters the inside of the eye along with the optic nerve and then divides to supply the entire inner retinal surface. Thus, to a great extent, the retina has its own blood supply independent of the other structures of the eye.

However, the outer layer of the retina is adherent to the *choroid*, which is a highly vascular tissue between the retina and the sclera. The outer layers of the retina, including the outer segments of the rods and cones, depend mainly on diffusion from the choroid vessels for their nutrition, especially for their oxygen.

Retinal Detachment. The neural retina occasionally detaches from the pigment epithelium. In some instances the cause of such detachment is injury to the eyeball that allows fluid or blood to collect between the retina and the pigment epithelium, but often it is also caused by contracture of fine collagenous fibrils in the vitreous humor, which pull the retina unevenly toward the interior of the globe.

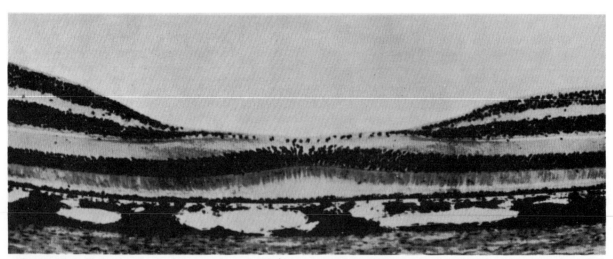

Figure 23–2. Photomicrograph of the macula and of the fovea in its center. Note that the inner layers of the retina are pulled to the side to decrease the interference with light transmission. (From Bloom and Fawcett: A Textbook of Histology. 10th ed. Philadelphia, W. B. Saunders Company, 1975; courtesy of H. Mizoguchi.)

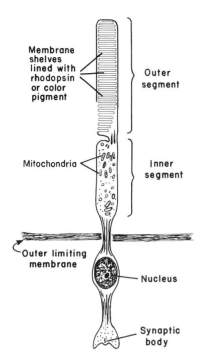

Figure 23–3. Schematic drawing of the functional parts of the rods and cones.

Fortunately, partly because of diffusion across the detachment gap and partly because of the independent blood supply to the retina through the retinal artery, the detached retina can resist degeneration for days and can become functional once again if surgically replaced in its normal relationship with the pigment epithelium. But, if not replaced soon, the retina finally does degenerate and is then unable to function even after surgical repair.

PHOTOCHEMISTRY OF VISION

Both the rods and cones contain chemicals that decompose on exposure to light and, in the process, excite the nerve fibers leading from the eye. The chemical in the *rods* is called *rhodopsin*, and the light-sensitive chemicals in the *cones* have compositions only slightly different from that of rhodopsin and are collectively called *iodopsin*.

In the present section we will discuss principally the photochemistry of rhodopsin, but we can apply almost exactly the same principles to the photochemistry of the iodopsin of the cones.

THE RHODOPSIN-RETINAL VISUAL CYCLE, AND EXCITATION OF THE RODS

Rhodopsin and Its Decomposition by Light Energy. The outer segment of the rod that projects into the pigment layer of the retina has a concentration of about 40 per cent of the light-sensitive pigment called *rhodopsin*, or *visual purple*. This substance is a combination of the protein *scotopsin* and the carotenoid pigment *retinal* (also called "retinene"). Furthermore, the retinal is a particular type called 11-*cis* retinal. This *cis* form of the retinal is

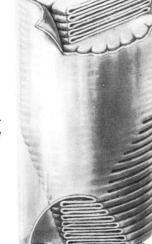

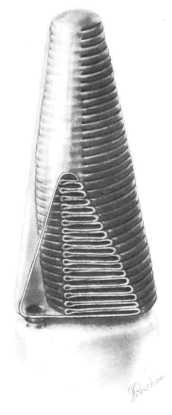

Figure 23–4. Membranous structures of the outer segments of a rod (left) and a cone (right). (Courtesy of Dr. Richard Young.)

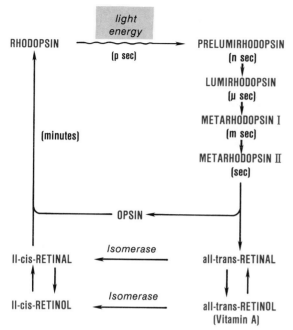

Figure 23–5. Photochemistry of the rhodopsin-retinal-vitamin A visual cycle.

important because only this form can combine with scotopsin to synthesize rhodopsin.

When light energy is absorbed by rhodopsin, the rhodopsin immediately begins to decompose, as shown at the top of Figure 23–5. The cause of this is photoactivation of electrons in the retinal portion of the rhodopsin, which leads to an instantaneous change (in the order of trillionths of a second) of the *cis* form of retinal into an all-*trans* form, which still has the same chemical structure as the *cis* form but has a different physical structure—a straight molecule rather than a curved molecule. Because the three-dimensional orientation of the reactive sites of the all-*trans* retinal no longer fits with that of the reactive sites on the protein scotopsin, it begins to pull away from the scotopsin. The immediate product is *prelumirhodopsin*, which is a partially split combination of the all-*trans* retinal and scotopsin. However, prelumirhodopsin is an extremely unstable compound and decays in nanoseconds to *lumirhodopsin*. This then decays in microseconds to *metarhodopsin I*, then in about a millisecond to *metarhodopsin II*, finally, much more slowly (in seconds) into the completely split products: *scotopsin* and *all-trans retinal*. During the first stages of splitting, the rods are excited and signals are transmitted into the central nervous system, as we shall discuss later.

Reformation of Rhodopsin. The first stage in reformation of rhodopsin, as shown in Figure 23–5, is to reconvert the all-*trans* retinal into 11-*cis* retinal. This process is catalyzed by the enzyme *retinal isomerase*. Once the 11-*cis* retinal is formed, it automatically recombines with the scotopsin to reform rhodopsin, an exergonic process (which means that it gives off energy). The product, rhodopsin,

is a stable compound until its decomposition is again triggered by absorption of light energy.

The Role of Vitamin A in the Formation of Rhodopsin. Note in Figure 23–5 that there is a second chemical route by which all-*trans* retinal can be converted into 11-*cis* retinal. This is by conversion of the all-*trans* retinal first into *all-trans retinol*, which is one form of vitamin A. Then, the all-*trans* retinol is converted into 11-*cis* retinol under the influence of the enzyme isomerase. And, finally the 11-*cis* retinol is converted into 11-*cis* retinal.

Vitamin A is present both in the cytoplasm of the rods and in the pigment layer of the retina as well. Therefore, vitamin A is normally always available to form new retinal when needed. On the other hand, when there is excess retinal in the retina, the excess is converted back into vitamin A, thus reducing the amount of light-sensitive pigment in the retina. We shall see later that this interconversion between retinal and vitamin A is especially important in long-term adaptation of the retina to different light intensities.

Night Blindness. Night blindness occurs in severe vitamin A deficiency. The simple reason for this is that not enough vitamin A is then available to form adequate quantities of retinal. Therefore, the amounts of rhodopsin that can be formed in the rods, as well as the amounts of color-photosensitive chemicals in the cones, are all depressed. This condition is called night blindness because the amount of light available at night is then too little to permit adequate vision, though in daylight the rods and cones can still be excited despite their reduction in photochemical substances.

For night blindness to occur, a person usually must remain on a vitamin A–deficient diet for months, mainly because large quantities of vitamin A are normally stored in the liver. However, once night blindness does develop, it can sometimes be completely cured in less than an hour by intravenous injection of vitamin A.

Excitation of the Rod When Rhodopsin Decomposes

Generation of the Rod Receptor Potential. Generation of the rod receptor potential is entirely different from the generation of receptor potentials in almost all other sensory receptors. That is, excitation of the rod causes *increased negativity* of the membrane potential, which is a state of *hyperpolarization*, rather than decreased negativity, which is the process of "depolarization" that is characteristic of almost all other sensory receptors.

But, how does the breakdown of rhodopsin cause hyperpolarization? The answer to this is that *when rhodopsin decomposes, it decreases the membrane conductance for sodium ions in the outer segment of the rod.* And this causes hyperpolarization of the entire rod membrane in the following way:

Figure 23–6 illustrates movement of sodium ions in a complete electrical circuit through the inner and outer segments of the rod. The inner segment continually pumps sodium from inside the rod to the outside, thereby creating a negative potential on the inside of the entire cell. However, the mem-

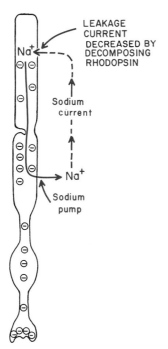

Figure 23–6. Theoretical basis for the generation of a hyperpolarization receptor potential caused by rhodopsin decomposition.

brane of the outer segment, in the *dark* state, is very leaky to sodium. Therefore, sodium continually leaks back to the inside of the rod and thereby neutralizes much of the negativity on the inside of the entire cell. Thus, under normal conditions, when the rod is not excited there is a reduced amount of electronegativity inside the membrane of the rod, normally about −30 millivolts.

When the rhodopsin in the outer segment of the rod is exposed to light and begins to decompose, however, this *decreases* the conductance of sodium to the interior of the rod even though sodium ions continue to be pumped out. Thus, more sodium ions now leave the rod than leak back in. Because these are positive ions, their loss from inside the rod creates increased negativity inside the membrane; and the greater the amount of light energy striking the rod, the greater the electronegativity—that is, the greater the degree of *hyperpolarization*. At maximum light intensity, the membrane potential approaches −90 millivolts, which is the equilibrium potential for potassium ions across the membrane.

Duration of the Receptor Potential and Logarithmic Relationship of the Receptor Potential to Light Intensity. When a sudden pulse of light strikes the retina, the transient hyperpolarization that occurs—that is, the receptor potential that occurs—lasts for about one twentieth to one half of a second, depending on the intensity of the light and other factors. Therefore, a visual image impinged on the retina for only a millionth of a second nevertheless can still cause the sensation of seeing the image sometimes for up to half a second.

Another characteristic of the receptor potential is that it is approximately proportional to the logarithm of the light intensity. This is exceedingly important, because it allows the eye to discriminate light intensities through a range many thousand times as great as would be possible otherwise.

The Mechanism by Which Rhodopsin Decomposition Decreases Membrane Sodium Conductance. Though it is now well known that the decomposition of rhodopsin by light causes decreased outer segment membrane conductance for sodium ions, the basic mechanism of this is still mainly theoretical. Two important theories are the following:

1. The discs inside the rods are actually large, flat vesicles, and inside these is a high concentration of calcium ions. It has been postulated that when the transmembrane rhodopsin molecule becomes activated by light, the breaking away of the retinal molecule from the scotopsin molecule opens a calcium channel through this scotopsin. Therefore, quantities of calcium ions discharge instantly from the vesicles into the cytoplasm of the outer segment. These calcium ions in turn diffuse to the cell membrane and bind with the inner surfaces of the membrane's sodium channels. This blocks the sodium channels and decreases the sodium conductance, thus leading to hyperpolarization.

2. Another theory is that light activation of the rhodopsin molecule triggers a sequence of chemical changes that causes closure of the sodium pores in the following way: (a) Splitting of the rhodopsin activates a phosphodiesterase. (b) The phosphodiesterase causes the breakdown of cyclic GMP. (c) The cyclic GMP normally functions in conjunction with a protein kinase to keep the sodium channels open. However, when light activation diminishes the quantity of cyclic GMP, this now makes it impossible to keep the sodium channels fully opened. Therefore, sodium conductance decreases.

Thus, it is not known exactly how light activation of rhodopsin decreases sodium conductance, but it is this decrease in sodium conductance that leads to the hyperpolarization, which is the receptor potential.

PHOTOCHEMISTRY OF COLOR VISION BY THE CONES

It was pointed out at the outset of this discussion that the photochemicals in the cones have almost exactly the same chemical composition as that of rhodopsin in the rods. The only difference is that the protein portions, the opsins, called *photopsins* in the cones, are different from the scotopsin of the rods. The retinal portions are exactly the same in the cones as in the rods. The color-sensitive pigments of the cones, therefore, are combinations of retinal and photopsins.

In the discussion of color vision later in the chapter, it will become evident that three different

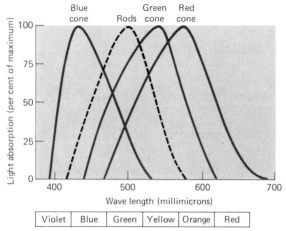

Figure 23–7. Light absorption by the respective pigments of the three color-receptive cones of the human retina. (Drawn from curves recorded by Marks, Dobelle, and MacNichol, Jr.: *Science, 143*:1181, 1964, and by Brown and Wald: *Science, 144*:45, 1964. Copyright 1964 by the American Association for the Advancement of Science.)

types of photochemicals are present in different cones, thus making these cones selectively sensitive to the different colors of blue, green, and red. These photochemicals are called respectively *blue-sensitive pigment, green-sensitive pigment*, and *red-sensitive pigment*. The absorption characteristics of the pigments in the three types of cones show peak absorbancies at light wavelengths respectively, of 445, 535, and 570 millimicrons. These are also the wavelengths for peak light sensitivity for each type of cone, which begins to explain how the retina differentiates the colors. The approximate absorption curves for these three pigments are shown in Figure 23–7. Also shown is the absorption curve for the rhodopsin of the rods, having a peak at 505 millimicrons.

AUTOMATIC REGULATION OF RETINAL SENSITIVITY—DARK AND LIGHT ADAPTATION

Relationship of Sensitivity to Pigment Concentration. The sensitivity of rods is approximately proportional to the antilogarithm of the rhodopsin concentration, and it is assumed that this relationship also holds true in the cones. Therefore, the sensitivity of the rods and cones can be altered up or down tremendously by only slight changes in concentrations of the photosensitive chemicals.

Light and Dark Adaptation. If a person has been in bright light for a long time, large proportions of the photochemicals in both the rods and cones have been reduced to retinal and opsins. Furthermore, most of the retinal of both the rods and cones has also been converted into vitamin A. Because of these two effects, the concentrations of the photosensitive chemicals are considerably reduced, and the sensitivity of the eye to light is even more reduced. This is called *light adaptation*.

On the other hand, if the person remains in darkness for a long time, essentially all the retinal and opsins in the rods and cones become converted into light-sensitive pigments. Furthermore, large amounts of vitamin A are converted into retinal, which is then changed into additional light-sensitive pigments, the final limit being determined by the amount of opsins in the rods and cones. Because of these two effects, the visual receptors gradually become so sensitive that even the minutest amount of light causes excitation. This is called *dark adaptation*.

Figure 23–8 illustrates the course of dark adaptation when a person is exposed to total darkness after having been exposed to bright light for several hours. Note that sensitivity of the retina is very low on first entering the darkness, but within 1 minute the sensitivity has increased tenfold—that is, the retina can respond to light of one tenth the previously required intensity. At the end of 20 minutes the sensitivity has increased about 6000-fold, and at the end of 40 minutes it has increased about 25,000-fold.

The resulting curve of Figure 23–8 is called the *dark adaptation curve*. Note, however, the inflection in the curve. The early portion of the curve is caused by adaptation of the cones, for these adapt much more rapidly than the rods because of a basic difference in the rate at which they resynthesize their photosensitive pigments. On the other hand, the cones do not achieve anywhere near the same degree of sensitivity as the rods. Therefore, despite rapid adaptation by the cones, they cease adapting after only a few minutes, whereas the slowly adapting rods continue to adapt for many minutes and even hours, their sensitivity increasing tremendously. However, a large share of the greater sensitivity of the rods is also caused by convergence of as many as 100 or more rods onto a single ganglion cell in the retina; these rods summate to increase their sensitivity, as will be discussed later in the chapter.

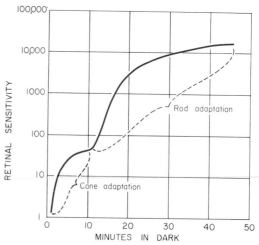

Figure 23–8. Dark adaptation, illustrating the relationship of cone adaptation to rod adaptation.

Other Mechanisms of Light and Dark Adaptation. In addition to adaptation caused by changes in concentrations of rhodopsin or color photochemicals, the eye has two other mechanisms for light and dark adaptation. The first of these is the *change in pupillary size*, which was discussed in the previous chapter. This can cause a degree of adaptation of approximately thirtyfold because of changes in the amount of light allowed through the pupillary opening.

The other mechanism is *neural adaptation*, involving the neurons in the successive stages of the visual chain in the retina itself. That is, when the light intensity first increases, the intensities of the signals transmitted by the bipolar cells, the horizontal cells, the amacrine cells, and the ganglion cells are all very intense. However, the intensities of these signals all decrease rapidly. Although the degree of this adaptation is only a fewfold rather than the many thousand-fold that occurs during adaptation of the photochemical system, this neural adaptation occurs in a fraction of a second, in contrast to the many minutes required for full adaptation by the photochemicals.

Value of Light and Dark Adaptation in Vision. Between the limits of maximal dark adaptation and maximal light adaptation, the eye can change its sensitivity to light by as much as 500,000 to 1,000,000 times, the sensitivity automatically adjusting to changes in illumination.

Since the registration of images by the retina requires detection of both dark and light spots in the image, it is essential that the sensitivity of the retina always be adjusted so that the receptors respond to the lighter areas but not to the darker areas. An example of maladjustment of the retina occurs when a person leaves a movie theater and enters the bright sunlight, for even the dark spots in the images then seem exceedingly bright, and, as a consequence, the entire visual image is bleached, having little contrast between its different parts. Obviously, this is poor vision, and it remains poor until the retina has adapted sufficiently that the darker spots of the image no longer stimulate the receptors excessively.

Conversely, when a person enters darkness, the sensitivity of the retina is usually so slight that even the light spots in the image cannot excite the retina. But, after dark adaptation, the light spots begin to register. As an example of the extremes of light and dark adaptation, the light intensity of the sun is approximately 30,000 times that of the moon; yet the eye can function well both in bright sunlight and in bright moonlight.

Fusion of Flickering Lights by the Retina

In a flickering light, the light intensity alternately increases and decreases rapidly. An instantaneous flash of light excites the visual receptors for as long as 0.05 to 0.5 second, and because of the *persistence* of excitation, rapidly successive flashes of light become *fused* together to give the appearance of being continuous. This effect is well known when one observes motion pictures or television. The images on the motion picture screen are flashed at a rate of 24 frames per second, while those of

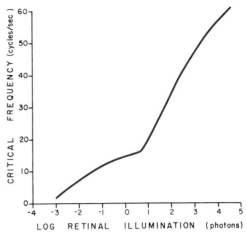

Figure 23–9. Relationship of intensity of illumination to the critical frequency for fusion.

the television screen are flashed at a rate of 60 frames per second. As a result, the images fuse together, and continuous motion is observed.

The frequency at which flicker fusion occurs, called the *critical frequency for fusion*, varies with the light intensity. Figure 23–9 illustrates the effect of intensity of illumination on the critical fusion frequency. At a low intensity, fusion results even when the rate of flicker is as low as 2 to 6 per second. However, in bright illumination, the critical frequency for fusion rises to as great as 60 flashes per second. This difference results at least partly from the fact that the cones, which operate mainly at high levels of illumination, can detect much more rapid alterations in illumination than can the rods, which are the important receptors in dim light.

COLOR VISION

From the preceding sections, we know that different cones are sensitive to different colors of light. The present section is a discussion of the mechanisms by which the retina detects the different gradations of color in the visual spectrum.

THE TRI-COLOR MECHANISM OF COLOR PERCEPTION

Many different theories have been proposed to explain the phenomenon of color vision, but they are all based on the well-known observation that the human eye can detect almost all gradations of colors when red, green, and blue monochromatic lights are appropriately mixed in different combinations.

The first important theory of color vision was that of Young, which was later expanded and given a more experimental basis by Helmholtz. Therefore, the theory is known as the *Young-Helmholtz theory*. According to this theory, there are three different types of cones, each of which responds maximally to a different color.

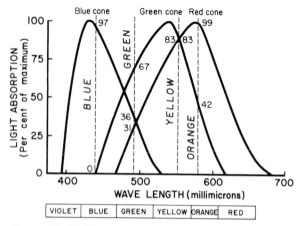

Figure 23–10. Demonstration of the degree of stimulation of the different color-sensitive cones by monochromatic lights of four separate colors: blue, green, yellow, and orange.

As time has gone by, the Young-Helmholtz theory has been expanded, and more details have been worked out. It now is generally accepted as the mechanism of color vision.

Spectral Sensitivities of the Three Types of Cones. On the basis of color vision tests, the spectral sensitivities of the three different types of cones in human beings have been proved to be essentially the same as the light absorption curves for the three types of pigment found in the respective cones. These were illustrated in Figure 23–7 and are also shown in Figure 23–10. These curves can readily explain almost all the phenomena of color vision.

Interpretation of Color in the Nervous System. Referring to Figure 23–10, one can see that an orange monochromatic light with a wavelength of 580 millimicrons stimulates the red cones to a stimulus value of approximately 99 (99 per cent of the peak stimulation at optimum wavelength), whereas it stimulates the green cones to a stimulus value of approximately 42 and the blue cones not at all. Thus, the ratios of stimulation of the three different types of cones in this instance are 99:42:0. The nervous system interprets this set of ratios as the sensation of orange. On the other hand, a monochromatic blue light with a wavelength of 450 millimicrons stimulates the red cones to a stimulus value of 0, the green cones to a value of 0, and the blue cones to a value of 97. This set of ratios—0:0:97—is interpreted by the nervous system as blue. Likewise, ratios of 83:83:0 are interpreted as yellow and 31:67:36, as green.

This scheme also shows how it is possible for a person to perceive a sensation of yellow when a red light and a green light are shone into the eye at the same time, for this stimulates the red and green cones approximately equally, which gives a sensation of yellow even though no wavelength of light corresponding to yellow is present.

Perception of White Light. Approximately equal stimulation of all the red, green, and blue cones gives one the sensation of seeing white. Yet there is no wavelength of light corresponding to white; instead, white is a combination of all the wavelengths of the spectrum. Furthermore, the sensation of white can be achieved by stimulating the retina with a proper combination of only three chosen colors that stimulate the respective types of cones approximately equally.

COLOR BLINDNESS

Red-Green Color Blindness. When a single group of color receptive cones is missing from the eye, the person is unable to distinguish some colors from others. As can be observed by studying Figure 23–10, if the red cones are missing, light of 525 to 675 millimicrons' wavelength can stimulate only the green-sensitive cones, so that the *ratio* of stimulation of the different cones does not change as the color changes from green all the way through the red spectrum. Therefore, within this wavelength range, all colors appear to be the same to this "color blind" person.

On the other hand, if the green-sensitive cones are missing, the colors in the range from green to red can stimulate only the red-sensitive cones, and the person again perceives only one color within these limits. Therefore, when either the red or green types of cones are lacking, the person is said to be "red-green" color blind. However, when one or more types of cones are abnormal but still function partially, a person has "color weakness," instead of color blindness.

The person with loss of red cones is called a *protanope*; his overall visual spectrum is noticeably shortened at the long wavelength end because of lack of the red cones. The color blind person who lacks green cones is called a *deuteranope*; this person has a perfectly normal visual spectral width because the absent green cones operate in the middle of the spectrum where red or blue cones also operate.

Blue Weakness. Occasionally, a person has "blue weakness," which results from diminished or absent blue receptors. If we observe Figure 23–10 still again, we can see that the blue cones are sensitive to a spectral range almost entirely different from that of both the red and green cones. Therefore, if the blue receptors are completely absent, the person has a greater preponderance of green, yellow, orange, and red in the visual spectrum than of blue, thus producing this rarely observed type of color weakness or blindness.

Tests for Color Blindness. Tests for color blindness depend on the person's ability to distinguish various colors from each other and also on his ability to judge correctly the degree of contrast between colors. For instance, to determine whether or not a person is red-green color blind, he may be given many small tufts of wool whose colors encompass the entire visual spectrum. He is then asked to place those tufts that have the same colors in the same piles. If he is not color blind, he recognizes immediately that all the tufts have slightly different colors; however, if he is red-green color blind, he places the red, orange, yellow, and yellow-green colors all together as having essentially the same color.

Color Test Charts. A rapid method for determining color blindness is based on the use of spot-charts such as those illustrated in Figure 23–11. These charts are arranged with a confusion of spots of several different colors. In the top chart, the normal person reads "74," while the red-green color blind person reads "21." In the bottom chart, the normal person reads "42," while the red blind protanope reads "2," and the green blind deuteranope reads "4."

If one will study these charts while at the same time observing the spectral sensitivity curves of the different cones in Figure 23–10, it can be readily understood how excessive emphasis can be placed on spots of certain colors by color blind persons in comparison with normal persons.

Genetics of Color Blindness. Color blindness is sex-linked and results from absence of appropriate color genes in the X chromosomes. This lack of color genes is a recessive trait; therefore, color blindness will not appear as long as another X chromosome carries the genes necessary for development of the respective color-receptive cones.

Because the male human being has only one X chromosome, all three color genes must be present in this single chromosome if he is not to be color blind. In

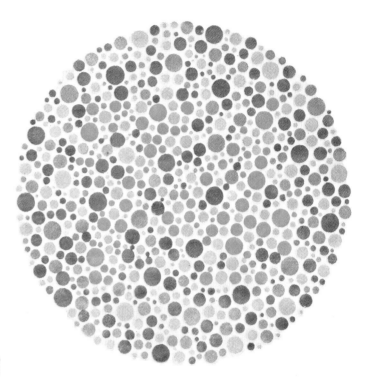

Figure 23–11. Two Ishihara charts. *Upper*: In this chart, the normal person reads "74," whereas the red-green color blind person reads "21." *Lower*: In this chart, the red-blind person (protanope) reads "2," while the green-blind person (deuteranope) reads "4." The normal person reads "42." (From Ishihara: Tests for Colour-Blindness. Tokyo, Kanehara and Co.)

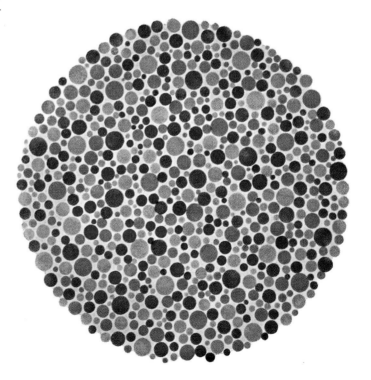

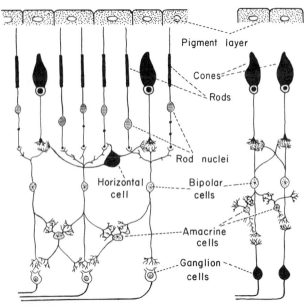

Figure 23–12. Neural organization of the retina: peripheral area to the left, foveal area to the right.

approximately 1 of every 50 times, the X chromosome lacks the red gene; in approximately 1 of every 16, it lacks the green gene; and, rarely, it lacks the blue gene. This means, therefore, that 2 per cent of all men are red color blind (protanopes) and 6 per cent are green color blind (deuteranopes), making a total of approximately 8 per cent who are red-green color blind. Because a female has two X chromosomes, red-green color blindness is a rare abnormality in the female.

NEURAL FUNCTION OF THE RETINA

NEURAL ORGANIZATION OF THE RETINA

The detailed anatomy of the retina was illustrated in Figure 23–1; Figure 23–12 illustrates the basic essentials of the retina's neural connections; to the left is the general organization of the neural elements in a peripheral retinal area and to the right in the foveal area. Note that in the peripheral region both rods and cones converge on *bipolar cells* which in turn converge on *ganglion cells*. In the fovea, where only cones exist, there is little convergence; instead, the cones are represented by approximately equal numbers of bipolar and ganglion cells.

Not emphasized in the figure is the fact that in both the outer and inner plexiform layers (where the neurons synapse with each other) are many lateral connections between the different neural elements. Many of these lateral connections are collateral branches of the dendrites and axons of the bipolar and ganglion cells. But, in addition, two special types of cells are present in the inner nuclear layer that transmits signals laterally: the *horizontal cell*, and the *amacrine cells*.

Each retina contains about 125 million rods and

5.5 million cones; yet, as counted with the light microscope, only 1,000,000 optic nerve fibers lead from the retina to the brain. Thus, an average of about 125 rods and 5 cones converge on each optic nerve fiber. However, there are major differences between the peripheral retina and the central retina, for nearer the fovea fewer and fewer rods and cones converge on each optic fiber, and the rods and cones both become slenderer. These two effects progressively increase the acuity of vision toward the central retina. In the very central portion, in the *fovea*, there are no rods at all. Also, the number of optic nerve fibers leading from this part of the retina is almost equal to the number of cones, as shown to the right in Figure 23–12. This mainly explains the high degree of visual acuity in the central portion of the retina in comparison with the very poor acuity in the peripheral portions.

Another difference between the peripheral and central portions of the retina is the considerably greater sensitivity of the peripheral retina to weak light. This results partly from the fact that as many as 300 rods converge on the same optic nerve fiber in the most peripheral portions of the retina; the signals from the rods summate to give intense stimulation of the peripheral ganglion cells. But, in addition, rods are more sensitive to weak light than are the cones because of intrinsic differences in the receptors themselves.

STIMULATION OF THE RODS AND CONES

Neither the rods nor the cones generate action potentials. Instead, the hyperpolarization receptor potentials generated in the outer segments of the rods and cones are transmitted through the bodies of these receptors to the *synaptic bodies* at their other ends by direct conduction of the electrical voltage itself; this is called *electrotonic conduction*. Then, at the synaptic body, the receptor potential controls the release of a transmitter substance the chemical nature of which is still not known. However, in the dark state, when the receptor is depolarized, the rate of transmitter release is greatest, and its release decreases markedly as the receptor becomes hyperpolarized in the full light condition. The transmitter in turn induces signals in the successive neurons, the bipolar and horizontal cells. The signals in both these cells are also transmitted by electrotonic conduction and not by action potentials.

STIMULATION OF THE BIPOLAR CELLS

The most direct pathway from the rods and cones to the ganglion cells is through the bipolar cells. However, there are two different types of bipolar cells, the *depolarizing bipolar cell* and the *hyperpolarizing bipolar cell*.

The depolarizing bipolar cell is stimulated by the rods and cones when they are exposed to light. The mechanism of this is peculiar in the following way: The transmitter substance from the rods and cones inhibits the depolarizing bipolar cell. Therefore, in the dark, when the rods and cones are secreting large quantities of the transmitter substance, the depolarizing bipolar cell is inhibited. But in the light state, the reduction of transmitter substance from the rods and cones now reduces the inhibition of the bipolar cell, allowing it to become *excited*.

The hyperpolarizing bipolar cell is excited, not inhibited, by the same transmitter from the rods and cones that inhibits the depolarizing cell because its receptors are of the excitatory variety, not the inhibitory variety. Therefore, in the light, exactly opposite events occur in the hyperpolarizing cell to those in the depolarizing cell. That is, the hyperpolarizing cell becomes inhibited.

Because of this difference between the two different types of bipolar cells, both positive signals and negative signals can be transmitted through different bipolar cells from the rods and cones to the amacrine and ganglion cells. (Both types of bipolar cells release an excitatory transmitter at their endings that causes excitation of the amacrine and ganglion cells.)

STIMULATION AND FUNCTION OF THE HORIZONTAL CELLS

The horizontal cells, illustrated to the left in Figure 23–12, connect laterally in the outer plexiform layer of the retina. The input to these cells is principally from the rods and cones; in turn, they excite the dendrites of bipolar cells located many microns laterally.

The horizontal cells respond to the transmitter from the rods and cones in the same manner as the depolarizing bipolar cells. That is, they are excited by light. However, they in turn release an inhibitory transmitter that inhibits the laterally displaced bipolar cells with which they connect. Therefore, the horizontal cells represent a *lateral inhibitory pathway* in the retina.

STIMULATION AND FUNCTION OF THE AMACRINE CELLS

The amacrine cells are excited by the bipolar cells and they in turn excite the ganglion cells. Many of their fiber pathways travel laterally in the inner plexiform layer of the retina so that this represents another pathway by which lateral signals can be transmitted, though this time the signals are excitatory in contrast to the inhibitory signals of the horizontal cells.

Perhaps the most important characteristic of the amacrine cells is that when they are stimulated by the bipolar cells, they at first respond very strongly, but the signal dies away to almost nothing in a fraction of a second. Therefore, it is believed that the amacrine cells send strong signals to the brain to indicate sudden changes in light intensity.

Another difference between amacrine cells and the bipolar and horizontal cells is that amacrine cells often transmit action potentials (but can transmit signals by electrotonic conduction as well); the significance of this difference is not known.

EXCITATION OF THE GANGLION CELLS

Spontaneous, Continuous Discharge of the Ganglion Cells. The ganglion cells transmit their signals through the optic nerve fibers to the brain in the form of action potentials. These cells, even when unstimulated, transmit continuous nerve impulses at an average rate of about 5 per second. The visual signal is superimposed onto this basic level of ganglion cell stimulation. It can be either an excitatory signal, with the number of impulses increasing to greater than 5 per second, or an inhibitory signal, with the number of nerve impulses decreasing to below 5 per second—often all the way to zero.

Summation at the Ganglion Cells of Signals from the Bipolar Cells, the Horizontal Cells, and the Amacrine Cells. The depolarizing bipolar cells transmit the main direct *excitatory* information from the rods and the cones to the ganglion cells: the hyperpolarizing bipolar cells and the horizontal cells transmit *inhibitory* information from laterally displaced rods and cones to surrounding bipolar cells and then to the ganglion cells; the amacrine cells seem to transmit direct but short-lived transient signals that signal a *change* in the level of illumination of the retina. Thus, each of these types of cells performs a separate function in stimulating the ganglion cells.

Also, there are at least three different types of ganglion cells, as we shall discuss in the following chapter. Some of these transmit very discrete signals from narrow groups of visual receptors. Others have widespreading dendritic trees that collect visual information from large areas of the retina and therefore transmit general information, such as luminosity or a sudden change in the visual scene, rather than transmitting the specific visual pattern.

DIFFERENT TYPES OF SIGNALS TRANSMITTED BY THE GANGLION CELLS THROUGH THE OPTIC NERVE

Transmission of Signals Depicting Contrasts in the Visual Scene—The Role of Lateral Inhibition

Most of the ganglion cells do not respond to the actual level of illumination of the scene; instead they respond only to contrast borders in the scene. Since it seems that this is the major means by which the form of the scene is transmitted to the brain, let us explain how this process occurs.

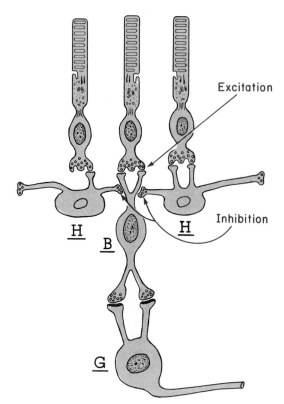

Figure 23–13. Typical arrangement of rods, horizontal cells (*H*), a bipolar cell (*B*), and a ganglion cell (*G*) in the retina, showing excitation at the synapses between the rods and the horizontal cells but inhibition between the horizontal cells and the bipolar cells.

When flat light is applied to the entire retina—that is, when all the photoreceptors are stimulated equally by the incident light—the contrast type of ganglion cell is neither stimulated nor inhibited. The reason for this is that the signals transmitted *directly* from the photoreceptors through the depolarizing bipolar cells are excitatory, whereas the signals transmitted *laterally* through the hyperpolarizing bipolar cells and horizontal cells are inhibitory. Thus, the direct excitatory signal through one pathway is likely to be completely neutralized by the inhibitory signals through the lateral pathways. One circuit for this is illustrated in Figure 23–13, which shows three photoreceptors; the central one of these receptors excites a depolarizing bipolar cell. However, the two receptors on either side are connected to the same bipolar cell through inhibitory horizontal cells that neutralize the direct excitatory signal if these receptors are also stimulated by light.

Now, let us examine what happens when a contrast border occurs in the visual scene. Referring again to Figure 23–13, let us assume that the central photoreceptor is stimulated by a bright spot of light while the two lateral receptors are in the dark. The bright spot of light will excite the direct pathway through the bipolar cell. Then, in addition, the fact that the two lateral photoreceptors are in the dark causes the two horizontal cells to be inhibited. In turn, these cells lose their inhibitory effect on the bipolar cell, and this allows still more excitation of the bipolar cell. Thus, when light is everywhere, the excitatory and inhibitory signals to the bipolar cells mainly neutralize each other, but where contrasts occur the signals through the direct and lateral pathways actually accentuate each other.

Thus, the mechanism of lateral inhibition functions in the eye in the same way that it functions in most other sensory systems as well—that is, to provide contrast detection and enhancement.

Detection of Instantaneous Changes in Light Intensity—The On-Off Response. Many of the ganglion cells are especially excited by *change* in light intensity. For instance, the upper tracing of Figure 23–14 shows that when the light was first turned on the ganglion cell became strongly excited for a fraction of a second, and then the level of excitation diminished. The bottom tracing shows that a second ganglion cell located in the dark area lateral to the spot of light was markedly inhibited at the same time because of lateral inhibition. Then when the light was turned off, exactly the opposite effects occurred. Thus, the responses of these two types of cells are called the "on-off" and the "off-on" responses.

This ability of the retina to detect and transmit signals related to *change* in light intensity is caused by a rapid phase of "adaptation" of some of the neurons in the visual chain. Since this effect is known to be extremely marked in the amacrine cells, it has been suggested that the amacrine cells are peculiarly adapted to detecting light intensity change.

This capability to detect change in light intensity is especially well developed in the peripheral retina. For instance, a minute gnat flying across the peripheral field of vision is instantaneously detected. On the other hand, the same gnat sitting quietly in the peripheral field of vision remains entirely below the threshold of visual detection.

Transmission of Color Signals by the Ganglion Cells. A single ganglion cell may be stimulated by a number of cones or by only a very few. When all three types of cones—the red, blue, and green types—all stimulate the same ganglion cell, the signal transmitted through the ganglion cell is the

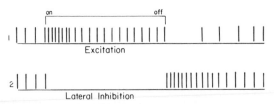

Figure 23–14. Responses of ganglion cells to light in (1) an area excited by a spot of light and (2) an area immediately adjacent to the excited spot; the ganglion cells in this area are inhibited by the mechanism of lateral inhibition. (Modified from Granit: Receptors and Sensory Perception: A Discussion of Aims, Means, and Results of Electrophysiological Research into the Process of Reception. Yale University Press, 1955.)

same for any color of the spectrum. Therefore, this signal plays no role in the detection of the different colors. Instead, it is a "white" signal.

On the other hand, many of the ganglion cells are excited by only one color type of cone but inhibited by a second type. For instance, this frequently occurs for the red and green cones, red causing excitation and green causing inhibition—or vice versa, that is, green causing excitation and red, inhibition. The same type of reciprocal effect also occurs between blue cones on the one hand and a combination of red and green cones on the other hand, giving a reciprocal excitation inhibition relationship between the blue and yellow colors.

The mechanism of this opposing effect of colors is the following: One color-type cone excites the ganglion cell by the direct excitatory route through a depolarizing bipolar cell, while the other color type inhibits the ganglion cell by the indirect inhibitory route through a horizontal cell or a hyperpolarizing bipolar cell.

The importance of these color-contrast mechanisms is that they represent a mechanism by which the retina itself begins to differentiate colors. Thus each color-contrast type of ganglion cell is excited by one color but inhibited by the "opponent color." Therefore, the process of color analysis begins in the retina and is not entirely a function of the brain.

REFERENCES

Allansmith, M. R.: The Eye and Immunology. St. Louis, C. V. Mosby, 1983.

Callender, R., and Honig, B.: Resonance Raman studies of visual pigments. *Annu. Rev. Biophys. Bioeng.*, 6:33, 1977.

Cervetto, L., and Fuortes, M. G. F.: Excitation and interactions in the retina. *Annu. Rev. Biophys. Bioeng.*, 7:229, 1978.

Chignell, A. H.: Retinal Detachment Surgery. New York, Springer-Verlag, 1979.

Cunha-Vaz, J. G. (ed.): The Blood-Retinal Barriers. New York, Plenum Press, 1980.

Davson, H.: The Physiology of the Eye, 3rd Ed. New York, Academic Press, 1972.

Daw, N. W.: Neurophysiology of color vision. *Physiol. Rev.*, 53:571, 1973.

DeValois, R. L., and Jacobs, G. H.: Neural mechanisms of color vision. *In* Darian-Smith, I. (ed.): Handbook of Physiology. Sec. 1, Vol. III. Bethesda, American Physiological Society, 1984, p. 525.

Dick, G. L.: Studies in Ocular Anatomy and Physiology. Kensington, N. S. W., New South Wales University Press, 1976.

Dowling, J. E., and Dubin, M. W.: The vertebrate retina. *In* Darian-Smith, I. (ed.): Handbook of Physiology. Sec. 1, Vol. III. Bethesda, American Physiological Society, 1984, p. 317.

Fatt, I.: Physiology of the Eye: An Introduction to the Vegetative Function. Boston, Butterworths, 1978.

Favreau, O. E., and Corballis, M. C.: Negative aftereffects in visual perception. *Sci. Am.*, 235(6):42, 1976.

Fine, B. S., and Yanoff, M.: Ocular Histology: A Text and Atlas. Hagerstown, Md., Harper & Row, 1979.

Freeman, R. D. (ed.): Developmental Neurobiology of Vision. New York, Plenum Press, 1979.

Friedlaender, M. H.: Allergy and Immunology of the Eye. Hagerstown, Md., Harper & Row, 1979.

Hillman, P., *et al.*: Transduction in invertebrate photoreceptors: Role of pigment bistability. *Physiol. Rev.*, 63:668, 1983.

Kaneko, A.: Physiology of the retina. *Annu. Rev. Neurosci.*, 2:169, 1979.

Kanski, J. J. (ed.): BIMR Ophthalmology. Vol. 1. Disorders of the Vitreous, Retina, and Choroid. Woburn, MA, Butterworths, 1983.

Kohner, E. M. (ed.): Diabetic Retinopathy. Boston, Little, Brown, 1978.

Land, E. H.: The retinex theory of color vision. *Sci. Am.*, 237(6):108, 1977.

MacNichol, E. F., Jr.: Three-pigment color vision. *Sci. Am.*, 211:48, 1964.

Marks, W. B., *et al.*: Visual pigments of single primate cones. *Science*, 143:1181, 1964.

Michael, C. R.: Color vision. *N. Engl. J. Med.*, 288:724, 1973.

Michaelson, I. C.: Textbook of the Fundus of The Eye. New York, Churchill Livingstone, 1980.

Ming, A. L. S., and Constable, I. J.: Colour Atlas of Ophthalmology. Boston, Houghton Mifflin, 1979.

Moses, R. A.: Adler's Physiology of the Eye; Clinical Application. 7th Ed. St. Louis, C. V. Mosby, 1981.

Padgham, C. A., and Saunders, J. E.: The Perception of Light and Color. New York, Academic Press, 1975.

Retina and Vitreous. Rochester, Minn., American Academy of Ophthalmology, 1978.

Rushton, W. A. H.: Visual pigments and color blindness. *Sci. Am.*, 232(3):64, 1975.

Schepens, C. L.: Retinal Detachment and Allied Diseases. Philadelphia, W. B. Saunders Co., 1983.

Sherman, S. M., and Spear, P. D.: Organization of visual pathways in normal and visually deprived cats. *Physiol. Rev.*, 62:738, 1982.

Wolf, G.: Multiple functions of vitamin A. *Physiol. Rev.*, 64:873, 1984.

Yannuzzi, L. A., *et al.* (eds.): The Macula: A Comprehensive Text and Atlas. Baltimore, Williams & Wilkins, 1978.

Young, R. W.: Proceedings: Biogenesis and renewal of visual cell outer segment membranes. *Exp. Eye Res.*, 18:215, 1974.

Zimmerman, T. J., *et al.*: Advances in ocular pharmacology. *Annu. Rev. Pharmacol. Toxicol.*, 20:415, 1980.

Zinn, K. M., and Marmor, M. F. (eds.): The Retinal Pigment Epithelium. Cambridge, Mass., Harvard University Press, 1979.

24

The Eye: III. Central Neurophysiology of Vision

THE VISUAL PATHWAY

Figure 24–1 illustrates the visual pathway from the two retinas to the *visual cortex*. After impulses leave the retinas they pass backward through the *optic nerves*. At the *optic chiasm* all the fibers from the nasal halves of the retinas cross to the opposite side where they join the fibers from the opposite temporal retinas to form the *optic tracts*. The fibers of each optic tract synapse in the *lateral geniculate body* and from here, the *geniculocalcarine fibers* pass through the *optic radiation*, or *geniculocalcarine tract*, to the *primary visual cortex* in the calcarine area of the occipital lobe.

In addition, visual fibers also pass to other areas of the brain: (1) from the optic tracts to the *suprachiasmatic nucleus of the hypothalamus*, presumably for controlling circadian rhythms; (2) into the *pretectal nuclei*, for control of fixation of the eyes on objects of importance and also for activating the pupillary light reflex; (3) into the *superior colliculus*, for control of bilateral simultaneous movement of the two eyes; and (4) into the *pulvinar* as a secondary visual pathway either directly from the optic tracts or indirectly from the superior colliculus.

THREE DIFFERENT TYPES OF RETINAL GANGLIAL CELLS AND THEIR PROJECTIONS

The ganglion cells of the retina are not all the same type either anatomically or functionally. They are mainly divided into three separate types: large, medium, and small.

About 55 per cent of the ganglion cells are of medium size, 10 to 15 microns in diameter. Each of these is excited by a small, circumscribed group of rods or cones or both. This is especially true of the ganglion cells in the foveal region where each one connects with only a few cones. These medium-sized ganglion cells then, after relaying their signals in the lateral geniculate body, transmit the visual pattern to the visual cortex.

The small ganglion cells, less than 10 microns in diameter and representing about 40 per cent of all the ganglion cells, have very thin dendrites that spread widely in the retina. In turn, their axons project directly to the superior colliculus and adjacent regions of the pretectal nuclei. These small ganglion cells are especially important for detecting movement in the visual image, and in response they cause turning of the eyes and head toward the moving object.

The very large ganglion cells, some having diameters as large as 35 microns, represent only 5 per cent of all the ganglion cells. They have a very broad dendritic field in the retina and therefore transmit general information into the visual pathway. They project to both the lateral geniculate body and to the superior colliculus.

Thus, specific features of visual information begin to be dissected from other features before the visual signals leave the retina; then the different types of information are transmitted through different pathways to different brain areas.

Function of the Lateral Geniculate Body

Each lateral geniculate body is located laterally at the dorsal end of the thalamus. In this body the *optic tract terminates*, and from here the visual signals are relayed through the *geniculocalcarine tract to the visual cortex*.

Each lateral geniculate body is composed of six nuclear layers. Layers 2, 3, and 5 (from ventral to dorsal) receive signals from the temporal portion of the ipsilateral retina, whereas layers 1, 4, and 6 receive signals that cross in the optic chiasm from the nasal retina of the opposite eye.

The respective retinal areas of the two eyes connect with neurons that are approximately superimposed over each other in the paired layers, and the layers in turn connect with each other by short axons. Therefore, with a little imagination, one can postulate that the adjacent layers of the lateral geniculate body perhaps play roles in two important processes: (1) *fusion of vision*, which means appropriate control of the directions of gaze of the two eyes so that the two retinal images will superimpose exactly onto each other, and (2) *stereoscopic depth perception*, which depends on comparing the visual images of the two eyes and determining their slight differences, as was discussed in Chapter 22.

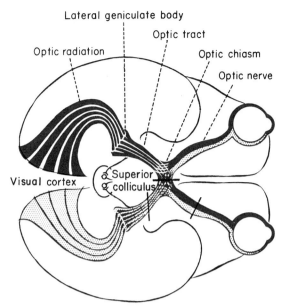

Figure 24–1. The visual pathways from the eyes to the visual cortex. (Modified from Polyak: The Retina. Chicago, University of Chicago Press.)

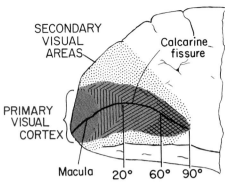

Figure 24–2. The visual cortex.

Relay Function of the Lateral Geniculate Body. The lateral geniculate body does not change the "pattern" of the visual image significantly as it relays this image from the retina to the visual cortex. Also, the neurons in the lateral geniculate body respond in almost the same manner as the medium-sized ganglion cells of the retina. That is, they respond very strongly to contrast borders in the retinal image, to spots of light, and to opponent colors.

It is not known why the lateral geniculate body has three entirely different pairs of neuronal layers. However, the signals in layers 1 and 2 are mainly related to black and white vision, whereas the color signals occur mainly in layers 3 and 4, and layers 5 and 6.

FUNCTION OF THE PRIMARY VISUAL CORTEX

The ability of the visual system to detect spatial organization of the visual scene—that is, to detect the forms of objects, brightness of the individual parts of the objects, shading, and so forth—depends on function of the *primary visual cortex,* the anatomy of which is illustrated in Figure 24–2. This area lies mainly in the calcarine fissure located bilaterally on the medial aspect of each occipital cortex. Specific points of the retina connect with specific points of the visual cortex, the right halves of the two respective retinas connecting with the right visual cortex and the left halves connecting with the left visual cortex. The macula is represented at the occipital pole of the visual cortex and the peripheral regions of the retina are represented in concentric circles farther and farther forward from the occipital pole. The upper portion of the retina is represented superiorly in the visual cortex, and the lower portion, inferiorly. Note the large area of cortex receiving signals from the macular region of the retina. It is in this region that the fovea is represented, which gives the highest degree of visual acuity. Based on foveal area, the fovea has 35 times as much representation in the primary visual cortex as do the peripheral portions of the retina.

DETECTION OF LINES AND BORDERS BY THE PRIMARY VISUAL CORTEX

If a person looks at a blank wall, only a few neurons of the primary visual cortex will be stimulated, whether the illumination of the wall is bright or weak. Therefore, the question must be asked: What does the visual cortex do? To answer this question, let us now place on the wall a large solid cross such as that illustrated to the left in Figure 24–3. To the right is illustrated the spatial pattern of the greater majority of the excited neurons that one finds in the visual cortex. *Note that the areas of excitation occur along the sharp borders of the visual pattern.* Thus, by the time the visual signal is recorded in the primary visual cortex, it is concerned mainly with the *contrasts* in the visual scene rather than with the flat areas. At each point in the visual scene where there is a change from dark to light or light to dark, the corresponding area of the primary visual cortex becomes stimulated. The intensity of

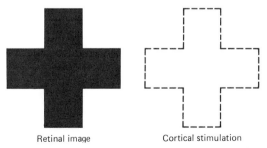

Retinal image   Cortical stimulation

Figure 24–3. Pattern of excitation occurring in the visual cortex in response to a retinal image of a dark cross.

stimulation is determined by the *gradient of contrast*. That is, the greater the sharpness in the contrast border and the greater the difference in intensities between the light and dark areas, the greater the degree of stimulation.

Thus, the *pattern of contrasts* in the visual scene is impressed upon the neurons of the visual cortex, and this pattern has a spatial orientation roughly the same as that of the retinal image.

Detection of Orientation of Lines and Borders—The Neuronal Columns

Not only does the visual cortex detect the *existence* of lines and borders in the different areas of the retinal image, but it also detects the *orientation* of each line or border—that is, whether it is a vertical or horizontal line or border, or lies at some degree of inclination. The mechanism of this effect is the following:

In each small area of the visual cortex the neurons are arranged in columns, each column containing many neurons and having a diameter of 200 to 500 microns, extending downward from the surface of the cortex through its six layers. The signals arriving in the cortex from the lateral geniculate body terminate in layer 4, and from here secondary signals spread upward or downward in the column.

Within each column of neurons, the neurons of layer 4 respond to lines that (1) are located at single positions on the retina and (2) are oriented in a specific direction. Thus, these neurons are line detectors that are both direction-specific and position-specific. They are called *simple cells*.

Detection of Line Orientation Even When the Line Is Displaced Laterally. As the signal progresses farther away from layer 4 of each column, some of the neurons now respond to lines still oriented in the same direction but not position-specific. That is, the line can be displaced laterally in either direction over a moderate distance, and still the neuron will be stimulated. Therefore, these cells are called *complex cells*.

Detection of Length of Lines. Many of the neurons in the outer layers of each column of cells are stimulated only by lines or borders *of specific lengths*. Thus, this is a still higher order for deciphering information from the visual scene; these neurons are called *hypercomplex cells*.

Changing Orientation of the Lines from One Column of Neurons to the Next. When one moves a recording electrode from one column of cells of the primary visual cortex to an adjacent column, it is seen that now a different orientation of lines is required to excite the column, usually rotated about 10 degrees from those of the first column. And, when going to the next column, the lines are rotated still another 10 degrees. Thus, the separate columns of cells detect images oriented in different directions.

The Neuronal Mechanism for Detecting Lines. The mechanism by which the neurons of the primary visual cortex detect lines rather than spots of light is believed to be the following: It is believed that each linear group of ganglion cells in the retina project their signals to a single "simple cell" in layer 4 of the primary visual cortex. When one ganglion cell of the group is stimulated but the rest are not, the signal intensity is not strong enough to excite the simple cell. However, when the entire group of ganglion cells in the linear sequence are stimulated, then the signal strength is great enough to excite the simple cell.

Now, if we remember that each excitatory ganglion cell of the retina is excited by light but is also excited by darkness falling on the retina to the sides of the ganglion cell, then it becomes clear that any contrast border in the visual image will cause double excitation of the linear group of ganglion cells—that is, (1) direct excitation caused by the light portion of the contrast border, and (2) excitation caused by lateral inhibition from the laterally placed dark portion of the retina. Thus, it is this organization of the neuronal connections from the ganglion cells of the retina that allows the simple cells of the primary visual cortex to detect lines.

In a similar manner, the complex cells and the hypercomplex cells are believed to receive converging excitatory and inhibitory neuronal signals from the lower order neurons, in this way deciphering more and more complex information from the scene.

ANALYSIS OF COLOR BY THE VISUAL CORTEX

Some of the columns of cells in the visual cortex respond specifically to colors rather than simply to lines. However, as is true in the retina and also in the lateral geniculate body, stimulation of the neurons in these columns usually requires contrasting opponent colors, especially the red-green opponent colors and the blue-yellow opponent colors. The deciphering of color information is believed also to become more complex at different levels of neuronal organization. In fact, full appreciation of color probably does not occur in the primary visual cortex alone, for it has recently been found in human beings that lesions on the ventral surface of the occipital lobe can cause lack of color reception. It is suggested, therefore, that this area might be a final region for color signal processing.

Interaction of Visual Signals from the Two Different Eyes in the Primary Visual Cortex. From our earlier description of the lateral geniculate body, it will be recalled that the visual signals from the two separate eyes are relayed through separate lateral geniculate body neuronal layers. These signals from the two eyes are still separated from each other when they arrive in the primary visual cortex. The cortex is interlaced with zebra-like stripes of neurons, each stripe about 0.5 mm wide; the signals from one eye enter every other stripe, and the signals from the other eye the opposite set of stripes. The signals from the two eyes remain separated from each other when they excite the layer 4 neurons; this is also true for excitation of almost all the simple cells that detect simple line orientation. However, by the time the complex, and especially the hypercomplex, cells are excited, many of the signals from the two separate eyes have by then begun to converge. As we shall see later in the chapter, when these signals are not "in register"—that is, not both excited or inhibited together—*interference patterns* develop and excite still other cells. It is presumed that these patterns are the basis for controlling fusion of the visual images from the two eyes, and they are likely also the basis of stereopsis.

PERCEPTION OF LUMINOSITY

Very little is known about the way in which the brain detects the level of luminosity. However, it is believed that this results at least partly from the effect that luminosity has of increasing the intensity of the visual contrasts caused by lines, borders, moving objects, and opponent colors in the visual scene. That is, the greater the light intensity, the greater are the degrees of contrast and therefore the more strongly the visual cortex is stimulated.

In addition, some of the ganglion cells of the retina do respond to luminosity, especially some of the very small ganglion cells. These transmit luminosity signals into the pretectal region of the brain stem to control the size of the pupil. It is possible that this same information is used to help the person appreciate the level of illumination.

EFFECT OF REMOVING THE PRIMARY VISUAL CORTEX

Removal of the primary visual cortex in the human being always causes loss of conscious vision. However, psychological studies have demonstrated that such persons can still react subconsciously to many aspects of vision, especially to changes in light intensity, and to crude aspects of form as well. The reactions include turning the eyes, turning the head, avoidance, and so on. In some low-level mammals a large share of the vision is still preserved even when the primary visual cortex is completely removed. This vision is believed to be subserved by neuronal pathways from the optic tracts to the superior colliculi and thence to the secondary visual cortical areas.

TRANSMISSION OF VISUAL INFORMATION INTO OTHER REGIONS OF THE CEREBRAL CORTEX

The primary visual cortex is located in the *calcarine fissure area*, mainly on the medial aspect of each hemi-

sphere but also spreading slightly over the occipital pole. It is known as *Brodmann area 17* of the cortex, and it is also called the *striate area* because of its striated appearance to the naked eye.

Signals from the striate area project laterally in the occipital cortex into area 18 and then into area 19, as illustrated in Figure 24–4. These areas are called the *secondary visual cortex*, the *peristriate area*, or *visual association areas*. In reality, they are simply the loci for additional processing of visual information.

The visual projection images in areas 18 and 19 are organized into columns of cells in the same manner as described earlier for the primary visual cortex. There are also as many as five different topographic representations of the visual field as found in the primary visual cortex. However, the neuronal cells are mainly of the *hypercomplex type* and respond to more complex patterns than do those in the primary visual cortex. Presumably, these progressively more complex interpretations eventually decode the visual information, giving the overall impression of the visual scene that the person is observing.

Projection of Visual Information into the Temporal Cortex. From areas 18 and 19, visual signals next proceed to the posterior portion of the temporal lobes, Brodmann areas 20 and 21. In these areas simple visual patterns such as lines, borders, angles, and so forth fail to cause excitation of specific neurons. The degree of integration of visual information at this level, such as interpretation of letters or words, is presumably much higher.

Effects of Destruction of the Secondary Visual Cortex. Human beings who have destructive lesions of any of the visual association areas, areas 18 and 19 in the occipital cortex or areas 20 and 21 in the temporal cortex, have difficulty with certain types of visual perception and visual learning. For instance, destruction in areas 18 and 19 generally makes it difficult to perceive form, such as shapes of objects, their sizes, and their meanings. It is believed that this type of lesion in the dominant hemisphere can cause the abnormality known as *dyslexia* or *word blindness*, which means that the person has difficulty understanding the meanings of words that are seen.

Destruction of the temporal projections of the visual system makes it especially difficult for animals, and presumably for human beings as well, to learn tasks that are based upon visual perceptions. For instance, a person might be able to see a plate of food perfectly well but be unable to utilize this visual information to direct a fork toward the food. Yet, when the person feels the plate with the hand, the fork can be directed accurately by stereotactic information from the somesthetic cortex.

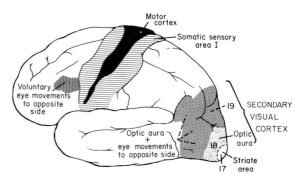

Figure 24–4. The visual association fields and the cortical areas for control of eye movements.

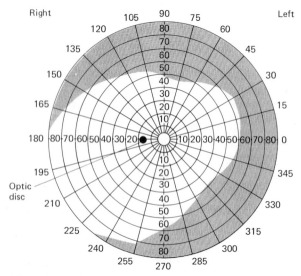

Figure 24–5. A perimetry chart, showing the field of vision for the left eye.

THE FIELDS OF VISION; PERIMETRY

The *field of vision* is the area seen by an eye at a given instant. The area seen to the nasal side is called the *nasal field of vision,* and the area seen to the lateral side is called the *temporal field of vision.*

To diagnose blindness in specific portions of the retinas, one charts the field of vision for each eye by a process known as *perimetry.* This is done by having the subject look with one eye toward a central spot directly in front of the eye. Then a small dot of light or a small object is moved back and forth in all areas of the field of vision, both laterally and nasally and upward and downward, and the person indicates when the spot of light or object can be seen and when it cannot. At the same time, a chart (Fig. 24–5) is made for the eye, showing the areas in which the subject can and cannot see the spot. Thus, the field of vision is plotted.

In all perimetry charts, a *blind spot* caused by lack of rods and cones in the retina over the *optic disc* is found approximately 15 degrees lateral to the central point of vision, as illustrated in the figure.

Abnormalities in the Fields of Vision. Occasionally blind spots are found in other portions of the field of vision besides the optic disc area. Such blind spots are called *scotomata;* they frequently result from allergic reactions in the retina or from toxic conditions, such as lead poisoning or even excessive use of tobacco.

Still another condition that can be diagnosed by perimetry is *retinitis pigmentosa.* In this disease, portions of the retina degenerate and excessive melanin pigment deposits in the degenerated areas. Retinitis pigmentosa generally causes blindness in the peripheral field of vision first and then gradually encroaches on the central areas.

Effect of Lesions in the Optic Pathway on the Fields of Vision. One of the most important uses of perimetry is for localization of lesions in the visual nervous pathway. Lesions in the optic nerve, in the optic chiasm, in the optic tract, and in the geniculocalcarine tract all cause blind areas in the visual fields, and the "patterns" of these blind areas often indicate the location of the lesion.

Destruction of an entire *optic nerve* obviously causes blindness of the respective eye. Destruction of the *optic chiasm,* as shown by the longitudinal line across the chiasm in Figure 24–1, prevents the passage of impulses from the nasal halves of the two retinae to the opposite optic tracts. Therefore, the nasal halves are both blinded, which means that the person is blind in both temporal fields of vision *because the image of the field of vision is inverted on the retina;* this condition is called *bitemporal hemianopsia.* Such lesions frequently result from tumors of the adenohypophysis pressing upward on the optic chiasm.

Interruption of an *optic tract,* which is also shown by a line in Figure 24–1, denervates the corresponding half of each retina on the same side as the lesion, and, as a result, neither eye can see objects to the opposite side. This condition is known as *homonymous hemianopsia.* Destruction of the *optic radiation* or the *visual cortex* of one side also causes homonymous hemianopsia. A common condition that destroys the visual cortex is thrombosis of the posterior cerebral artery, which infarcts the occipital cortex except for the foveal area, thus often sparing central vision.

One can differentiate a lesion in the optic tract from a lesion in the geniculocalcarine tract or visual cortex by determining whether impulses can still be transmitted into the pretectal nuclei to initiate a pupillary light reflex.

EYE MOVEMENTS AND THEIR CONTROL

To make use of the abilities of the eye, almost equally as important as the system for interpretation of the visual signals from the eyes is the cerebral control system for directing the eyes toward the object to be viewed.

Muscular Control of Eye Movements. The eye movements are controlled by three separate pairs of muscles, shown in Figure 24–6: (1) the *medial* and *lateral recti,* (2) the *superior* and *inferior recti,* and (3) the *superior* and *inferior obliques.* The medial and lateral recti contract reciprocally to move the eyes from side to side. The superior and inferior recti contract reciprocally to move the eyes upward or downward. And the oblique muscles function

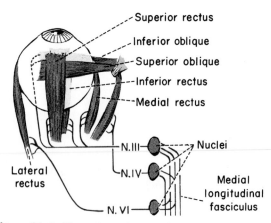

Figure 24–6. The extraocular muscles of the eye and their innervation.

mainly to rotate the eyeballs to keep the visual fields in the upright position.

Neural Pathways for Control of Eye Movements. Figure 24–6 also illustrates the nuclei of the third, fourth, and sixth cranial nerves and their innervation of the ocular muscles. Shown, too, are the interconnections among these three nuclei through the *medial longitudinal fasciculus.* Either by way of this fasciculus or by way of other closely associated pathways, each of the three sets of muscles to each eye is *reciprocally* innervated so that one muscle of the pair relaxes while the other contracts.

Figure 24–7 illustrates cortical control of the oculomotor apparatus, showing spread of signals from the occipital visual areas through occipitotectal and occipitocollicular tracts into the pretectal and superior colliculus areas of the brain stem. In addition, a frontotectal tract passes from the frontal cortex into the pretectal area. From both the pretectal and the superior colliculus areas, the oculomotor control signals then pass to the nuclei of the oculomotor nerves. Strong signals are also transmitted into the oculomotor system from the vestibular nuclei by way of the medial longitudinal fasciculus.

FIXATION MOVEMENTS OF THE EYES

Perhaps the most important movements of the eyes are those that cause the eyes to "fix" on a discrete portion of the field of vision.

Fixation movements are controlled by two different neuronal mechanisms. The first of these allows the person to move his eyes voluntarily to find the object upon which he wishes to fix his vision; this is called the *voluntary fixation mechanism.* The second is an involuntary mechanism that holds the eyes firmly on the object once it has been found; this is called the *involuntary fixation mechanism.*

The voluntary fixation movements are controlled by a small cortical field located bilaterally in the premotor cortical regions of the frontal lobes, as illustrated in Figure 24–7. Bilateral dysfunction or destruction of these areas makes it difficult or almost impossible for the person to "unlock" the eyes from one point of fixation and then move them to another point. It is usually necessary for the person to blink eyes or put a hand over the eyes for a short time, which then allows the eyes to be moved.

On the other hand, the fixation mechanism that causes the eyes to "lock" on the object of attention once it is found is controlled by the *secondary visual area of the occipital cortex*—mainly area 19—which is also illustrated in Figure 24–7. When this area is destroyed bilaterally, an animal has difficulty keeping its eyes directed toward a given fixation point or becomes completely unable to do so.

To summarize, the posterior eye fields automatically "lock" the eyes on a given spot of the visual field and thereby prevent movement of the image across the retina. To unlock this visual fixation, voluntary impulses must be transmitted from the "voluntary" eye fields located in the frontal areas.

Mechanism of Fixation. Visual fixation results from a negative feedback mechanism that prevents the object of attention from leaving the foveal portion of the retina. The eyes even normally have three types of continuous but almost imperceptible movements: (1) a *continuous*

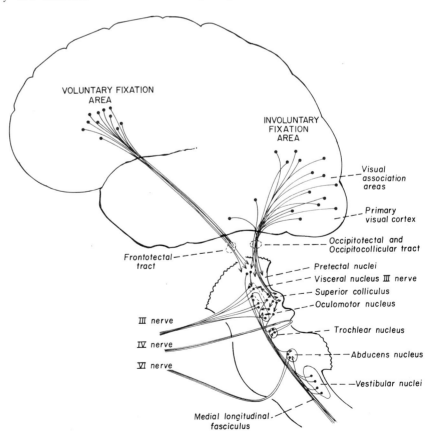

Figure 24–7. Neural pathways for control of conjugate movement of the eyes.

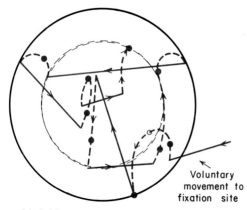

Voluntary
movement to
fixation site

Figure 24–8. Movements of a spot of light on the fovea, showing sudden "flicking" movements to move the spot back toward the center of the fovea whenever it drifts to the foveal edge. (The dashed lines represent slow movements, and the solid lines represent sudden flicking movements.) (Modified from Whitteridge: Handbook of Physiology. Vol. 2, Sec. 1. Baltimore, Williams & Wilkins, 1960, p. 1089.)

tremor at a rate of 30 to 80 cycles per second caused by successive contractions of the motor units in the ocular muscles, (2) a *slow drift* of the eyeballs in one direction or another, and (3) sudden *flicking movements* which are controlled by the involuntary fixation mechanism. When a spot of light has become fixed on the foveal region of the retina, the tremorous movements cause the spot to move back and forth at a rapid rate across the cones, and the drifting movements cause it to drift slowly across the cones. However, each time the spot of light drifts as far as the edge of the fovea, a sudden reflex reaction occurs, producing a flicking movement that moves the spot away from this edge back toward the center. Thus, whenever the image drifts away from the point of fixation, an automatic response moves the image back toward the central portion of the fovea. These drifting and flicking motions are illustrated in Figure 24–8, which shows by the dashed lines the slow drifting across the retina and by the solid lines the flicks that keep the image from leaving the foveal region.

Fixation of the Eyes on Important Visual Highlights— Role of the Superior Colliculi. The eyes have an automatic capability for instantaneously *fixing* on an important highlight in the visual field. However, this capability is mostly lost when the superior colliculi are destroyed. The signals for fixation originate in the visual areas of the occipital cortex, primarily in the secondary visual areas, then pass to the superior colliculi, probably from there to reticular areas around the oculomotor nuclei, and thence into the motor nuclei themselves.

Function of the Superior Colliculi in Turning of the Eyes or the Head Toward a Visual Disturbance. The superior colliculi are also important in causing sudden turning of the eyes to the side when a flash of light or some other sudden visual disturbance occurs on that side. In addition, signals are transmitted from the superior colliculi through the medial longitudinal fasciculus to other areas of the brain stem to cause turning of the whole head and perhaps even of the whole body toward the direction of the light. Other types of disturbances besides visual disturbances, such as strong sounds or even stroking the side of the body, will cause similar turning of the eyes, head, and body if the superior colliculi are intact. This effect, also, is absent or severely

disturbed when the superior colliculi are destroyed. Therefore, it is frequently said that the superior colliculi play an important role in orienting the eyes, the head, and the body with respect to external signals—visual signals, auditory signals, somatic signals, and perhaps even others.

Saccadic Movement of the Eyes. When the visual scene is moving continually before the eyes, such as when a person is riding in a car or turning around, the eyes fix on one highlight after another in the visual field, jumping from one to the next at a rate of two to three jumps per second. The jumps are called *saccades*, and the movements are called *opticokinetic movements.* The saccades occur so rapidly that not more than 10 per cent of the total time is spent in moving the eyes, 90 per cent of the time being allocated to the fixation sites. Also, the brain suppresses the visual image during the saccades so that one is completely unconscious of the movements from point to point.

Saccadic Movements During Reading. During the process of reading, a person usually makes several saccadic movements of the eyes for each line. In this case the visual scene is not moving past the eyes, but the eyes are trained to scan across the visual scene to extract the important information. Similar saccades occur when a person observes a painting, except that the saccades occur in one direction after another from one highlight of the painting to another, then another, and so forth.

Fixation on Moving Objects—"Pursuit Movements." The eyes can also remain fixed on a moving object, which is called *pursuit movement.* A highly developed cortical mechanism automatically detects the course of movement of an object and then gradually develops a similar course of movement of the eyes. For instance, if an object is moving up and down in a wavelike form at a rate of several times per second, the eyes at first may be completely unable to fixate on it. However, after a second or so the eyes begin to jump coarsely in approximately the same pattern of movement as that of the object. Then after a few more seconds, the eyes develop progressively smoother and smoother movements and finally follow the course of movement almost exactly. This represents a high degree of automatic, subconscious computational ability by the cerebral cortex.

Vestibular Control of Eye Movements. Another type of eye movement is elicited by stimulation of the vestibular apparatus. The vestibular nuclei are connected directly with the brainstem nuclei that control ocular movements, and, whenever the head is accelerated in a vertical, longitudinal, lateral or angular direction, an immediate compensatory motion of the eyes occurs in the opposite direction. This allows the eyes to remain fixed on an object of attention despite rapid movements of the body or head.

Vestibular control of the eyes is especially valuable when a person is subjected to jerky motions of the body. For instance, when a person with bilateral destruction of the vestibular apparatuses rides over rough roads, fixing the eyes on the road or on any horizontal scene is extremely difficult. The opticokinetic type of movement is not capable of keeping the eyes fixed under such conditions because it has a latent period of about one-fifth second before the direction of movement of the visual scene can be detected and followed by the eyes. On the other hand, the vestibular type of eye movement has a short latent period, measured in thousandths of a second rather than one-fifth second.

Pathological Nystagmus. Occasionally, abnormalities

occur in the control system for eye movements that cause continuous nystagmus (back and forth movements) despite the fact that neither the visual scene nor the body is moving. This is likely to occur when one of the vestibular apparatuses is damaged or when severe damage is sustained in the deep nuclei of the cerebellum. This was discussed further in Chapter 17.

Another pathological type of eye movement that is sometimes called nystagmus occurs when the foveal regions of the two eyes have been destroyed or when the vision in these areas is greatly weakened. In such a condition the eyes attempt to fix the object of attention on the foveae but always overshoot the mark because of foveal insensitivity. Therefore, they oscillate back and forth but never achieve foveal fixation.

FUSION OF THE VISUAL IMAGES

To make the visual perceptions more meaningful and also to aid in depth perception by the mechanism of stereopsis, which was discussed in Chapter 22, the visual images in the two eyes normally *fuse* with each other on "corresponding points" of the two retinas.

The visual cortex plays a very important role in fusion. It was pointed out earlier in the chapter that corresponding points of the two retinas transmit visual signals to different neuronal layers of the lateral geniculate body, and these signals in turn are relayed to parallel stripes of neurons in the visual cortex. Interactions occur between the stripes of cortical neurons; these cause *interference patterns of excitation* in some of the local neuronal cells when the two visual images are not precisely "in register"—that is, not precisely fused. This excitation presumably provides the signal that is transmitted to the oculomotor apparatus to cause convergence or divergence or rotation of the eyes so that fusion can be re-established. Once the corresponding points of the retinas are precisely in register with each other, the excitation of the specific cells in the visual cortex disappears.

The Neural Mechanism for Stereopsis. The visual images that appear on the retina during the process of stereopsis were discussed in Chapter 22. It was pointed out that because the two eyes are a little more than 2 inches apart the images on the two retinas are not exactly the same. The closer the object is to the eye the greater is the disparity between the two images. Consequently, it is impossible for all corresponding points in the visual image to be in complete register at the same time. Furthermore, the nearer the object is to the eye, the less the degree of register. Here again, specific cells in the primary visual cortex are believed to become excited in the areas of the visual field where highlights are out of register. Presumably, this excitation is the source of the signals for detection of the distance of the object in front of the eyes; this mechanism is called *stereopsis.*

Strabismus. Strabismus, which is also called *squint* or *cross-eyedness,* means lack of fusion of the eyes in one or more of the coordinates described above. Three basic types of strabismus are illustrated in Figure 24–9: *horizontal strabismus, vertical strabismus,* and *torsional strabismus.* However, combinations of two or even of all three of the different types of strabismus often occur.

Strabismus is perpetuated by an abnormal "set" of the fusion mechanism of the visual system. That is, in the early efforts of the child to fixate the two eyes on the same object, one of the eyes fixates satisfactorily while

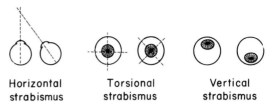

Horizontal strabismus   Torsional strabismus   Vertical strabismus

Figure 24–9. The three basic types of strabismus.

the other fails to fixate, or they both fixate satisfactorily but never simultaneously. Soon, the patterns of conjugate movements of the eyes become abnormally "set" so that the eyes never fuse.

Frequently, some abnormality of the eyes contributes to the failure of the two eyes to fixate on the same point. For instance, if at birth one eye has poor vision in comparison with the other, the good eye tends to fixate on the object of attention while the poor eye might never do so. Also, in hypermetropic infants, intense impulses must be transmitted to the ciliary muscles to focus the eyes, and some of these impulses overflow into the oculomotor nuclei to cause simultaneous convergence of the eyes, as will be discussed later. As a result, the child's fusion mechanism becomes "set" for continual inward deviation of the eyes.

Suppression of Visual Image from a Repressed Eye. In many patients with strabismus the eyes alternate in fixing on the object of attention. However, in other patients, one eye alone is used all the time while the other eye becomes repressed and is never used for vision. The vision in the repressed eye develops only slightly, usually remaining 20/400 or less. If the dominant eye then becomes blinded, vision in the repressed eye can develop only to a slight extent in the adult but far more in young children. This illustrates that visual acuity is highly dependent on proper development of the central synaptic connections from the eyes.

AUTONOMIC CONTROL OF ACCOMMODATION AND PUPILLARY APERTURE

The Autonomic Nerves to the Eyes. The eye is innervated by both parasympathetic and sympathetic fibers, as illustrated in Figure 24–10. The parasympathetic preganglionic fibers arise in the *Edinger-Westphal nucleus* (the visceral nucleus of the third nerve) and then pass in the *third nerve* to the *ciliary ganglion,* which lies about 1 centimeter behind the eye. Here the preganglionic fibers synapse with postganglionic parasympathetic neurons that, in turn, send fibers through the *ciliary nerves* into the eyeball. These nerves excite the ciliary muscle and the sphincter of the iris.

The sympathetic innervation of the eye originates in the *intermediolateral horn cells* of the first thoracic segment of the spinal cord. From here, sympathetic fibers enter the sympathetic chain and pass upward to the *superior cervical ganglion* where they synapse with postganglionic neurons. Fibers from these spread along the carotid artery and successively

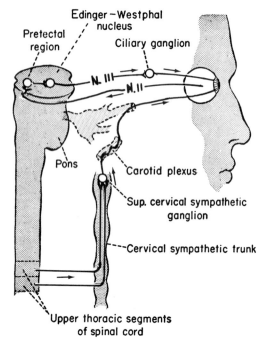

Figure 24–10. Autonomic innervation of the eye, showing also the reflex arc of the light reflex. (Modified from Ranson and Clark: Anatomy of the Nervous System. Philadelphia, W. B. Saunders Company, 1959.)

smaller arteries until they reach the eye. There the sympathetic fibers innervate the radial fibers of the iris as well as several extraocular structures around the eye, which are discussed shortly in relation to Horner's syndrome. Also, they supply very weak innervation to the ciliary muscle.

CONTROL OF ACCOMMODATION (FOCUSING THE EYES)

The accommodation mechanism—that is, the mechanism that focuses the lens system of the eye—is essential for a high degree of visual acuity. Accommodation results from contraction or relaxation of the ciliary muscle, contraction causing increased strength of the lens system, as explained in Chapter 22, and relaxation causing decreased strength. The question that must be answered now is: How does a person adjust accommodation to keep the eyes in focus all the time?

Accommodation of the lens is regulated by a negative feedback mechanism that automatically adjusts the focal power of the lens for the highest degree of visual acuity. When the eyes have been fixed on some far object and then suddenly fix on a near object, the lens accommodates for maximum acuity of vision usually within one second. Though the precise control mechanism that causes this rapid and accurate focusing of the eye is still unclear, some of the known features of the mechanism are the following:

First, when the eyes suddenly change the dis-

tance of the fixation point, the lens always changes its strength in the proper direction to achieve a new state of focus. In other words, the lens *does not hunt* back and forth on the two sides of focus in an attempt to find the focus.

Second, different types of clues that can help the lens change its strength in the proper direction include the following: (1) *Chromatic aberration* appears to be important. That is, the red light rays focus slightly posteriorly to the blue light rays. The eyes appear to be able to detect which of these two types of rays is in better focus, and this clue relays information to the accommodation mechanism whether to make the lens stronger or weaker. (2) When the eyes fixate on a near object they also converge toward each other. The neural mechanisms for *convergence cause a simultaneous signal to strengthen the lens of the eye.* (3) *Since the fovea is a depressed area, the clarity of focus in the depth of the fovea versus the clarity of focus on the edges will be different.* It has been suggested that this also gives clues as to which way the strength of the lens needs to be changed. (4) It has been found that *the degree of accommodation of the lens oscillates slightly* all of the time, at a frequency up to two times per second. It has been suggested that the visual image becomes clearer when the oscillation of the lens strength is in the appropriate direction and poorer when the lens strength is in the wrong direction. This could give a rapid cue as to which way the strength of the lens needs to change to provide appropriate focus.

It is presumed that the cortical areas that control accommodation closely parallel those that control fixation movements of the eyes, with final integration of the visual signals in areas 18 and 19 and transmission of motor signals to the ciliary muscle through the pretectal area and Edinger-Westphal nucleus.

CONTROL OF THE PUPILLARY DIAMETER

Stimulation of the parasympathetic nerves excites the pupillary sphincter, thereby decreasing the pupillary aperture; this is called *miosis*. On the other hand, stimulation of the sympathetic nerves excites the radial fibers of the iris and causes pupillary dilatation, which is called *mydriasis*.

The Pupillary Light Reflex. When light is shone into the eyes the pupils constrict, a reaction that is called the *pupillary light reflex*. The neuronal pathway for this reflex is illustrated in Figure 24–10. When light impinges on the retina, the resulting impulses pass through the optic nerves and optic tracts to the pretectal nuclei. From here, impulses pass to the *Edinger-Westphal nucleus* and finally back through the *parasympathetic nerves* to constrict the sphincter of the iris. In darkness, the reflex becomes inhibited, which results in dilatation of the pupil.

The function of the light reflex is to help the eye

adapt extremely rapidly to changing light conditions, the importance of which was explained in relation to retinal adaptation in the previous chapter. The limits of pupillary diameter are about 1.5 mm on the small side and 8 mm on the large side. Therefore, the range of light adaptation that can be effected by the pupillary reflex is about 30 to 1.

Pupillary Reflexes in Central Nervous System Disease. Certain central nervous system diseases block the transmission of visual signals from the retinas to the Edinger-Westphal nucleus. Such blocks frequently occur as a result of *central nervous system syphilis, alcoholism, encephalitis,* or so forth. The block usually occurs in the pretectal region of the brain stem, though it can also result from destruction of the small afferent fibers in the optic nerves.

The nerve fibers to the Edinger-Westphal nucleus from the pretectal area are of the inhibitory type. Therefore, when they are blocked, the nucleus becomes chronically active, causing the pupils thereafter to remain partially constricted in addition to their failure to respond to light.

When the light reflex is lost, the pupils can still constrict an additional amount if the Edinger-Westphal nucleus is stimulated through some other pathway. For instance, when the eyes fixate on a near object, the signals that cause accommodation of the lens (and also those that cause convergence of the two eyes) cause a mild degree of pupillary constriction at the same time. This is called the *accommodation reflex.* Such a pupil that fails to respond to light but does respond to accommodation and also is very small (an *Argyll Robertson pupil*) is an important diagnostic sign of central nervous system disease—very often syphilis.

Horner's Syndrome. The sympathetic nerves to the eye are occasionally interrupted, and this interruption frequently occurs in the cervical sympathetic chain. This results in *Horner's syndrome,* which consists of the following effects: First, because of interruption of fibers to the pupillary dilator muscle, the pupil remains persistently constricted to a smaller diameter than that of the pupil of the opposite eye. Second, the superior eyelid droops because this eyelid is normally maintained in an open position during the waking hours partly by contraction of a smooth muscle embedded in the lid and innervated by the sympathetics. Therefore, destruction of the sympathetics makes it impossible to open the superior eyelid nearly as widely as normally. Third, the blood vessels on the corresponding side of the face and head become persistently dilated. And, fourth, sweating cannot occur on the side of the face and head affected by Horner's syndrome.

REFERENCES

Anderson, D. R.: Testing the Field of Vision. St. Louis, C. V. Mosby, 1983.

Bishop, P. O.: Processing of visual information within the retinostriate system. *In* Darian-Smith, I. (ed.): Handbook of Physiology. Sec. 1, Vol. III. Bethesda, American Physiological Society, 1984, p. 341.

Bizzi, E.: Eye-head coordination. *In* Brooks, V. B. (ed.): Handbook of Physiology. Sec. 1, Vol. II. Bethesda, American Physiological Society, 1981, p. 1321.

Buttner, E. J. (ed.): Neuroanatomy of the Oculomotor System. New York, Elsevier Science Publishing Co., 1984.

DeValois, R. L., and Jacobs, G. H.: Neural mechanisms of color vision. *In* Darian-Smith, I. (ed.): Handbook of Physiology. Sec. 1, Vol. III. Bethesda, American Physiological Society, 1984, p. 525.

Fraser, S. E., and Hunt, R. K.: Retinotectal specificity: Models and experiments in search of a mapping function. *Annu. Rev. Neurosci.,* 3:319, 1980.

Fregnac, Y., and Imbert, M.: Development of neuronal selectivity in primary visual cortex of cat. *Physiol. Rev.,* 64:325, 1984.

Gilbert, C. D.: Microcircuitry of the visual cortex. *Annu. Rev. Neurosci.,* 6:217, 1983.

Hubbell, W. L., and Bownds, M. D.: Visual transduction in vertebrate photoreceptors. *Annu. Rev. Neurosci.,* 2:17, 1979.

Hubel, D. H., and Wiesel, T. N.: Receptive fields of cells in striate cortex of very young, visually inexperienced kittens. *J. Neurophysiol.,* 26:994, 1963.

Hubel, D. H., and Wiesel, T. N.: Cortical and callosal connections concerned with vertical meridian of visual fields in the cat. *J. Neurophysiol.,* 30:1561, 1967.

Hubel, D. H., and Wiesel, T. N.: Brain mechanisms of vision. *Sci. Am.,* 241(3):150, 1979.

Mitchell, D. E., and Timney, B.: Postnatal development of function in the mammalian visual system. *In* Darian-Smith, I. (ed.): Handbook of Physiology. Sec. 1, Vol. III. Bethesda, American Physiological Society, 1984, p. 507.

Moses, R. A.: Adler's Physiology of the Eye; Clinical Application. 7th Ed. St. Louis, C. V. Mosby, 1981.

Poggio, G. F., and Poggio, T.: The analysis of stereopsis. *Annu. Rev. Neurosci.,* 7:379, 1984.

Robinson, D. A.: Control of eye movements. *In* Brooks, V. B. (ed.): Handbook of Physiology. Sec. 1, Vol. II. Bethesda, American Physiological Society, 1981, p. 1275.

Schiller, P. H.: The superior colliculus and visual function. *In* Darian-Smith, I. (ed.): Handbook of Physiology. Sec. 1, Vol. III. Bethesda, American Physiological Society, 1984, p. 457.

Schor, C. M. (ed.): Vergence Eye Movements. Basic and Clinical Aspects. Woburn, MA, Butterworth, 1982.

Sherman, S. M., and Spear, P. D.: Organization of visual pathways in normal and visually deprived cats. *Physiol. Rev.,* 62:738, 1982.

Simpson, J. I.: The accessory optic system. *Annu. Rev. Neurosci.,* 7:13, 1984.

Song, P.-S.: Protozoan and related photoreceptors: Molecular aspects. *Annu. Rev. Biophys. Bioeng.,* 12:35, 1983.

Sterling, P.: Microcircuitry of the cat retina. *Annu. Rev. Neurosci.,* 6:149, 1983.

Walsh, T. J.: Neuro-Ophthalmology: Clinical Signs and Symptoms. Philadelphia, Lea & Febiger, 1978.

Woolsey, C. N. (ed.): Cortical Sensory Organization. Multiple Visual Areas. Clifton, NJ, Humana Press, 1981.

Wurtz, R. H., and Albano, J. E.: Visual-motor function of the primate superior colliculus. *Annu. Rev. Neurosci.,* 3:189, 1980.

25

The Sense of Hearing

The purpose of the present chapter is to describe and explain the mechanism by which the ear receives sound waves, discriminates their frequencies, and finally transmits auditory information into the central nervous system.

THE TYMPANIC MEMBRANE AND THE OSSICULAR SYSTEM

CONDUCTION OF SOUND FROM THE TYMPANIC MEMBRANE TO THE COCHLEA

Figure 25–1 illustrates the *tympanic membrane* (commonly called the *eardrum)* and the *ossicular system,* which conducts sound through the middle ear. The tympanic membrane is cone-shaped, with its concavity facing downward and outward toward the auditory canal. Attached to the very center of the tympanic membrane is the *handle* of the *malleus.* At its other end the malleus is tightly bound to the *incus* by ligaments so that whenever the malleus moves the incus moves with it. The opposite end of the incus in turn articulates with the stem of the *stapes,* and the *faceplate* of the stapes lies against the membranous labyrinth in the opening of the oval window where sound waves are conducted into the inner ear, the *cochlea.*

The ossicles of the middle ear are suspended by ligaments in such a way that the combined malleus and incus act as a single lever having its fulcrum approximately at the border of the tympanic membrane. The large *head* of the malleus, which is on the opposite side of the fulcrum from the handle, almost exactly balances the other end of the lever.

The articulation of the incus with the stapes causes the stapes to push forward on the cochlear fluid every time the handle of the malleus moves inward and to pull backward on the fluid every time the malleus moves outward, which promotes inward and outward motion of the faceplate at the oval window.

The handle of the malleus is constantly pulled inward by the *tensor tympani muscle,* which keeps the tympanic membrane tensed. This allows sound vibrations on *any* portion of the tympanic membrane to be transmitted to the malleus, which would not be true if the membrane were lax.

Impedance Matching by the Ossicular System. The amplitude of movement of the stapes faceplate with each sound vibration is only three fourths as much as the amplitude of the handle of the malleus. Therefore, the ossicular lever system does not amplify the movement distance of the stapes, as is commonly believed. Instead, the system actually reduces the amplitude but increases the *force* of movement about 1.3 times. However, the surface area of the tympanic membrane is approximately 55 square millimeters, whereas the surface area of the stapes averages 3.2 square millimeters. This 17-fold difference times the 1.3-fold ratio of the lever system allows all the energy of a sound wave impinging on the tympanic membrane to be applied to the small faceplate of the stapes, causing approximately 22 times as much *pressure* on the fluid of the cochlea as is exerted by the sound wave against the tympanic membrane. Since fluid has far greater inertia than air, it is easily understood that increased amounts of pressure are needed to cause vibration in the fluid. Therefore, the tympanic membrane and ossicular system provide *impedance matching* between the sound waves in air and the sound vibrations in the fluid of the cochlea. Indeed, the impedance matching is about 50 to 75 per cent of perfect for sound frequencies between 300 and 3000 cycles per second, which allows almost full utilization of the energy in the incoming sound waves.

In the absence of the ossicular system and tympanum, sound waves can travel directly through the air of the middle ear and can enter the cochlea at the oval window. However, the sensitivity for hearing is then 15 to 20 decibels less than for ossicular transmission—equivalent to a decrease from a loud voice to a very low voice level.

Attenuation of Sound by Contraction of the Stapedius and Tensor Tympani Muscles. When loud sounds are transmitted through the ossicular system into the central nervous system, a reflex occurs after a latent period of 40 to 80 milliseconds to cause contraction of the *stapedius* and *tensor tympani muscles.* The tensor tympani muscle pulls the handle of the malleus inward while the stapedius muscle pulls the stapes outward. These two forces oppose each other and thereby cause the entire ossicular system to develop a high degree of rigidity, thus greatly reducing the ossicular conduction of low frequency

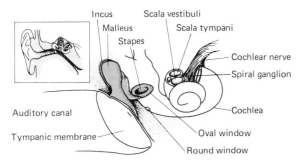

Figure 25–1. The tympanic membrane, the ossicular system of the middle ear, and the inner ear.

sound, mainly frequencies below 1000 cycles per second.

This *attenuation reflex* can reduce the intensity of sound transmission by as much as 30 to 40 decibels, which is about the same difference as that between a loud voice and the sound of a whisper. The function of this mechanism is probably twofold:

1. To *protect* the cochlea from damaging vibrations caused by excessively loud sound. It is mainly low frequency sounds (the ones that are attenuated) that are frequently loud enough to damage the basilar membrane of the cochlea. Unfortunately, because of the 40 or more millisecond latency for reaction of the reflex, the sudden, loud, thunderous sounds that result from explosions can still cause extensive cochlear damage.

2. To *mask* low frequency sounds in loud environments. This usually removes a major share of the background noise and allows a person to concentrate on sounds above 1000 cycles per second frequency. It is in this upper frequency range that most of the pertinent information in voice communication is transmitted.

Another function of the tensor tympani and stapedius muscles is to decrease a person's hearing sensitivity to his or her own speech. This effect is activated by collateral signals transmitted to these muscles at the same time that the brain activates the voice mechanism.

TRANSMISSION OF SOUND THROUGH BONE

Because the inner ear, the *cochlea*, is embedded in a bony cavity in the temporal bone called the bony labyrinth, vibrations of the entire skull can cause fluid vibrations in the cochlea itself. Therefore, under appropriate conditions, a tuning fork or an electronic vibrator placed on any bony protuberance of the skull causes the person to hear the sound. Unfortunately, the energy available even in very loud sound in the air is not sufficient to cause hearing through the bone except when a special electromechanical sound-transmitting device is applied directly to the bone, usually to the mastoid process.

THE COCHLEA

FUNCTIONAL ANATOMY OF THE COCHLEA

The cochlea is a system of coiled tubes, shown in Figure 25–1 and in cross section in Figures 25–2 and 25–3. It is comprised of three different tubes coiled side by side: the *scala vestibuli*, the *scala media*, and the *scala tympani*. The scala vestibuli and scala media are separated from each other by *Reissner's membrane* (also called the *vestibular membrane*), and the scala tympani and scala media are separated from each other by the *basilar membrane*. On the surface of the basilar membrane lies a structure, the *organ of Corti*, which contains a series of mechanically sensitive cells, the *hair cells*. These are the receptive end-organs that generate nerve impulses in response to sound vibrations.

Figure 25–4 diagrams the functional parts of the uncoiled cochlea for conduction of sound vibrations. First, note that Reissner's membrane is missing from this figure. This membrane is so thin and so easily moved that it does not obstruct the passage of sound vibrations from the scala vestibuli into the scala media at all. Therefore, so far as the conduction of sound is concerned, the scala vestibuli and scala media are considered to be a single chamber. The importance of Reissner's membrane is to maintain a special fluid in the scala media that is required for normal function of the sound-receptive hair cells, as discussed later in the chapter.

Sound vibrations enter the scala vestibuli from the faceplate of the stapes at the oval window. The faceplate covers this window and is connected with the window's edges by a relatively loose annular ligament so that it can move inward and outward with the sound vibrations. Inward movement causes the fluid to move into the scala vestibuli and scala media, which immediately increases the pressure in the entire cochlea.

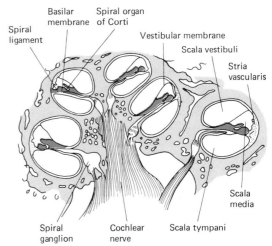

Figure 25–2. The cochlea. (From Goss, C. M. [ed.]: Gray's Anatomy of the Human Body. Philadelphia, Lea & Febiger.)

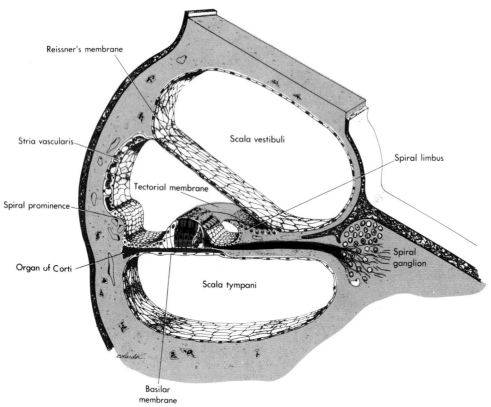

Figure 25–3. A section through one of the turns of the cochlea. (Drawn by Sylvia Colard Keene. From Bloom and Fawcett: A Textbook of Histology. Philadelphia, W. B. Saunders Company, 1975.)

Note in Figure 25–4 that the distal ends of the scala vestibuli and scala tympani open into each other through an opening at the apex of the cochlea called the *helicotrema*. If the stapes moves inward *very slowly,* fluid from the scala vestibuli is pushed through the helicotrema into the scala tympani, and the fluid in the scala tympani then moves backward toward the base of the cochlea where it causes the membrane of the round window to bulge outward. However, if the stapes vibrates inward and outward rapidly, the fluid simply does not have time to pass all the way through the helicotrema to the round window, and then back again to the oval window between each two successive vibrations. Instead, the fluid wave takes a shortcut through the basilar membrane, causing it to bulge back and forth between the scala vestibuli and the scala tympani with each sound vibration. We shall see later that each frequency of sound causes a different "pattern" of vibration in the basilar membrane and that this is the important means by which the sound frequencies are discriminated from each other.

The Basilar Membrane and Resonance in the Cochlea. The basilar membrane is a fibrous membrane that separates the scala media and the scala tympani. It contains 20,000 to 30,000 *basilar fibers* that project from the bony center of the cochlea, the *modiolus,* toward the outer wall. These fibers are stiff, elastic, reedlike structures that are fixed at their basal ends but not at their distal ends except

that the distal ends are embedded in the loose basilar membrane. Because the fibers are stiff and also free at one end, they can vibrate like reeds of a harmonica.

The lengths of the basilar fibers increase progressively as one goes from the base of the cochlea to its apex, from a length of approximately 0.04 mm near the oval and round windows to 0.5 mm at the helicotrema, a 12-fold increase in length.

The diameters of the fibers, on the other hand, decrease from the base to the helicotrema, so that their overall stiffness decreases more than 100-fold. As a result, the stiff, short fibers near the base of the cochlea have a tendency to vibrate at a high frequency, whereas the long, limber fibers near the helicotrema have a tendency to vibrate at a low frequency.

In addition to the differences in stiffness of the basilar fibers, they are also differently "loaded" by the fluid mass of the cochlea. That is, when a fiber vibrates back and forth, all the fluid between the vibrating fiber and the oval and round windows must also move back and forth at the same time. For a fiber vibrating near the base of the cochlea (near the two windows), the total mass of moving fluid is slight in comparison with that for a fiber vibrating near the helicotrema. This difference, too, favors high frequency vibration near the windows and low frequency vibration near the tip of the cochlea.

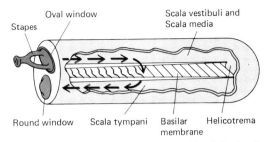

Figure 25–4. Movement of fluid in the cochlea following forward thrust of the stapes.

Thus, high frequency resonance of the basilar membrane occurs near the base, and low frequency resonance occurs near the apex because of (1) difference in stiffness of the fibers and (2) difference in "loading."

TRANSMISSION OF SOUND WAVES IN THE COCHLEA—THE "TRAVELING WAVE"

If the foot of the stapes moves inward instantaneously, the round window must also bulge outward instantaneously because the cochlea is bounded on all sides by bony walls. Since the fluid will not have time to move all the way from the oval window through the helicotrema to the round window, the initial effect is to cause the basilar membrane at the very base of the cochlea to bulge in the direction of the round window. However, the elastic tension that is built up in the basilar fibers as they bend toward the round window initiates a wave that "travels" along the basilar membrane toward the helicotrema, as illustrated in Figure 25–5. Figure 25–5A shows movement of a high frequency wave down the basilar membrane; Figure 25–5B, a medium frequency wave; and Figure 25–5C, a very low frequency wave. Movement of the wave along the basilar membrane is comparable to the movement of a pressure wave along the arterial walls, or it is also comparable to the wave that travels along the surface of a pond.

Pattern of Vibration of the Basilar Membrane for Different Sound Frequencies. Note in Figure 25–5 the different patterns of transmission for sound waves of different frequencies. Each wave is relatively weak at the outset but becomes strong when it reaches that portion of the basilar membrane that has a natural resonant frequency equal to the respective sound frequency. At this point the basilar membrane can vibrate back and forth with such great ease that the energy in the wave is completely dissipated. Consequently, the wave ceases at this point and fails to travel the remaining distance along the basilar membrane. Thus, a high frequency sound wave travels only a short distance along the basilar membrane before it reaches its resonant point and dies out; a medium frequency sound wave travels about halfway and then dies out; and,

finally, a very low frequency sound wave travels the entire distance along the membrane.

Another feature of the traveling wave is that it travels fast along the initial portion of the basilar membrane but progressively more slowly as it goes farther and farther into the cochlea. The cause of this is the high coefficient of elasticity of the basilar fibers near the stapes and a progressively decreasing coefficient farther along the membrane. This rapid initial transmission of the wave allows the high frequency sounds to travel far enough into the cochlea to spread out and separate from each other on the basilar membrane. Without this spread, all the high frequency waves would be bunched together within the first millimeter or so of the basilar membrane, and their frequencies could not be discriminated one from the other.

Amplitude Pattern of Vibration of the Basilar Membrane. The dashed curves of Figure 25–6A show the position of a sound wave on the basilar membrane when the stapes (a) is all the way inward, (b) has moved back to the neutral point, (c) is all the way outward, and (d) has moved back again to the neutral point but is moving inward. The shaded area around these different waves shows the maximum extent of vibration of the basilar membrane during a complete vibratory cycle. This is the amplitude pattern of vibration of the basilar membrane for this particular sound frequency.

Figure 25–6B shows the amplitude patterns of vibration for different frequencies, showing that the maximum amplitude for 8000 cycles occurs near the base of the cochlea, whereas that for frequencies less than 200 cycles per second is all the way at the tip of the basilar membrane near the helicotrema.

Note in Figure 25–6B that the basal end of the

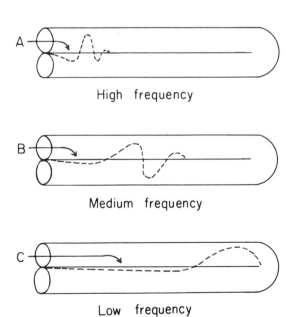

Figure 25–5. "Traveling waves" along the basilar membrane for high, medium, and low frequency sounds.

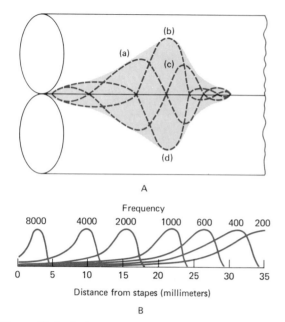

A

B

Figure 25–6. *A*, Amplitude pattern of vibration of the basilar membrane for a medium frequency sound. *B*, Amplitude patterns for sounds of all frequencies between 200 and 8000 per second, showing the points of maximum amplitude (the resonance points) on the basilar membrane for the different frequencies.

basilar membrane vibrates weakly for all frequencies. However, beyond the resonant area for each given frequency, the vibration of the basilar membrane cuts off sharply. The principal method by which sound frequencies, especially those above 200 cycles per second, are discriminated from each other is based on the "place" of maximum stimulation of the nerve fibers from the organ of Corti lying on the basilar membrane, as will be explained in the following section.

FUNCTION OF THE ORGAN OF CORTI

The organ of Corti, illustrated in Figures 25–2, 25–3, and 25–7, is the receptor organ that generates nerve impulses in response to vibration of the basilar membrane. Note that the organ of Corti lies on the surface of the basilar fibers and basilar membrane. The actual sensory receptors in the organ of Corti are two types of *hair cells*, a single row of *internal hair cells*, numbering about 3500 and measuring about 12 microns in diameter, and three to four rows of *external hair cells*, numbering about 20,000 and having diameters of only about 8 microns. The bases and sides of the hair cells synapse with a network of cochlear nerve endings. These lead to the *spiral ganglion of Corti*, which lies in the modiolus (the center) of the cochlea. The spiral ganglion in turn sends axons into the *cochlear nerve* and thence into the central nervous system at the level of the upper medulla. The relationship of the organ of Corti to the spiral ganglion and to the cochlear nerve is illustrated in Figure 25–2.

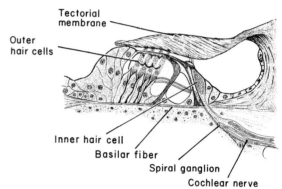

Figure 25–7. The organ of Corti, showing especially the hair cells and the tectorial membrane against the projecting hairs.

Excitation of the Hair Cells. Note in Figure 25–7 that minute hairs, or cilia, project upward from the hair cells and either touch or are embedded in the surface gel coating of the *tectorial membrane* which lies above the cilia in the scala media. These hair cells are similar to the hair cells found in the macula and cristae ampullaris of the vestibular apparatus, which were discussed in Chapter 16. Bending of the hairs in one direction depolarizes the hair cells, and this in turn excites the nerve fibers synapsing with their bases.

Figure 25–8 illustrates the mechanism by which vibration of the basilar membrane excites the hair endings. This shows that the upper ends of the hair cells are fixed tightly in a very rigid structure composed of a flat plate called the *reticular lamina* supported by triangular *rods of Corti* that in turn are attached tightly to the basilar fibers. Therefore, the basilar fiber, the rods of Corti, and the reticular lamina all move as a rigid unit.

Upward movement of the basilar fiber rocks the reticular lamina upward and *inward*. Then, when the basilar membrane moves downward, the reticular lamina rocks downward and *outward*. The inward and outward motion causes the hairs to shear back and forth against the tectorial membrane, thus exciting the cochlear nerve fibers whenever the basilar membrane vibrates.

Mechanism by Which the Hair Cells Excite the Nerve Fibers—Receptor Potentials. Back-and-forth bending of the hairs causes alternate changes in the

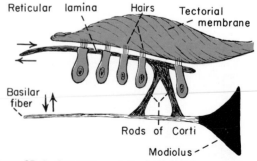

Figure 25–8. Stimulation of the hair cells by the to-and-fro movement of the hairs in the tectorial membrane.

electrical potential across the hair cell membrane. This alternating potential is the *receptor potential* of the hair cell, and it in turn stimulates the cochlear nerve endings that terminate on the hair cells.

When the basilar fiber bends toward the scala vestibuli (in the upward direction in Figure 25–8), the hair cell becomes depolarized, and it is this depolarization that generates action potentials in the nerve fiber. When the basilar fiber moves in the opposite direction, the hair cell becomes hyperpolarized, and the number of action potentials decreases.

The Endocochlear Potential. To explain even more fully the electrical potentials generated by the hair cells, we need to explain still another electrical phenomenon called the endocochlear potential: The scala media is filled with a fluid called *endolymph* in contradistinction to the *perilymph* present in the scala vestibuli and scala tympani. The scala vestibuli and scala tympani in most young children and in some adults communicate directly with the subarachnoid space around the brain, so that the perilymph is almost identical with cerebrospinal fluid. On the other hand, the endolymph that fills the scala media is an entirely different fluid probably secreted by the *stria vascularis*, a highly vascular area on the outer wall of the scala media. Endolymph contains a very high concentration of potassium and a very low concentration of sodium, which is exactly opposite to the perilymph.

An electrical potential of approximately +80 millivolts exists all the time between the endolymph and the perilymph, with positivity inside the scala media and negativity outside. This is called the *endocochlear potential*, and it is believed to be generated by continual secretion of positive potassium ions into the scala media by the stria vascularis.

The importance of the endocochlear potential is that the tops of the hair cells project through the reticular lamina into the endolymph of the scala media while perilymph bathes the lower bodies of the hair cells. Furthermore, the hair cells have a negative intracellular potential of −70 millivolts with respect to the perilymph, but −150 millivolts with respect to the endolymph at their upper surfaces where the hairs project into the endolymph. It is believed that this high electrical potential at the hair border of the cell greatly sensitizes the cell, thereby increasing its ability to respond to slight movement of the hairs.

DETERMINATION OF SOUND FREQUENCY—THE "PLACE" PRINCIPLE

From earlier discussions in this chapter it is already apparent that low frequency sounds cause maximal activation of the basilar membrane near the apex of the cochlea, sounds of high frequency activate the basilar membrane near the base of the cochlea, and intermediate frequencies activate the membrane at intermediate distances between these two extremes. Furthermore, there is spatial organization of the cochlear nerve fibers from the cochlea to the cochlear nuclei in the brain stem, with the fibers from each respective area of the basilar membrane terminating in a corresponding area of the cochlear nuclei. We shall see later that this spatial organization continues all the way up the brain stem to the cerebral cortex. The recording of signals from the auditory tracts in the brain stem and from the auditory receptive fields in the cerebral cortex shows that specific neurons are activated by specific sound frequencies. Therefore, the major method used by the nervous system to detect different frequencies is to determine the position along the basilar membrane that is most stimulated. This is called the *place principle* for determination of frequency (or of sound "pitch").

Yet, referring again to Figure 25–6, one can see that the distal end of the basilar membrane at the helicotrema is stimulated by all sound frequencies below 200 cycles per second. Therefore, it has been difficult to understand from the place principle how one can differentiate between very low sound frequencies. It is postulated that these low frequencies are discriminated mainly by the so-called *frequency principle*. That is, the low frequency sounds cause volleys of impulses at the same low frequencies to be transmitted by the cochlear nerve into the cochlear nuclei. And it is believed that the cochlear nuclei then distinguish the different frequencies. In fact, destruction of the entire apical half of the cochlea, which destroys the basilar membrane where all the lower frequency sounds are normally detected, still does not completely eliminate the discrimination of low frequency sounds.

DETERMINATION OF LOUDNESS

Loudness is determined by the auditory system in at least three different ways: First, as the sound becomes louder, the amplitude of vibration of the basilar membrane and hair cells also increases so that the hair cells excite the nerve endings at more rapid rates. Second, as the amplitude of vibration increases, it causes more and more of the hair cells on the fringes of the resonating portion of the basilar membrane to become stimulated, thus causing *spatial summation* of impulses—that is, transmission through many nerve fibers, rather than through a few. Third, certain hair cells do not become stimulated until the vibration of the basilar membrane reaches a relatively high intensity, and it is believed that stimulation of these cells in some way apprises the nervous system that the sound is then very loud.

Detection of Changes in Loudness—The Power Law. It was pointed out in Chapter 12 that a person interprets changes in intensity of sensory stimuli approximately in proportion to a power function of the actual intensity. In the case of sound, the interpreted sensation changes approximately in proportion to the cube root of the actual sound intensity. To express this another way, the ear can discriminate differences in sound intensity from the softest whisper to the loudest possible noise, representing an *approximate one trillion times* increase in sound energy or one million times increase in amplitude of movement of the basilar membrane. Yet the ear interprets this much difference in sound level as approximately a 10,000-fold change. Thus, the scale of intensity is greatly "compressed" by the sound perception mechanisms of the auditory system. This obviously allows a person to interpret differences in sound intensities over an extremely wide range, a far broader range than would be possible were it not for compression of the scale.

The Decibel Unit. Because of the extreme changes in sound intensities that the ear can detect and discriminate, sound intensities are usually expressed in terms of the logarithm of their actual intensities. A 10-fold increase in sound energy (or a $\sqrt{10}$-fold increase in sound pressure, because energy is proportional to the square of pressure) is called 1 *bel,* and 0.1 bel is called 1 *decibel.* One decibel represents an actual increase in sound energy of 1.26 times.

Another reason for using the decibel system in expressing changes in loudness is that, in the usual sound intensity range for communication, the ears can barely distinguish approximately a 1 decibel *change* in sound intensity.

The "Zero" Decibel Reference Level. The usual method for expressing the intensity of sound is to state the pressure difference between the peak of the sound compression wave and the trough of the wave. A pressure difference of *0.0002 dyne per square centimeter* is considered by audiologists to be unit intensity, and this is expressed as *zero decibels* when converted to the decibel scale. This sound level is also approximately the minimum that can be detected by the normal ear at the optimal frequency of 3000 cycles per second.

Threshold for Hearing Sound at Different Frequencies. Figure 25–9 shows the energy threshold at which sounds of different frequencies can barely be heard by the ear. This figure illustrates that a 3000 cycle per second sound can be heard even when its intensity is as low as 70 decibels below 1 dyne/cm² sound pressure level, which is one ten-millionth microwatt/cm². On the other hand, a 100 cycle per second sound can be detected only if its intensity is 10,000 times as great as this.

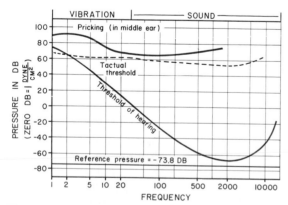

Figure 25–9. Relationship of the threshold of hearing and the threshold of somesthetic perception to the sound energy level at each sound frequency. (Modified from Stevens and Davis: Hearing. John Wiley & Sons.)

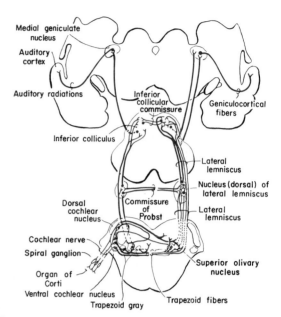

Figure 25–10. The auditory pathway. (Modified from Crosby, Humphrey, and Lauer: Correlative Anatomy of the Nervous System. New York, The Macmillan Co.)

Frequency Range of Hearing. The frequencies of sound that a young person can hear, before aging has occurred in the ears, is generally stated to be between 20 and 20,000 cycles per second. However, referring again to Figure 25–9, we see that the sound range depends to a great extent on intensity. If the intensity is 60 decibels below the 1 dyne/cm² sound pressure level, the sound range is 500 to 5000 cycles per second, and only with intense sounds can the complete range of 20 to 20,000 cycles be achieved. In old age, the frequency range falls to 50 to 8000 cycles per second or less, as is discussed later in the chapter.

CENTRAL AUDITORY MECHANISMS

THE AUDITORY PATHWAY

Figure 25–10 illustrates the major auditory pathways. It shows that nerve fibers from the *spiral ganglion of Corti* enter the *dorsal* and *ventral cochlear nuclei* located in the upper part of the medulla. At this point, all the fibers synapse, and second order neurons pass mainly to the opposite side of the brain stem through the *trapezoid body* to the *superior olivary nucleus.* However, other second order fibers also pass ipsilaterally to the superior olivary nucleus on the same side. From the superior olivary nucleus the auditory pathway then passes upward through the *lateral lemniscus,* and many of the fibers terminate in the *nucleus of the lateral lemniscus.* Many bypass this nucleus and pass on to the inferior colliculus where most terminate; a few pass on without terminating to higher levels. A few fibers cross from the nucleus of the lateral lemniscus through the *commissure of Probst* to the contralateral nucleus, and still other fibers cross through the *inferior collicular commissure* from one inferior colliculus to the other. From the inferior colliculus, the pathway passes to the *medial geniculate nucleus,* where all the fibers synapse. From here, the auditory pathway proceeds by way of the *auditory radiation* to the *auditory cortex* located mainly in the superior gyrus of the temporal lobe.

Several points of importance in relation to the auditory pathway should be noted. First, signals from both ears are transmitted through the pathways of both sides of the brain with only slight preponderance of transmission in the contralateral pathway. In at least three different places in the brain stem crossing-over occurs between the two pathways: (1) in the trapezoid body, (2) in the commissure of Probst, and (3) in the commissure connecting the two inferior colliculi.

Second, many collateral fibers from the auditory tracts pass directly into the *reticular activating system of the brain stem*. This system projects diffusely upward into the cerebral cortex and downward into the spinal cord. Other collaterals go to the *vermis of the cerebellum*, which is activated instantaneously in the event of a sudden noise.

Third, a high degree of spatial orientation is maintained in the fiber tracts from the cochlea all the way to the cortex. In fact, there are three different spatial representations of sound frequencies in the cochlear nuclei, two representations in the inferior colliculi, one precise representation for discrete sound frequencies in the auditory cortex, and at least five other less precise representations in the auditory cortex and auditory association areas.

Firing Rates at Different Levels of the Auditory Pathway. Single nerve fibers entering the cochlear nuclei from the eighth nerve can fire at rates up to at least 1000 per second, the rate being determined mainly by the loudness of the sound. At low sound frequencies, the nerve impulses are usually synchronized with the sound waves but they do not necessarily occur with every wave.

In the auditory tracts of the brain stem, the firing is usually no longer synchronized with the sound frequency except at sound frequencies below 200 cycles per second. And above the level of the inferior colliculi, even this synchronization is mainly lost. These findings demonstrate that the sound signals are not transmitted unchanged directly from the ear to the higher levels of the brain; instead, information from the sound signals begins to be dissected from the impulse traffic at levels as low as the cochlear nuclei. We will have more to say about this later, especially in relation to perception of direction from which sound comes.

Another significant feature of the auditory pathways is that low rates of impulse firing continue even in the absence of sound all the way from the cochlear nerve fibers to the auditory cortex. When the basilar membrane moves toward the scala vestibuli, the impulse traffic increases; and when the basilar membrane moves toward the scala tympani, the impulse traffic decreases. Thus, the presence of this background signal allows information to be transmitted from the basilar membrane when the membrane moves in either direction: positive information in one direction and negative information in the opposite direction. Were it not for the background signal, only the positive half of the information could be transmitted. This type of so-called "carrier wave" method for transmitting information is utilized in many parts of the brain, as has been discussed in several of the preceding chapters.

Discriminatory Functions of the Auditory Relay Nuclei. Cats and even monkeys can detect very low intensity sound even when the cerebral cortex is removed bilaterally, which indicates that the nuclei in the brain stem and thalamus can perform many auditory functions without the cerebral cortex. However, discrimination of tonal patterns, sound sequences, and direction from which the sound is coming are considerably impaired. In human beings, *bilateral* destruction of the cortical auditory centers may give a different picture: it is said to cause severe hearing loss but, unfortunately, this has not been studied adequately.

FUNCTION OF THE CEREBRAL CORTEX IN HEARING

The projection of the auditory pathway to the cerebral cortex is illustrated in Figure 25–11, which shows that the auditory cortex lies principally on the *supratemporal plane of the superior temporal gyrus* but also extends over the *lateral border of the temporal lobe*, over much of the *insular cortex*, and even into the most lateral portion of the *parietal operculum*.

Two separate areas are shown in Figure 25–11: the *primary auditory cortex* and the *auditory association cortex* (also called the *secondary auditory cortex*). The primary auditory cortex is directly excited by projections from the medial geniculate body, while the auditory association areas are excited secondarily by impulses from the primary auditory cortex and by projections from thalamic association areas adjacent to the medial geniculate body.

Locus of Sound Frequency Perception in the Primary Auditory Cortex. At least six different *tonotopic maps* have been found in the primary auditory cortex and auditory association areas. In

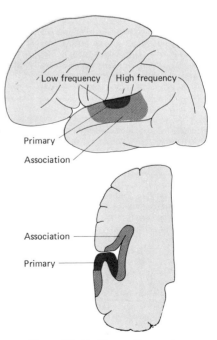

Figure 25–11. The auditory cortex.

each of these maps, high frequency sounds excite neurons at one end of the map while low frequency sounds excite the neurons at the opposite end. In most, the low frequency sounds are located anteriorly, as shown in Figure 25–11, and the high frequency sounds posteriorly. However, this is not true for all the maps. The question that one must ask is why does the auditory cortex have so many different tonotopic maps? The answer is presumably that each of the separate areas dissects out some specific feature of the sounds. For instance, one of the large maps in the primary auditory cortex almost certainly discriminates the sound frequencies themselves and gives the person the psychic sensation of sound pitches. Another one of the maps probably is used to detect the direction from which the sound comes.

The frequency range to which each individual neuron in the auditory cortex responds is much narrower than that in the cochlear and brain stem relay nuclei. Referring back to Figure 25–6B, we note that the basilar membrane near the base of the cochlea is stimulated by all frequency sounds, and in the cochlear nuclei this same breadth of sound representation is found. Yet by the time the excitation has reached the cerebral cortex, most sound-responsive neurons respond only to a narrow range of frequencies rather than a broad range. Therefore, somewhere along the pathway, processing mechanisms "sharpen" the frequency response. It is believed that this sharpening effect is caused mainly by the phenomenon of lateral inhibition, which was discussed in Chapter 11 in relation to mechanisms for transmitting information in nerves. That is, stimulation of the cochlea at one frequency causes inhibition of signals caused by sound frequencies on either side of the stimulated frequency, this resulting from collateral fibers angling off the primary signal pathway and exerting inhibitory influences on adjacent pathways. The same effect has also been demonstrated to be important in sharpening patterns of somesthetic images, visual images, and other types of sensations.

A large share of the neurons in the auditory cortex, especially in the auditory association cortex, do not respond to specific sound frequencies in the ear. It is believed that these neurons "associate" different sound frequencies with each other or associate sound information with information from other sensory areas of the cortex. Indeed, the parietal portion of the auditory association cortex partly overlaps somatic sensory area II, which could provide easy opportunity for association of auditory information with somatic sensory information.

Discrimination of Sound "Patterns" by the Auditory Cortex. Complete bilateral removal of the auditory cortex does not prevent an animal from detecting sounds or reacting in a crude manner to the sounds. However, it does greatly reduce or sometimes even abolish its ability to discriminate different sound pitches and especially *patterns of sound*. For instance, an animal that has been trained to recognize a combination or sequence of tones, one following the other in a particular pattern, loses this ability when the auditory cortex is destroyed, and, furthermore, it cannot relearn this type of response. Therefore, the auditory cortex is important in the discrimination of *tonal* and *sequential sound patterns*.

In the human being, lesions affecting the auditory association areas but not affecting the primary auditory cortex do not decrease the person's full capability to hear and differentiate sound tones and to interpret at least simple patterns of sound. However, he or she will often be unable to interpret the *meaning* of the sound heard. For instance, lesions in the posterior portion of the superior temporal gyrus, which is Wernicke's area and is also part of the auditory association cortex, often make it impossible for the person to interpret the meanings of words even though he hears them perfectly well and can even repeat them. These functions of the auditory association areas and their relationship to the overall intellectual functions of the brain were discussed in detail in Chapter 18.

DISCRIMINATION OF DIRECTION FROM WHICH SOUND EMANATES

A person determines the direction from which sound emanates by two principal mechanisms: (1) by the time lag between the entry of sound into one ear and into the opposite ear and (2) by the difference between the intensities of the sounds in the two ears. The first mechanism functions best for frequencies below 3000 cycles per second, and the intensity mechanism operates best at higher frequencies because the head acts as a sound barrier at these frequencies. The time lag mechanism discriminates direction much more exactly than the intensity mechanism, for the time lag mechanism does not depend on extraneous factors but only on an exact interval of time between two acoustical signals. If a person is looking straight toward the sound, the sound reaches both ears at exactly the same instant, while, if the right ear is closer to the sound than the left ear, the sound signals from the right ear enter the brain ahead of those from the left ear.

Neural Mechanisms for Detecting Sound Direction. Destruction of the auditory cortex on both sides of the brain, in either human beings or lower mammals, causes loss of almost all ability to detect the direction from which sound comes. Yet, the mechanism for this detection process begins in the superior olivary nuclei, even though it requires the neural pathways all the way from these nuclei to the cortex for interpretation of the signals. The mechanism is believed to be the following:

First, the superior olivary nucleus is divided into two sections, the *medial superior olivary nucleus* and the *lateral superior olivary nucleus*. The lateral nucleus is concerned with detecting the direction from which the sound is coming by the *difference in intensities of the sound* reaching the two ears, presumably by simply comparing the two intensities and sending an appropriate signal to the auditory cortex to estimate the direction.

The *medial superior olivary nucleus*, on the other hand, has a very specific mechanism for *detecting the time-lag between acoustic signals entering the two ears*. This nucleus contains large numbers of neurons that have two major dendrites, one projecting to the right and the other to the left. The acoustical signal from the right ear impinges on the right dendrite and the signal from the left ear impinges on the left dendrite. The intensity of excitation of each of these neurons is highly sensitive to a specific time-lag between the two acoustical signals from the two ears. That is, the neurons near one border of the nucleus respond maximally to a short time-lag; whereas those near the opposite border respond to a very long time-lag; and those between, to intermediate time-lags. Thus, a spatial pattern of neuronal stimulation develops in the medial superior olivary nucleus, with sound from directly in front of the head stimulating one set of olivary neurons maximally and sounds from different side angles stimulating other sets of neurons maximally. This spatial orientation of signals is then transmitted all the way to the auditory cortex where sound direction is determined by the locus in the cortex that is stimulated maximally. It is believed that the signals for determining sound direction are transmitted through a different pathway and that this pathway terminates in the cerebral cortex in a different locus from the transmission pathway and termination locus for the tonal patterns of sound.

This mechanism for detection of sound direction indicates again how information in sensory signals is dissected out as the signals pass through different levels of neuronal activity. In this case, the "quality" of sound direction is separated from the "quality" of sound tones at the level of the superior olivary nuclei.

CENTRIFUGAL CONDUCTION OF IMPULSES FROM THE CENTRAL NERVOUS SYSTEM

Retrograde pathways have been demonstrated at each level of the nervous system from the auditory cortex to the cochlea. The final pathway is mainly from the superior olivary nucleus to the organ of Corti.

These retrograde fibers are inhibitory. Indeed, direct stimulation of discrete points in the olivary nucleus have been shown to inhibit specific areas of the organ of Corti, reducing their sound sensitivities as much as 15 to 20 decibels. One can readily understand how this could allow a person to direct attention to sounds of particular qualities while rejecting sounds of other qualities. This is readily demonstrated when one listens to a single instrument in a symphony orchestra.

HEARING ABNORMALITIES

TYPES OF DEAFNESS

Deafness is usually divided into two types: first, that caused by impairment of the cochlea or auditory nerve, which is usually classed under the heading "nerve deafness," and, second, that caused by impairment of the middle ear mechanisms for transmitting sound into the cochlea, which is usually called "conduction deafness." Obviously, if either the cochlea or the auditory nerve is completely destroyed the person is permanently deaf. However, if the cochlea and nerve are still intact but the ossicular system has been destroyed or ankylosed ("frozen" in place by fibrosis or calcification), sound waves can still be conducted into the cochlea by means of bone conduction.

The Audiometer. To determine the nature of hearing disabilities, the audiometer is used. This is simply an earphone connected to an electronic oscillator capable of emitting pure tones ranging from low frequencies to high frequencies. Based on previous studies of normal persons, the instrument is calibrated so that the zero intensity level of sound at each frequency is the loudness that can barely be heard by the normal person. However, a calibrated volume control can increase or decrease the loudness of each tone above or below the zero level. If the loudness of a tone must be increased to 30 decibels above normal before it can be heard, the person is said to have a *hearing loss* of 30 decibels for that particular tone.

In performing a hearing test using an audiometer, one tests approximately 8 to 10 frequencies covering the auditory spectrum, and the hearing loss is determined for each of these frequencies. Then the so-called "audiogram" is plotted as shown in Figures 25–12 and 25–13, depicting the hearing loss for each of the frequencies in the auditory spectrum.

The audiometer, in addition to being equipped with an earphone for testing air conduction by the ear, is also equipped with an electronic vibrator for testing bone conduction from the mastoid process into the cochlea.

The Audiogram in Nerve Deafness. In nerve deafness—this term including damage to the cochlea, to the auditory nerve, or to the central nervous system circuits from the ear—the person has decreased or total loss of ability to hear sound as tested by both the air conduction apparatus and the bone conduction apparatus. An audiogram de-

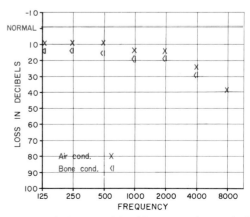

Figure 25–12. Audiogram of the old-age type of nerve deafness.

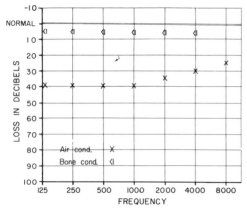

Figure 25–13. Audiogram of deafness resulting from middle ear sclerosis.

picting partial nerve deafness is illustrated in Figure 25–12. In this figure the deafness is mainly for high frequency sound. Such deafness could be caused by damage to the base of the cochlea. This type of deafness occurs to some extent in almost all older persons.

Other patterns of nerve deafness frequently occur as follows: (1) deafness for low frequency sounds caused by excessive and prolonged exposure to very loud sounds (the rock band or the jet airplane engine) because low frequency sounds are usually louder and more damaging to the organ of Corti, and (2) deafness for all frequencies caused by drug sensitivity of the organ of Corti, especially sensitivity to some antibiotics such as streptomycin, kanamycin, and chloramphenicol.

The Audiogram in Conduction Deafness. A second and frequent type of deafness is that caused by fibrosis of the middle ear following repeated infection in the middle ear or fibrosis occurring in the hereditary disease called *otosclerosis.* In this instance the sound waves cannot be transmitted easily through the ossicles from the tympanic membrane to the oval window. Figure 25–13 illustrates an audiogram from a person with "middle ear deafness" of this type. In this case the bone conduction is essentially normal, but air conduction is greatly depressed at all frequencies, more so at the low frequencies. In this type of deafness, the faceplate of the stapes frequently becomes "ankylosed" by bony overgrowth to the edges of the oval window. In this case, the person becomes totally deaf for air conduction, but can be made to hear again almost normally by removing the stapes and replacing it with a minute Teflon or metal prosthesis that transmits the sound from the incus to the oval window.

REFERENCES

Aitkin, L. M.: Tonotopic organization at higher levels of the auditory pathway. *Int. Rev. Physiol.*, 10:249, 1976.

Aitkin, L. M. *et al.*: Central neural mechanisms of hearing. *In* Darian-Smith, I. (ed.): Handbook of Physiology. Sec. 1, Vol. III. Bethesda, American Physiological Society, 1984, p. 675.

Ballenger, J. J. (ed.): Diseases of the Nose, Throat, Ear, Head, and Neck. Philadelphia, Lea & Febiger, 1985.

Beagley, H. A. (ed.): Auditory Investigation: The Scientific and Technological Basis. New York, Oxford University Press, 1979.

Becker, W.: Atlas of Ear, Nose and Throat Diseases, Including Bronchoesophagology. Philadelphia, W. B. Saunders Company, 1984.

Bench, J., and Bamford, J. (eds.): Speech-Hearing Tests and the Spoken Language of Hearing-Impaired Children. New York, Academic Press, 1979.

Brugge, J. F., and Geisler, C. D.: Auditory mechanisms of the lower brainstem. *Annu. Rev. Neurosci.*, 1:363, 1978.

Busnel, R., and Fish, J. F. (eds.): Animal Sonar Systems. New York, Plenum Press, 1979.

Carterette, E. C., and Friedman, M. P.: Hearing. New York, Academic Press, 1978.

Dallos, P.: Peripheral mechanisms of hearing. *In* Darian-Smith, I. (ed.): Handbook of Physiology. Sec. 1, Vol. III. Bethesda, American Physiological Society, 1984, p. 595.

Davis, H.: Biophysics and physiology of the inner ear. *Physiol. Rev.*, 37:1, 1957.

Evans, E. F., and Wilson, J. P. (eds.): Psychophysics and Physiology of Hearing. New York, Academic Press, 1977.

Green, D. M., and Wier, C. C.: Auditory perception. *In* Darian-Smith, I. (ed.): Handbook of Physiology. Sec. 1, Vol. III. Bethesda, American Physiological Society, 1984, p. 557.

Guth, P. S., and Melamed, B.: Neurotransmission in the auditory system: A primer for pharmacologists. *Annu. Rev. Pharmacol. Toxicol.*, 22:383, 1982.

Harris, J. D.: The Electrophysiology and Layout of the Auditory Nervous System. Indianapolis, The Bobbs-Merrill Co., 1974.

Heasley, B. E.: Auditory Processing Disorders and Remediation, 2nd Ed. Springfield, Ill., Charles C Thomas, 1980.

Hudspeth, A. J.: Mechanoelectrical transduction by hair cells in the acousticolateralis sensory system. *Annu. Rev. Neurosci.*, 6:187, 1983.

Imig, T. J., and Morel, A.: Organization of the thalamocortical auditory system in the cat. *Annu. Rev. Neurosci.*, 6:95, 1983.

Kay, R. H.: Hearing of modulation in sounds. *Physiol. Rev.*, 62:894, 1982.

Kiang, N. Y. S.: Peripheral neural processing of auditory information. *In* Darian-Smith, I. (ed.): Handbook of Physiology. Sec. 1, Vol. III. Bethesda, American Physiological Society, 1984, p. 639.

Masterton, R. B., and Imig, T. J.: Neural mechanisms of sound localization. *Annu. Rev. Physiol.*, 46:275, 1984.

Naunton, R. F., and Fernandez, C. (eds.): Evoked Electrical Activity in the Auditory Nervous System. New York, Academic Press, 1978.

Rhode, W. S.: Cochlear mechanics. *Annu. Rev. Physiol.*, 46:231, 1984.

Rosenblum, E. H.: Fundamentals of Hearing for Health Professionals. Boston, Little, Brown, 1979.

Rubel, E. W.: Ontogeny of auditory system function. *Annu. Rev. Physiol.*, 46:213, 1984.

Sachs, M. B.: Neural coding of complex sounds: Speech. *Annu. Rev. Physiol.*, 46:261, 1984.

Sataloff, J., *et al.*: Hearing Loss, 2nd Ed. Philadelphia, J. B. Lippincott Co., 1980.

Scheich, O. C. H., and Schreiner, C. (eds.): Hearing Mechanisms and Speech. New York, Springer-Verlag, 1979.

Schneiderman, C. R.: Basic Anatomy and Physiology in Speech and Hearing. San Diego, College-Hill Press, 1984.

Simmons, J. A., and Kick, S. A.: Physiological mechanisms for spatial filtering and image enhancement in the sonar of bats. *Annu. Rev. Physiol.*, 46:599, 1984.

Singh, R. P.: Anatomy of Hearing and Speech. New York, Oxford University Press, 1980.

Skinner, P. H., and Shelton, R. L.: Speech, Language, and Hearing: Normal Processes and Disorders. Reading, Mass., Addison-Wesley Publishing Co., 1978.

Stevens, S. S.: Hearing. Its Psychology and Physiology. New York, Acoustical Society of America, 1983.

Van Hattum, R. J.: Communication Disorders. New York, The Macmillan Co., 1980.

Weiss, T. F.: Relation of receptor potentials of cochlear hair cells to spike discharges of cochlear neurons. *Annu. Rev. Physiol.*, 46:247, 1984.

Wever, E. G., and Lawrence, M.: Physiological Acoustics. Princeton, Princeton University Press, 1954.

Woolsey, D. N. (ed.): Cortical Sensory Organization. Multiple Auditory Areas. Clifton, NJ, Humana Press, 1982.

26

The Chemical Senses—Taste and Smell

THE SENSE OF TASTE

Taste is mainly a function of the *taste buds* in the mouth, but it is common experience that one's sense of smell also contributes strongly to taste perception. In addition, the texture of food, as detected by tactual senses of the mouth, and the presence of such elements in the food as pepper, which stimulate pain endings, greatly condition the taste experience. The importance of taste lies in the fact that it allows a person to select food in accord with desires and perhaps also in accord with the needs of the tissues for specific nutritive substances.

On the basis of psychological studies, there are generally stated to be four *primary* sensations of taste: *sour, salty, sweet, and bitter.* Yet we know that a person can perceive literally hundreds of different tastes. These are all supposed to be combinations of the four primary sensations in the same manner that all the colors of the spectrum are combinations of three primary color sensations, as described in Chapter 23.

THE PRIMARY SENSATIONS OF TASTE

The Sour Taste. The sour taste is caused by acids, and the intensity of the taste sensation is approximately proportional to the logarithm of the *hydrogen ion concentration.* That is, the more acidic the acid, the stronger becomes the sensation.

The Salty Taste. The salty taste is elicited by ionized salts. The quality of the taste varies somewhat from one salt to another because the salts also elicit other taste sensations besides saltiness. The cations of the salts are mainly responsible for the salty taste, but the anions also contribute to a lesser extent.

The Sweet Taste. The sweet taste is not caused by any single class of chemicals. A list of some of the types of chemicals that cause this taste includes sugars, glycols, alcohols, aldehydes, ketones, amides, esters, amino acids, sulfonic acids, halo-genated acids, and inorganic salts of lead and beryllium. Note specifically that most of the substances that cause a sweet taste are organic chemicals. It is especially interesting that very slight changes in the chemical structure, such as addition of a simple radical, can often change the substance from sweet to bitter.

The third column of Table 26–1 shows the relative intensities of taste of certain substances that cause the sweet taste. *Sucrose,* which is common table sugar, is considered to have an index of 1. Note that one of the substances has a sweet index 5000 times as great as that of sucrose. However, this extremely sweet substance, known as *P-4000,* is unfortunately extremely toxic and therefore cannot be used as a sweetening agent. *Saccharin,* on the other hand, is also more than 600 times as sweet as common table sugar, and since it is not toxic (except that it might be mildly carcinogenic), it can be used as a sweetening agent.

The Bitter Taste. The bitter taste, like the sweet taste, is not caused by any single type of chemical agent, but, here again, the substances that give the bitter taste are almost entirely organic substances. Two particular classes of substances are especially likely to cause bitter taste sensations: (1) long chain organic substances containing nitrogen and (2) alkaloids. The alkaloids include many of the drugs used in medicines such as quinine, caffeine, strychnine, and nicotine.

Some substances that at first taste sweet have a bitter aftertaste. This is true of saccharin, which makes this substance objectionable to some people. Some substances have a sweet taste on the front of the tongue, where taste buds with special sensitivity to the sweet taste are principally located, and a bitter taste on the back of the tongue, where taste buds more sensitive to the bitter taste are located.

The bitter taste, when it occurs in high intensity, usually causes the person or animal to reject the food. This is undoubtedly an important purposive function of the bitter taste sensation because many of the deadly toxins found in poisonous plants are alkaloids, and these all cause intensely bitter taste.

Table 26–1. RELATIVE TASTE INDICES OF DIFFERENT SUBSTANCES

Sour Substances	Index	Bitter Substances	Index	Sweet Substances	Index	Salty Substances	Index
Hydrochloric acid	1	Quinine	1	Sucrose	1	NaCl	1
Formic acid	1.1	Brucine	11	1-propoxy-2-amino-		NaF	2
Chloracetic acid	0.9	Strychnine	3.1	4-nitrobenzene	5000	CaCl$_2$	1
Acetyllactic acid	0.85	Nicotine	1.3	Saccharin	675	NaBr	0.4
Lactic acid	0.85	Phenylthiourea	0.9	Chloroform	40	NaI	0.35
Tartaric acid	0.7	Caffeine	0.4	Fructose	1.7	LiCl	0.4
Malic acid	0.6	Veratrine	0.2	Alanine	1.3	NH$_4$Cl	2.5
Potassium H tartrate	0.58	Philocarpine	0.16	Glucose	0.8	KCl	0.6
Acetic acid	0.55	Atropine	0.13	Maltose	0.45		
Citric acid	0.46	Cocaine	0.02	Galactose	0.32		
Carbonic acid	0.06	Morphine	0.02	Lactose	0.3		

(From Derma: *Proc. Oklahoma Acad. Sci.*, 27:9, 1947; and Pfaffman: Handbook of Physiology. Sec., I, Vol. I. Baltimore, Williams & Wilkins, 1959, p. 507.)

Threshold for Taste

The threshold for stimulation of the sour taste by hydrochloric acid averages 0.0009 N; for stimulation of the salty taste by sodium chloride, 0.01 M; for the sweet taste by sucrose, 0.01 M; and for the bitter taste by quinine, 0.000008 M. Note especially how much more sensitive is the bitter taste sense than all the others, which would be expected since this sensation provides an important protective function.

Table 26–1 gives the relative taste indices (the reciprocals of the taste thresholds) of different substances. In this table, the intensities of the four different primary sensations of taste are referred, respectively, to the intensities of taste of hydrochloric acid, quinine, sucrose, and sodium chloride, each of which is considered to have a taste index of 1.

Taste Blindness. Many persons are taste blind for certain substances, especially for different types of thiourea compounds. A substance used frequently by psychologists for demonstrating taste blindness is *phenylthiocarbamide*, for which approximately 15 to 30 per cent of all people exhibit taste blindness, the exact percentage depending on the method of testing and the concentration of the substance.

THE TASTE BUD AND ITS FUNCTION

Figure 26–1 illustrates a taste bud, which has a diameter of about 1/30 millimeter and a length of

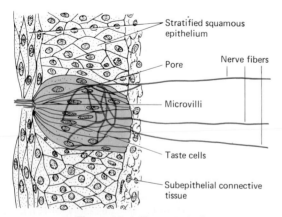

Figure 26–1. The taste bud.

Labels: Stratified squamous epithelium; Pore; Nerve fibers; Microvilli; Taste cells; Subepithelial connective tissue

about 1/16 millimeter. The taste bud is composed of about 40 modified epithelial cells, some of which are supporting cells called *sustentacular cells* and others are *taste cells*. The taste cells are continually being replaced by mitotic division from the surrounding epithelial cells so that some are young cells and others are mature cells that lie toward the center of the bud and soon disintegrate. The life span of each taste cell is about ten days in lower mammals but is unknown for the human being.

The outer tips of the taste cells are arranged around a minute *taste pore*, shown in Figure 26–1. From the tip of each cell, several *microvilli*, or *taste hairs*, about 2 to 3 microns in length and 0.1 to 0.2 micron in width, protrude outward into the taste pore to approach the cavity of the mouth. These microvilli are believed to provide the receptor surface for taste.

Interwoven among the taste cells is a branching terminal network of several *taste nerve fibers* that are stimulated by the taste cells. Some of these fibers invaginate into folds of the taste cell membranes, so that there is extremely intimate contact between the taste cells and the nerves.

An interesting feature of the taste buds is that they completely degenerate when the taste nerve fibers are destroyed. Then, if the taste fibers regrow to the epithelial surface of the mouth, the local epithelial cells regroup themselves to form new taste buds. This illustrates the important principle of "tropic" function of nerve fibers in certain parts of the body. The cause of the tropism is unknown, but it has been postulated to be a protein tropic factor secreted by the nerve endings.

Location of the Taste Buds. The taste buds are found on three of four different types of papillae of the tongue, as follows: (1) A large number of taste buds are on the walls of the troughs that surround the circumvallate papillae, which form a V line toward the posterior of the tongue. (2) Moderate numbers of taste buds are on the fungiform papillae over the front surface of the tongue. (3) Moderate numbers are on the foliate papillae located in the folds along the lateral surfaces of the tongue. Additional taste buds are located on the palate and a few on the tonsillar pillars and at other points around the nasopharynx. Adults have approximately 10,000 taste buds, and children a few more. Beyond the age of 45 years many taste buds rapidly degenerate, causing the taste sensation to become progressively less critical.

Especially important in relation to taste is the tendency for taste buds subserving particular primary sensations of taste to be located in special areas. The sweet and salty tastes are located *principally* on the tip of the tongue, the sour taste on the two lateral sides of the tongue, and the bitter taste on the circumvallate papillae on the posterior tongue.

Specificity of Taste Buds for the Primary Taste Stimuli. Psychological tests using different types of taste stimuli carefully applied to individual taste buds, one at a time, have suggested that we have four distinctly different varieties of taste buds, each sensitive for only one type of taste. Yet, microelectrode studies from single taste buds while they are stimulated successively by the four different primary taste stimuli have shown that most of them can be excited by two, three, or even four of the primary taste stimuli, though usually with one or two of these predominating.

Regardless of the degree of specificity of the individual taste buds for different taste sensations, one can well understand that the hundreds of different types of tastes that we experience result from different quantitative degrees of stimulation of the four primary sensations of taste, as well as simultaneous stimulation of smell in the nose and tactile and pain nerve endings in the mouth.

Mechanism of Stimulation of Taste Buds. *The Receptor Potential.* The membrane of the taste cell, like that of other sensory receptor cells, is negatively charged on the inside with respect to the outside. Application of a taste substance to the taste hairs causes partial loss of this negative potential—that is, the taste cell is *depolarized*. The decrease in potential, within a wide range, is approximately proportional to the logarithm of concentration of the stimulating substance. This change in potential in the taste cell is the *receptor potential* for taste.

The mechanism by which the stimulating substance reacts with the taste hairs to initiate the receptor potential is unknown. It is believed by some physiologists that the substance is simply adsorbed to receptors on the membrane surface of the taste hair and that this adsorption changes the physical characteristics of the hair membrane. This in turn makes the taste cell more permeable to sodium ions and thus depolarizes the cell. The substance is gradually washed away from the taste hair by the saliva, thus removing the taste stimulus. Supposedly, the type or types of receptor in each taste hair determine the types of taste that will elicit responses.

Generation of Nerve Impulses by the Taste Bud. Most of the taste nerve fiber endings are encased by folds of the taste cell membranes. In some way not understood the receptor potentials of the taste cells generate impulses in the taste fibers, perhaps by secreting a chemical transmitter that in turn stimulates the nerve endings.

On first application of the taste stimulus, the rate of discharge of the nerve fibers rises to a peak in a small fraction of a second, but then it adapts within the next 2 seconds back to a lower steady level. Thus, a strong immediate signal is transmitted by the taste nerve, and a weaker continuous signal is transmitted as long as the taste bud is exposed to the taste stimulus.

TRANSMISSION OF TASTE SIGNALS INTO THE CENTRAL NERVOUS SYSTEM

Figure 26–2 illustrates the neuronal pathways for transmission of taste signals from the tongue and pharyngeal region into the central nervous system. Taste impulses from the anterior two thirds of the tongue pass first into the *fifth nerve* and then through the *chorda tympani* into the *facial nerve*, thence into the *tractus solitarius* in the brain stem. Taste sensations from the circumvallate papillae on the back of the tongue and from other posterior regions of the mouth are transmitted through the *glossopharyngeal nerve* also into the *tractus solitarius* but at a slightly lower level. Finally, a few taste signals are transmitted into the *tractus solitarius* from the base of the tongue and other parts of the pharyngeal region by way of the *vagus nerve*.

All taste fibers synapse in the *nuclei of the tractus solitarius* and send second order neurons to a small area of the *thalamus* located slightly medial to the thalamic terminations of the facial regions of the dorsal column–medial lemniscal system. From the thalamus, third order neurons are transmitted to the *lower tip of the postcentral gyrus in the parietal cortex* where it curls deep into the sylvian fissure. This lies in close association with, or even superimposed on, the tongue area of somatic area I. Third order neurons also project to the nearby *opercular-insular area*, located deep in the sylvian fissure as well.

From this description of the taste pathways, it

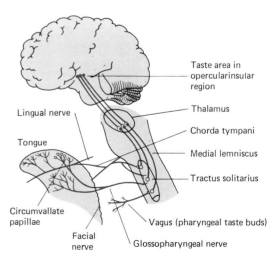

Figure 26–2. Transmission of taste impulses into the central nervous system.

immediately becomes evident that they parallel closely the somatic pathways from the tongue.

Taste Reflexes. From the tractus solitarius a large number of impulses are transmitted directly into the *superior* and *inferior salivatory nuclei*, and these in turn transmit impulses to the submandibular, sublingual, and parotid glands to help control the secretion of saliva during the ingestion of food.

Adaptation of Taste. Everyone is familiar with the fact that taste sensations adapt rapidly, often with almost complete adaptation within a minute or so of continuous stimulation. Yet, from electrophysiological studies of taste nerve fibers, it seems that the taste buds themselves do not adapt enough to account for all or even most of the taste adaptation. The first burst of impulses from the taste bud allows one to detect extremely minute concentrations of taste substances, but normal concentrations of taste substances cause a weaker prolonged discharge of the taste fibers. Therefore, the progressive adaptation that occurs in the sensation of taste has been postulated to occur in the central nervous system itself, though the mechanism and site of this are not known. If this is true, it is a mechanism different from that of most other sensory systems, which adapt mainly at the receptors.

SPECIAL ATTRIBUTES OF THE TASTE SENSE

Affective Nature of Taste. *Pleasantness* and *unpleasantness* are called the "affective" attributes of a sensation. Figure 26–3 illustrates the affective effects of different types of taste at different concentrations of the stimulating substances, showing, strangely enough, that the sweet taste is likely to be unpleasant at a very low concentration but very pleasant at high concentrations. The other types of taste, on the other hand, are likely to be pleasant at low concentrations but exceedingly unpleasant at high concentrations. This is particularly true of the bitter taste.

Importance of the Sense of Smell in Taste. Persons

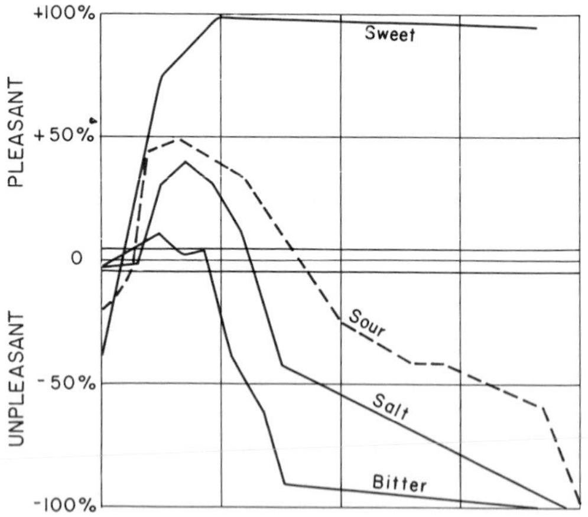

Figure 26–3. The affective nature of the different primary sensations of taste at progressively increasing degrees of taste stimulus. (From Engel, *in* Woodworth and Schlosberg: Experimental Psychology. New York, Holt, Rinehart & Winston, Inc. Reprinted with permission of CBS College Publishing.)

with severe colds frequently state that they have lost their sense of taste. However, on testing, the taste sensations are found to be completely normal. This illustrates that much of what we call taste is actually smell. Odors from the food can pass upward into the nasopharynx, often stimulating the olfactory system thousands of times as strongly as the taste system. For instance, if the olfactory system is intact, alcohol can be "tasted" in 1/25,000 the concentration required when the olfactory system is not intact.

Taste Preference and Control of the Diet. Taste preferences mean simply that an animal will choose certain types of food in preference to others, and it automatically uses this to help control the type of diet it eats. Furthermore, its taste preferences often change in accord with the needs of the body for certain specific substances. The following experimental studies illustrate this ability of an animal to choose food in accord with the need of its body: First, adrenalectomized animals automatically select drinking water with a high concentration of sodium chloride in preference to pure water, and this in many instances is sufficient to supply the needs of the body and prevent death as a result of salt depletion. Second, an animal injected with excessive amounts of insulin develops a depleted blood sugar, and it automatically chooses the sweetest food from among many samples. Third, parathyroidectomized animals automatically choose drinking water with a high concentration of calcium chloride.

These same phenomena are also observed in many instances of everyday life. For instance, the salt licks of the desert region are known to attract animals from far and wide, and even the human being rejects any food that has an unpleasant affective sensation, which certainly in many instances protects our bodies from undesirable substances.

The phenomenon of taste preference almost certainly results from some mechanism located in the central nervous system and not from a mechanism in the taste buds themselves, though it is true that the taste buds often do become sensitized to the needed nutrient. An important reason for believing taste preference to be mainly a central phenomenon is that previous experience with unpleasant or pleasant tastes plays a major role in determining one's different taste preferences. For instance, if a person becomes sick immediately after eating a particular type of food, the person generally develops a negative taste preference, or taste aversion, for that particular food thereafter; the same effect can be demonstrated in animals.

THE SENSE OF SMELL

Smell is the least understood sense. This results partly from the location of the olfactory membrane high in the nose where it is difficult to study and partly from the fact that the sense of smell is a subjective phenomenon that cannot be studied with ease in lower animals. Still another complicating problem is the fact that the sense of smell is almost rudimentary in the human being in comparison with that of some lower animals.

THE OLFACTORY MEMBRANE

The olfactory membrane lies in the superior part of each nostril, as illustrated in Figure 26–4. Medi-

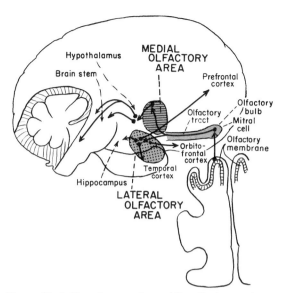

Figure 26-4. Neural connections of the olfactory system.

ally it folds downward over the surface of the septum, and laterally it folds over the superior turbinate and even over a small portion of the upper surface of the middle turbinate. In each nostril the olfactory membrane has a surface area of approximately 2.4 square centimeters.

The Olfactory Cells. The receptor cells for the smell sensation are the *olfactory cells*, which are actually bipolar nerve cells derived originally from the central nervous system itself. There are about 100 million of these cells in the olfactory epithelium interspersed among *sustentacular cells*, as shown in Figure 26-5. The mucosal end of the olfactory cell forms a knob from which 6 to 12 *olfactory hairs*, or *cilia*, 0.3 micron in diameter and 50 to 80 microns in length, project into the mucus that coats the inner surface of the nasal cavity. These projecting olfactory cilia form a dense mat in the mucus, and it is these cilia that react to odors in the air and then stimulate the olfactory cells, as discussed later. Spaced among the olfactory cells in the olfactory membrane are many small *glands of Bowman* that

secrete mucus onto the surface of the olfactory membrane.

STIMULATION OF THE OLFACTORY CELLS

The Necessary Stimulus for Smell. We do not know what it takes chemically to stimulate the olfactory cells. Yet we do know the physical characteristics of the substances that cause olfactory stimulation: First, the substance must be volatile so that it can be sniffed into the nostrils. Second, it must be at least slightly water-soluble so that it can pass through the mucus to the olfactory cells. And, third, it must also be lipid-soluble, presumably because the olfactory cilia are composed principally of lipid materials.

Regardless of the basic mechanism by which the olfactory cells are stimulated, it is known that they become stimulated only when air blasts upward into the superior region of the nose. Therefore, smell occurs in cycles along with the inspirations, which indicates that the olfactory receptors respond in milliseconds to the volatile agents. Because smell intensity is exacerbated by blasting air through the upper reaches of the nose, the sensitivity of smell can be greatly increased by the well-known sniffing technique.

Receptor Potentials in Olfactory Cells. The olfactory cells react to olfactory stimuli in the same manner that most other sensory receptors react to their specific stimuli; that is, by depolarizing the cell and thus creating a receptor potential. This in turn initiates nerve impulses in the olfactory nerve fibers. An experiment that demonstrates this property of the olfactory receptors is the following: An electrode is placed on the surface of the olfactory membrane, and its electrical potential with respect to the remainder of the body is recorded. When an odorous substance is blown into the nostril, the surface potential becomes negative and remains negative as long as the odorous air continues to pass through the nostril. This electrical recording is called the *electro-olfactogram*, and it is believed to result from summation of receptor potentials developed in the receptor olfactory cells.

Over a wide range, both the amplitude of the electro-olfactogram and the rate of olfactory nerve impulses are approximately proportional to the logarithm of the stimulus strength, which illustrates that the olfactory receptors tend to obey principles of transduction similar to those of other sensory receptors.

Adaptation. The olfactory receptors adapt approximately 50 per cent in the first second or so after stimulation. Thereafter, they adapt very little and very slowly. Yet we all know from our own experience that smell sensations adapt almost to extinction within a minute or so after one enters a strongly odorous atmosphere. Since this psychological adaptation is far greater than the degree of adaptation of the receptors themselves, it is almost certain that the adaptation occurs in the central nervous system, which has also been postulated to be the locus of much of the adaptation for taste sensations. The neuronal mechanism for this adaptation could be the following: Large numbers of centrifugal nerve fibers pass from the olfactory

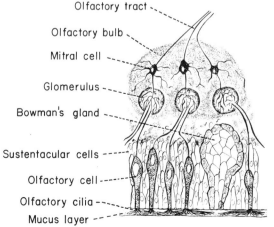

Olfactory tract

Olfactory bulb

Mitral cell

Glomerulus

Bowman's gland

Sustentacular cells

Olfactory cell

Olfactory cilia

Mucus layer

Figure 26-5. Organization of the olfactory membrane.

regions of the brain backward along the olfactory tract and terminate on special inhibitory cells in the olfactory bulb, the *granule cells*. It is postulated that after the onset of an olfactory stimulus the central nervous system gradually develops a strong inhibitory signal to suppress transmission of the signal through the olfactory bulb.

Search for the Primary Sensations of Smell. Most physiologists are convinced that the many smell sensations are subserved by a few rather discrete primary sensations, in the same way that taste is subserved by sour, sweet, bitter, and salty sensations. But, thus far, only minor success has been achieved in classifying the primary sensations of smell. Yet, on the basis of psychological tests and action potential studies from various points in the olfactory nerve pathways, it has been postulated that about seven different primary classes of olfactory stimulants preferentially excite separate olfactory cells. These classes of olfactory stimulants are characterized as follows:

1. Camphoraceous
2. Musky
3. Floral
4. Pepperminty
5. Ethereal
6. Pungent
7. Putrid

However, it is unlikely that this list actually represents the true primary sensations of smell, even though it does illustrate the results of one of the many attempts to classify them. Indeed, several clues in recent years have indicated that there may be as many as *50* or more primary sensations of smell—a marked contrast to only *three* primary sensations of color detected by the eyes and only *four* primary sensations of taste detected by the tongue. For instance, persons have been found who have *odor blindness* for single substances; and such discrete odor blindness has been identified for more than 50 different substances. Since it is presumed that odor blindness for each substance represents a lack of the appropriate receptor cell for that substance, it is postulated that the sense of smell might be subserved by 50 or more primary smell sensations.

Mechanism for Excitation of the Olfactory Cells. The basic mechanism by which the olfactory cells are stimulated is not known, but two principal theories have been proposed. One of these is a *physical theory* which suggests that it is the physical shapes of the odor molecules that determine which olfactory cells will be stimulated, but the evidence for this theory is weak. The second theory, a *chemical theory*, is much more likely to be correct. This theory assumes that the odor molecules bind chemically to protein *receptors* in the membranes of the olfactory cilia. The type of receptor in each olfactory cell determines the type of stimulant that will excite the cell. The reaction between the stimulant and the receptor supposedly increases the permeability of the olfactory ciliary membrane, and this in turn creates the receptor potential in the olfactory cell that generates impulses in the olfactory nerve fibers.

Affective Nature of Smell. Smell, equally as much as taste, has the affective qualities of either pleasantness or unpleasantness. Because of this, smell is as important as, if not more important than, taste in the selection of food. Indeed, a person who has previously eaten food that has disagreed with him is often nauseated by even the smell of that same type of food on a second occasion. Other types of odors that have proved to be unpleasant in the past may also provoke a disagreeable feeling; on the other hand, perfume of the right quality can wreak havoc with masculine emotions. In addition, in some lower animals odors are the primary excitant of sexual drive.

Threshold for Smell. One of the principal characteristics of smell is the minute quantity of the stimulating agent in the air often required to effect a smell sensation. For instance, the substance *methyl mercaptan* can be smelled when only 1/25,000,000,000 milligram is present in each milliliter of air. Because of this low threshold, this substance is mixed with natural gas to give the gas an odor that can be detected when it leaks from a gas pipe.

Measurement of Smell Threshold. One of the problems in studying smell has been difficulty in obtaining accurate measurements of the threshold stimulus required to induce smell. The simplest technique is simply to allow a person to sniff different substances in the usual manner of smelling. Indeed, some investigators feel that this is as satisfactory as almost any other procedure. However, to eliminate variations from person to person, more objective methods have been developed: One of these has been to place a box containing the volatilized agent over the subject's head. Appropriate precautions are taken to exclude odors from the person's own body. The person is allowed to breathe naturally, but the volatilized agent is distributed evenly in the air that is breathed.

Gradations of Smell Intensities. Though the threshold concentrations of substances that evoke smell are extremely slight, concentrations only 10 to 50 times above the threshold values often evoke maximum intensity of smell. This is in contrast to most other sensory systems of the body, in which the ranges of detection are tremendous—for instance, 500,000 to 1 in the case of the eyes and 1,000,000,000,000 to 1 in the case of the ears. This perhaps can be explained by the fact that smell is concerned more with detecting the presence or absence of odors than with quantitative detection of their intensities.

TRANSMISSION OF SMELL SIGNALS INTO THE CENTRAL NERVOUS SYSTEM

The function of the central nervous system in olfaction is almost as vague as the function of the peripheral receptors. However, Figures 26–4 and 26–5 illustrate the general plan for transmission of olfactory signals into the central nervous system. Figure 26–5 shows a number of separate *olfactory cells* sending axons into the *olfactory bulb* to end on *dendrites from mitral cells* in a structure called the *glomerulus*. Approximately 25,000 axons enter each glomerulus and synapse with about 25 mitral cells that in turn send signals into the brain. Also in the glomerulus are about 60 smaller cells, the *tufted cells*, that send signals to the brain as well—perhaps to the older portions of the olfactory nervous system.

Figure 26–4 shows the major pathways for transmission of olfactory signals from the mitral and tufted cells into the brain. The fibers from the cells travel through the olfactory tract and terminate either primarily or after relay neurons in two principal areas of the brain called the *medial olfactory area* and the *lateral olfactory area*, respectively. The medial olfactory area is composed of a group of nuclei located in the midportion of the brain anterior to the hypothalamus. This group includes the *olfactory nucleus*, the *olfactory tubercle*, parts of the *hypothalamus*, and other adjacent areas.

The lateral olfactory area is composed mainly of the *prepyriform* and *pyriform cortex* and part of the *amygdaloid nuclei*.

Secondary olfactory tracts pass from both the medial and lateral olfactory areas into many other portions of the *limbic system* and into associated regions of the *thalamus* and *brain stem nuclei*.

The lateral olfactory area, especially part of the *amygdala* and the overlying cortex, the *pyriform* and *prepyriform* areas, is believed to be responsible for the more complex aspects of olfaction, such as association of olfactory sensations with somatic, visual, tactile, and other types of sensation. These regions of the brain, operating in association with other areas of the cortex located more anteriorly in the *uncus*, *orbitofrontal cortex*, and *frontal cortex*, are probably responsible for a person's specific appetites for certain types of foods. For instance, it might be in these areas that one develops special likes or dislikes for certain foods depending upon previous experience with the foods.

The *pyriform area* of the temporal cortex is frequently considered to be the *primary olfactory cortex*. It is particularly interesting that this is the only part of the entire cerebral cortex that receives primary sensory signals that are not relayed through the thalamus.

Complete removal of the lateral olfactory area hardly affects the primitive responses to olfaction, such as licking the lips, salivation, and other feeding responses caused by the smell of food or such as the various emotions associated with smell. On the other hand, its removal does abolish the more complicated conditioned reflexes that depend on olfactory stimuli.

Centrifugal Control of Activity in the Olfactory Bulb by the Central Nervous System. Many nerve fibers originating in the olfactory portions of the brain pass in the backward direction in the olfactory tract to the olfactory bulb, that is, "centrifugally" from the brain to the periphery. These terminate on the very large number of small *granule cells* located in the center of the bulb. These in turn send short, inhibitory *dendrites* to the mitral and tufted cells. As discussed earlier, it is believed that this inhibitory feedback to the olfactory bulb might be a method for central adaptation of olfaction to the different odors. It might also be a means for helping sharpen one's specific capability of distinguishing one odor from another.

Electrical Activity in the Olfactory Nerves and Tracts. The olfactory receptors in the olfactory epithelium, even normally, send impulses at a slow rate of 1 to 3 pulses per second. Most odors increase the impulse traffic, but a few actually inhibit it. A strong olfactory signal can increase the impulse rate to a maximum of about 20 per second.

Electrophysiological studies show that the mitral and tufted cells are also continually active. Superimposed on this background are increases or decreases in impulse traffic caused by different odors. Thus, the olfactory stimuli *modulate* the frequency of impulses in the olfactory system and in this way transmit the olfactory information.

REFERENCES

Alberts, J. R.: Producing and interpreting experimental olfactory deficits. *Physiol. Behav.*, 12:657, 1974.

Dastoli, F. R.: Taste receptor proteins. *Life Sci.*, 14:1417, 1974.

Denton, D. A.: Salt appetite. In Code, C. F., and Heidel, W. (eds.): Handbook of Physiology. Sec. 6, Vol. 1. Baltimore, Williams & Wilkins, 1967, p. 433.

Douek, E.: The Sense of Smell and Its Abnormalities. New York, Churchill Livingstone, 1974.

Hodgson, E. S.: Taste receptors. *Sci. Am.*, 204:135, 1961.

Kare, M. R.,. and Maller, O.: The Chemical Sense and Nutrition. Baltimore, The Johns Hopkins Press, 1967.

Kashara, Y. (ed.): Proceedings of the Seventeenth Japanese Symposium on Taste and Smell. Arlington, VA, IRL Press, 1984.

Lat, J.: Self-selection of dietary components. In Code, C. F., and Heidel, W. (eds.): Handbook of Physiology. Sec. 6, Vol. 1. Baltimore, Williams & Wilkins, 1967, p. 367.

McBurney, D. H.: Taste and olfaction: Sensory discrimination. In Darian-Smith, I. (ed.): Handbook of Physiology. Sec. 1, Vol. III. Bethesda, American Physiological Society, 1984, p. 1067.

Moulton, D. G., and Beidler, L. M.: Structure and function in the peripheral olfactory system. *Physiol. Rev.*, 47:1, 1967.

Norgren, R.: Central neural mechanisms of taste. In Darian-Smith, I. (ed.): Handbook of Physiology. Sec. 1, Vol. III. Bethesda, American Physiological Society, 1984, p. 1087.

Oakley, B., and Benjamin, R. M.: Neural mechanisms of taste. *Physiol. Rev.*, 46:173, 1966.

Ohloff, G., and Thomas, A. F. (eds.): Gustation and Olfaction. New York, Academic Press, 1971.

Shepherd, G. M.: The olfactory bulb: A simple system in the mammalian brain. In Brookhart, J. M., and Mountcastle, V. B. (eds.): Handbook of Physiology. Sec. 1, Vol. 1. Baltimore, Williams & Wilkins, 1977, p. 945.

Takagi, S. F.: The olfactory nervous system of the Old World monkey. *Jpn. J. Physiol.*, 34:561, 1984.

Todd, J. H.: The chemical language of fishes. *Sci. Am.*, 224:98, 1971.

Wenzel, B. M., and Sieck, M. H.: Olfaction. *Annu. Rev. Physiol.*, 28:381, 1966.

Zotterman, Y.: Olfaction and Taste. New York, The Macmillan Co., 1963.

VI

NERVOUS CONTROL OF BODY FUNCTIONS

27

Nervous Regulation of the Circulation and of Respiration

Because the nervous system is the major overall controller of our bodily activities, it is equally as important to understand the ways in which the nervous system interfaces with the peripheral parts of the body as to understand the nervous system itself. Therefore, the remaining chapters of this text will help to explain some of the more important ways in which the nervous system controls what we call the *vegetative functions* of the body, meaning the life processes of the body, such as the control of arterial pressure, respiration, gastrointestinal function, body temperature, and even sexual functions.

The present chapter will address the control of the circulation and respiration.

NERVOUS REGULATION OF THE CIRCULATION

The circulation is regulated partly by nonnervous mechanisms that are intrinsic to the circulation itself and partly by extrinsic mechanisms, especially by the nervous system. The intrinsic mechanisms consist of such functions as intrinsic control of rhythmicity within the heart muscle itself and local control of blood flow by each tissue of the body when the tissue needs more or less nutrients.

Nervous control of the circulation has two very important features: First, nervous regulation can function extremely rapidly, some of the nervous effects beginning to occur within 1 second and reaching full development within 5 to 30 seconds. Second, the nervous system provides a means for controlling large parts of the circulation simultaneously, often in spite of the effect that this has on the blood flow to individual tissues. For instance, when it is important to raise the arterial pressure temporarily, the nervous system can arbitrarily cut off, or at least greatly decrease, blood flow to major segments of the circulation despite the fact that the local blood flow regulatory mechanisms oppose this.

AUTONOMIC CONTROL OF THE CIRCULATION

The autonomic nervous system was discussed in detail in Chapter 21. However, it is so important to the regulation of the circulation that its specific anatomical and functional characteristics relating to the circulation deserve special attention here.

By far the most important part of the autonomic nervous system for regulation of the circulation is the *sympathetic nervous system*. The *parasympathetic nervous system* is important only for its regulation of heart function, as we shall see later in the chapter.

The Sympathetic Nervous System. Figure 27–1 illustrates the anatomy of sympathetic nervous control of the circulation. Sympathetic vasomotor nerve fibers leave the spinal cord through all the thoracic and the first one to two lumbar spinal nerves. These pass into the sympathetic chain and thence by two routes to the blood vessels throughout the body: (1) through specific *sympathetic nerves* that innervate mainly the internal viscera, and (2) through the *spinal nerves* that innervate mainly the peripheral areas. The precise pathways of these fibers in the spinal cord and in the sympathetic chains were discussed in Chapter 21.

Sympathetic Innervation of the Vasculature. Figure 27–2 illustrates the distribution of sympathetic nerve fibers to the blood vessels and shows that all the vessels except the capillaries, precapillary sphincters, and most of the metarterioles are innervated.

The innervation of the small arteries and arterioles allows sympathetic stimulation to increase the *resistance* and thereby to change the rate of blood flow through the tissues. The innervation of large vessels, particularly of the veins, makes it possible for sympathetic stimulation to change the volume of these vessels and thereby to alter the volume of the peripheral circulatory system, which can translocate blood into the heart and thereby play a major role in the regulation of cardiovascular function, as we shall see later in this chapter.

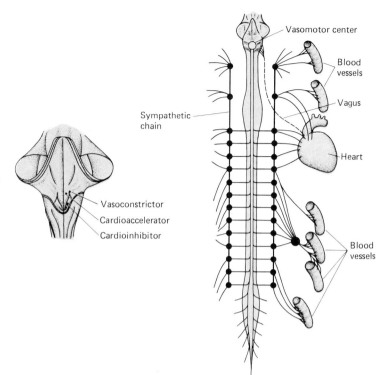

Figure 27–1. The vasomotor center and its control of the circulatory system through the sympathetic nerves and through the vagus nerves to the heart, which are part of the parasympathetic nervous system.

Sympathetic Nerve Fibers to the Heart. In addition to sympathetic nerve fibers supplying the blood vessels, other sympathetic fibers go to the heart, as was discussed in Chapter 9. It will be recalled that sympathetic stimulation markedly increases the activity of the heart, increasing the heart rate, and enhancing its strength of pumping.

Parasympathetic Control of Heart Function, Especially Heart Rate. Though the parasympathetic nervous system is exceedingly important for many other autonomic functions of the body, it plays only a minor role in regulation of the circulation. Its only really important circulatory effect is its control of heart rate by way of parasympathetic fibers carried to the heart in the vagus nerves, shown in Figure 27–1 by the dotted line from the medulla directly to the heart. The parasympathetics also have a slight

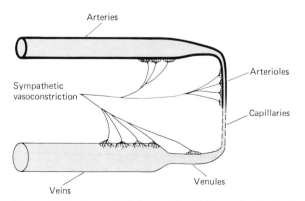

Figure 27–2. Sympathetic innervation of the systemic circulation.

effect on control of cardiac contractility; however, this effect is far overshadowed by the sympathetic nervous system's control of contractility.

The effects of parasympathetic stimulation on heart function were discussed in detail in Chapter 9. Principally, parasympathetic stimulation causes a marked *decrease* in heart rate and a slight decrease in contractility.

The Sympathetic Vasoconstrictor System and Its Control by the Central Nervous System

The sympathetic nerves carry both vasoconstrictor and vasodilator fibers, but by far the most important of these are the *sympathetic vasoconstrictor* fibers. Sympathetic vasoconstrictor fibers are distributed to essentially all segments of the circulation. However, this distribution is greater in some tissues than in others. It is less potent in both skeletal and cardiac muscle and in the brain, whereas it is powerful in the kidneys, the gut, the spleen, and the skin.

The Vasomotor Center and Its Control of the Vasoconstrictor System—Vasomotor Tone. Located bilaterally in the reticular substance of the medulla and the lower third of the pons, as illustrated in Figure 27–3, is an area called the *vasomotor center*. This center transmits impulses downward through the cord and thence through the sympathetic vasoconstrictor fibers to all or almost all the blood vessels of the body.

Though the total organization of the vasomotor

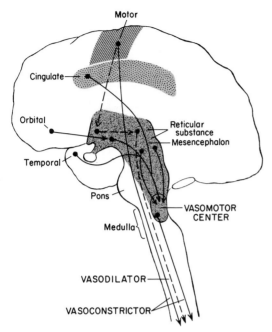

Figure 27–3. Areas of the brain that play important roles in the nervous regulation of the circulation. The dashed lines represent inhibitory pathways.

center is still unclear, recent experiments have made it possible to identify certain important areas in the center, as follows:

1. A *vasoconstrictor area*, called area "C-1," located bilaterally in the anterolateral portions of the upper medulla and lower pons. The neurons in this area secrete *norepinephrine*; their fibers are distributed throughout the cord where they excite the vasoconstrictor neurons of the sympathetic nervous system.

2. A *vasodilator area*, called area "A-1," located bilaterally in the anterolateral portions of the lower half of the medulla. The neurons in this area also secrete norepinephrine, but their fibers project up-

ward to the vasoconstrictor area (A-1) and inhibit the vasoconstrictor activity of that area, thus causing vasodilation.

3. A *sensory area*, located bilaterally in the *tractus solitarius* in the posterolateral portions of the medulla and lower pons. The neurons of this area receive nerve signals mainly from the vagus and glossopharyngeal nerves, and the output signals from the sensory area then help control the activities of both the vasoconstrictor and vasodilator areas, thus providing sensory control of many of the vasomotor center's activities.

Under normal conditions, the vasoconstrictor area of the vasomotor center transmits signals continuously to the sympathetic vasoconstrictor nerve fibers, causing continuous slow firing of these fibers at a rate of about one half to two impulses per second. This continual firing is called *sympathetic vasoconstrictor tone*. These impulses maintain a partial state of contraction in the blood vessels, a state called *vasomotor tone*.

Figure 27–4 demonstrates the significance of vasoconstrictor tone. In the experiment illustrated by this figure, total spinal anesthesia was administered to an animal, which completely blocked all transmission of nerve impulses from the central nervous system to the periphery. As a result, the arterial pressure fell from 100 to 50 mm Hg, illustrating the effect of loss of vasoconstrictor tone throughout the body. A few minutes later a small amount of the hormone norepinephrine was injected intravenously. As this hormone was transported in the blood to all the blood vessels, the vessels once again became constricted, and the arterial pressure rose to a level even greater than normal for a minute or two until the norepinephrine was destroyed.

Control of Heart Activity by the Vasomotor Center. At the same time that the vasomotor center is controlling the degree of vascular constriction, it

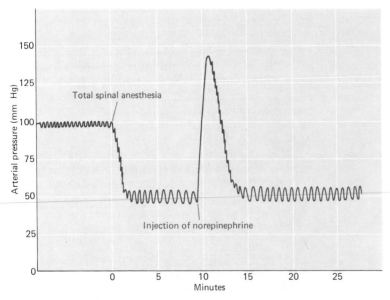

Figure 27–4. Effect of total spinal anesthesia on the arterial pressure, showing a marked fall in pressure resulting from loss of vasomotor tone.

also controls heart activity. The lateral portions of the vasomotor center transmit excitatory impulses through the sympathetic nerve fibers to the heart to increase heart rate and contractility, while the medial portion of the vasomotor center, which lies in immediate apposition to the *dorsal motor nucleus of the vagus nerve*, transmits impulses through the vagus nerve to the heart to decrease heart rate. Therefore, the vasomotor center can either increase or decrease heart activity, this ordinarily increasing at the same time that vasoconstriction occurs throughout the body and ordinarily decreasing at the same time that vasoconstriction is inhibited. However, these interrelationships are not invariable, because some signals that pass down the vagus nerves to the heart can bypass the vasomotor center.

Control of the Vasomotor Center by Higher Nervous Centers. Large numbers of areas throughout the *reticular substance* of the *pons, mesencephalon,* and *diencephalon* can either excite or inhibit the vasomotor center. This reticular substance is illustrated in Figure 27–3 by the diffuse shaded area. In general, the more lateral and superior portions of the reticular substance cause excitation, while the more medial and inferior portions cause inhibition.

The *hypothalamus* plays a special role in the control of the vasoconstrictor system, for it can exert powerful excitatory or inhibitory effects on the vasomotor center. The *posterolateral portions* of the hypothalamus cause mainly excitation, while the *anterior part* can cause mild excitation or inhibition, depending on the precise part of the anterior hypothalamus stimulated.

Many different parts of the *cerebral cortex* can also excite or inhibit the vasomotor center. Stimulation of the *motor cortex*, for instance, excites the vasomotor center because of impulses transmitted downward into the hypothalamus and thence to the vasomotor center. Also, stimulation of the *anterior temporal lobe*, the *orbital areas of the frontal cortex*, the *anterior part of the cingulate gyrus*, the *amygdala*, the *septum*, and the *hippocampus* can all either excite or inhibit the vasomotor center, depending on the precise portion of these areas that is stimulated and upon the intensity of the stimulus.

Thus, widespread areas of the brain can have profound effects on the vasomotor center and in turn on the sympathetic vasoconstrictor system of the body, either further enhancing the degree of vasoconstriction or causing vasodilatation by inhibiting the vasoconstrictor tone.

Norepinephrine—The Sympathetic Vasoconstrictor Transmitter Substance. The substance secreted at the endings of the vasoconstrictor nerves is norepinephrine. Norepinephrine acts directly on the so-called "alpha" receptors of the vascular smooth muscle to cause vasoconstriction, as was discussed in Chapter 21.

The Adrenal Medullae and Their Relationship to the Sympathetic Vasoconstrictor System. Sympathetic impulses are transmitted to the adrenal medullae at the same time that they are transmitted to all the blood vessels. These impulses cause the medullae to secrete both epinephrine and norepinephrine into the circulating blood, as was described in Chapter 21. These two hormones are carried in the bloodstream to all parts of the body, where they act directly on the blood vessels usually to cause vasoconstriction, but sometimes the epinephrine induces vasodilatation because it has a potent "beta" receptor stimulatory effect, which often dilates vessels, as was also discussed in Chapter 21.

"PATTERNS" OF CIRCULATORY RESPONSES ELICITED BY DIFFERENT CENTRAL NERVOUS SYSTEM CENTERS

Stimulation of the Vasomotor Center—The Mass Action Effect. Stimulation of the lateral portions of the vasomotor center causes widespread activation of the vasoconstrictor fibers throughout the body, while stimulation of the medial portions of the vasomotor center causes widespread *inhibition of vasoconstriction*. In many conditions the entire vasomotor center acts as a unit, stimulating at the same time all the body's vasoconstrictors and the heart itself, as well as stimulating the adrenal medullae to secrete epinephrine and norepinephrine that circulate in the blood to excite the circulation still further. The results of this "mass action" are threefold: First, the peripheral resistance increases in most parts of the circulation, thereby elevating the arterial pressure. Second, the capacity vessels, particularly the veins, are excited, which greatly decreases their capacity; this forces increased quantities of blood into the heart, thereby increasing the cardiac output. Third, the heart is strongly stimulated so that it can handle the increased cardiac output.

Thus, the overall effect of this "mass action" is to prepare the circulation for increased delivery of blood flow to the body.

Stimulation of the Hypothalamus—The "Alarm" Pattern. Under normal conditions, the hypothalamus probably does not transmit large numbers of impulses into the sympathetic vascular control system. However, on occasion the hypothalamus becomes strongly stimulated and can then activate either the vasoconstrictor or the vasodilator systems or both of them together.

Diffuse stimulation of the hypothalamus (or of closely allied areas such as the septum) activates the vasodilator system to the muscles, thereby increasing the blood flow through the muscles; at the same time it causes intense vasoconstriction throughout the remainder of the body and an intense increase in heart activity. The arterial pressure rises, the cardiac output increases, the heart rate increases, and the circulation is ready to supply nutrients to the muscles if needed. Also, impulses are transmitted simultaneously throughout the central nervous system to cause a state of generalized excitement and attentiveness, these often increasing to such a pitch that the overall pattern of the reaction is that of *alarm*, sometimes also called the *defense pattern*.

Thus, the "alarm" pattern contains all the ingredients of the "mass action" pattern as well as the elements of muscle vasodilation and extreme psychic excitement. This pattern seems to have the purposeful effect of preparing the animal or person to perform on a second's notice whatever activity is required.

The "Motor" Pattern of Circulatory Stimulation. When the motor cortex transmits signals to the skeletal muscle to cause motor activities, it also sends signals to the circulatory system to cause the following effects: First, it excites the alarm system just described, and this generally activates the heart and increases arterial pressure, making the circulatory system ready to supply increased blood flow to the muscles. This effect also causes vasoconstriction in most nonmuscular parts of the body, such as the kidneys, the skin, and the gut, thereby forcing a larger share of the blood flow through the active muscles. Second, impulses pass directly from the motor cortex to the sympathetic neurons of the spinal cord. These enhance the vasoconstriction in the nonmuscular parts of the body, thereby raising the arterial pressure still more and helping to increase muscle blood flow. They possibly also inhibit the vasoconstrictor nerves to the excited muscles.

The motor pattern of circulatory response can also be elicited by stimulation of several areas of the reticular substance in the brain stem. Stimulation of one of these areas, the *fields of Forel*, elicits a response almost precisely the same as that caused by direct activation of the motor cortex. Therefore, it is possible, if not likely, that this area of the reticular substance plays a major role in control of the circulatory system in exercise.

Emotional Fainting—Vasovagal Syncope. A particularly interesting circulatory reaction occurs in persons who faint because of intense emotional experiences. In this condition, the muscle vasodilator system becomes powerfully activated so that blood flow through the muscles increases severalfold. Intense vagal stimulation of the heart also occurs, causing the heart rate to slow markedly. This overall effect is called *vasovagal syncope.* The arterial pressure falls instantly, which in turn reduces the blood flow to the brain and causes the person to lose consciousness. It is probable, therefore, that emotional fainting results from powerful stimulation of the anterior hypothalamic vasodilator center.

REFLEX CONTROL OF ARTERIAL PRESSURE

THE ARTERIAL BARORECEPTOR CONTROL SYSTEM—BARORECEPTOR REFLEXES

By far the best known of the mechanisms for arterial pressure control is the *baroreceptor reflex.* Basically, this reflex is initiated by stretch receptors, called either *baroreceptors* or *pressoreceptors,* located in the walls of the large systemic arteries. A rise in pressure stretches the baroreceptors and causes them to transmit signals into the central nervous system, and "feedback" signals are then sent back through the autonomic nervous system to the circulation to reduce arterial pressure downward toward the normal level.

Physiologic Anatomy of the Baroreceptors, and Their Innervation. Baroreceptors are spray-type nerve endings lying in the walls of the arteries; they are stimulated when stretched. A few baroreceptors are located in the wall of almost every large artery of the thoracic and neck regions; but, as illustrated in Figure 27–5, baroreceptors are extremely abundant in the wall of each internal carotid artery

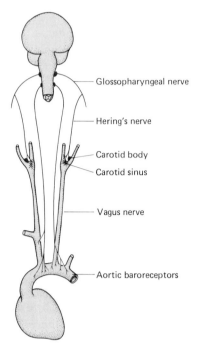

Figure 27–5. The baroreceptor system.

slightly above the carotid bifurcation, an area known as the *carotid sinus,* and in the wall of the aortic arch.

Figure 27–5 also shows that signals are transmitted from each carotid sinus through the very small *Hering's nerve* to the glossopharyngeal nerve and thence to the *tractus solitarius* in the medullary area of the brain stem. Signals from the arch of the aorta are transmitted through the vagus nerves also into this area of the medulla. Hering's nerve is especially important in physiologic experiments because baroreceptor impulses can be recorded from it with ease.

Response of the Baroreceptors to Pressure. Figure 27–6 illustrates the effect of different arterial pressures on the rate of impulse transmission in a Hering's nerve. Note that the carotid sinus baroreceptors are not stimulated at all by pressures between 0 and 60 mm Hg, but above 60 mm Hg they respond progressively more and more rapidly and reach a maximum at about 180 mm Hg. The responses of the aortic baroreceptors are similar to those of the carotid receptors, except that they respond, in general, at pressure levels about 30 mm Hg higher.

Note especially that the increase in number of impulses for each unit change in arterial pressure, expressed as $\Delta I/\Delta P$ in the figure, is greatest at a pressure level near the normal mean arterial pressure. That is, in the normal operating range of arterial pressure, even a slight change in pressure causes strong autonomic reflexes to readjust the arterial pressure back toward normal. Thus, the baroreceptor feedback mechanism functions most effectively in the very pressure range where it is most needed.

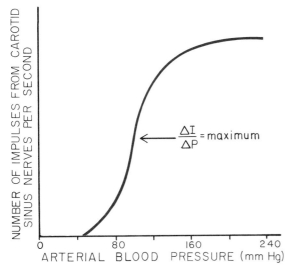

Figure 27-6. Response of the baroreceptors at different levels of arterial pressure.

The baroreceptors respond extremely rapidly to changes in arterial pressure; in fact, the rate of impulse firing increases during systole and decreases again during diastole. Furthermore, the baroreceptors *respond much more to a rapidly changing pressure* than to a stationary pressure. That is, if the mean arterial pressure is 150 mm Hg but at that moment is rising rapidly, the rate of impulse transmission may be as much as twice that when the pressure is stationary at 150 mm Hg. On the other hand, if the pressure is falling, the rate might be as little as one quarter that for the stationary pressure.

The Reflex Initiated by the Baroreceptors. After the baroreceptor signals have entered the tractus solitarius of the medulla, secondary signals *inhibit the vasoconstrictor center* of the medulla and *excite the vagal center*. The net effects are (1) *vasodilatation* throughout the peripheral circulatory system, and (2) *decreased heart rate* and *strength of heart contraction*. Therefore, excitation of the baroreceptors by pressure in the arteries reflexly *causes the arterial pressure to decrease* because of both a decrease in peripheral resistance and a decrease in cardiac output. Conversely, low pressure has opposite effects, reflexly causing the pressure to rise back toward normal.

Figure 27-7 illustrates a typical reflex change in arterial pressure caused by occluding the common carotid arteries. This reduces the carotid sinus pressure; as a result, the baroreceptors become inactive and lose their inhibitory effect on the vasomotor center. The vasomotor center then becomes much more active than usual, causing the arterial pressure to rise and to remain elevated during the ten minutes that the carotids are occluded. Removal of the occlusion allows the pressure to fall immediately to slightly below normal as a momentary overcompensation and then to return to normal in another minute or so.

Function of the Baroreceptors During Changes in Body Posture. The ability of the baroreceptors to maintain relatively constant arterial pressure is extremely important when a person sits or stands after having been lying down. Immediately upon standing, the arterial pressure in the head and upper part of the body obviously tends to fall, and marked reduction of this pressure can cause loss of consciousness. Fortunately, however, the falling pressure at the baroreceptors elicits an immediate reflex, resulting in strong sympathetic discharge throughout the body, and this minimizes the decrease in pressure in the head and upper body.

The "Buffer" Function of the Baroreceptor Control System. Because the baroreceptor system opposes increases and decreases in arterial pressure, it is often called a *pressure buffer system*, and the nerves from the baroreceptors are called *buffer nerves*.

Figure 27-8 illustrates the importance of this buffer function of the baroreceptors. The upper record in this figure shows an arterial pressure recording for two hours from a normal dog and the lower record from a dog whose baroreceptor nerves from both the carotid sinuses and the aorta had previously been removed. Note the extreme variability of pressure in the denervated dog caused by simple events of the day such as lying down, standing, excitement, eating, defecation, noises, and so forth.

Thus, one can see the extreme variability of pressure in the absence of the arterial baroreceptor system.

In summary, we can state that the primary purpose of the arterial baroreceptor system is to reduce the daily variation in arterial pressure to about one half to one third of that which would occur were the baroreceptor system not present.

Unimportance of the Baroreceptor System for Long-Term Regulation of Arterial Pressure—Adaptation of the Baroreceptors. The baroreceptor control system is probably of little or no importance in long-term regulation of arterial pressure for a very simple reason: The baroreceptors themselves adapt in one to two days to whatever pressure level they are exposed to. That is, if the pressure rises

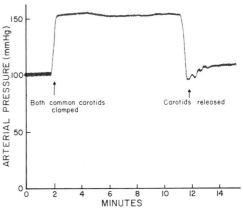

Figure 27-7. Typical carotid sinus reflex effect on arterial pressure caused by clamping both common carotids (after the two vagus nerves have been cut).

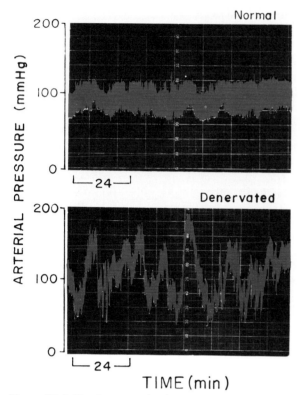

Figure 27–8. Two-hour records of arterial pressure in a normal dog (above) and in the same dog (below) several weeks after the baroreceptors had been denervated. (From Cowley, Liard, and Guyton: *Circ. Res.*, 32:564, 1973. By permission of the American Heart Association, Inc.)

from the normal value of 100 mm Hg to 200 mm Hg, extreme numbers of baroreceptor impulses are at first transmitted. During the next few seconds, the rate of firing diminishes considerably; then it diminishes very slowly during the next one to two days, at the end of which time the rate will have returned essentially to the normal level despite the fact that the arterial pressure remains 200 mm Hg. Conversely, when the arterial pressure falls to a very low value, the baroreceptors at first transmit no impulses at all, but gradually over a day or days the rate of baroreceptor firing returns again to the original control level.

This adaptation of the baroreceptors obviously prevents the baroreceptor reflex from functioning as a control system to buffer arterial pressure changes that last longer than a few days at a time. In fact, referring again to Figure 27–8, one can see that the average arterial pressure over any prolonged period of time is almost exactly the same whether the baroreceptors are present or not. This illustrates the *unimportance of the baroreceptor system for long-term regulation of the arterial pressure* even though it is a potent mechanism for preventing the rapid changes of arterial pressure that occur moment by moment or hour by hour. Instead, prolonged regulation of arterial pressure requires other control systems, principally the renal-body fluid-pressure control system (along with its associated hormonal mechanisms).

THE CNS ISCHEMIC RESPONSE— CONTROL OF ARTERIAL PRESSURE BY THE VASOMOTOR CENTER IN RESPONSE TO DIMINISHED BRAIN BLOOD FLOW

Normally, most nervous control of blood pressure is achieved by reflexes originating in the baroreceptors, the chemoreceptors, and the low pressure receptors, all of which are located in the peripheral circulation outside the brain. However, when blood flow to the vasomotor center in the lower brain stem becomes decreased enough to cause nutritional deficiency, a condition called *ischemia*, the neurons in the vasomotor center itself respond directly to the ischemia and become strongly excited. When this occurs, the systemic arterial pressure often rises to a level as high as the heart can possibly pump. This effect is believed to be caused by failure of the slowly flowing blood to carry carbon dioxide away from the vasomotor center; the local concentration of carbon dioxide then increases greatly and has an extremely potent effect in stimulating the sympathetic nervous system. It is possible that other factors, such as the buildup of lactic acid and other acidic substances, also contribute to the marked stimulation of the vasomotor center and to the elevation in pressure. This arterial pressure elevation in response to cerebral ischemia is known as the *central nervous system ischemic response* or simply *CNS ischemic response*.

The magnitude of the ischemic effect on vasomotor activity is tremendous; it can elevate the mean arterial pressure for as long as ten minutes sometimes to as high as 270 mm Hg. *The degree of sympathetic vasoconstriction caused by intense cerebral ischemia is often so great that some of the peripheral vessels become totally or almost totally occluded.* The kidneys, for instance, will entirely cease their production of urine because of arteriolar constriction in response to the sympathetic discharge. Therefore, *the CNS ischemic response is one of the most powerful of all the activators of the sympathetic vasoconstrictor system.*

Importance of the CNS Ischemic Response as a Regulator of Arterial Pressure. Despite the extremely powerful nature of the CNS ischemic response, it does not become very active until the arterial pressure falls far below normal, down to 60 mm Hg and below, reaching its greatest degree of stimulation at a pressure of 15 to 20 mm Hg. Therefore, it is not one of the mechanisms for regulating normal arterial pressure. Instead, it operates principally as an *emergency arterial pressure control system that acts rapidly and extremely powerfully to prevent further decrease in arterial pressure whenever blood flow to the brain decreases dangerously close to the lethal level.* It is sometimes called the "last ditch stand" pressure control mechanism.

NERVOUS CONTROL OF BODY WATER AND BODY FLUID OSMOLALITY

Another important function of the nervous system in controlling the overall environment of the body is its capability to control the amount of water in the body. This is achieved by two separate centers located in the anterior and lateral hypothalamus: (1) A center for controlling the rate of excretion of water by the kidneys and (2) a center for controlling the rate of intake of water by mouth. The first of these centers is called the *antidiuretic center* because it controls the secretion of the hormone *antidiuretic hormone*, which in turn acts on the kidneys to reduce water excretion, thus retaining water in the body. The second of these centers is the *thirst* center, which controls one's drive to drink liquids.

At the same time that the nervous system controls total body water, it also controls the concentration of the dissolved constituents in both the extracellular and intracellular fluid. The normal concentration of these fluids is about 300 mOsm of solute in each liter of fluid. In the extracellular fluid, almost half of these milliosmoles are comprised of sodium ions, and most of the remaining one half are negative ions that balance the sodium ions. Therefore, the total osmolality of the fluids is mainly determined either directly or indirectly by the sodium concentration itself.

The basic stimulus to the receptors in both the antidiuretic center and the thirst center is the osmolality of the extracellular fluid, but since this is determined almost entirely by the sodium ion concentration, these receptors are in effect sodium receptors as well and can be called either *osmoreceptors* or *osmosodium receptors*. When the osmolality of the extracellular fluid becomes too great, this activates the antidiuretic system to retain water and the thirst system to increase water intake, thus diluting the fluids and correcting the hyperosmotic state. Conversely, a hypo-osmotic state inactivates the antidiuretic mechanism as well as thirst, so that excessive amounts of water are now excreted in the urine and at the same time the person drinks little if any water, until the hypo-osmotic state is corrected. In the following sections we will explain these two nervous mechanisms for body water control.

THE OSMOSODIUM RECEPTOR–ANTIDIURETIC HORMONE FEEDBACK CONTROL SYSTEM

Figure 27–9 illustrates the osmosodium receptor–antidiuretic hormone system for control of ex-

tracellular fluid sodium concentration and osmolality. It is a typical feedback control system that operates by the following steps: (1) An increase in osmolality (mainly excess sodium and the negative ions that go with it) excites *osmoreceptors* located in the supraoptic nuclei of the hypothalamus. (2) Excitation of the supraoptic nuclei causes the posterior pituitary gland to release *antidiuretic hormone*. (3) The antidiuretic hormone increases the permeability of the late distal tubules, the collecting tubules, and the collecting ducts, as explained in the previous chapter, and therefore *causes increased conservation of water by the kidneys.* (4) The conservation of water but *loss of sodium and other osmolar substances in the urine* causes dilution of the sodium and other substances in the extracellular fluid, thus correcting the initial, excessively concentrated extracellular fluid.

Conversely, when the extracellular fluid becomes too dilute (hypo-osmotic), less antidiuretic hormone is formed, and excess water is lost in comparison with the extracellular fluid solutes, thus concentrating the body fluids back toward normal.

The Osmoreceptors (or Osmosodium Receptors). Located in the supraoptic nuclei of the anterior hypothalamus, shown in Figure 27–10, are specialized neuronal cells called *osmoreceptors*. These respond to changes in osmolality of the extracellular fluid. When the osmolality of the extracellular fluid becomes low, osmosis of water occurs into the osmoreceptors, causing them to swell. This decreases their rate of impulse discharge. Conversely, increased osmolality in the extracellular fluid pulls water out of the osmoreceptors, causing them to shrink and thereby to increase their rate of discharge.

The osmoreceptors respond to changes in extracellular fluid sodium concentration but very little to changes in potassium concentration and only slightly to changes in urea and glucose concentrations. Therefore, it must be emphasized again that, for all practical purposes, *the osmoreceptors are actually sodium concentration receptors*—hence the name *osmosodium receptors.*

The impulses from the osmoreceptors are trans-

Figure 27–9. Control of extracellular fluid osmolality and sodium ion concentration by the osmosodium receptor-antidiuretic hormone feedback control system.

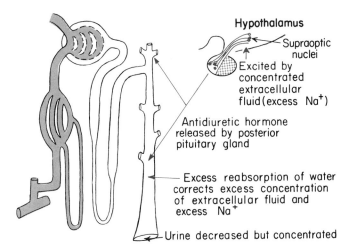

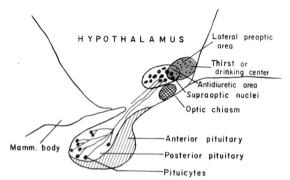

Figure 27–10. The supraopticopituitary antidiuretic system and its relationship to the thirst center in the hypothalamus.

mitted from the supraoptic nuclei through the pituitary stalk into the posterior pituitary gland where they promote the release of antidiuretic hormone (ADH). Signals from the volume receptors in the heart as well as from the baroreceptors also help to control antidiuretic hormone secretion; this is in addition to the effect of changes in extracellular fluid osmolality in controlling its secretion. Figure 27–11 illustrates quantitatively the effects of these two separate stimuli on the concentration of ADH ("arginine vasopressin") in the plasma. The open circles show the effect of plasma osmolality, illustrating that an increase in plasma osmolality of about 6 per cent will increase the plasma ADH concentration to 10 to 20 times normal. The effect of decreased blood volume is illustrated by the solid circles, showing that relatively little increase in antidiuretic hormone concentration occurs until the blood volume is decreased more than 5 to 10 per cent. Since this much decrease occurs only when a

person bleeds severely, one can see that normally antidiuretic hormone secretion is controlled almost entirely by the changes in plasma osmolality.

Summary of the Antidiuretic Hormone Mechanism for Controlling Extracellular Fluid Osmolality and Extracellular Fluid Sodium Concentration. From these discussions, we can reiterate once again the importance of the antidiuretic hormone mechanism for controlling at the same time both extracellular fluid osmolality and extracellular fluid sodium concentration. That is, an increase in sodium concentration causes almost an exactly parallel increase in osmolality, which in turn excites the osmoreceptors of the hypothalamus. These receptors then cause the secretion of antidiuretic hormone, which markedly increases the reabsorption of water in the renal tubules. Consequently, very little water is lost into the urine, but the urinary solutes continue to be lost. Therefore, the relative proportion of water in the extracellular fluid increases, whereas the proportion of solutes decreases. In this way, the sodium ion concentration of the extracellular fluid, and the osmolality as well, decrease toward the normal level. This is a very powerful mechanism for controlling both the extracellular fluid osmolality and the extracellular fluid sodium concentration.

THIRST AND ITS ROLE IN CONTROLLING SODIUM CONCENTRATION AND EXTRACELLULAR FLUID OSMOLALITY

The phenomenon of thirst is equally as important for regulating body water, sodium concentration, and osmolality as is the osmoreceptor-renal mechanism discussed above, because the amount of water in the body at any one time is determined by the balance between both *intake* and *output* of water. Thirst, the primary regulator of the intake of water, is defined as the *conscious desire for water*.

Neural Integration of Thirst— The "Thirst" Center

Referring again to Figure 27–10, one sees a small area located slightly anterior to the supraoptic nuclei in the lateral preoptic area of the hypothalamus, which is called the *thirst center*. Electrical stimulation of this center by implanted electrodes causes an animal to begin drinking within seconds and to continue drinking until the electrical stimulus is stopped. Also, injection of hypertonic salt solutions into the area, which causes osmosis of water out of the neuronal cells, thus shrinking the cells, also causes drinking. Thus, the neuronal cells of the thirst center function in almost the same way as the osmoreceptors of the supraoptic nuclei.

An increase in osmotic pressure of the cerebrospinal fluid in the third ventricle has essentially the same effect of promoting thirst as an increase in the osmotic pressure of the circulating extracellular fluid. Therefore, it has been suggested that the

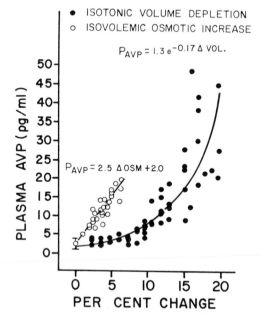

Figure 27–11. Effect of changes in plasma osmolality or blood volume on the level of plasma ADH (arginine vasopressin-AVP). (From Dunn, et al.: *J. Clin. Invest.*, 52:3212, 1973.)

primary site for detecting changes in osmolality might be at the surface of the third ventricle and that appropriate signals are then transmitted to the thirst center to cause drinking. However, the importance of this is still debated.

Basic Stimulus for Exciting the Thirst Center— Intracellular Dehydration. Any factor that will cause *intracellular dehydration* will in general cause the sensation of thirst. The most common cause of this is increased osmolar concentration of the extracellular fluid, especially increased sodium concentration, which causes osmosis of fluid from the neuronal cells of the thirst center. However, another important cause is excessive loss of potassium from the body, which reduces the intracellular potassium of the thirst cells and therefore decreases their volume.

Temporary Relief of Thirst Caused by the Act of Drinking

A thirsty person receives relief from thirst immediately after drinking water, even before the water has been absorbed from the gastrointestinal tract. In fact, in persons who have an esophageal opening to the exterior so that the water is lost to the outside and never goes into the gastrointestinal tract, partial relief of thirst still occurs following the act of drinking, but this relief is only temporary, and the thirst returns after 15 or more minutes. If the water does enter the stomach, distension of the stomach and other portions of the upper gastrointestinal tract provides still further temporary relief from thirst. For instance, simple inflation of a balloon in the stomach can relieve thirst for 5 to 30 minutes.

One might wonder what the value of this temporary relief from thirst could be, but there is good reason for its occurrence. After a person has drunk water, as long as one half to one hour may be required for all the water to be absorbed and distributed throughout the body. Were the thirst sensation not temporarily relieved after drinking water, the person would continue to drink more and more. When all this water should finally become absorbed, the body fluids would be far more diluted than normal, and an abnormal condition opposite to that which the person was attempting to correct would have been created. It is well known that a thirsty animal almost never drinks more than the amount of water needed to relieve its state of dehydration. Indeed, it is uncanny that the animal usually drinks almost exactly the right amount.

Role of Thirst in Controlling Extracellular Fluid Osmolality and Sodium Concentration

Threshold for Drinking—The Tripping Mechanism. The kidneys are continually excreting fluid; also water is lost by evaporation from the skin and lungs. Therefore, a person is continually being dehydrated, causing the volume of extracellular fluid to decrease and its concentration of sodium and other osmolar elements to rise. When the sodium concentration rises approximately 2 mEq/liter above normal (or the osmolality rises approximately 4 mOsm/liter above normal) the drinking mechanism becomes "tripped"; that is, the person then reaches a level of thirst that is strong enough to activate the necessary motor effort to cause drinking. This is called the *threshold for drinking*. The person ordinarily drinks precisely the required amount of fluid to bring the extracellular fluids back to normal—that is, to a state of *satiety*. Then the process of dehydration and sodium concentration begins again, and after a period of time the drinking act is tripped again, the process continuing on and on indefinitely.

In this way, both the sodium concentration and the osmolality of the extracellular fluid are very precisely controlled.

COMBINED ROLES OF THE ANTIDIURETIC AND THIRST MECHANISMS FOR CONTROL OF EXTRACELLULAR FLUID SODIUM CONCENTRATION AND OSMOLALITY

When either the antidiuretic hormone mechanism or the thirst mechanism fails, the other ordinarily can still control both sodium concentration and extracellular fluid osmolality with reasonable effectiveness. On the other hand, if both of them fail simultaneously, neither sodium nor osmolality is then adequately controlled.

Figure 27–12 illustrates dramatically the overall

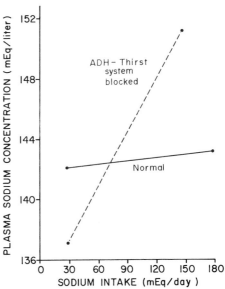

Figure 27–12. Effect on the extracellular fluid sodium concentration in dogs caused by tremendous changes in sodium intake (1) under normal conditions, and (2) after the antidiuretic hormone and thirst feedback systems had been blocked. This figure shows lack of sodium ion control in the absence of these systems. (Courtesy of Dr. David B. Young.)

capability of the ADH-thirst system to control extracellular fluid sodium concentration. This figure demonstrates the ability of the same animal to control its extracellular fluid sodium concentration in two different conditions: (1) in the normal state, and (2) after both the antidiuretic hormone and thirst mechanisms had been blocked. Note that in the normal animal (the solid curve) a sixfold increase in sodium intake caused the sodium concentration to change only two thirds of 1 per cent (from 142 mEq/liter to 143 mEq/liter)—an excellent degree of sodium concentration control. Now note the dashed curve of the figure, which shows the change in sodium concentration when the ADH-thirst system was blocked. In this case, the sodium concentration increased 10 per cent with only a fivefold increase in sodium intake (a change in sodium concentration from 137 mEq/liter to 151 mEq/liter), which is an extreme change in sodium concentration when one realizes that the normal sodium concentration rarely rises or falls more than 1 per cent from day to day.

Therefore, the major feedback mechanism for control of sodium concentration (and also for extracellular osmolality) is the ADH-thirst mechanism. In the absence of this mechanism there is no feedback mechanism that will cause the body to increase water ingestion or water conservation by the kidneys when excess sodium enters the body. Therefore, the sodium concentration simply increases.

REGULATION OF RESPIRATION

The nervous system adjusts the rate of alveolar ventilation almost exactly to the demands of the body so that the blood oxygen pressure (Po_2) and carbon dioxide pressure (Pco_2) are hardly altered even during strenuous exercise or other types of respiratory stress.

This section describes the operation of this neurogenic system for regulation of respiration.

THE RESPIRATORY CENTER

The "respiratory center" is composed of several widely dispersed groups of neurons located *bilaterally* in the medulla oblongata and pons, as illustrated in Figure 27–13. It is divided into three major collections of neurons: (1) a *dorsal respiratory group*, located in the dorsal portion of the medulla, which mainly causes inspiration, (2) a *ventral respiratory group*, located in the ventrolateral part of the medulla, which can cause either expiration or inspiration depending upon which neurons in the group are stimulated, and (3) the *pneumotaxic center*, located dorsally in the superior portion of the pons, which helps control both the rate and pattern of breathing. The dorsal respiratory group of neurons plays the fundamental role in the control of respiration. Therefore, let us discuss its function first.

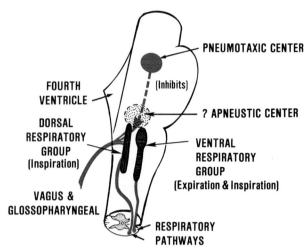

Figure 27–13. Organization of the respiratory center.

The Dorsal Respiratory Group of Neurons

The dorsal respiratory group of neurons extends approximately the entire length of the medulla. Either all or most of its neurons are located within the *nucleus of the tractus solitarius,* though additional neurons in the adjacent reticular substance of the medulla probably also play important roles in respiratory control. The nucleus of the tractus solitarius is also the sensory termination of both the vagal and glossopharyngeal nerves, which transmit sensory signals into the respiratory center from the peripheral chemoreceptors, the baroreceptors, and several different types of receptors in the lung. All the signals from these peripheral areas help in the control of respiration, as we shall discuss in subsequent sections of this chapter.

The Inspiratory Function of the Dorsal Respiratory Group of Neurons. Stimulation of the neurons in the dorsal respiratory group always causes inspiration, never expiration. However, it will be recalled that normal quiet respiration is caused almost entirely, if not entirely, by contraction of the inspiratory muscles. Then expiration is caused passively by elastic recoil of the distended chest and lungs.

Rhythmical Inspiratory Discharges from the Dorsal Respiratory Group. The basic rhythm of respiration is generated in the dorsal respiratory group of neurons. Even when all the peripheral nerves entering the medulla are sectioned and also the brain stem is transected both above and below the medulla, this group of neurons still emits repetitive bursts of inspiratory action potentials. Unfortunately, though, the basic cause of these repetitive discharges is still unknown. In primitive animals, neural networks have been found in which activity of one set of neurons excites a second set, which in turn inhibits the first. Then after a period of time the mechanism repeats itself, continuing throughout the life of the animal. Therefore, most respiratory physiologists believe that some similar network of neurons located within the medulla, probably involving not only the dorsal respiratory group but adjacent areas of the medulla as well, is responsible for the basic rhythm of respiration.

The Inspiratory "Ramp" Signal. The nervous signal that is transmitted to the inspiratory muscles is not an instantaneous burst of action potentials. Instead, in normal respiration, it begins very weakly at first and increases steadily in a ramp fashion for about 2 seconds. Then, it abruptly ceases for approximately the next 3 seconds, then begins again for still another cycle, and again and again. Thus, the inspiratory signal is said to be a *ramp signal.* The obvious advantage of this is that it causes a steady increase in the volume of the lungs during inspiration, rather than inspiratory gasps.

There are two ways in which the inspiratory ramp is controlled:

1. Control of the rate of increase of the ramp signal, so that during very active respiration the ramp increases rapidly and therefore fills the lungs rapidly as well.

2. Control of the limiting point at which the ramp suddenly ceases. This is the usual method for controlling the rate of respiration; that is, the earlier the ramp ceases, the shorter the duration of inspiration, and for reasons not presently understood this also shortens the duration of expiration. Thus, the rate of respiration is increased.

The Pneumotaxic Center—Its Function in Limiting the Duration of Inspiration and Increasing Respiratory Rate

The pneumotaxic center, located dorsally in the *nucleus parabrachialis* of the upper pons, transmits impulses continuously to the inspiratory area. The primary effect of these is to control the "switch-off" point of the inspiratory ramp, thus controlling the duration of the filling phase of the lung cycle. When the pneumotaxic signals are strong, inspiration might last for as little as 0.5 second, but when weak, the inspiratory ramp might continue to rise for perhaps as long as 5 to 10 seconds, thus filling the lungs with a great excess of air.

Therefore, the function of the pneumotaxic center is primarily to limit inspiration. However, this has a secondary effect on the rate of breathing because limitation of inspiration also shortens the entire period of respiration. Thus, a strong pneumotaxic signal can increase the rate of breathing up to 30 to 40 breaths per minute, whereas a weak pneumotaxic signal may reduce the rate to only a few breaths per minute.

Limitation of Inspiration by Lung Inflation Signals—The Hering-Breuer Inflation Reflex

Located in the walls of the bronchi and bronchioles throughout the lungs are *stretch receptors* that transmit signals through the *vagi* into the dorsal respiratory group of neurons when the lungs become overstretched. These signals affect inspiration in much the same way as signals from the pneumotaxic center; that is, they limit the duration of inspiration. Therefore, when the lungs become overly inflated, the stretch receptors activate an appropriate feedback response that "switches off" the inspiratory ramp and thus limits further inspiration. This is called the *Hering-Breuer inflation reflex.* This reflex also increases the rate of respiration because of the reduced period of inspiration, the same as is true for signals from the pneumotaxic center.

However, in human beings, the Hering-Breuer reflex probably is not activated until the tidal volume increases to greater than approximately 1.5 liters. Therefore, this reflex appears to be mainly a protective mechanism for preventing excess lung inflation rather than an important ingredient in the normal control of ventilation.

The Ventral Respiratory Group of Neurons—Its Function in Both Inspiration and Expiration

Located about 5 mm anterior and lateral to the dorsal respiratory group of neurons is still another group, the ventral respiratory group, that is important during more active breathing. These neurons, like the dorsal respiratory group, also are present in the entire length of the medulla and are found mainly in the *nucleus ambiguus* rostrally and the *nucleus retroambiguus* caudally. The function of this area differs from that of the dorsal respiratory group in several important ways:

1. The neurons of the ventral respiratory group remain almost totally inactive during normal, quiet respiration. Furthermore, there is no evidence that the ventral respiratory neurons participate in the basic rhythmic oscillation that controls respiration.

2. When the respiratory drive for increased pulmonary ventilation becomes greater than normal, respiratory signals then spill over into the ventral respiratory neurons from the basic oscillating mechanism of the dorsal respiratory area. As a consequence, the ventral respiratory area then contributes its share to the respiratory drive as well.

3. Electrical stimulation of some of the neurons in the ventral group causes inspiration whereas stimulation of others causes expiration. Therefore, these neurons contribute to both inspiration and expiration. However, they are especially important in providing the powerful expiratory forces during expiration. Thus, this area operates more or less as an overdrive mechanism when high levels of pulmonary ventilation are required.

Possibility of an "Apneustic Center" in the Lower Pons

To add to the confusion of our knowledge about respiratory center function, there is another strange center in the lower part of the pons, called the *apneustic center*. However, its function can be demonstrated only when the vagus nerves to the medulla have been sectioned and when the connections from the pneumotaxic center have also been blocked by transecting the pons in its midregion. Then the apneustic center of the lower pons sends signals to the dorsal respiratory group of neurons that prevent the "switch-off" of the inspiratory ramp signal. Therefore, the ramp continues for as long as 10 to 20 seconds, thus greatly overfilling the lungs. Consequently, the lungs become inflated near maximum, and only occasional short expiratory gasps occur.

The function of the apneustic center might be to provide extra drive to inspiration, but the pneumotaxic center and the stretch signals from the vagi normally override this excessive inspiratory drive and therefore allow normal respiration.

CONTROL OF OVERALL RESPIRATORY CENTER ACTIVITY

Up to this point we have discussed the basic mechanisms for causing inspiration and expiration, but it is also important to know how the overall level of respiratory center activity is controlled to match the ventilatory needs of the body. For example, during very heavy exercise, the rates of oxygen utilization and carbon dioxide formation are often increased to as much as 20 times normal, requiring commensurate increases in pulmonary ventilation. This is achieved in two different ways: (1) By feedback excitation of respiratory center activity in response to changes in chemical composition of the blood, especially its concentrations of carbon dioxide, hydrogen ions, and oxygen. (2) By excitatory signals from other parts of the nervous system; such signals are especially important during exercise.

The major purpose of the remainder of this chapter is to discuss this control of ventilation in response to the needs of the body.

CHEMICAL CONTROL OF RESPIRATION

The ultimate goal of respiration is to maintain proper concentrations of oxygen, carbon dioxide, and hydrogen ions in the body fluid. It is fortunate, therefore, that respiratory activity is highly responsive to changes in any one of these.

Excess carbon dioxide or hydrogen ions affect respiration mainly by excitatory effects on the respiratory center itself, causing greatly increased strength of both the inspiratory and expiratory signals to the respiratory muscles. The resulting increase in ventilation increases the elimination of carbon dioxide from the blood; this also removes

hydrogen ions from the blood because decreased carbon dioxide also decreases the blood carbonic acid.

Oxygen, on the other hand, does not have a significant *direct* effect on the respiratory center of the brain in controlling respiration. Instead, it acts either entirely or almost entirely on peripheral chemoreceptors located in the carotid and aortic bodies, and these in turn transmit appropriate nervous signals to the respiratory center for control of respiration.

Let us discuss first the stimulation of the respiratory center itself by carbon dioxide and hydrogen ions.

DIRECT CHEMICAL CONTROL OF RESPIRATORY CENTER ACTIVITY BY CARBON DIOXIDE AND HYDROGEN IONS

The Chemosensitive Area of the Respiratory Center. Thus far, we have discussed mainly three different areas of the respiratory center: the dorsal respiratory group of neurons, the ventral respiratory group, and the pneumotaxic center. However, it is believed that none of these are affected directly by changes in blood carbon dioxide concentration or hydrogen ion concentration. Instead, a very sensitive *chemosensitive* area, illustrated in Figure 27–14, is located bilaterally only a few microns beneath the surface of the medulla ventral to the entry of the glossopharyngeal and vagal nerves into the medulla. This area is highly sensitive to changes in either blood CO_2 or hydrogen ion concentration, and it in turn excites the other portions of the respiratory center. It has especially potent effects on increasing the degree of activity of the inspiratory center, increasing both the rate of rise of the inspiratory ramp signal and also the intensity of the

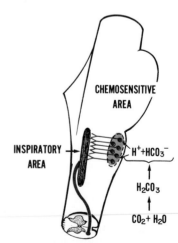

Figure 27–14. Stimulation of the inspiratory area by the *chemosensitive area* located bilaterally in the medulla, lying only a few microns beneath the ventral medullary surface. Note also that hydrogen ions stimulate the chemosensitive area, whereas mainly carbon dioxide in the fluid gives rise to the hydrogen ions.

signal. This in turn has an automatic secondary effect of increasing the frequency of the respiratory rhythm.

Response of the Chemosensitive Neurons to Hydrogen Ions—The Primary Stimulus

The sensor neurons in the chemosensitive area are especially excited by hydrogen ions; in fact, it is believed that hydrogen ions are perhaps the only important direct stimulus for these neurons. Unfortunately, though, hydrogen ions do not easily cross either the blood-brain barrier or the blood–cerebrospinal fluid barrier. For this reason, changes in hydrogen ion concentration in the blood actually have considerably less effect in stimulating the chemosensitive neurons than do changes in carbon dioxide, even though carbon dioxide stimulates these neurons indirectly, as will be explained below.

Effect of Blood Carbon Dioxide on Stimulating the Chemosensitive Area

Though carbon dioxide has very little direct effect in stimulating the neurons in the chemosensitive area, it does have a very potent indirect effect. It does this by reacting with the water of the tissues to form carbonic acid. This in turn dissociates into hydrogen and bicarbonate ions; the hydrogen ions then have a potent direct stimulatory effect. These effects are illustrated in Figure 27–14.

But, why is it that blood CO_2 has a more potent effect to stimulate the chemosensitive neurons than do blood hydrogen ions? The answer is that hydrogen ions, as noted above, pass through both the blood-brain barrier and the blood-cerebrospinal fluid barrier only very poorly whereas carbon dioxide passes through both these barriers almost as if they did not exist. Consequently, whenever the blood carbon dioxide concentration increases, so also does the P_{CO_2} in both the interstitial fluid of the medulla and also in the cerebrospinal fluid. And, in both of these fluids the carbon dioxide immediately reacts with the water to form hydrogen ions. Thus, paradoxically, more hydrogen ions are released into the respiratory chemosensitive sensory area when the blood carbon dioxide concentration increases than when the blood hydrogen ion concentration increases. For this reason, respiratory center activity is affected considerably more by changes in blood carbon dioxide than by changes in blood hydrogen ions, a fact that we will subsequently discuss quantitatively.

Decrease in the Effect of Blood CO_2 on Respiratory Activity in One to Two Days. The stimulatory effect of increased carbon dioxide on respiration reaches its peak within a few minutes after an increase in blood P_{CO_2}. Thereafter, the stimulation gradually declines for the next one to two days to as little as one fifth the initial effect. The cause of this decreasing stimulation is not known, but one

suggestion is that it results from readjustment of the bicarbonate ion concentration in the respiratory center or in the cerebrospinal fluid or both. The bicarbonate ions in turn would combine with the excess hydrogen ions, thus reducing the hydrogen ion concentration and simultaneously reducing the respiratory drive.

Therefore, a change in blood carbon dioxide concentration has a very potent *acute* effect on controlling respiration but only a weak *chronic* effect after a few days' adaptation.

Quantitative Effects of Blood P_{CO_2} and Hydrogen Ion Concentration on Alveolar Ventilation

Figure 27–15 illustrates quantitatively the approximate effects of blood P_{CO_2} and blood pH (which is an inverse measure of hydrogen ion concentration) on alveolar ventilation. Note the marked increase in ventilation caused by the increase in P_{CO_2}. But note also the much smaller effect of increased hydrogen ion concentration (that is, decreased pH).

Finally, note that this *difference* in stimulation of ventilation is especially great in the normal P_{CO_2} and pH ranges: P_{CO_2}s between 30 and 50 mm Hg and pHs between 7.5 and 7.3. Therefore, from a practical point, changes in blood carbon dioxide play by far the greater role in the normal minute-by-minute control of pulmonary ventilation.

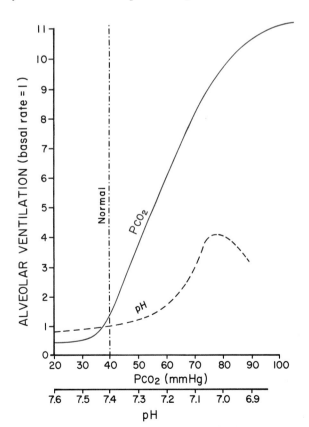

Figure 27–15. Effects of increased arterial P_{CO_2} and decreased arterial pH on the rate of alveolar ventilation.

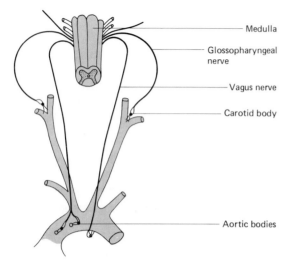

Figure 27–16. Respiratory control by the carotid and aortic bodies.

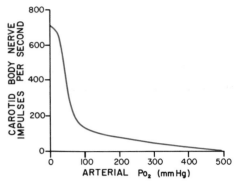

Figure 27–17. Effect of arterial P_{O_2} on impulse rate from the carotid body of a cat. (Curve drawn from data from several sources, but primarily from Von Euler.)

Value of Carbon Dioxide as a Regulator of Alveolar Ventilation. Since carbon dioxide is one of the end-products of metabolism, its concentration in the body fluids greatly affects the chemical reactions of the cells and also affects the tissue pH. For these reasons, the tissue fluid P_{CO_2} must be regulated exactly, and the respiratory system is the only effective means that the body has to control the blood and tissue P_{CO_2}. Therefore, stimulation of the respiratory center by carbon dioxide provides the necessary feedback mechanism for regulation of the concentration of carbon dioxide throughout the body. That is, an increase in respiratory center P_{CO_2} causes the respiratory system to eliminate the excess carbon dioxide. Thus, the respiratory center maintains the P_{CO_2} of the tissue fluids at a relatively constant level and, therefore, might well be called a "carbon dioxide pressostat."

THE PERIPHERAL CHEMORECEPTOR SYSTEM FOR CONTROL OF RESPIRATORY ACTIVITY—ROLE OF OXYGEN IN RESPIRATORY CONTROL

Aside from the direct sensitivity of the respiratory center itself to CO_2 and hydrogen ions, special chemical receptors called *chemoreceptors,* located outside the central nervous system, are also responsive to changes in oxygen, carbon dioxide, and hydrogen ion concentrations. These transmit signals to the respiratory center to help regulate respiratory activity.

The chemoreceptors are located in the *carotid* and *aortic bodies,* which are illustrated in Figure 27–16 along with their afferent nerve connections to the respiratory center. The *carotid bodies* are located bilaterally in the bifurcations of the common carotid arteries, and their afferent nerve fibers pass through

Hering's nerves to the *glossopharyngeal nerves* and thence to the dorsal respiratory area of the medulla. The *aortic bodies* are located along the arch of the aorta; their afferent nerve fibers pass through the *vagi* to the dorsal respiratory area. Each of these chemoreceptor bodies receives a special blood supply through a minute artery directly from the adjacent arterial trunk.

Stimulation of the Chemoreceptors by Decreased Arterial Oxygen. Changes in arterial oxygen concentration have *no* direct stimulatory effect on the respiratory center itself, but when the oxygen concentration in the arterial blood falls below normal, the chemoreceptors become strongly stimulated. This effect is illustrated in Figure 27–17, which shows the relationship between *arterial* P_{O_2} and rate of nerve impulse transmission from a carotid body. Note that the impulse rate is particularly sensitive to changes in arterial P_{O_2} in the range between 60 and 30 mm Hg, which is the range in which the arterial hemoglobin saturation with oxygen decreases rapidly.

Quantitative Effect of Low Blood P_{O_2} on Alveolar Ventilation

Low blood P_{O_2} normally will not increase alveolar ventilation significantly until the alveolar P_{O_2} falls almost to one half normal. This is illustrated in Figure 27–18. The lowermost curve of this figure shows that changing the alveolar arterial P_{O_2} from

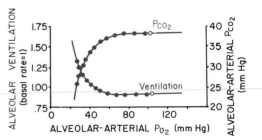

Figure 27–18. Effect of arterial P_{O_2} on alveolar ventilation and on the subsequent decrease in arterial P_{CO_2}. (From Gray: Pulmonary Ventilation and Its Physiological Regulation. Charles C Thomas.)

the normal value of slightly more than 100 mm Hg down to about 60 mm Hg has an imperceptible effect on ventilation. But, then, as the P_{O_2} falls still further, down to 40 and then to 30 mm Hg, alveolar ventilation increases 1.5– to 1.7-fold. However, contrast this rather feeble increase in alveolar ventilation to the fourfold increase caused by decreasing blood pH or the elevenfold increase caused by increasing the P_{CO_2}. Thus, it is clear that the normal effect of changes in blood P_{O_2} on respiratory activity is very slight, especially when compared with the effect of P_{CO_2}.

Cause of the Poor Response of Respiration to Low P_{O_2}—The Opposing Effects of the P_{CO_2} and pH Regulatory Mechanisms. The cause of the poor effect of P_{O_2} changes on respiratory control is *opposition* caused by *both* the carbon dioxide and the hydrogen ion control mechanisms. This phenomenon can be explained by referring again to Figure 27–18. The increase in ventilation that does occur when the P_{O_2} falls expels carbon dioxide from the blood and therefore decreases the P_{CO_2}, which is also illustrated in the figure; at the same time it also decreases the hydrogen ion concentration. Therefore, two powerful respiratory inhibitory effects are caused: (1) diminished carbon dioxide and (2) diminished hydrogen ions. These two exert inhibitory effects that oppose the excitatory effect of the diminished oxygen. As a result, they keep the decreased oxygen from causing a marked increase in ventilation until the P_{O_2} falls to 20 to 40 mm Hg, a range that is incompatible with life for more than a few minutes. Therefore, the maximum effect of decreased alveolar oxygen on alveolar ventilation, in the range compatible with life, is normally only about a 66 per cent increase.

Thus, one can see that during normal respiration the P_{CO_2} and pH feedback control mechanisms are extremely powerful in relation to the P_{O_2} feedback control. Indeed, under normal conditions the P_{O_2} mechanism is of almost no significance in the control of respiration.

Yet, under some abnormal conditions the P_{CO_2} and hydrogen ion concentrations *increase at the same time that the arterial P_{O_2} decreases.* Under these conditions, all three of the feedback mechanisms support each other, and the P_{O_2} mechanism then exerts its full share of respiratory stimulation, sometimes becoming even more potent as a controller of respiration than the P_{CO_2} and hydrogen ion mechanisms.

Effects of the Oxygen-Lack Mechanism at High Altitudes. When a person first ascends to high altitudes (or in any other way is exposed to a rarefied atmosphere), the diminished oxygen in the air stimulates the oxygen lack control system of respiration. The respiration at first increases to a maximum of about two thirds above normal, which is a comparatively slight increase. Once again, the cause of this slight increase is the tremendous opposition effects of the carbon dioxide and hydrogen ion control mechanisms on the oxygen lack mechanism.

However, over several days, the respiratory center gradually becomes "adapted" to the diminished carbon dioxide, as explained earlier in the chapter, so that its opposition effect to the oxygen control is gradually lost, and alveolar ventilation then rises to as high as five to seven times normal. This is part of the acclimatization that occurs as a person slowly ascends a mountain, thus allowing the person to adjust respiration gradually to a level fitted for the higher altitude.

REGULATION OF RESPIRATION DURING EXERCISE

In strenuous exercise, oxygen utilization and carbon dioxide formation can increase as much as twentyfold. Yet, alveolar ventilation ordinarily increases almost exactly in step with the increased level of metabolism, as illustrated in Figure 27–19. Therefore, the blood P_{O_2}, P_{CO_2}, and pH all remain *almost exactly normal.*

In trying to analyze the factors that cause increased ventilation during exercise, one is tempted immediately to ascribe this increase to the chemical alterations in the body fluids during exercise, including increase of carbon dioxide, increase of hydrogen ions, and decrease of oxygen. However, this is not valid, for measurements of arterial P_{CO_2}, pH, and P_{O_2} show that none of these usually changes significantly and certainly not enough to account for more than a small percentage of the increase in ventilation. Indeed, even if a very high P_{CO_2} should develop during exercise, this still would be sufficient to account for only two thirds of the increased ventilation of heavy muscular exercise, for, as shown in Figure 27–20, the minute respiratory volume in exercise is about 50 per cent greater than that which can be effected by maximal carbon dioxide stimulation.

Therefore, the question must be asked: What is it during exercise that causes the intense ventila-

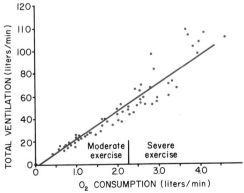

Figure 27–19. Effect of exercise on oxygen consumption and ventilatory rate. (From Gray: Pulmonary Ventilation and Its Physiological Regulation. Charles C Thomas.)

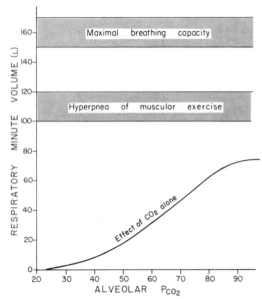

Figure 27–20. Relationship of hyperpnea caused by muscular exercise to that caused by increased alveolar P_{CO_2}. (Modified from Comroe: The Lung: Clinical Physiology and Pulmonary Function Tests. Chicago, Year Book Medical Publishers.)

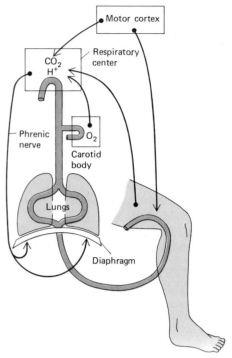

Figure 27–21. The different factors that enter into regulation of respiration during exercise.

tion? This question has not been definitively answered, but at least two different effects seem to be predominantly concerned:

1. The brain, on transmitting impulses to the contracting muscles, is believed to transmit collateral impulses into the brain stem to excite the respiratory center. This is analogous to the stimulatory effect of the higher centers of the brain on the vasomotor center of the brain stem during exercise, causing a rise in arterial pressure as well as an increase in ventilation.

2. During exercise, the body movements, especially of the limbs, are believed to increase pulmonary ventilation by exciting joint proprioceptors that then transmit excitatory impulses to the respiratory center. The reason for believing this is that even passive movements of the limbs often increase pulmonary ventilation severalfold.

It is possible that still other factors are also important in increasing pulmonary ventilation during exercise. For instance, some experiments even suggest that hypoxia developing in the muscles during exercise elicits afferent nerve signals to the respiratory center to excite respiration. However, since the increase in ventilation begins immediately upon the initiation of exercise, most of the increase in respiration probably results from the two neurogenic factors noted above, namely *stimulatory impulses from the higher centers of the brain* and *proprioceptive stimulatory reflexes*.

Interrelationship Between Chemical Factors and Nervous Factors in the Control of Respiration During Exercise. Figure 27–21 illustrates the different factors that operate in the control of respiration during exercise, showing two neurogenic factors: (1) direct stimulation of the respiratory center by

signals from the motor cortex, and (2) indirect stimulation by proprioceptors. It shows also the three humoral factors of carbon dioxide, hydrogen ions, and oxygen.

When a person exercises, usually the nervous factors stimulate the respiratory center almost exactly the proper amount to supply the extra oxygen requirements for the exercise and to expel off the extra carbon dioxide. But, occasionally, the nervous signals are either too strong or too weak in their stimulation of the respiratory center. Then, the chemical factors play a very significant role in bring-

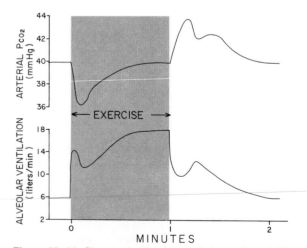

Figure 27–22. Changes in alveolar ventilation and arterial P_{CO_2} during a 1-minute period of exercise and also following termination of the exercise. (Extrapolated to the human being from data in dogs; from Bainton: *J. Appl. Physiol., 33*:778, 1972.)

ing about the final adjustment in respiration required to keep the carbon dioxide and hydrogen ion concentrations of the body fluids as nearly normal as possible. This effect is illustrated in Figure 27–22, which shows changes in alveolar ventilation and in arterial P_{CO_2} during a one-minute period of exercise and then for another minute after the exercise is over. Note that the alveolar ventilation increases without an initial increase in arterial P_{CO_2}; this increase is caused by a stimulus that originates in the brain at the same time that the brain excites the muscles.

Often, the increase in alveolar ventilation at the onset of ventilation is so great that it actually *decreases* arterial P_{CO_2} below normal, as shown in the figure, even though the exercising muscles are beginning to form large amounts of carbon dioxide. The reason for this is that the ventilation forges ahead of the buildup of carbon dioxide in the blood. Thus, the brain provides an "anticipatory" stimulation of respiration at the onset of exercise, causing excessive alveolar ventilation even before this is needed. However, after about 30 to 40 seconds, the amount of carbon dioxide released into the blood from the muscles approximately matches the increased rate of ventilation. Then the arterial P_{CO_2} returns essentially to normal and no longer is a significant factor in controlling the ventilation. Thereafter, it is then mainly the nervous signals that drive the respiration, not the chemical signals.

To summarize, at the onset of exercise, an anticipatory signal from the brain initiates an immediate increase in alveolar ventilation; sometimes the increase is too much, sometimes too little. However, within less than one minute, the chemical feedback factors (mainly arterial P_{CO_2}) make additional adjustments, either upward or downward, to balance the rate of alveolar ventilation with the rate of metabolism in the body. Yet, on the average, because of the direct brain stimulus to respiration, the final levels of P_{CO_2}, H^+ concentration, and P_{O_2} in the arterial blood are very near normal during exercise—sometimes slightly above normal and sometimes slightly below normal.

Now for a final comment regarding the brain factor for stimulation of respiration during exercise: Many experiments indicate that this brain factor is partly if not entirely a learned response. That is, with repeated periods of exercise of the same degree of strenuousness, the brain seems to become progressively more able to establish the proper amount of brain signal to maintain the chemical factors at their normal levels during exercise. Therefore, there is much reason to believe that some of the higher centers of learning in the brain are important in this brain factor—probably even the cerebral cortex. Indeed, when a person is anesthetized, so that the higher brain centers become nonfunctional, respiration is then controlled almost entirely by the chemical factors.

REFERENCES

THE CIRCULATION

Abboud, F. M., and Thames, M. D.: Interaction of cardiovascular reflexes in circulatory control. *In* Shepherd, J. T., and Abboud, F. M. (eds.): Handbook of Physiology. Sec. 2, Vol. III. Bethesda, American Physiological Society, 1983, p. 675.

Antonaccio, M. J. (ed.): Cardiovascular Pharmacology. New York, Raven Press, 1984.

Brezenoff, H. E., and Giuliano, R.: Cardiovascular control by cholinergic mechanisms in the central nervous system. *Annu. Rev. Pharmacol. Toxicol.*, 22:341, 1982.

Burattini, R., and Borgdorff, P.: Closed-loop baroreflex control of total peripheral resistance in the cat: Identification of gains by aid of a model. *Cardiovasc. Res.*, 18:715, 1984.

Coleridge, H. M., and Coleridge, J. C. G.: Cardiovascular afferents involved in regulation of peripheral vessels. *Annu. Rev. Physiol.*, 42:413, 1980.

Conway, J.: Hemodynamic aspects of essential hypertension in humans. *Physiol. Rev.*, 64:617, 1984.

Cowley, A. W., Jr., and Guyton, A. C.: Baroreceptor reflex contribution in angiotension-II-induced hypertension. *Circulation*, 50:61, 1974.

Cushing, H.: Concerning a definite regulatory mechanism of the vasomotor center which controls blood pressure during cerebral compression. *Bull. Johns Hopkins Hosp.*, 12:290, 1901.

Dampney, R. A., *et al.*: Identification of cardiovascular cell groups in the brain stem. *Clin. Exp. Hypertens.*, 6:205, 1984.

Donald, D. E., and Shepherd, J. T.: Autonomic regulation of the peripheral circulation. *Annu. Rev. Physiol.*, 42:429, 1980.

Folkow, B.: Physiological aspects of primary hypertension. *Physiol. Rev.*, 62:347, 1982.

Guyton, A. C.: Acute hypertension in dogs with cerebral ischemia. *Am. J. Physiol.*, 154:45, 1948.

Guyton, A. C.: Arterial Pressure and Hypertension. Philadelphia, W. B. Saunders Co., 1980.

Herd, J. A.: Cardiovascular response to stress in man. *Annu. Rev. Physiol.*, 46:177, 1984.

Hilton, S. M., and Spyer, K. M.: Central nervous regulation of vascular resistance. *Annu. Rev. Physiol.*, 42:399, 1980.

Krieger, E. M.: Time course of baroreceptor resetting in acute hypertension. *Am. J. Physiol.*, 218:484, 1970.

Mancia, G., and Mark, A. L.: Arterial baroreflexes in humans. *In* Shepherd, J. T., and Abboud, F. M. (eds.): Handbook of Physiology. Sec. 2, Vol. III. Bethesda, American Physiological Society, 1983, p. 755.

Randall, W. C. (ed.): Nervous Control of Cardiovascular Function. New York, Oxford University Press, 1984.

Rowell, L. B.: Reflex control of regional circulations in humans. *J. Autonom. Nerv. Syst.*, 11:101, 1984.

Sagawa, K.: Baroreflex control of systemic arterial pressure and vascular bed. *In* Shepherd, J. T., and Abboud, F. M. (eds.): Handbook of Physiology. Sec. 2, Vol. III. Bethesda, American Physiological Society, 1983, p. 453.

Stephenson, R. B.: Modification of reflex regulation of blood pressure by behavior. *Annu. Rev. Physiol.*, 46:133, 1984.

Uther, J. B., and Guyton, A. C.: Cardiovascular regulation following changes in central nervous perfusion pressure in the unanesthetized rabbit. *Aust. J. Exp. Biol. Med. Sci.*, 51:295, 1973.

THE RESPIRATION

Bainton, C. R.: Effect of speed versus grade and shivering on ventilation in dogs during active exercise. *J. Appl. Physiol.*, 33:778, 1972.

Cohen, M. I.: Central determinants of respiratory rhythm. *Annu. Rev. Physiol.*, 43:91, 1981.

Eldridge, F. L., and Millhorn, D. E.: Central regulation of respiration by endogenous neurotransmitters and neuromodulators. *Annu. Rev. Physiol.*, 43:121, 1981.

Eyzaguirre, C., *et al.*: Arterial chemoreceptors. *In* Shepherd, J. T., and Abboud, F. M. (eds.): Handbook of Physiology. Sec. 2, Vol. III. Bethesda, American Physiological Society, 1983, p. 557.

Flenley, D. C., and Warren, P. M.: Ventilatory responses to O_2 and CO_2 during exercise. *Annu. Rev. Physiol.*, 45:415, 1983.

Jansen, A. H., and Chernick, V.: Development of respiratory control. Physiol. Rev., 63:437, 1983.

Kalia, M. P.: Anatomical organization of central respiratory neurons. *Annu. Rev. Physiol.*, 43:105, 1981.

Mitchell, R. A., and Berger, A. J.: Neural regulation of respiration. *Am. Rev. Resp. Dis.*, 111:206, 1975.

Pack, A. I.: Sensory inputs to the medulla. *Annu. Rev. Physiol.*, 43:73, 1981.

Rigatto, H.: Control of ventilation in the newborn. *Annu. Rev. Physiol.*, 46:661, 1984.

Schlaefke, M. E. (ed.): Central Neurone Environment and the Control Systems of Breathing and Circulation. New York, Springer-Verlag, 1983.

Von Euler, C., and Lagercrantz, H. (eds.): Central Nervous Control Mechanisms in Breathing. New York, Pergamon Press, 1980.

Whipp, B. J.: Ventilatory control during exercise in humans. *Annu. Rev. Physiol.*, 45:393, 1983.

28

Regulation of Gastrointestinal Function, Micturition, Food Intake, and Body Temperature

INNERVATION OF THE GUT— THE "ENTERIC" NERVOUS SYSTEM

The gastrointestinal tract has an intrinsic nervous system of its own, called the *enteric nervous system*, that begins in the esophagus and extends all the way to the anus. This system controls most gastrointestinal functions, especially gastrointestinal movements and secretion. On the other hand, both parasympathetic and sympathetic nervous signals to the gastrointestinal tract from the brain can strongly alter the degree of activity of this enteric nervous system.

THE MYENTERIC PLEXUS AND THE SUBMUCOSAL PLEXUS

The enteric nervous system is composed principally of two layers of neurons and appropriate connecting fibers: the outer layer, called the *myenteric plexus* or *Auerbach's plexus*, lies between the longitudinal and circular muscular layers; the inner layer, called the *submucosal plexus* or *Meissner's plexus*, lies in the submucosa. The myenteric plexus controls mainly the *gastrointestinal movements*, whereas the submucosal plexus is important in controlling *secretion* and *blood flow* and also subserves many *sensory functions*, receiving signals principally from the gut epithelium and from stretch receptors in the gut wall.

Most often, stimulation of the myenteric plexus increases the motor activity of the gut, causing four principal effects: (1) increased tonic contraction, or "tone," of the gut wall, (2) increased intensity of the rhythmic contractions, (3) slightly increased rate of rhythmic contraction, and (4) increased velocity of conduction of excitatory waves along the gut wall. On the other hand, some myenteric plexus fibers are inhibitory rather than excitatory; these fibers secrete an inhibitory transmitter, possibly VIP

(vasoactive intestinal polypeptide) or some other peptide. A large share of the excitatory fibers are *cholinergic*—that is, they secrete *acetylcholine*, though some secrete other excitatory transmitters. Transmitters that have been identified in the enteric plexuses, though their functions are mainly unknown, include *ATP, substance P, enkephalin, somatostatin, serotonin, bombesin,* and *neurotensin*.

AUTONOMIC CONTROL OF THE GASTROINTESTINAL TRACT

The gastrointestinal tract receives extensive parasympathetic and sympathetic innervation that is capable of altering the overall activity of the entire gut or of specific parts of it.

Parasympathetic Innervation. The parasympathetic supply to the gut is divided into *cranial* and *sacral divisions*, which were discussed in Chapter 21. Except for a few parasympathetic fibers to the mouth and pharyngeal regions of the alimentary tract, the cranial parasympathetics are transmitted almost entirely in the *vagus nerves*. These fibers provide extensive innervation to the esophagus, stomach, pancreas, and first half of the large intestine (but rather little innervation to the small intestine). The sacral parasympathetics originate in the second, third, and fourth sacral segments of the spinal cord and pass through the *pelvic nerves* to the distal half of the large intestine. The sigmoidal, rectal, and anal regions of the large intestine are considerably better supplied with parasympathetic fibers than are the other portions. These fibers function especially in the defecation reflexes, which are discussed later in the chapter.

The postganglionic neurons of the parasympathetic system are mainly located in the myenteric and submucosal plexuses, so that stimulation of the parasympathetic nerves causes a general increase in activity of the entire enteric nervous system. This in turn enhances the activity of most gastrointestinal functions, but not all, for some of the enteric neurons are inhibitory and therefore inhibit certain of the functions.

Sympathetic Innervation. The sympathetic fibers to the gastrointestinal tract originate in the spinal cord between the segments T-8 and L-2. The preganglionic fibers, after leaving the cord, enter the sympathetic chains and pass through the chains to outlying ganglia, such as the *celiac ganglion* and various *mesenteric ganglia*. Here, the postganglionic neuron bodies are located, and postganglionic fibers spread from them along with the blood vessels to all parts of the gut, terminating principally on neurons in the enteric nervous system. The sympathetics innervate essentially all portions of the gastrointestinal tract rather than being more extensively supplied to the most orad and most analward portions as is true of the parasympathetics. The sympathetic nerve endings secrete *norepinephrine*.

In general, stimulation of the sympathetic nervous system inhibits activity in the gastrointestinal tract, causing effects essentially opposite to those of the parasympathetic system. It exerts its effects in two different ways: (1) to a slight extent by the direct effect of the norepinephrine on the smooth muscle to inhibit this activity (except the muscularis mucosa, which it excites), and (2) to a major extent by an inhibitory effect of the norepinephrine on the neurons of the enteric nervous system. Thus, strong stimulation of the sympathetic system can totally block movement of food through the gastrointestinal tract.

Afferent Nerve Fibers Entering the Enteric Plexus. Many afferent nerve fibers arise in the gut. Some of these have their cell bodies in the enteric nervous system itself. These nerves can be stimulated by (1) irritation of the gut mucosa, (2) excessive distension of the gut, or (3) the presence of specific chemical substances in the gut. Signals transmitted through these fibers can cause excitation or, under some conditions, inhibition of intestinal movements or intestinal secretion.

In addition to the afferent fibers that terminate in the enteric nervous system, still two other types of afferent fibers are associated with this system. One of these has its cell bodies in the enteric nervous system but sends its axons through the extrinsic nerves to terminate in the *prevertebral sympathetic ganglia*, that is, in the *celiac, mesenteric,* and *hypogastric ganglia*. The other type of afferent fibers has its cell bodies in the dorsal root ganglia of the spinal cord or in the cranial nerve ganglia; these fibers transmit their signals directly into the spinal cord or brain stem, traveling in the same nerve trunks along with the sympathetic or parasympathetic nerves. For example, 80 per cent of the nerve fibers in the vagus nerves are afferent rather than efferent. These fibers transmit afferent signals into the medulla, which in turn initiates many vagal efferent signals returning to the gastrointestinal tract to control many of its functions.

The Gastrointestinal Reflexes. The anatomical arrangement of the enteric nervous system and its connections with the sympathetic and parasympathetic systems supports three different types of gastrointestinal reflexes that are essential to gastrointestinal control. These are:

(1) *Reflexes that occur entirely within the enteric nervous system.* These include reflexes that control gastrointestinal secretion, peristalsis, mixing contractions, local inhibitory effects, and so forth.

(2) *Reflexes from the gut to the prevertebral sympathetic ganglia and then back to the gastrointestinal tract.* These reflexes transmit signals for long distances in the gastrointestinal tract, such as signals from the stomach to cause evacuation of the colon (the gastrocolic reflex), signals from the colon and small intestine to inhibit stomach motility and stomach secretion (the enterogastric reflexes), and reflexes from the colon to inhibit emptying of ileal contents into the colon (the colonoileal reflex).

(3) *Reflexes from the gut to the spinal cord or brain stem and then back to the gastrointestinal tract.* These include especially reflexes from the stomach and duodenum to the brain stem and back to the stomach to control gastric motor and secretory activity; pain reflexes that cause general inhibition throughout the gastrointestinal tract; and defecation reflexes that produce the powerful colonic, rectal, and abdominal contractions required for defecation (the defecation reflexes).

FUNCTIONAL TYPES OF MOVEMENTS IN THE GASTROINTESTINAL TRACT

Two basic types of movements occur in the gastrointestinal tract: (1) *mixing movements*, which keep the intestinal contents thoroughly mixed at all times, and (2) *propulsive movements*, which cause food to move forward along the tract at an appropriate rate for digestion and absorption.

THE MIXING MOVEMENTS

In most parts of the alimentary tract, the mixing movements are caused by either *peristaltic contractions* or *local constrictive contractions of small segments of the gut wall*. These movements are modified in different parts of the gastrointestinal tract for proper performance of the respective activities of each part.

THE PROPULSIVE MOVEMENTS— PERISTALSIS

The basic propulsive movement of the gastrointestinal tract is *peristalsis*, which is illustrated in Figure 28–1. A contractile ring appears around the gut and then moves forward; this is analogous to putting one's fingers around a thin distended tube, then constricting the fingers and moving forward along the tube. Obviously, any material in front of the contractile ring is pushed forward.

Peristalsis is an inherent property of many syncytial smooth muscle tubes; stimulation at any point

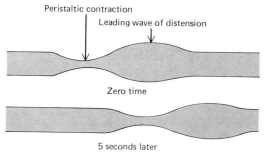

Peristaltic contraction

Leading wave of distension

Zero time

5 seconds later

Figure 28–1. Peristalsis.

can cause a contractile ring to spread along the tube. Thus, peristalsis occurs in (a) the gastrointestinal tract, (b) the bile ducts, (c) other glandular ducts throughout the body, (d) the ureters, and (e) many other smooth muscle tubes of the body.

The usual stimulus for peristalsis is *distension*. That is, if a large amount of food collects at any point in the gut, the distension stimulates the gut wall 2 to 3 cm above this point, and a contractile ring appears that initiates a peristaltic movement. Other stimuli that can initiate peristalsis include irritation of the epithelium lining the gut and extrinsic nervous signals that excite the gut.

Function of the Myenteric Plexus in Peristalsis. Peristalsis occurs only weakly, if at all, in portions of the gastrointestinal tract that have congenital absence of the myenteric plexus. Also, it is greatly depressed or completely blocked in the entire gut when the person is treated with atropine to paralyze the cholinergic nerve endings of the myenteric plexus. Therefore, *effectual* peristalsis requires an active myenteric plexus.

Analward Peristaltic Movements. Peristalsis, theoretically, can occur in either direction from a stimulated point, but it normally dies out rapidly in the orad direction while continuing for a considerable distance analward. The exact cause of this directional transmission of peristalsis has never been ascertained, though it probably results mainly from the fact that the myenteric plexus itself is "polarized" in the anal direction, which can be explained as follows:

The Peristaltic Reflex and the "Law of the Gut." When a segment of the intestinal tract is excited by distension and thereby initiates peristalsis, the contractile ring for causing the peristalsis begins slightly on the orad side of the distended segment; then it moves toward the distended segment, thus pushing the intestinal contents in the anal direction. At the same time, the gut sometimes relaxes several centimeters downstream toward the anus, which is called "receptive relaxation," thus allowing the food to be propelled more easily analward than in the orad direction.

This complex pattern, consisting of contraction of the gut above the point of distension and relaxation below, does not occur in the absence of the myenteric plexus. Therefore, the complex is frequently

called the *myenteric reflex*, or it is also called simply the *peristaltic reflex*. And the peristaltic reflex plus the analward direction of movement of the peristalsis is called the "law of the gut."

INGESTION OF FOOD

The amount of food that a person ingests is determined principally by the intrinsic desire for food called *hunger*. The type of food that a person preferentially seeks is determined by *appetite*. These mechanisms in themselves are extremely important automatic regulatory systems for maintaining an adequate nutritional supply for the body.

MASTICATION (CHEWING)

The teeth are admirably designed for chewing, the anterior teeth (incisors) providing a strong cutting action and the posterior teeth (molars) a grinding action. All the jaw muscles working together can close the teeth with a force as great as 55 pounds on the incisors and 200 pounds on the molars. When this is applied to a small object, such as a small seed between the molars, the actual force *per square inch of contact* may be several thousand pounds.

Most of the muscles of chewing are innervated by the motor branch of the 5th cranial nerve, and the chewing process is controlled by nuclei in the hindbrain. Stimulation of the reticular formation near the hindbrain centers for taste can cause continual rhythmic chewing movements. Also, stimulation of areas in the hypothalamus, amygdala, and even in the cerebral cortex near the sensory areas for taste and smell can cause chewing.

Much of the chewing process is caused by the *chewing reflex*, which may be explained as follows: The presence of a bolus of food in the mouth causes reflex inhibition of the muscles of mastication, which allows the lower jaw to drop. The drop in turn initiates a stretch reflex of the jaw muscles that leads to *rebound* contraction. This automatically raises the jaw to cause closure of the teeth, but it also compresses the bolus again against the linings of the mouth, which inhibits the jaw muscles once again, allowing the jaw to drop and rebound another time, and this is repeated again and again.

Chewing of the food is important for digestion of all foods, but it is especially important for most fruits and raw vegetables, because these have undigestible cellulose membranes around their nutrient portions which must be broken before the food can be utilized. Chewing aids in the digestion of food for the following simple reason: Since the *digestive enzymes act only on the surfaces of food particles*, the rate of digestion is highly dependent on the total surface area exposed to the intestinal secretions. Also, grinding the food to a very fine

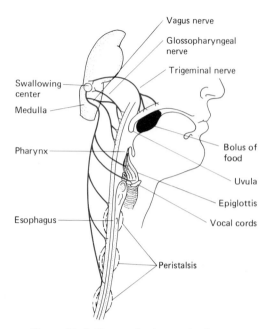

Figure 28–2. The swallowing mechanism.

particulate consistency prevents excoriation of the gastrointestinal tract and increases the ease with which food is emptied from the stomach into the small intestine and thence into all succeeding segments of the gut.

SWALLOWING (DEGLUTITION)

Swallowing is a complicated mechanism, principally because the pharynx most of the time subserves several other functions besides swallowing and is converted for only a few seconds at a time into a tract for propulsion of food. It is especially important that respiration not be seriously compromised during swallowing.

In general, swallowing can be divided into (1) the *voluntary stage*, which initiates the swallowing process, (2) the *pharyngeal stage*, which is involuntary and constitutes the passage of food through the pharynx into the esophagus, and (3) the *esophageal stage*, another involuntary phase which promotes passage of food from the pharynx to the stomach.

Voluntary Stage of Swallowing. When the food is ready for swallowing, it is "voluntarily" squeezed or rolled posteriorly in the mouth by pressure of the tongue upward and backward against the palate, as shown in Figure 28–2. Thus, the tongue forces the bolus of food into the pharynx. From here on, the process of swallowing becomes entirely, or almost entirely, automatic and ordinarily cannot be stopped.

Pharyngeal Stage of Swallowing. When the bolus of food is pushed backward in the mouth, it stimulates *swallowing receptor areas* all around the opening of the pharynx, especially on the tonsillar pillars, and impulses from these pass to the brain stem to initiate a series of automatic pharyngeal muscular contractions as follows:

1. The soft palate is pulled upward to close the posterior nares, in this way preventing reflux of food into the nasal cavities.

2. The palatopharyngeal folds on either side of the pharynx are pulled medialward to approximate each other. In this way these folds form a sagittal slit through which the food must pass into the posterior pharynx. This slit performs a selective action, allowing food that has been masticated properly to pass with ease while impeding the passage of large objects. Since this stage of swallowing lasts less than 1 second, any large object is usually impeded too much to pass through the pharynx into the esophagus.

3. The vocal cords of the larynx are strongly approximated, and the hyoid bone and larynx are pulled upward and anteriorly by the neck muscles, causing the epiglottis to swing backward over the superior opening of the larynx. Both these effects prevent passage of food into the trachea. Especially important is the approximation of the vocal cords, but the epiglottis helps to prevent food from ever getting as far as the vocal cords. Destruction of the vocal cords or of the muscles that approximate them can cause strangulation. On the other hand, removal of the epiglottis usually does not cause serious debility in swallowing.

4. The upward movement of the larynx also stretches the opening of the esophagus. At the same time, the upper 3 to 4 centimeters of the esophagus, an area called the *upper esophageal sphincter*, the *pharyngoesophageal sphincter*, or the *cricopharyngeal muscle*, relaxes, thus allowing food to move easily and freely from the posterior pharynx into the upper esophagus. This sphincter, between swallows, remains tonically and strongly contracted, thereby preventing air from going into the esophagus during respiration. The upward movement of the larynx also lifts the glottis out of the main stream of food flow so that the food usually passes on either side of the epiglottis rather than over its surface; this adds still another protection against passage of food into the trachea.

5. At the same time that the larynx is raised and the pharyngoesophageal sphincter is relaxed, the superior constrictor muscle of the pharynx contracts, giving rise to a rapid peristaltic wave passing downward over the middle and inferior pharyngeal muscles and into the esophagus, which also propels the food into the esophagus.

To summarize the mechanics of the pharyngeal stage of swallowing—the trachea is closed, the esophagus is opened, and a fast peristaltic wave originating in the pharynx then forces the bolus of food into the upper esophagus, the entire process occurring in 1 to 2 seconds.

Nervous Control of the Pharyngeal Stage of Swallowing. The most sensitive tactile areas of the pharynx for initiation of the pharyngeal stage of swallowing lie in a ring around the pharyngeal opening, with greatest sensitivity in the tonsillar pillars. Impulses are transmitted from these areas through the sensory portions of the trigeminal and glossopharyngeal nerves into a region of the medulla oblongata closely associated with the *tractus solitarius* which receives essentially all sensory impulses from the mouth.

The successive stages of the swallowing process are then automatically controlled in orderly sequence by neuronal areas distributed throughout the reticular substance of the medulla and lower portion of the pons. The sequence of the swallowing reflex is the same from one swallow to the next, and the timing of the entire cycle also remains constant from one swallow to the next. The areas in the medulla and lower pons that control swallowing are collectively called the *deglutition* or *swallowing center*.

The motor impulses from the swallowing center to the pharynx and upper esophagus that cause swallowing are transmitted by the 5th, 9th, 10th, and 12th cranial nerves and even a few of the superior cervical nerves.

In summary, the pharyngeal stage of swallowing is principally a reflex act. It is almost never initiated by direct stimuli to the swallowing center from higher regions of the central nervous system. Instead, it is almost always initiated by voluntary movement of food into the back of the mouth, which, in turn, elicits the swallowing reflex.

Effect of the Pharyngeal Stage of Swallowing on Respiration. The entire pharyngeal stage of swallowing occurs in less than 1 to 2 seconds, thereby interrupting respiration for only a fraction of a usual respiratory cycle. The swallowing center specifically inhibits the respiratory center of the medulla during this time, halting respiration at any point in its cycle to allow swallowing to proceed. Yet, even while a person is talking, swallowing interrupts respiration for such a short time that it is hardly noticeable.

Esophageal Stage of Swallowing. The esophagus functions primarily to conduct food from the pharynx to the stomach, and its movements are organized specifically for this function.

Normally the esophagus exhibits two types of peristaltic movements—*primary peristalsis* and *secondary peristalsis*. Primary peristalsis is simply a continuation of the peristaltic wave that begins in the pharynx and spreads into the esophagus during the pharyngeal stage of swallowing. This wave passes all the way from the pharynx to the stomach in approximately 8 to 10 seconds. However, food swallowed by a person who is in the upright position is usually transmitted to the lower end of the esophagus even more rapidly than the peristaltic wave itself, in about 5 to 8 seconds, because of the additional effect of gravity pulling the food downward. If the primary peristaltic wave fails to move all the food that has entered the esophagus into the

stomach, secondary peristaltic waves, generated by the enteric nervous system of the esophagus, result from distension of the esophagus by the retained food. These waves are essentially the same as the primary peristaltic waves, except that they originate in the esophagus itself rather than in the pharynx. Secondary peristaltic waves continue to be initiated until all the food has emptied into the stomach.

The peristaltic waves of the esophagus are initiated by vagal reflexes that are part of the overall swallowing mechanism. These reflexes are transmitted through *vagal afferent fibers* from the esophagus to the medulla and then back again to the esophagus through *vagal efferent fibers*.

The musculature of the pharynx and the upper quarter of the esophagus is striated muscle, and, therefore, the peristaltic waves in these regions are controlled only by skeletal nerve impulses in the glossopharyngeal and vagus nerves. In the lower two thirds of the esophagus, the musculature is smooth, but this portion of the esophagus is also strongly controlled by the vagus nerves acting through their connections with the enteric nervous system. However, when the vagus nerves to the esophagus are sectioned, the myenteric nerve plexus of the esophagus becomes excitable enough after several days to cause secondary peristaltic waves even without support from the vagal reflexes. Therefore, following paralysis of the swallowing reflex, food forced into the upper esophagus and then pulled by gravity to the lower esophagus still passes readily into the stomach.

Receptive Relaxation of the Stomach. As the esophageal peristaltic wave passes toward the stomach, a wave of relaxation, transmitted through myenteric inhibitory neurons, precedes the constriction. Furthermore, the entire stomach and, to a lesser extent, even the duodenum become relaxed as this wave reaches the lower end of the esophagus. Especially important, also, is relaxation of the gastroesophageal sphincter at the juncture between the esophagus and the stomach. In other words, the constrictor and the stomach are prepared ahead of time to receive food being propelled down the esophagus during the swallowing act.

NERVOUS CONTROL OF FOOD MOVEMENT THROUGH THE STOMACH, SMALL INTESTINE, AND COLON

Movement of food through the stomach, small intestine, and colon is caused by various forms of peristaltic propulsive movements. Most of these movements are controlled by the enteric nervous system of the gastrointestinal wall. That is, when a segment of bowel becomes overfilled, the stretch of the nerve endings elicits a local peristaltic reflex, as explained earlier in the chapter, causing propulsion of the food forward.

In general, parasympathetic stimulation by way

of the vagi and sacral nerves increases the rate of peristalsis, and sympathetic stimulation normally inhibits it.

Intrinsic GI Reflexes That Inhibit Rate of Food Movement. At several points in the gastrointestinal tract special reflex mechanisms prevent too rapid movement of food along the gstrointestinal tract. For instance, when the stomach empties too much food into the upper portions of the small intestine, stretch of the intestinal walls transmits signals backwards along the myenteric plexus to the stomach to inhibit its peristaltic movements. This obviously allows the small intestine to receive food at a rate slow enough for it to process the food appropriately. Another reflex occurs from the colon to the lower end of the small intestine; when the colon becomes overfilled, myenteric reflex signals inhibit peristalsis in the small intestine and thereby prevent movement of the intestinal contents into the colon at a rate more rapid than these can be processed.

DEFECATION

Most of the time, the rectum is empty of feces. This results partly from the fact that a weak functional sphincter exists approximately 20 cm from the anus at the juncture between the sigmoid and the rectum. There is also a sharp angulation here that contributes additional resistance to filling of the rectum. However, when a mass movement forces feces into the rectum the desire for defecation is normally initiated, including reflex contraction of the rectum and relaxation of the anal sphincters.

Continual dribble of fecal matter through the anus is prevented by tonic constriction of (1) the *internal anal sphincter*, a circular mass of smooth muscle that lies immediately inside the anus, and (2) the *external anal sphincter*, composed of striated voluntary muscle that both surrounds the internal sphincter and also extends distal to it; the external sphincter is controlled by nerve fibers in the pudendal nerve, which is part of the somatic nervous system and therefore is under voluntary, conscious control.

The Defecation Reflexes. Ordinarily, defecation is initiated by *defecation reflexes*, which can be described as follows: When the feces enter the rectum, distension of the rectal wall initiates afferent signals that spread through the *myenteric plexus* to initiate peristaltic waves in the descending colon, sigmoid, and rectum, forcing feces toward the anus. As the peristaltic wave approaches the anus, the internal anal sphincter is inhibited by inhibitory nerves, and if the external anal sphincter is relaxed, defecation will occur. This overall effect is called the *intrinsic defecation reflex* of the colon itself.

However, the intrinsic defecation reflex itself is usually weak, and to be effective in causing defecation it must be fortified by another type of defecation reflex, a *parasympathetic defecation reflex* that involves the sacral segments of the spinal cord, as

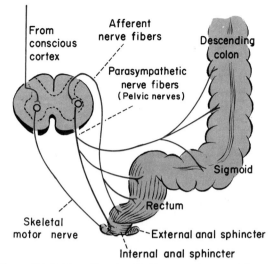

Figure 28–3. The afferent and efferent pathways of the parasympathetic mechanism for enhancing the defecation reflex.

illustrated in Figure 28–3. When the afferent fibers in the rectum are stimulated, signals are transmitted into the spinal cord and thence, reflexly, back to the descending colon, sigmoid, rectum, and anus by way of parasympathetic nerve fibers in the *pelvic nerves*. These parasympathetic signals greatly intensify the peristaltic waves as well as relaxing the internal anal sphincter and convert the intrinsic defecation reflex from an ineffectual weak movement into a powerful process of defecation that is sometimes effective in emptying the large bowel in one movement all the way from the splenic flexure to the anus. Also, the afferent signals entering the spinal cord initiate other effects, such as taking a deep breath, closure of the glottis, and contraction of the abdominal muscles to force the fecal contents of the colon downward, at the same time causing the pelvic floor to extend downward and to pull outward on the anus to evaginate the feces.

However, despite the defecation reflexes other effects are also necessary before actual defecation occurs, because relaxation of the internal sphincter and forward movement of feces toward the anus normally initiates an instantaneous contraction of the external sphincter, which still temporarily prevents defecation. Except in babies and mentally inept persons, the conscious mind then takes over voluntary control of the external sphincter and either inhibits it to allow defecation to occur or further contracts it if the moment is not socially acceptable for defecation. If the external sphincter is kept contracted, the defecation reflexes die out after a few minutes, and they remain quiescent for several hours or until additional amounts of feces enter the rectum.

When it becomes convenient for the person to defecate, the defecation reflexes can sometimes be excited by taking a deep breath to move the diaphragm downward and then contracting the abdominal muscles to increase the pressure in the abdomen, thus forcing fecal contents into the rectum to elicit new reflexes. Unfortunately, reflexes initiated in this way are never as effective as those that arise naturally, for which reason people who too often inhibit their natural reflexes are likely to become severely constipated.

In the newborn baby and in some persons with transected spinal cords, the defecation reflexes cause automatic emptying of the lower bowel without the normal control exercised through contraction of the external anal sphincter.

AUTONOMIC CONTROL OF GASTROINTESTINAL SECRETION

The nervous sytem of the gastrointestinal tract not only controls peristaltic movement of food but also controls secretion by many of the gastrointestinal glands, especially salivary secretion in the mouth, gastric juice secretion in the stomach, and mucus secretion in the distal colon and in the sigmoid.

Nervous Regulation of Salivary Secretion

Figure 28–4 illustrates the nervous pathways for regulation of salivation, showing that the salivary glands are controlled mainly by *parasympathetic nervous signals* from the *salivatory nuclei*. The salivatory nuclei are located approximately at the juncture of the medulla and pons and are excited by both taste and tactile stimuli from the tongue and other areas of the mouth. Many taste stimuli, especially the sour taste, elicit copious secretion of saliva—often as much as 5 to 8 ml per minute or 8 to 20 times the basal rate of secretion. Also, certain tactile stimuli, such as the presence of smooth objects in the mouth (a pebble, for instance), cause marked

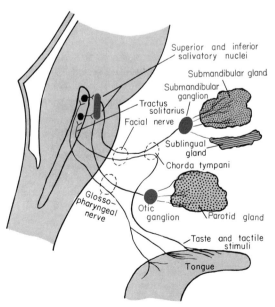

salivation, while rough objects cause less salivation and occasionally even inhibit salivation.

Salivation can also be stimulated or inhibited by impulses arriving in the salivatory nuclei from higher centers of the central nervous system. For instance, when a person smells or eats favorite foods, salivation is greater than when disliked food is smelled or eaten. The *appetite area* of the brain that partially regulates these effects is located in close proximity to the parasympathetic centers of the anterior hypothalamus, and it functions to a great extent in response to signals from the taste and smell areas of the cerebral cortex or amygdala.

Finally, salivation also occurs in response to reflexes originating in the stomach and upper intestines—particularly when very irritating foods are swallowed or when a person is nauseated because of some gastrointestinal abnormality. The swallowed saliva presumably helps to remove the irritating factor in the gastrointestinal tract by diluting or neutralizing the irritant substances.

REGULATION OF GASTRIC SECRETION BY NERVOUS AND HORMONAL MECHANISMS

Gastric secretion is regulated by both nervous and hormonal mechanisms; nervous regulation is effected through the parasympathetic fibers of the vagus nerves as well as through local enteric nervous system reflexes, and hormonal regulation takes place mainly in response to the hormone *gastrin*. Thus, regulation of gastric secretion is different from the regulation of salivary secretion, which is effected entirely by nervous mechanisms.

Vagal Stimulation of Gastric Secretion

Nervous signals to cause gastric secretion originate in the dorsal motor nuclei of the vagi and pass via the vagus nerves to the enteric nervous system of the stomach wall and thence to the oxyntic glands. In response, these glands secrete vast quantities of both pepsin and acid, but with a higher proportion of pepsin than in gastric juice elicited in other ways. Also, vagal signals to all the mucus-secreting glands and epithelial lining cells cause increased mucus secretion as well.

Still another effect of vagal stimulation is to cause the antral part of the stomach mucosa to secrete the hormone *gastrin*. As will be explained in the following paragraphs, this hormone then acts on the gastric glands to cause additional flow of highly acidic gastric juice. Thus, vagal stimulation excites stomach secretion both directly by stimulation of the gastric glands and indirectly through the gastrin mechanism.

Stimulation of Gastric Secretion by Gastrin

When food enters the stomach, it causes the antral portion of the stomach mucosa to secrete the

Figure 28–4. Nervous regulation of salivary secretion.

hormone gastrin. This hormone is secreted by *gastrin cells,* also called *G cells,* in the pyloric glands and to a lesser extent in the proximal glands (Brunner's glands) of the duodenum. Gastrin is a large peptide secreted in two forms, a large form called *G-34,* containing 34 amino acids, and a smaller form, *G-17,* containing 17 amino acids. Though both of these are important, the smaller form is more abundant.

The food causes release of this hormone in two ways: (1) The actual bulk of the food distends the stomach, and this causes the hormone gastrin to be released from the antral mucosa. (2) Certain substances called secretagogues—such as food extractives, partially digested proteins, alcohol (in low concentration), caffeine, and so forth—also cause gastrin to be liberated from the antral mucosa.

Both of these stimuli—the distension and the chemical action of the secretagogues—elicit gastrin release by means of a local nerve reflex. That is, they stimulate sensory nerve fibers in the stomach epithelium which in turn synapse with the enteric nervous system. This then transmits efferent signals to the gastrin cells, causing them to secrete the gastrin. Therefore, any factor that blocks this reflex will also block the formation of gastrin. For instance, anesthetization of the gastric mucosa to block the sensory stimuli will prevent gastrin release; administration of atropine, which blocks the action on the gastrin cells of the acetylcholine released by the enteric nerves, will also prevent gastrin release.

Gastrin is absorbed into the blood and carried to the oxyntic glands in the body of the stomach where it stimulates mainly the oxyntic cells but to a lesser extent the peptic cells, also. The oxyntic cells increase their rate of hydrochloric acid secretion as much as eightfold, and the peptic cells increase their rate of enzyme secretion two- to fourfold.

The rate of secretion in response to gastrin is somewhat less than to vagal stimulation, 200 ml per hour in contrast to about 500 ml per hour, indicating that the gastrin mechanism is a less potent acute mechanism for stimulation of stomach secretion than is vagal stimulation. However, the gastrin mechanism usually continues for several hours in contrast to a much shorter period of time for vagal stimulation. Therefore, as a whole, it is likely that the gastrin mechanism is equally as important as, if not more important than, the vagal mechanism for control of gastric secretion. Yet, when both of these work together, the total secretion is much greater than the sum of the individual secretions caused by each of the two mechanisms. In other words, *the two mechanisms multiply each other rather than simply add to each other.*

Feedback Inhibition of Gastric Acid Secretion. When the acidity of the gastric juices increases to a pH of 2.0, the gastrin mechanism for stimulating gastric secretion becomes totally blocked. This effect probably results from two different factors. First, greatly enhanced acidity depresses or blocks the extraction of gastrin itself from the antral mucosa. Second, the acid seems to cause a nervous reflex that inhibits gastric acid secretion.

Obviously, this feedback inhibition of the gastric glands plays an important role in protecting the stomach against excessively acid secretions, which would readily cause peptic ulceration. In addition to this protective effect, the feedback mechanism is also important in maintaining optimal pH for function of the peptic enzymes in the digestive process, because whenever the pH rises above 2.5 to 3.5, gastrin begins to be secreted again and more acid is secreted.

NERVOUS CONTROL OF SECRETION IN THE SMALL AND LARGE INTESTINES

The intestinal mucosa contains several million minute tubular glands each a millimeter or so in length. In addition, mucous cells line the entire inner surface of the intestinal tract from the small intestine to the anus and secrete intestinal mucus. Both the tubular glands and the mucous cells are controlled almost entirely by local control mechanisms within the gastrointestinal tract itself and only to a very slight extent by the parasympathetic and sympathetic nerves.

The mucous cells respond mainly to direct contact with the intestinal contents; the mucus that they secrete serves as a lubricant for movement of the intestinal matter along the intestinal tube. The tubular glands, on the other hand, secrete large amounts of electrolytic solution that provides a vehicle for moving food along the intestinal tract. Also, this fluid serves as a transport medium for absorbing the digestive products from the food. The tubular glands are controlled by both hormonal and nervous stimuli. The hormonal stimuli are similar to the stimulation of the gastric mucosa by gastrin, though the hormones responsible are relatively uncharted. The nervous stimuli control intestinal secretion through local enteric nervous reflexes. As the food passes through the intestines, either contact with the epithelial surfaces or the action of chemical substances from the foods elicits local nerve signals that excite the submucosal and myenteric plexuses, and these in turn stimulate the tubular glands. This enteric reflex mechanism is probably responsible for most of the intestinal secretion.

MICTURITION

Micturition is the process by which the urinary bladder empties when it becomes filled. Basically the bladder (1) progressively fills until the tension in its walls rises above a threshold value, at which time (2) a nervous reflex called the "micturition reflex" occurs that either causes micturition or, if it fails in this, at least arouses a conscious desire to urinate.

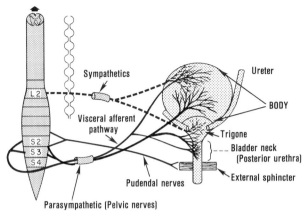

Figure 28–5. The urinary bladder and its innervation.

Innervation of the Bladder. The principal nerve supply to the bladder, illustrated in Figure 28–5, is by way of the *pelvic nerves*, which connect with the spinal cord through the sacral plexus, mainly connecting with cord segments S-2 and S-3. Coursing through the pelvic nerves are both *sensory nerve fibers* and *motor fibers*. The sensory fibers mainly detect the degree of stretch of the bladder walls. Stretch signals from the bladder neck are especially strong and are mainly responsible for initiating the reflexes that cause bladder emptying.

The motor nerve fibers transmitted in the pelvic nerves are *parasympathetic fibers*. These terminate on ganglion cells located in the wall of the bladder. Short postganglionic nerves then innervate the *detrusor muscle*.

Aside from the pelvic nerves, two other types of innervation are important to bladder function. Most important are the motor fibers transmitted through the *pudendal nerve* to the *external bladder sphincter*. These are somatic nerve fibers that innervate the skeletal muscle of this sphincter. In addition, the bladder receives sympathetic innervation from the sympathetic chain through the hypogastric nerves, connecting mainly with the L-2 segment of the spinal cord. These sympathetic fibers probably stimulate mainly the blood vessels and have very little to do with bladder contraction. Some sensory nerve fibers also pass by way of the sympathetic nerves and may be important for the sensation of fullness and perhaps pain in some instances.

THE MICTURITION REFLEX

As the bladder fills, many *micturition contractions* begin to appear. These are the result of a stretch reflex initiated by stretch receptors in the bladder wall, especially by the receptors in the bladder neck when this neck begins to fill with urine at the higher bladder pressures. *Sensory signals* are conducted to the sacral segments of the cord through the *pelvic nerves* and then back again to the bladder through the *parasympathetic fibers* in these same nerves.

Once a micturition reflex begins, it is "self-regenerative." That is, initial contraction of the bladder further activates the receptors to cause still further increase in afferent impulses from the bladder, which causes further increase in reflex contraction of the bladder, the cycle thus repeating itself again and again until the bladder has reached a strong degree of contraction. Then, after a few seconds to more than a minute, the reflex begins to fatigue, and the regenerative cycle of the micturition reflex ceases, allowing rapid reduction in bladder contraction. In other words, the micturition reflex is a single complete cycle of (1) progressive and rapid increase in pressure, (2) a period of sustained pressure, and (3) return of the pressure to the basal tonic pressure of the bladder. Once a micturition reflex has occurred and has not succeeded in emptying the bladder, the nervous elements of this reflex usually remain in an inhibited state for at least a few minutes to sometimes as long as an hour or more before another micturition reflex occurs. However, as the bladder becomes more and more filled, micturition reflexes occur more and more often and more and more powerfully.

Once the micturition reflex becomes powerful enough and the fluid pressure in the bladder great enough to force the bladder neck open despite the tonic contraction of the bladder neck muscle, stretch of the neck not only greatly exacerbates the intensity of the micturition reflex itself but causes still another reflex as well. This reflex passes to the sacral portion of the spinal cord and then back through the *pudendal nerve* to the *external sphincter* to inhibit it. If this inhibition is more potent than the voluntary constrictor signals from the brain, then urination will occur. If not, urination still will not occur until the bladder fills still more and the micturition reflex becomes more powerful.

Control of Micturition by the Brain. The micturition reflex is a completely automatic cord reflex, but it can be inhibited or facilitated by centers in the brain. These include strong *facilitatory and inhibitory centers in the brain stem*, probably located in the pons, and several *centers located in the cerebral cortex* that are mainly inhibitory but can at times become excitatory.

The micturition reflex is the basic cause of micturition, but the higher centers normally exert final control of micturition by the following means:

1. The higher centers keep the micturition reflex partially inhibited all the time except when it is desired to micturate.

2. The higher centers prevent micturition, even if a micturition reflex occurs, by continual tonic contraction of the external bladder sphincter until a convenient time presents itself.

3. When the time to urinate arrives, the cortical centers can (a) facilitate the sacral micturition centers to help initiate a micturition reflex, and (b) inhibit the external urethral sphincter so that urination can occur. However, even more important, voluntary urination is usually initiated in the following way: First, the person contracts his abdominal muscles, which increases the pressure of the urine in the bladder. At the same time, the pelvic floor muscles are relaxed, which lengthens the bladder neck and allows extra urine to enter the neck under pressure, thus stretching its walls. This then excites the stretch receptors, which excites the micturition reflex and simultaneously inhibits the external urethral sphincter. Ordinarily, all the urine will then be emptied, with rarely more than 5 to 10 milliliters left in the bladder.

REGULATION OF FOOD INTAKE

Hunger. The term hunger means a craving for food, and it is associated with a number of objective sensations. For instance, in a person who has not had food for many hours, the stomach undergoes intense rhythmic contractions called *hunger contractions*. These cause a tight or gnawing feeling in the pit of the stomach and sometimes actually cause pain called *hunger pangs*. In addition to the hunger pangs, the hungry person also becomes more tense and restless than usual.

Some physiologists actually define hunger as the tonic contractions of the stomach. However, even after the stomach is completely removed, the psychic sensations of hunger still occur, and craving for food still makes the person search for an adequate food supply.

Appetite. The term appetite is often used in the same sense as hunger except that it usually implies desire for specific types of food instead of food in general. Therefore, appetite helps a person choose the quality of food to eat.

Satiety. Satiety is the opposite of hunger. It means a feeling of fulfillment in the quest for food. Satiety usually results from a filling meal, particularly when the person's nutritional storage depots, the adipose tissue and the glycogen stores, are already filled.

NEURAL CENTERS FOR REGULATION OF FOOD INTAKE

Hunger and Satiety Centers. Stimulation of the *lateral hypothalamus* causes an animal to eat voraciously, which is called *hyperphagia*. On the other hand, stimulation of the *ventromedial nuclei of the hypothalamus* causes complete satiety, and, even in the presence of highly appetizing food, the animal will still refuse to eat, which is *aphagia*. Conversely, destructive lesions of the two respective areas cause results exactly opposite to those caused by stimulation. That is, ventromedial lesions cause voracious and continued eating until the animal becomes extremely obese, sometimes as large as four times normal size. And lesions of the lateral hypothalamic nuclei cause complete lack of desire for food and progressive inanition of the animal. Therefore, we can label the lateral nuclei of the hypothalamus as a *hunger center* or *feeding center*, and we can label the ventromedial nuclei of the hypothalamus as a *satiety center*.

The feeding center operates by directly exciting the emotional drive to search for food (while also stimulating other emotional drives as well—see Chapters 20 and 21). On the other hand, it is believed that the satiety center operates primarily by inhibiting the feeding center.

Other Neural Centers That Enter into Feeding. If the brain is sectioned below the hypothalamus but above the mesencephalon, the animal can still perform the basic mechanical features of the feeding process. It can salivate, lick its lips, chew food, and swallow. Therefore, *the actual mechanics of feeding are controlled by centers in the brain stem*. The function of the hypothalamus in feeding, then, is to control the quantity of food intake and to excite the lower centers to activity.

Higher centers than the hypothalamus also play important roles in the control of feeding, particularly in the control of appetite. These centers include especially the *amygdala* and the *cortical areas of the limbic system*, all of which are closely coupled with the hypothalamus. It will be recalled from the discussion of the sense of smell that portions of the amygdala are a major part of the olfactory nervous system. Destructive lesions in the amygdala have demonstrated that some of its areas greatly increase feeding, while others inhibit feeding. In addition, stimulation of some areas of the amygdala elicits the mechanical act of feeding. However, the most important effect of destruction of the amygdala on both sides of the brain is a "psychic blindness" in the choice of foods. In other words, the animal (and presumably the human being as well) loses or at least partially loses the mechanism of appetite control of type and quality of food that it eats.

The cortical regions of the limbic system, including the infraorbital regions, the hippocampal gyrus, and the cingulate gyrus, all have areas that when stimulated can either increase or decrease feeding activities. These areas seem especially to play a role in the animal's drive to search for food when it is hungry. It is presumed that these centers are also responsible, probably operating in association with the amygdala and hypothalamus, for determining the quality of food that is eaten. For instance, a previous unpleasant experience with almost any type of food often destroys a person's appetite for that food thenceforth.

FACTORS THAT REGULATE FOOD INTAKE

We can divide the regulation of food into (1) *nutritional regulation*, which is concerned primarily with maintenance of normal quantities of nutrient stores in the body, and (2) *alimentary regulation*, which is concerned primarily with the immediate effects of feeding on the alimentary tract and is sometimes called *peripheral regulation* or *short-term regulation*.

Nutritional Regulation. An animal that has been starved for a long time and is then presented with unlimited food eats a far greater quantity than does an animal that has been on a regular diet. Conversely, an animal that has been force-fed for several weeks eats little when allowed to eat according to its own desires. Thus, the feeding center in the hypothalamus is geared to the nutritional status of the body. Some of the nutritional factors that control the degree of activity of the feeding center are the following:

Availability of Glucose to the Body Cells—The Glucostatic Theory of Hunger and of Feeding Regulation. It has long been known that a decrease in blood glucose concentration is associated with development of hunger, which has led to the so-called *glucostatic theory of hunger and of feeding regulation:* When the blood glucose level falls too low, this automatically causes the animal to increase its feeding, which eventually returns the glucose concentration back toward normal. Two other observations also support the glucostatic theory: (1) An increase in blood glucose level increases the measured electrical activity in the satiety center in the ventromedial nuclei of the hypothalamus and simultaneously decreases the electrical activity in the feeding center of the lateral nuclei. (2) Chemical studies show that the ventromedial nuclei (the satiety center) concentrate glucose while other areas of the hypothalamus fail to concentrate glucose; therefore, it is assumed that glucose acts by increasing the degree of satiety.

Effect of Blood Amino Acid Concentration on Feeding. An increase in amino acid concentration in the blood also reduces feeding, and a decrease enhances feeding. In general, though, this effect is not as powerful as the glucostatic mechanism.

Effect of Fat Metabolites on Feeding—Long-Term Regulation. The overall degree of feeding varies almost inversely with the amount of adipose tissue in the body. That is, as the quantity of adipose tissue increases, the rate of feeding decreases. Therefore, many physiologists believe that *long-term regulation* of feeding is controlled mainly by fat metabolites of undiscovered nature. This is called the "lipostatic" theory of feeding regulation. In support of this is the fact that the long-term average concentration of free fatty acids in the blood is directly proportional to the quantity of adipose tissue in the body. Therefore, it is likely that the free fatty acids or some other similar fat metabolites act in the same manner as glucose and amino acids to cause a negative feedback regulatory effect on feeding. It is also possible, if not probable, that this is the most important long-term regulator of feeding.

Interrelationship Between Body Temperature and Food Intake. When an animal is exposed to cold, it tends to overeat; when exposed to heat, it tends to undereat. This is caused by interaction within the hypothalamus between the temperature-regulating system (discussed later in this chapter) and the food intake-regulating system. It is important because increased food intake in the cold animal increases its metabolic rate and provides increased fat for insulation, both of which tend to correct the cold state.

Summary of Long-Term Regulation. Even though our information on the different feedback factors in long-term feeding regulation is imprecise, we can make the following general statement: When the nutrient stores of the body fall below normal, the feeding center of the hypothalamus becomes highly active, and the person exhibits increased hunger; on the other hand, when the nutrient stores are abundant, the person loses the hunger and develops a state of satiety.

Alimentary Regulation (Short-Term, Nonmetabolic Regulation). The degree of hunger or satiety at different times of the day depends to a great extent on habit. For instance, normally, people have the habit of eating three meals a day, and, if they miss one, they are likely to develop a state of hunger at mealtime despite completely adequate nutritional stores in their tissues. But, in addition to habit, several other short-term physiological stimuli—mainly related to the alimentary tract—can alter one's desire for food for several hours at a time, as follows:

Gastrointestinal Filling. When the gastrointestinal tract becomes distended, especially the stomach or the duodenum, inhibitory signals temporarily suppress the feeding center, thereby reducing the desire for food. This effect probably depends mainly on sensory signals transmitted through the vagi, but part of the effect still persists after the vagi and the sympathetic nerves from the upper gastrointestinal tract have been severed. Therefore, somatic sensory signals from the stretched abdomen might also play a role. And, recently it has been found that hormonal feedback also suppresses feeding, for *cholecystokinin* that is released in response mainly to fat entering the duodenum has a strong effect on inhibition of further eating.

Obviously, these mechanisms are of particular importance in bringing one's feeding to a halt during a heavy meal.

Metering of Food by Head Receptors. When a person with an esophageal fistula is fed large quantities of food, even though this food is immediately lost again to the exterior, the degree of hunger is decreased after a reasonable quantity of food has passed through the mouth. This effect occurs despite the fact that the gastrointestinal tract does not become the least bit filled. Therefore, it is postulated that various "head factors" relating to feeding, such as chewing, salivation, swallowing, and tasting, "meter" the food as it passes through the mouth, and after a certain amount has passed through, the hypothalamic feeding center becomes inhibited. However, the inhibition caused by this metering mechanism is considerably less intense and less lasting, usually enduring only 20 to 40 minutes, than is the inhibition caused by gastrointestinal filling.

Importance of Having Both Long- and Short-term Regulatory Systems for Feeding. The long-term regulatory system, especially the lipostatic feedback mechanism, obviously helps an animal maintain constant stores of nutrients in its tissues, preventing these from becoming too low or too high. On the other hand, the short-term regulatory stimuli make the animal feed only when the gastrointestinal tract is receptive to food. Thus, food passes through its gastrointestinal tract fairly continuously so that its digestive, absorptive, and storage mechanisms can all work at a steady pace rather than only when the animal needs food for energy.

OBESITY

Energy Input Versus Energy Output. When greater quantities of energy (in the form of food) enter the body than are expended, the body weight increases. Therefore, obesity is obviously caused by excess energy input over energy output. For each 9.3 calories of excess energy entering the body, 1 gram of fat is stored.

Excess energy input occurs *only during the developing phase of obesity*, and once a person has become obese, all that is required to remain obese is that the energy input equal the energy output. For the person to reduce in weight, the input must be *less* than the output. Indeed, studies of obese persons have shown that the intake of food of most of them in the static stage of obesity (after the obesity has already been attained) is approximately the same as that for normal persons.

Effect of Muscular Activity on Energy Output. About one third of the energy used each day by the normal person goes into muscular activity, and in the laborer as much as two thirds or occasionally three fourths is used in this way. Since muscular activity is by far the most important means by which energy is expended in the body, it is frequently said that obesity results from *too high a ratio of food intake to daily exercise.*

Abnormal Feeding Regulation as a Pathological Cause of Obesity

We have already emphasized that the rate of feeding is normally regulated in proportion to the nutrient stores in the body. When these stores begin to approach an optimal level in a normal person, feeding is automatically reduced to prevent overstorage. However, in many obese persons this is not true, for feeding does not slacken until body weight is far above normal. Therefore, in effect, obesity is often caused by an abnormality of the feeding regulatory mechanism. This can result from either psychogenic factors that affect the regulation or actual abnormalities of the hypothalamus itself.

Psychogenic Obesity. Studies of obese patients show that a large proportion of obesity results from psychogenic factors. Perhaps the most common psychogenic factor contributing to obesity is the prevalent idea that healthy eating habits require three meals a day and that each meal must be filling. Many children are forced into this habit by overly solicitous parents, and the children continue to practice it throughout life. In addition, persons are known often to gain large amounts of weight during or following stressful situations, such as the death of a parent, a severe illness, or even mental depression. It seems that eating is often a means of release from tension.

Hypothalamic Abnormalities as a Cause of Obesity. In the preceding discussion of feeding regulation, it was pointed out that lesions in the ventromedial nuclei of the hypothalamus cause an animal to eat excessively and become obese. It has also been discovered that such lesions are associated with excess insulin production, which in turn increases fat deposition. Also, many persons with hypophysial tumors that encroach on the hypothalamus develop progressive obesity, illustrating that obesity in the human being, too, can definitely result from damage to the hypothalamus.

Yet, in the normal obese person hypothalamic damage is almost never found. Nevertheless, it is possible that the functional organization of the feeding center is differ-

ent in the obese person from that of the nonobese person. For instance, a normally obese person who has reduced to normal weight by strict dietary measures usually develops hunger that is demonstrably far greater than that of the normal person. This indicates that the "set-point" of the obese person's feeding center is at a much higher level of nutrient storage than that of the normal person.

REGULATION OF BODY TEMPERATURE—THE "HYPOTHALAMIC THERMOSTAT"

Figure 28–6 illustrates approximately what happens to the temperature of the nude body after a few hours' exposure to *dry* air ranging from 30° to 170° F. Obviously, the precise dimensions of this curve vary, depending on the movement of air, the amount of moisture in the air, and even the nature of the surroundings. However, in general, between approximately 60° and 130° F in dry air the nude body is capable of maintaining indefinitely a normal body core temperature somewhere between 97° and 100° F.

The temperature of the body is regulated almost entirely by nervous feedback mechanisms, and almost all of these operate through *temperature-regulating centers* located in the *hypothalamus*. However, for these feedback mechanisms to operate, there must also exist temperature detectors, discussed next, to determine when the body temperature becomes either too hot or too cold.

Thermostatic Detection of Temperature in the Hypothalamus—Role of the Preoptic Area

In recent years, experiments have been performed in which minute areas in the brain have been either heated or cooled by use of a so-called

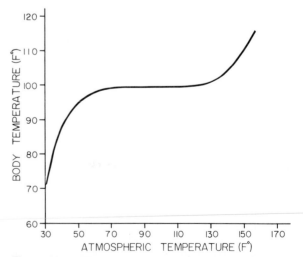

Figure 28–6. Effect of high and low atmospheric temperature for several hours' duration on the internal body temperature, showing that the internal body temperature remains stable despite wide changes in atmospheric temperature.

thermode. This small, needle-like device is heated by electrical means or by passing hot water through it, or it is cooled by cold water. The principal area in the brain in which heat from a thermode affects body temperature control is the preoptic area of the hypothalamus, and to a lesser extent the adjacent regions of the anterior hypothalamus.

Using the thermode, the preoptic area of the hypothalamus has been found to contain large numbers of heat-sensitive neurons that seem to function as temperature sensors for controlling body temperature. These neurons increase their firing rate as the temperature rises, the rate sometimes increasing as much as tenfold with an increase in body temperature of 10° C.

In addition to the heat-sensitive neurons, a few cold-sensitive neurons have also been found in the hypothalamus, in the septum, and in the reticular substance of the midbrain, all of which increase their rate of firing when exposed to cold. Also, still other neurons change their rates of firing in response to signals transmitted to the brain from cold and warmth receptors in the skin and certain deep tissues of the body. These signals are believed to interact with those from both the heat- and cold-sensitive neurons of the hypothalamus to provide the very effective temperature control system of the body.

When the preoptic area is heated, the skin immediately breaks out into a profuse sweat while at the same time the skin blood vessels over the entire body become greatly vasodilated. Thus, this is an immediate reaction to cause the body to lose heat, thereby helping to return the body temperature toward the normal level. In addition, excess body heat production is inhibited. Therefore, it is clear that the preoptic area of the hypothalamus has the capability of serving as a thermostatic body temperature control center.

Detection of Temperature by Receptors in the Skin and Deep Body Tissues

Though the signals generated by the temperature receptors of the hypothalamus are extremely powerful in controlling body temperature, temperature receptors in other parts of the body also play important roles in temperature regulation. This is especially true of temperature receptors in the skin and in a few specific deep tissues of the body.

It will be recalled from the discussion of sensory receptors in Chapter 13 that the skin is endowed with both *cold* and *warmth* receptors. However, there are far more cold receptors than warmth receptors; in fact, ten times as many in many parts of the skin. Therefore, peripheral detection of temperature mainly concerns detecting cool and cold instead of warm temperatures.

When the skin is chilled over the entire body, immediate reflex effects are invoked to increase the temperature of the body in several ways: (1) by providing a strong stimulus to cause shivering, with resultant increase in the rate of body heat production, (2) by inhibiting the process of sweating if this should be occurring, and (3) by promoting skin vasoconstriction to diminish the transfer of body heat to the skin.

The deep body temperature receptors are found only in certain parts of the body, mainly in the *spinal cord*, in the *abdominal viscera*, and in or around the *great veins*. However, these deep receptors function differently from the skin receptors, for they are exposed to the body core temperature rather than the body surface temperature. Yet, like the skin temperature receptors, they mainly detect cold rather than warmth. It is probable that both the skin and the deep body receptors are concerned with preventing hypothermia—that is, preventing low body temperatures.

Integration of the Temperature Signals in the Posterior Hypothalamus

Even though a large share of the signals for temperature detection arise in peripheral receptors, these signals help control body temperature mainly through the hypothalamus. However, the area of the hypothalamus that they stimulate is not the preoptic area but instead an area located bilaterally in the posterior hypothalamus approximately at the level of the mammary bodies. The thermostatic signals from the preoptic area are also transmitted into this posterior hypothalamus area. Here the signals from the preoptic area and the signals from the body periphery are combined to provide the heat-producing or heat-losing reactions of the body.

The overall heat-controlling mechanism of the hypothalamus is called the *hypothalamic thermostat.*

NEURONAL EFFECTOR MECHANISMS THAT DECREASE OR INCREASE BODY TEMPERATURE

When the hypothalamic thermostat detects that the body temperature is either too hot or too cold, it institutes appropriate temperature-decreasing or temperature-increasing procedures. The student is familiar with most of these from personal experience, but special features are the following:

Temperature-Decreasing Mechanisms

The thermostatic system employs three important mechanisms to reduce body heat when the temperature becomes too great:

1. *Vasodilatation.* In almost all areas of the body the skin blood vessels are intensely dilated. This is caused by *inhibition of the sympathetic centers in the posterior hypothalamus that cause vasoconstriction.* Full vasodilatation can increase the rate of heat transfer to the skin as much as eightfold.

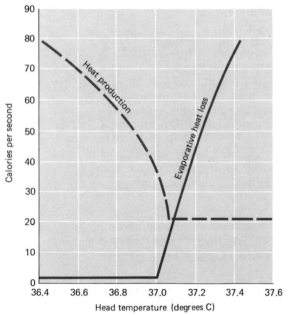

Figure 28–7. Effect of hypothalamic temperature on (1) evaporative heat loss from the body and (2) heat production caused primarily by muscular activity and shivering. This figure demonstrates the extremely critical temperature level at which increased heat loss begins and increased heat production stops. (Drawn from data in Benzinger, Kitzinger, and Pratt, in Hardy [ed.]: Temperature, Part 3, p. 637. Reinhold Publishing Corp.)

2. *Sweating.* The effect of increased temperature on sweating is illustrated by the solid curve in Figure 28–7, which shows a sharp increase in the rate of evaporative heat loss resulting from sweating when the body core temperature rises above the critical temperature level of 37° C (98.6° F). An additional 1° C increase in body temperature causes enough sweating to remove ten times the basal rate of body heat production.

3. *Decrease in heat production.* Those mechanisms that cause excess heat production, such as shivering and chemical thermogenesis, are strongly inhibited.

Temperature-Increasing Mechanisms

When the body is too cold, the temperature control system institutes exactly opposite procedures. These are:

1. *Skin vasoconstriction throughout the body.* This is caused by stimulation of the posterior hypothalamic sympathetic centers.

2. *Piloerection.* Piloerection means hairs "standing on end." Sympathetic stimulation causes the arrector pili muscles attached to the hair follicles to contract, which brings the hairs to an upright stance. This is not important in the human being, but in lower animals upright projection of the hairs allows them to entrap a thick layer of "insulator air" next to the skin so that the transfer of heat to the surroundings is greatly depressed.

3. *Increase in heat production.* Heat production by the metabolic systems is increased by promoting

(a) shivering, (b) sympathetic excitation of heat production, and (c) thyroxine secretion. These require additional explanation, as follows:

Hypothalamic Stimulation of Shivering. Located in the dorsomedial portion of the posterior hypothalamus near the wall of the third ventricle is an area called the *primary motor center for shivering.* This area is normally inhibited by signals from the heat center in the preoptic thermostatic area but is excited by cold signals from the skin and spinal cord. Therefore, as illustrated by the dashed curve in Figure 28–7, this center becomes activated when the body temperature falls even a fraction of a degree below a critical temperature level. It then transmits signals that cause shivering through bilateral tracts down the brain stem, into the lateral columns of the spinal cord, and, finally, to the anterior motor neurons. These signals are nonrhythmic and do not cause the actual muscle shaking. Instead, they increase the tone of the skeletal muscles throughout the body. When the tone rises above a certain critical level, shivering begins. This probably results from feedback oscillation of the muscle spindle stretch reflex mechanism, which was discussed in Chapter 15. During maximum shivering, body heat production can rise to as high as four to five times normal.

Sympathetic "Chemical" Excitation of Heat Production. It was pointed out in Chapter 21 that either sympathetic stimulation or circulating norepinephrine and epinephrine in the blood can cause an immediate increase in the rate of cellular metabolism; this effect is called *chemical thermogenesis,* and it results at least partially from the ability of norepinephrine and epinephrine to uncouple oxidative phosphorylation, as a result of which more oxidation of foodstuffs must occur to produce the energy required for normal function of the body. Therefore, the rate of cellular metabolism increases.

The degree of chemical thermogenesis that occurs in an animal is almost directly proportional to the amount of *brown* fat that exists in the animal's tissues. This is a type of fat that contains large numbers of mitochondria in its cells, and these cells are supplied by a strong sympathetic innervation.

The process of acclimatization greatly affects the intensity of chemical thermogenesis; some animals that have been exposed for several weeks to a very cold environment exhibit as much as a 100 to 500 per cent increase in heat production when acutely exposed to cold, in contrast to the unacclimatized animal, which responds with an increase of perhaps one third as much.

In adult human beings, who have almost no brown fat, it is rare that chemical thermogenesis increases the rate of heat production more than 10 to 15 per cent. However, in infants, who *do* have a small amount of brown fat in the interscapular space, chemical thermogenesis can increase the rate of heat production as much as 100 per cent, which is probably a very important factor in maintaining normal body temperature in the neonate.

Increased Thyroxine Output as a Cause of Increased Heat Production. Cooling the preoptic area of the hypothalamus also increases the production of the neurosecretory hormone *thyrotropin-releasing hormone* by the hypothalamus. This hormone is carried by way of the hypothalamic portal veins to the anterior pituitary gland where it stimulates the secretion of thyroid-stimulating hormone. Thyroid-stimulating hormone, in turn, stimulates increased output of thyroxine by the thyroid gland. The increased thyroxine increases the rate of cellular metabolism throughout the body, which is yet another mechanism of *chemical thermogenesis.* However, this increase in metabolism does not occur immediately but requires several weeks for the thyroid gland to hypertrophy before it reaches its new level of thyroxine secretion.

Exposure of animals to extreme cold for several weeks can cause their thyroid glands to increase in size as much as 20 to 40 per cent. However, human beings rarely allow themselves to be exposed to the same degree of cold as that to which animals have been subjected. Therefore, we still do not know, quantitatively, how important the thyroid method of adaptation to cold is in the human being. Yet, isolated measurements have shown that military personnel residing for several months in the Arctic develop increased metabolic rates; Eskimos also have abnormally high basal metabolic rates. Also, the continuous stimulatory effect of cold on the thyroid gland can probably explain the much higher incidence of toxic thyroid goiters in persons living in colder climates than in those living in warmer climates.

THE FEEDBACK GAIN FOR BODY TEMPERATURE CONTROL

Feedback gain is a measure of the effectiveness of a control system. In the case of body temperature control, it is important for the internal body temperature to change as little as possible despite marked changes in the environmental temperature, and the gain of the temperature control system is approximately equal to the ratio of the change in environmental temperature to the change in body temperature that this causes. Experiments have shown that the body temperature of man changes about 1° C for each 25° to 30° C change in environmental temperature. Therefore, the feedback gain of the hypothalamic thermostat mechanism for control of body temperature averages about 27, which is an extremely high gain for a biological control system (the baroreceptor arterial pressure control system, for instance, has a gain of less than 2).

BEHAVIORAL CONTROL OF BODY TEMPERATURE

Aside from the thermostatic mechanism for body temperature control, the body has still another temperature-controlling mechanism that is even more potent than all the previously cited mechanisms together. This is behavioral control of temperature, which can be explained as follows: Whenever the internal body temperature becomes too high, signals from the thermostatic brain areas give the person a psychic sensation of being overheated. Conversely, whenever the body becomes too cold, signals from the skin and probably also from the deep body receptors elicit the feeling of cold discomfort. Therefore, the person makes appropriate environmental adjustments to re-establish comfort. This is a much more powerful system of body temperature control than most physiologists have recognized in the past. Indeed, for people, this is the only really effective mechanism for body heat control in severely cold environs.

The obvious types of behavioral adjustments include selecting appropriate clothing, moving the body to a different environmental setting, increasing the delivery of heat or cold from appropriate heaters or air conditioners, and so forth.

It is important to note that many other of our body's control systems utilize similar behavior mechanisms to achieve highly refined degrees of control. For instance, even respiration is controlled to a great extent in this way—that is, when people perceive that they are being subjected to air hunger, they consciously breathe more to make up the deficit. Therefore, it is not valid to think of the body's homeostatic control systems as operating only in the subconscious portions of the brain.

FEVER

Fever, which means a body temperature above the normal range, may be caused by abnormalities in the brain itself or by toxic substances that affect the temperature-regulating centers. Some causes of fever are presented in Figure 28–8. These include

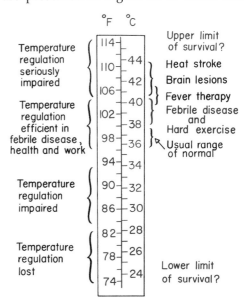

Figure 28–8. Body temperatures under different conditions. (From DuBois: Fever. Charles C Thomas.)

bacterial diseases, brain tumors, and environmental conditions that may terminate in heat stroke.

Resetting the Hypothalamic Thermostat in Febrile Diseases—Effect of Pyrogens

Many proteins, breakdown products of proteins, and certain other substances, especially lipopolysaccharide toxins secreted by bacteria, can cause the set-point of the hypothalamic thermostat to rise. Substances that cause this effect are called *pyrogens*. It is pyrogens secreted by toxic bacteria or pyrogens released from degenerating tissues of the body that cause fever during disease conditions. When the set-point of the hypothalamic thermostat becomes increased to a higher level than normal, all the mechanisms for raising the body temperature are brought into play, including heat conservation and increased heat production. Within a few hours after the thermostat has been set to a higher level, the body temperature also approaches this level.

Mechanism of Action of Pyrogens in Causing Fever—Role of "Endogenous Pyrogen." Experiments in animals have shown that most pyrogens, when injected into the hypothalamus, can act directly on the hypothalamic thermostat to increase its set-point, though many pyrogens require several hours of latent period before causing this effect. However, many of the bacterial pyrogens, especially the *endotoxins* from gram-negative bacteria, can also cause very severe fever acting in an indirect manner rather than directly on the hypothalamus.

When bacteria or breakdown products of bacteria are present in the tissues or in the blood, these are *phagocytized by the blood leukocytes and the tissue macrophages*. Both these types of cells in turn digest the bacterial products and then release into the body fluids a substance called *leukocyte pyrogen* or *endogenous pyrogen*. This endogenous pyrogen, on reaching the hypothalamus, immediately produces fever, increasing the body temperature in as little as 8 to 10 minutes. As little as one ten millionth of a gram of endotoxin lipopolysaccharide acting in this manner in concert with the blood leukocytes and the tissue macrophages can cause fever. The amount of endogenous pyrogen that is formed in response to the lipopolysaccharide to cause the fever is only a few nanograms.

Several recent experiments have suggested that endogenous pyrogen causes fever by first inducing the formation of *prostaglandin E$_1$* in the local cells of the hypothalamus; the prostaglandin E$_1$ in turn elicits the fever reaction. When prostaglandin formation is blocked by drugs, the fever is either completely abrogated or at least reduced. In fact, this may be the explanation for the manner in which aspirin reduces the degree of fever, because aspirin impedes the formation of prostaglandins. It also would explain why aspirin does not lower the body temperature in a normal person, because a normal person does not have any endogenous pyrogen

affecting the hypothalamus. Drugs such as aspirin that reduce the level of fever are called *antipyretics*.

Fever Caused by Brain Lesions. When a brain surgeon operates in the region of the hypothalamus, this almost invariably causes severe fever, though rarely the opposite effect occurs, thus illustrating both the potency of the hypothalamic thermostat mechanism for body temperature control and also the ease with which abnormalities of the hypothalamus can alter the set-point of the thermostat. Another condition that frequently causes prolonged high temperature is compression of the hypothalamus by brain tumors.

Characteristics of Febrile Conditions

Chills. When the set-point of the hypothalamic thermostat is suddenly changed from the normal level to a higher than normal value as a result of tissue destruction, pyrogenic substances, or dehydration, the body temperature usually takes several hours to reach the new temperature set-point. Figure 28–9 illustrates this, showing the effect of suddenly increasing the set-point to a level of 103° F. Because the blood temperature is less than the set-point of the hypothalamic thermostat, the usual responses that cause elevation of body temperature occur. During this period the person experiences chills and feels extremely cold, even though his or her body temperature may already be above normal. Also, the skin is cold because of vasoconstriction, and the person shakes all over because of shivering. Chills continue until the body temperature reaches the hypothalamic setting of 103° F. Then, when the temperature of the body reaches this value, the person no longer experiences chills but instead feels neither cold nor hot. As long as the factor that is causing the hypothalamic thermostat to be set at this high value continues its effect, the body temperature is regulated more or less in the normal manner but at the high temperature set-point level.

The Crisis, or "Flush." If the factor that is causing the high temperature is suddenly removed, the set-

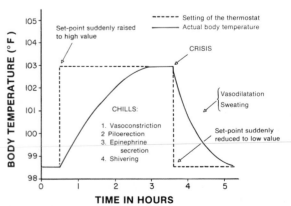

Figure 28–9. Effects of changing the setting of the "hypothalamic thermostat."

point of the hypothalamic thermostat is suddenly reduced to a lower value—perhaps even back to the normal level, as illustrated in Figure 28–9. In this instance, the body temperature is still 103° F, but the hypothalamus is attempting to regulate the temperature to 98.6° F. This situation is analogous to excessive heating of the preoptic area, which causes intense sweating and sudden development of a hot skin because of vasodilatation everywhere. This sudden change of events in a febrile disease is known as the "crisis" or, more appropriately, the "flush." In olden days, before the advent of antibiotics, the crisis was always awaited, for once this occurred the doctor knew immediately that the patient's temperature would soon be falling, which is called *defervescence*.

REFERENCES

GASTROINTESTINAL MOTILITY

Gabella, G.: Structural apparatus for force transmission in smooth muscle. *Physiol. Rev.,* 64:455, 1984.

Hunt, J. N.: Mechanisms and disorders of gastric emptying. *Ann. Rev., Med.,* 34:219, 1983.

Klimov, P. K.: Behavior of the organs of the digestive system. *Neurosci. Behav. Physiol.,* 14:333, 1984.

Luschei, E. S., and Goldberg, L. J.: Neural mechanisms of mandibular control: mastication and voluntary biting. *In* Brooks, V. B. (ed.): Handbook of Physiology, Sec. 1, Vol. II. Bethesda, American Physiological Society, 1981, p. 1237.

Miller, A. J.: Deglutition. *Physiol. Rev.,* 62:129, 1982.

Weems, W. A.: The intestine as a fluid propelling system. *Ann. Rev. Physiol.,* 43:9, 1981.

Wood, J. D.: Intrinsic neural control of intestinal motility. *Ann. Rev. Physiol.,* 43:33, 1981.

GASTROINTESTINAL SECRETION

Burnham, D. B., and Williams, J. A.: Stimulus-secretion coupling in pancreatic acinar cells. *J. Pediatr. Gastroenterol. Nutr.,* 3 (Suppl. 1):S1, 1984.

Ginsberg, B. L., and House, C. R.: Stimulus-response coupling in gland cells. *Ann. Rev. Biophys. Bioeng.,* 90:55, 1980.

Shepherd, A. P.: Local control of intestinal oxygenation and blood flow. *Ann. Rev. Physiol.,* 44:13, 1982.

Soll, A., and Walsh, J. H.: Regulation of gastric acid secretion. *Annu. Rev. Physiol.,* 41:35, 1979.

Williams, J. A.: Regulatory mechanisms in pancreas and salivary acini. *Annu. Rev. Physiol.,* 46:361, 1984.

MICTURITION

Charlton, C. A.: The Urological System. New York, Churchill Livingstone, Inc., 1983.

FOOD INTAKE

Anderson, K. E., *et al.*: Nutrient regulation of chemical metabolism in humans. *Fed. Proc.,* 44:130, 1985.

Baile, C. A., and Forbes, J. M.: Control of feed intake and regulation of energy balance in ruminants. *Physiol. Rev.,* 54:160, 194.

Magnen, J. L.: Body energy balance and food intake: A neuroendocrine regulatory mechanism. *Physiol. Rev.,* 63:314, 1983.

Oomura, Y., and Yoshimatsu, H.: Neural network of glucose monitoring system. *J. Auton. Nerv. Syst.,* 10:359, 1984.

Storlien, L. H.: The role of the ventromedial hypothalamic area in periprandial glucoregulation. *Life Sci.,* 360:505, 1985.

TEMPERATURE REGULATION

Benzinger, T. H.: Heat regulation: Homeostasis of central temperature in man. *Physiol. Rev.,* 49:61, 1969.

Crawshaw, L. I.: Temperature regulation in vertebrates. *Annu. Rev. Physiol.,* 42:43, 1980.

Galanter, E.: Detection and discrimination of environmental change. *In* Darian-Smith, I. (ed.): Handbook of Physiology. Sec. 1, Vol. III. Bethesda, American Physiological Society, 1984, p. 103.

Hales, J. E. (ed.): Thermal Physiology. New York, Raven Press, 1984.

Hardy, J. D.: Physiology of temperature regulation. *Physiol. Rev.,* 41:521, 1961.

Hensel, H.: Neural processes in thermoregulation. *Physiol. Rev.,* 53:948, 193.

Quinton, P. M.: Sweating and its disorders. *Annu. Rev. Med.,* 34:453, 1983.

29

Hypothalamic and Pituitary Control of Hormones and Reproduction

One of the means by which the nervous system controls bodily acitivity is by increasing or decreasing the secretion of many of the body's hormones. In previous chapters we have already discussed part of this function, such as control of the secretion of epinephrine and norepinephrine by the autonomic nervous system and control of different local hormones in the gastrointestinal tract.

In this chapter we will discuss a much more global means by which the nervous system controls the secretion of hormones by most of the body's endocrine glands. These hormones in turn control many if not most of the body's metabolic functions as well as reproduction.

The nervous system's central control area for this global system is the *hypothalamus,* which controls the secretions of at least eight important hormones by the pituitary gland. These pituitary hormones in turn control the secretion of still other hormones by the thyroid gland, the adrenal glands, and the ovaries or testes. The function of the hypothalamus, and therefore its control effects on this pyramidal hormonal system, is itself controlled by nerve signals from almost all other parts of the brain, especially signals elicited by such subconscious nervous effects as the emotions, sex drives, body temperature, hunger, thirst, and even the crying of a baby.

It will not be possible to describe in the limited pages of this text this entire system and its multiple effects on the body. Yet, in this chapter we will discuss the most important features of the system, (1) the relationship of the hypothalamus to the pituitary gland and (2) the neurohormonal factors that promote the onset of reproduction.

THE PITUITARY GLAND AND ITS RELATION TO THE HYPOTHALAMUS

The *pituitary gland* (Fig. 29–1), also called the *hypophysis,* is a small gland—about 1 cm in diameter and 0.5 to 1 gram in weight—that lies in the *sella*

turcica at the base of the brain and is connected with the hypothalamus by the *pituitary* (or *hypophysial) stalk.* Physiologically, the pituitary gland is divisible into two distinct portions: the *anterior pituitary,* also known as the *adenohypophysis,* and the *posterior pituitary,* also known as the *neurohypophysis.* Between these is a small, relatively avascular zone called the *pars intermedia,* which is almost absent in the human being while much larger and much more functional in some lower animals.

Embryologically, the two portions of the pituitary originate from different sources, the anterior pituitary from *Rathke's pouch,* which is an embryonic invagination of the pharyngeal epithelium, and the posterior pituitary from an outgrowth of the hypothalamus. The origin of the anterior pituitary from the pharyngeal epithelium explains the epithelioid nature of its cells, while the origin of the posterior pituitary from neural tissue explains the presence of large numbers of glial-type cells in this gland.

Six very important hormones plus several less important ones are secreted by different types of cells in the anterior pituitary, and two important hormones are secreted by the posterior pituitary. The hormones of the anterior pituitary play major roles in the control of metabolic functions throughout the body, as shown in Figure 29–2. (1) *Growth hormone* promotes growth by affecting many metabolic functions throughout the body, especially protein formation. (2) *Adrenocorticotropin* controls the secretion of some of the adrenocortical hormones, which in turn affect the metabolism of glucose, proteins, and fats. (3) *Thyroid-stimulating hormone* controls the rate of secretion of thyroxine by the thyroid gland, and thyroxine in turn controls the rates of most chemical reactions of the entire body. (4) *Prolactin* promotes mammary gland development and milk production. And two separate gonadotropic hormones, (5) *follicle-stimulating hormone* and (6) *luteinizing hormone,* control growth of the gonads as well as their reproductive activities.

The two hormones secreted by the posterior pi-

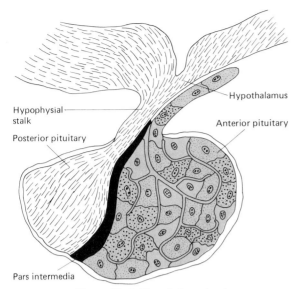

Figure 29–1. The pituitary gland.

tuitary play other roles. (1) *Antidiuretic hormone* (also called *vasopressin*) controls the rate of water excretion into the urine and in this way helps control the concentration of water in the body fluids. (2) *Oxytocin* helps deliver milk from the glands of the breast to the nipples during suckling, and possibly helps in the delivery of the baby at the end of gestation.

CONTROL OF PITUITARY SECRETION BY THE HYPOTHALAMUS

Almost all secretion by the pituitary is controlled by either hormonal or nervous signals from the hypothalamus. Indeed, when the pituitary gland is removed from its normal position beneath the hypothalamus and transplanted to some other part of the body, its rates of secretion of the different hormones (except for prolactin) fall to low levels—in the case of some of the hormones, almost to zero.

Secretion from the posterior pituitary is controlled by nerve fibers originating in the hypothalamus and terminating in the posterior pituitary. In contrast, secretion by the anterior pituitary is controlled by hormones called *hypothalamic releasing* and *inhibitory hormones* (or *factors*) secreted within the hypothalamus itself and then conducted to the anterior pituitary through minute blood vessels called *hypothalamic-hypophysial portal vessels*. In the anterior pituitary these releasing and inhibitory hormones act on the glandular cells to control their secretion. This system of control will be discussed in detail later in the chapter.

The hypothalamus receives signals from almost all possible sources in the nervous system. Thus, when a person is exposed to pain, a portion of the pain signal is transmitted into the hypothalamus. Likewise, when a person experiences some power-

ful depressing or exciting thought, a portion of the signal is transmitted into the hypothalamus. Olfactory stimuli denoting pleasant or unpleasant smells transmit strong signal components directly and through the amygdaloid nuclei into the hypothalamus. *Even the concentrations of nutrients, electrolytes, water, and various hormones* in the blood excite or inhibit various portions of the hypothalamus. Thus, the hypothalamus is a collecting center for information concerned with the internal well-being of the body, and in turn much of this information is used to control secretions of the many globally important pituitary hormones.

THE HYPOTHALAMIC-HYPOPHYSIAL PORTAL SYSTEM

The anterior pituitary is a highly vascular gland with extensive capillary sinuses among the glandular cells. Almost all the blood that enters these sinuses passes first through a capillary bed in the tissue of the lower tip of the hypothalamus and then through small *hypothalamic-hypophysial portal vessels* into the anterior pituitary sinuses. Thus, Figure 29–3 illustrates a small artery supplying the lowermost portion of the hypothalamus called the *median eminence* that connects inferiorly with the pituitary stalk. Small blood vessels project into the substance of the median eminence and then return to its surface, coalescing to form the hypothalamic-hypophysial portal vessels. These in turn pass downward along the pituitary stalk to supply blood to the anterior pituitary sinuses.

Secretion of Hypothalamic Releasing and Inhibitory Hormones into the Median Eminence. Special neurons in the hypothalamus synthesize and secrete hormones called *hypothalamic releasing* and *inhibitory hormones* (or *releasing* and *inhibitory factors*)

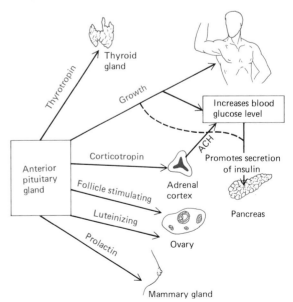

Figure 29–2. Metabolic functions of the anterior pituitary hormones.

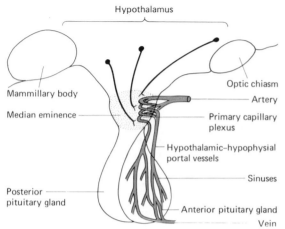

Figure 29–3. The hypothalamic-hypophysial portal system.

that control the secretion of the anterior pituitary hormones. These neurons originate in various parts of the hypothalamus and send their nerve fibers into the median eminence and the tuber cinereum, the hypothalamic tissue that extends into the pituitary stalk. The endings of these fibers are different from most endings in the central nervous system in that their function is not to transmit signals from one neuron to another but merely to secrete the hypothalamic releasing and inhibitory hormones (factors) into the tissue fluids. These hormones are immediately absorbed into the capillaries of the hypothalamic-hypophysial portal system and carried directly to the sinuses of the anterior pituitary gland.

(To avoid confusion, the student needs to know the difference between a "factor" and a "hormone." A substance that has the actions of a hormone but that has not been purified and identified as a distinct chemical compound is called a *factor*. Once it has been so identified it is thereafter known as a *hormone* instead of simply a factor.)

Function of the Releasing and Inhibitory Hormones. The function of the releasing and inhibitory hormones is to control the secretion of the anterior pituitary hormones. For each type of anterior pituitary hormone there is usually a corresponding hypothalamic releasing hormone; for some of the anterior pituitary hormones there is also a corresponding hypothalamic inhibitory factor. For most of the anterior pituitary hormones it is the releasing hormone that is important; but, for prolactin, an inhibitory hormone probably exerts most control. The hypothalamic releasing and inhibitory hormones (or factors) that are of major importance are:

1. *Thyroid-stimulating hormone releasing hormone* (TRH), which causes release of thyroid-stimulating hormone

2. *Corticotropin-releasing factor* (CRF), which causes release of adrenocorticotropin

3. *Growth hormone releasing hormone* (GHRH), which causes release of growth hormone, and

growth hormone inhibitory hormone (GHIH), which is the same as the hormone *somatostatin* and which inhibits the release of growth hormone

4. *Luteinizing hormone releasing hormone* (LRH), which causes release of both luteinizing hormone and follicle-stimulating hormone—this hormone is also called *gonadotropin-releasing hormone* (GnRH)

5. *Prolactin inhibitory factor* (PIF), which causes inhibition of prolactin secretion

In addition to these more important hypothalamic hormones, still another excites the secretion of prolactin, and several hypothalamic inhibitory hormones inhibit some of the other anterior pituitary hormones.

Specific Areas in the Hypothalamus That Control Secretion of Particular Hypothalamic Releasing and Inhibitory Factors. All or most of the hypothalamic hormones are secreted at nerve endings in the median eminence before being transported to the anterior pituitary gland. Electrical stimulation of this region excites these nerve endings and therefore causes release of essentially all the hypothalamic factors. However, the neuronal cell bodies that give rise to these median eminence nerve endings are located in other discrete areas of the hypothalamus or in closely related areas of the basal brain. Unfortunately, the specific loci of the neuronal cell bodies that form the different hypothalamic releasing or inhibitory hormones are so incompletely known that it would be misleading to attempt a delineation here.

Other Hypothalamic Substances That May Have Hormonal Effects. Multiple other substances, especially many small peptides, are found in the neurons of the hypothalamus. However, functions for these as hormones are only speculative. Yet, because they are of research interest, they are listed here: (1) *substance P*, (2) *neurotensin*, (3) *angiotensin II*, (4) *enkephalins*, (5) *endorphins*, (6) *vasoactive inhibitory polypeptide*, and (7) *cholecystokinin-8*. Many of these same substances are also found in neurons elsewhere in the brain, suggesting that they may function as neurotransmitters both in the hypothalamus and elsewhere. In addition, some of them are in the neurons of the enteric nervous system of the gastrointestinal tract, functioning there also as neurotransmitters and possibly as hormones released into the circulating blood from the nerve endings.

PHYSIOLOGICAL FUNCTIONS OF THE ANTERIOR PITUITARY HORMONES

All the major anterior pituitary hormones besides growth hormone exert their principal effects by stimulating target glands—such as the thyroid gland, the adrenal cortex, the ovaries, the testicles, and the mammary glands. We will discuss briefly the functions of four of the pituitary hormones, *growth hormone, thyroid-stimulating hormone, adrenocorticotropin,* and *prolactin.* The functions of the two gonadotropic hormones, *luteinizing hormone* and *follicle-stimulating hormone*, will be discussed later in this chapter.

GROWTH HORMONE

Growth hormone is secreted by the anterior pituitary gland throughout the entire life of a person. Its rate of secretion is controlled by *growth hormone–releasing hormone*, which is formed in the hypothalamus and transmitted to the anterior pituitary gland through the hypothalamic-hypophysial portal system.

Growth hormone has two major functions: The first of these is to promote growth of the infant into the child and then of the child into the adult. One of the growth-promoting effects is to cause growth of the bones, thus making the skeleton grow progressively longer and longer. However, the body stops increasing in height at adolescence because the long bones of the body then lose their capability for growth, not because of cessation of production of growth hormone. In addition to causing the bones to grow, this hormone promotes growth of essentially all other tissues of the body.

The second function of growth hormone is to control several of the metabolic functions of the body. Though these have not been defined in great detail, it is clear that growth hormone is essential for protein formation and for its maintenance in essentially all cells of the body. This, presumably, is the principal cause of growth. Growth hormone also enhances fat utilization but at the same time decreases carbohydrate use by the cells.

When growth hormone is not secreted by the anterior pituitary gland of a child, growth fails to occur, and the result is a so-called *pituitary dwarf* who retains childish features and often attains a height no greater than two to three feet. On the other hand, excess production of growth hormone by the anterior pituitary gland, caused usually by a tumor of the pituitary's growth hormone–producing cells, will cause the person to become a *giant*.

THYROID–STIMULATING HORMONE AND ITS CONTROL OF THYROID GLAND SECRETION

The thyroid gland secretes two hormones, *thyroxin* and *diiodothyronine*, that are very important in controlling the overall rate of metabolism of almost all tissues of the body—that is in controlling how rapidly the chemical reactions occur in all the tissues. When the rate of metabolism is great, a large amount of heat is also formed in the body, so that these thyroid hormones also play an important role in controlling body temperature.

Control of thyroid hormone secretion is vested in the hypothalamus and anterior pituitary gland. The hypothalamus secretes *thyroid-stimulating hormone–releasing hormone*. This then passes by way of the hypothalamic-hypophysial portal system to the anterior pituitary gland where it causes the release of *thyroid-stimulating hormone;* the thyroid-stimulating hormone, in turn, is carried to the thyroid gland in the blood and is the controller of the secretion of the thyroid hormones. Therefore, damage to either the hypothalamus or the anterior pituitary gland, especially the latter, can greatly reduce the rate of production of the thyroid hormones.

In the absence of the thyroid hormones, the person develops *hypothyroidism,* in which all the bodily activities become very sluggish, and the person often becomes obese. On the other hand, overactivity of the hypothalamus or anterior pituitary gland can cause *hyperthyroidism,* in which the bodily functions become greatly overactive. Many of the body's tissues can actually be seriously damaged because of this overactivity. The person also is very excitable and nervous. Hyperthyroidism is often caused by psychic stress that elicits excessive signals through the hypothalamus.

Fortunately, in the normal person there is a feedback mechanism for control of thyroid secretion. That is, when thyroid secretion becomes too great, the hypothalamic-pituitary control system itself becomes inhibited, thus returning the body to normal thyroid secretion.

ADRENOCORTICOTROPIN AND ITS CONTROL OF THE ADRENOCORTICAL HORMONES

Each person has two adrenal glands, lying respectively on top of the superior poles of the two kidneys. The cortical portions of these glands secrete several different steroid hormones, the two most important of which are *cortisol* and *aldosterone*. The rate of secretion of aldosterone is controlled mainly by such factors as plasma potassium ion concentration and by the hormone angiotensin. On the other hand, the secretion of cortisol by the adrenal cortex is controlled almost entirely by the rate of secretion of adrenocorticotropin by the anterior pituitary. And the rate of secretion of adrenocorticotropin is itself controlled by *corticotropin-releasing hormone*, which is formed in the hypothalamus and transported to the pituitary gland through the hypothalamic-hypophysial portal system.

Cortisol has powerful controlling effects on many metabolic functions of the body, including protein metabolism, carbohydrate metabolism, and fat metabolism. For instance, it has an opposite effect on protein metabolism to that of growth hormone—that is, it reduces the amount of protein in most of the tissues. In doing so, it releases amino acids into the circulating blood that can be used elsewhere in the body when they are required to repair damaged tissues. For this reason as well as others, cortisol is a very valuable hormone to help the body resist tissue destruction during stress. Cortisol also enhances the conversion of amino acids into carbohydrates, which in turn are used for energy. It increases the utilization of fats for energy as well.

The hypothalamic control of cortisol secretion is especially important. Within minutes after a person experiences serious physical stress, such as a broken bone, excessive heat, hemorrhage, or almost any other life-threatening occurrence, the level of cortisol circulating in the body fluids increases many times, sometimes 20-fold or more. And the cortisol in turn plays a very significant role in helping the cells resist the destructive effects of the stress.

PROLACTIN AND ITS CONTROL OF MILK SECRETION

Under normal conditions, the rate of prolactin secretion is relatively slight. However, during pregnancy its secretion increases progressively until it becomes about ten times normal by the time the baby is born. The prolactin helps to promote growth of protein tissues in the fetus. But its most important function is its ability to cause development of the breasts during pregnancy and to cause milk secretion after birth of the baby.

Even though prolactin stimulates development of the breasts during pregnancy, the large quantities of estrogens and progesterone that are secreted by the placenta during pregnancy inhibit milk production until the baby is born. But after birth, when the placenta is no longer available to secrete the estrogens and progesterone, the prolactin then causes rapid secretion of milk by the breasts. Furthermore, everytime the baby suckles a breast, nerve signals pass from the breast, up the spinal cord, and into the hypothalamus to cause an increase in prolactin secretion and therefore production of more milk.

The hypothalamus controls prolactin secretion somewhat differently from the way that it controls the secretion of other anterior pituitary hormones. It does so by an inhibitory hormone, *prolactin inhibitory hormone,* rather than by a releasing hormone. That is, the hypothalamus normally secretes an excess of prolactin inhibitory hormone, which keeps the rate of secretion of prolactin at a relatively low level. However, during pregnancy and during periods of milk production, the hypothalamus *decreases* its rate of formation of prolactin inhibitory hormone, in this way allowing increased production of prolactin.

Because of the essential role of the hypothalamus in milk secretion, strong psychic stimuli, particularly emotional states of anguish, can actually cause the mother's milk-secreting apparatus to dry up.

THE POSTERIOR PITUITARY GLAND AND ITS RELATION TO THE HYPOTHALAMUS

The *posterior pituitary gland,* also called the *neurohypophysis,* is composed mainly of glial-like cells called *pituicytes.* However, the pituicytes do not secrete hormones; they act simply as a supporting structure for large numbers of *terminal nerve fibers* and *terminal nerve endings* from nerve tracts that originate in the *supraoptic* and *paraventricular nuclei* of the hypothalamus, as shown in Figure 29–4. These tracts pass to the neurohypophysis through the *pituitary stalk* (hypophysial stalk). The nerve endings are bulbous knobs that lie on the surfaces of capillaries onto which they secrete the two posterior pituitary hormones: (1) *antidiuretic hormone* (ADH), also called *vasopressin,* and (2) *oxytocin.*

If the pituitary stalk is cut near the pituitary gland, leaving the entire hypothalamus intact, the posterior pituitary hormones continue, after a transient decrease for a few days, to be secreted almost normally, but they are then secreted by the cut ends of the fibers within the hypothalamus and not by the nerve endings in the posterior pituitary. The reason for this is that the hormones are initially synthesized in the cell bodies of the supraoptic and paraventricular nuclei and are then transported in combination with "carrier" proteins called *neurophysins* down to the nerve endings in the posterior pituitary gland, requiring about a week to reach the gland.

ADH is formed primarily in the supraoptic nuclei, whereas oxytocin is formed primarily in the paraventricular nuclei. However, each of these two nuclei can synthesize approximately one sixth as much of the second hormone as of its primary hormone.

Under resting conditions, large quantities of both ADH and oxytocin accumulate in large secretory granules in the nerve endings of the posterior pituitary gland, still loosely bound with their respective neurophysins. Then, when nerve impulses are transmitted downward along the fibers from

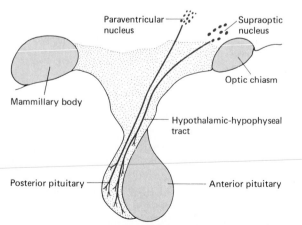

Figure 29–4. Hypothalamic control of the posterior pituitary.

the supraoptic or paraventricular nuclei, the hormone is immediately released from the nerve endings by the usual secretory mechanism of *exocytosis* and is absorbed into adjacent capillaries. Both the neurophysin and the hormone are secreted together, but since they are only loosely bound to each other, it is believed that the hormone separates almost immediately. The neurophysin has no known function after leaving the nerve terminals.

FUNCTION OF THE POSTERIOR PITUITARY HORMONES:

Antidiuretic Hormone. The function of antidiuretic hormone was discussed in detail in Chapter 27. It was pointed out that special neuronal cells called osmoreceptors located in the supraoptic nucleus are stimulated when the osmotic concentration of the extracellular fluids becomes too great. These cells then secrete antidiuretic hormone at their endings in the posterior pituitary gland. The antidiuretic hormone in turn acts on the tubules of the kidneys to cause increased water reabsorption, which retains water in the body fluids while allowing sodium and other dissolved substances to be excreted into the urine. Over a period of hours to days by this process the body fluids are diluted and their osmotic concentration returns to normal.

Oxytocin. The hormone oxytocin powerfully stimulates the pregnant uterus, especially so toward the end of gestation. Therefore, many physiologists believe that this hormone is at least partially responsible for causing birth. In fact, in a hypophysectomized animal, the duration of labor is prolonged. Also, the amount of oxytocin in the plasma increases during the latter stages of labor. And, finally, stimulation of the cervix in a pregnant animal elicits nerve signals that pass through the hypothalamus to the posterior pituitary gland to cause increased secretion of oxytocin.

Therefore, there are many reasons to believe that the intense stretching of the cervix of the uterus during labor elicits nervous reflexes which excite the anterior hypothalamus to cause increased secretion of the hormone oxytocin. The oxytocin in turn supposedly promotes additional contraction of the uterus, which expels the baby much more rapidly than would otherwise occur. In other words, once labor begins, this oxytocin feedback mechanism helps to create a cycle of progressively increasing uterine contractions that ordinarily will not stop until the baby is delivered.

Effect of oxytocin on milk ejection. Oxytocin also plays an important role in the process of lactation, a role that is far more certain than its possible role in the delivery of the baby. In lactation, oxytocin causes milk to be expressed from the alveoli of the breasts into the ducts that lead to the nipple. This makes the milk available to the baby by suckling.

This mechanism works as follows: The suckling stimuli on the nipple cause signals to be transmitted through sensory nerves to the brain. The signals pass upward through the brain stem and finally reach the oxytocin neurons in the paraventricular and supraoptic nuclei in the hypothalamus, to cause release of oxytocin. The oxytocin then is carried by the blood to the breasts. Here it causes contraction of *myoepithelial cells* that lie outside of and form a lattice-work around the alveoli of the mammary glands. In less than a minute after the beginning of suckling, milk begins to flow. Therefore, this mechanism is frequently called *milk let-down* or *milk ejection.*

CONTROL OF MALE SEXUAL FUNCTIONS BY THE GONADOTROPIC HORMONES— FSH AND LH

The anterior pituitary gland secretes two major gonadotropic hormones: (1) *follicle-stimulating hormone* (FSH); and (2) *luteinizing hormone* (LH). These are glycoprotein hormones that play major roles in the control of both male and female sexual function.

Regulation of Testosterone Production by LH. Testosterone is produced by the interstitial cells of Leydig only when the testes are stimulated by LH from the pituitary gland, and the quantity of testosterone secreted increases approximately in direct proportion to the amount of LH available.

Injection of purified LH into a child causes fibroblasts in the interstitial areas of the testes to develop into interstitial cells of Leydig, though mature Leydig cells are not normally found in the child's testes until after the age of approximately 10 years. Also, simultaneous administration of *prolactin* (another pituitary hormone that is closely associated with the gonadotropic hormones) greatly potentiates the effect of LH in promoting testosterone production.

Regulation of Pituitary Secretion of LH and FSH by the Hypothalamus

The gonadotropins, like corticotropin and thyrotropin, are secreted by the anterior pituitary gland mainly in response to nervous activity in the hypothalamus. For instance, in the female rabbit, coitus with a male rabbit elicits nervous activity in the hypothalamus that in turn stimulates the anterior pituitary to secrete FSH and LH. These hormones then cause rapid ripening of follicles in the rabbit's ovaries, followed a few hours later by ovulation.

Many other types of nervous stimuli are also known to affect gonadotropin secretion. For instance, in sheep, goats, and deer, nervous stimuli in response to changes in weather and amount of light in the day increase the quantities of gonadotropins during one season of the year, the mating season, thus allowing birth of the young during an appropriate period for survival. Also, psychic stimuli can affect fertility of the male animal, as exemplified by the fact that transporting a bull under uncomfortable conditions can often cause almost complete temporary sterility. In the human being, too, it is known that various psychic stimuli feeding into the hypothalamus can cause marked excitatory or inhibitory effects on gonadotropin secretion, in this way sometimes greatly altering the degree of fertility.

Luteinizing Hormone Releasing Hormone (LHRH), the Hypothalamic Hormone That Stimulates Gonadotropin Secretion. In both the male and the female the hypothalamus controls gonadotropin secretion by way of the hypothalamic-hypophysial portal system, as was discussed earlier in the chapter. Though there are two different gonadotropic hormones, luteinizing hormone and follicle-stimulating hormone, only one hypothalamic-releasing hormone has been discovered; this is *luteinizing hormone releasing hormone* (LHRH). Though this hormone has an especially strong effect on inducing luteinizing hormone secretion by the anterior pituitary gland, it has a potent effect in causing follicle-stimulating hormone secretion as well. For this reason it is often also called *gonadotropin-releasing hormone.*

LHRH plays a similar role in controlling gonadotropin secretion in the female, where the interrelationships are far more complex. Therefore, its nature and its functions will be discussed in much more detail later in the chapter.

Reciprocal Inhibition of Hypothalamic-Anterior Pituitary Secretion of Gonadotropic Hormones by Testicular Hormones. *Feedback Control of Testosterone Secretion.* Injection of testosterone into either a male or a female animal strongly inhibits the secretion of luteinizing hormone but only slightly inhibits the secretion of the follicle-stimulating hormone. This inhibition depends on normal function of the hypothalamus; therefore, it is quite clear that the following negative feedback control system operates continuously to control very precisely the rate of testosterone secretion:

1. The hypothalamus secretes *luteinizing hormone releasing hormone,* which stimulates the anterior pituitary gland to secrete *luteinizing hormone.*

2. Luteinizing hormone in turn stimulates *hyperplasia of the Leydig cells* of the testes and also stimulates production of *testosterone* by these cells.

3. The testosterone in turn feeds back negatively to the hypothalamus, inhibiting production of luteinizing hormone releasing hormone. This obviously limits the rate at which testosterone will be produced. On the other hand, when testosterone production is too low, lack of inhibition of the hypothalamus leads to subsequent return of testosterone secretion to the normal level.

Feedback Control of Spermatogenesis—Role of "Inhibin." It is known, too, that spermatogenesis by the testes inhibits the secretion of FSH. Con-

versely, failure of spermatogenesis causes markedly increased secretion of FSH; this is especially true when the seminiferous tubules are destroyed, including destruction of the Sertoli cells in addition to the germinal cells. Therefore, it is believed that the Sertoli cells secrete a hormone that has a direct inhibitory effect mainly on the anterior pituitary gland (but perhaps slightly on the hypothalamus as well) to inhibit the secretion of FSH. A glycoprotein hormone having a molecular weight between 10,000 and 30,000 called *inhibin* has been isolated from cultured Sertoli cells and is probably responsible for most of the feedback control of FSH secretion and of spermatogenesis. This feedback cycle is the following:

1. Follicle-stimulating hormone stimulates the Sertoli cells that provide nutrition for the developing spermatozoa.

2. The Sertoli cells release inhibin that in turn feeds back negatively to the anterior pituitary gland to inhibit the production of FSH. Thus, this feedback cycle maintains a constant rate of spermatogenesis, without underproduction or overproduction, that is required for male reproductive function.

Puberty and Regulation of Its Onset

Initiation of the onset of puberty has long been a mystery. In the earliest history of humanity, the belief was simply that the testicles "ripened" at this time. With the discovery of the gonadotropins, ripening of the anterior pituitary gland was considered responsible. Now it is known from experiments in which both testicular and pituitary tissues have been transplanted from infant animals into adult animals that both the testes and the anterior pituitary of the infant are capable of performing adult functions if appropriately stimulated. Therefore, it is now certain that *during childhood the hypothalamus simply does not secrete LHRH.*

For reasons not understood, some maturation process in the brain causes the hypothalamus to begin secreting LHRH at the time of puberty. This secretion will not occur if the neuronal connections between the hypothalamus and other parts of the brain are not intact. Therefore, the present belief is that the maturation process probably occurs elsewhere in the brain instead of in the hypothalamus. One suggested locus is the amygdala.

REGULATION OF THE FEMALE MONTHLY RHYTHM—INTERPLAY BETWEEN THE OVARIAN AND HYPOTHALAMIC-PITUITARY HORMONES

Function of the Hypothalamus in the Regulation of Gonadotropin Secretion–Luteinizing Hormone Releasing Hormone (LHRH). As was pointed out earlier in the chapter, secretion of most of the anterior pituitary hormones is controlled by releasing hormones formed in the hypothalamus and transported to the anterior pituitary gland by way of the hypothalamic-hypophysial portal system. In the case of the gonadotropins, at least one releasing factor, *luteinizing hormone releasing hormone (LHRH)*, is important. This has been purified and has been found to be a decapeptide having the following formula:

GLU-HIS-TRP-SER-TYR-GLY-LEU-ARG-
PRO-GLY-NH₂

Though some research workers believe that another substance similar to this, called follice-stimulating hormone releasing hormone (FSHRH), is also formed in the hypothalamus, the purified LHRH has been found to cause release not only of luteinizing hormone but also of follicle-stimulating hormone. Therefore, since there is reason to believe that this decapeptide is in reality both LHRH and FSHRH combined in the same molecule, it is often called simply *gonadotropin-releasing hormone (GnRH)*.

Hypothalamic Centers for Stimulating Release of LHRH. Several different areas that profoundly influence the rate of secretion of the hypothalamic gonadotropin-releasing hormone LHRH have been found in the hypothalamus. In monkeys—and presumably in people—the midbasal region of the hypothalamus is the area most importantly involved. In lower animals, the area around the infundibulum causes a continuous tonic secretion of gonadotropin-releasing hormone, while two other areas modulate the rate of release. These areas are (1) a center in the preoptic area that causes cyclic variation in the secretory rate and (2) a center in the posterior hypothalamus that allows the psychic attitude of the animal to enhance or decrease the secretion of gonadotropin-releasing hormone.

Effect of Psychic Factors on the Female Sexual Cycle. It is well known that the young woman on first leaving home to go to college almost as often as not experiences disruption or irregularity of the female sexual cycle. Likewise, serious stresses of almost any type can interfere with the cycle. Finally, in many lower animals no ovulation occurs at all until after copulation; the sexual excitation attendant to the sexual act initiates a sequence of events that leads first to secretion in the hypothalamus of LHRH, then to secretion of the anterior pituitary gonadotropins, and finally to ovarian secretion of the female sex hormones and to ovulation. It is these effects that are believed to be mediated through the posterior hypothalamic center for modulating the output of LHRH.

Negative Feedback Effect of Estrogen, Progesterone, and Inhibin on Secretion of Follicle-Stimulating Hormone and Luteinizing Hormone. Estrogen in small amounts and progesterone in large amounts inhibit the production of FSH and LH. Both these

feedback effects seem to operate on the hypothalamus and the anterior pituitary gland as well.

In addition to the feedback effects of estrogen and progesterone, still another hormone also seems to be involved. This is *inhibin,* which is secreted along with the steroid sex hormones by the ovaries in the same way that the Sertoli cells secrete this same hormone in the male testes. This inhibin has the same effect in the female as in the male of inhibiting the secretion of FSH by the anterior pituitary gland, and LH also to a lesser extent. Therefore, it is believed that inhibin might be especially important in causing the decrease in secretion of FSH and LH toward the end of the female sexual month.

Positive Feedback Effect of Estrogen Before Ovulation—The Preovulatory Luteinizing Hormone Surge. For reasons not completely understood, the anterior pituitary gland secretes greatly increased amounts of LH for a period of about one day beginning 24 to 48 hours before ovulation. This effect is illustrated in Figure 29–5. The figure shows a much smaller preovulatory surge of FSH as well.

Experiments have shown that infusion of estrogen into a female for a period of two to three days during the first half of the ovarian cycle will cause rapidly accelerating growth of the ovarian follicles and also rapidly accelerating secretion of ovarian estrogens. During this period the secretion of both the follicle-stimulating hormone and luteinizing hormone by the anterior pituitary gland is at first suppressed slightly. Then abruptly the secretion of luteinizing hormone increases about eightfold and that of follicle-stimulating hormone about twofold. The cause of this abrupt increase in secretion of the gonadotropins is not known. It has been suggested that estrogen at this point in the cycle has a peculiar *positive feedback effect* to stimulate pituitary secretion of the gonadotropins; this is in sharp contrast to its normal negative feedback effect that occurs during

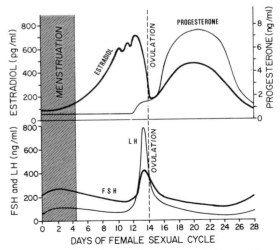

Figure 29–5. Approximate plasma concentrations of the gonadotropins and ovarian hormones during the normal female sexual cycle.

the remainder of the female monthly cycle. Since the granulosa cells of the follicles begin to secrete increasing quantities of progesterone a day or so prior to the preovulatory LH surge, it has also been suggested that this might be the factor that stimulates the excess LH secretion.

Without the normal preovulatory surge of luteinizing hormone, ovulation will not occur.

FEEDBACK OSCILLATION OF THE HYPOTHALAMIC-PITUITARY-OVARIAN SYSTEM

Now, after discussing much of the known information about the interrelationships of the different components of the female hormonal system, we can digress from the area of proven fact into the realm of speculation and attempt to explain the feedback oscillation that controls the rhythm of the female sexual cycle. It seems to operate in approximately the following sequence of three successive events:

1. The Postovulatory Secretion of the Ovarian Hormones and Depression of Gonadotropins. The easiest part of the cycle to explain is the events that occur during the postovulatory phase—between ovulation and the beginning of menstruation. During this time the corpus luteum in the ovary secretes large quantities of both progesterone and estrogen and probably the hormone inhibin as well. All these hormones together have a combined negative feedback effect on the anterior pituitary gland and the hypothalamus to cause strong suppression of both FSH and LH, decreasing these to their lowest levels at about three to four days before the onset of menstruation. These effects are illustrated in Figure 29–5.

2. The Follicular Growth Phase. Two to three days before menstruation the corpus luteum involutes, and the secretion of estrogen, progesterone, and inhibin decreases to a low ebb. This releases the hypothalamus and anterior pituitary from the feedback effect of these hormones, and a day or so later, at about the time that menstruation begins, FSH increases two- to threefold; then several days after menstruation begins, LH secretion increases about twofold as well. These hormones initiate new ovarian follicular growth and progressive increase in the secretion of estrogen, reaching a peak estrogen secretion at about 12.5 to 13 days after the onset of menstruation. During the first 11 to 12 days of this follicular growth the rates of secretion of the gonadotropins FSH and LH decrease; then this decrease reverses suddenly, followed by a rapid increase in secretion of both these hormones, leading to the preovulatory surge of LH and ovulation.

3. Preovulatory Surge of LH and FSH; Ovulation. At approximately 11.5 to 12 days after the onset of menstruation, the decline in secretion of FSH and LH comes to an abrupt halt. It is believed that the high level of estrogens at this time (or the beginning secretion of progesterone by the follicles) causes a positive feedback effect on the hypothalamus and anterior pituitary, as explained earlier, which leads to a terrific surge of secretion of LH and to a lesser extent of FSH. Whatever the cause of this preovulatory LH and FSH surge, the LH leads to both ovulation and subsequent conversion of the ovulated follicle into the *corpus luteum*, a highly secretory body that secretes large quantities of both estrogen and progesterone. Thus, the hormonal system begins a new round of the cycle until the next ovulation.

PUBERTY AND MENARCHE

Puberty means the onset of adult sexual life, and menarche means the onset of menstruation. The period of puberty is caused by a gradual increase in gonadotropic hormone secretion by the pituitary, beginning approximately in the eighth year of life, and usually culminating in the onset of menstruation between the ages of 11 and 16 years.

In the female, as in the male, the infantile pituitary gland and ovaries are capable of full function if appropriately stimulated. However, as is also true in the male and for reasons not yet understood, the hypothalamus does not secrete luteinizing hormone releasing hormone during childhood. Experiments have shown that the hypothalamus itself is perfectly capable of secreting this hormone, but there is lack of the appropriate signal from some other brain area to cause the secretion. Therefore, it is now believed that the onset of puberty is initiated by some maturation process occurring elsewhere in the brain besides the hypothalamus, perhaps somewhere in the limbic system.

Figure 29–6 illustrates (1) the increasing levels of estrogen secretion at puberty, (2) the cyclic variation during the monthly sexual cycles, (3) the further increase in estrogen secretion during the first few years of sexual life, (4) then progressive decrease in estrogen secretion toward the end of sexual life, and (5) finally almost no estrogen secretion beyond the menopause.

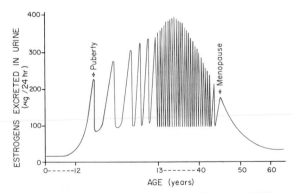

Figure 29–6. Estrogen secretion throughout sexual life.

THE MENOPAUSE

At the age of 45 to 50 years the sexual cycles usually become irregular, and ovulation fails to occur during many of the cycles. After a few months to a few years, the cycles cease altogether, as illustrated in Figure 29–6. This period during which the cycles cease and the female sex hormones diminish rapidly to almost none at all is called the *menopause.*

The cause of the menopause is "burning out" of the ovaries. Throughout a woman's sexual life about 450 of the primordial follicles grow into vesicular follicles and ovulate, while literally thousands of the ova degenerate. At the age of about 45 years only a few primordial follicles still remain to be stimulated by FSH and LH, and the production of estrogens by the ovary decreases as the number of primordial follicles approaches zero (also illustrated in Figure 29–6). When estrogen production falls below a critical value, the estrogens can no longer inhibit the production of FSH and LH; nor can they cause an ovulatory surge of LH and FSH to cause oscillatory cycles.

THE MALE SEXUAL ACT

NEURONAL STIMULUS FOR PERFORMANCE OF THE MALE SEXUAL ACT

The most important source of sensory impulses for initiating the male sexual act is the glans penis, for the glans contains a highly organized sensory end-organ system that transmits into the central nervous system a special modality of sensation called *sexual sensation.* The massaging action of intercourse on the glans stimulates the sensory end-organs, and the sexual sensations in turn pass through the pudendal nerve, thence through the sacral plexus into the sacral portion of the spinal cord, and finally up the cord to undefined areas of the cerebrum. Impulses may also enter the spinal cord from areas adjacent to the penis to aid in stimulating the sexual act. For instance, stimulation of the anal epithelium, the scrotum, and perineal structures in general can all send signals into the cord which add to the sexual sensation. Sexual sensations can even originate in internal structures, such as irritated areas of the urethra, the bladder, the prostate, the seminal vesicles, the testes, and the vas deferens. Indeed, one of the causes of "sexual drive" is probably overfilling of the sexual organs with secretions. Infection and inflammation of these sexual organs sometimes cause almost continual sexual desire, and "aphrodisiac" drugs, such as cantharides, increase the sexual desire by irritating the bladder and urethral mucosa.

The Psychic Element of Male Sexual Stimulation. Appropriate psychic stimuli can greatly enhance the ability of a person to perform the sexual act. Simply thinking sexual thoughts or even dreaming that the act of intercourse is being performed can cause the male sexual act to occur and to culminate in ejaculation. Indeed, *nocturnal emissions* during dreams occur in many males during some stages of sexual life, especially during the teens.

Integration of the Male Sexual Act in the Spinal Cord. Though psychic factors usually play an important part in the male sexual act and can actually initiate or inhibit it, the cerebrum is probably not absolutely necessary for its performance, because appropriate genital stimulation can cause ejaculation in some animals and occasionally in a human being after their spinal cords have been cut above the lumbar region. Therefore, the male sexual act results from inherent reflex mechanisms integrated in the sacral and lumbar spinal cord, and these mechanisms can be initiated by either psychic stimulation or actual sexual stimulation.

STAGES OF THE MALE SEXUAL ACT

Erection; Role of the Parasympathetic Nerves. Erection is the first effect of male sexual stimulation, and the degree of erection is proportional to the degree of stimulation, whether this be psychic or physical.

Erection is caused by parasympathetic impulses that pass from the sacral portion of the spinal cord through the nervi erigentes to the penis. These parasympathetic impulses dilate the arteries of the penis, thus allowing arterial blood to build up under high pressure in the *erectile tissue* of the penis, illustrated in Figure 29–7. This erectile tissue is nothing more than large, cavernous, venous sinusoids, which are normally relatively empty but which become dilated tremendously when arterial blood flows into them under pressure, since the venous outflow is partially occluded. Also, the erectile bodies, especially the two corpora cavernosa, are surrounded by strong fibrous coats; therefore, high pressure within the sinusoids causes ballooning of the erectile tissue to such an extent that the penis becomes hard and elongated.

Lubrication, a Parasympathetic Function. During sexual stimulation, the parasympathetic impulses, in addition to promoting erection, cause the urethral glands and the bulbourethral glands to secrete mucus. This mucus flows through the urethra during intercourse to aid in the lubrication of coitus. However, most of the lubrication of coitus is provided by the female sexual organs rather than by the

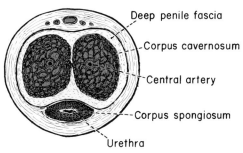

Figure 29–7. Erectile tissue of the penis.

male. Without satisfactory lubrication, the male sexual act is rarely successful because unlubricated intercourse causes grating, painful sensations which inhibit rather than excite sexual sensations.

Emission and Ejaculation; Function of the Sympathetic Nerves. Emission and ejaculation are the culmination of the male sexual act. When the sexual stimulus becomes extremely intense, the reflex centers of the spinal cord begin to emit *sympathetic impulses* that leave the cord at L-1 and L-2 and pass to the genital organs through the hypogastric plexus to initiate emission, the forerunner of ejaculation.

Emission is believed to begin with contraction of the vas deferens and the ampulla, causing the expulsion of sperm into the internal urethra. Then contractions of the muscular coat of the prostate gland followed lastly by contraction of the seminal vesicles expel prostatic fluid and seminal fluid, forcing the sperm forward. All these fluids mix in the internal urethra with the mucus already secreted by the bulbo-urethral glands to form the semen. The process to this point is *emission*.

The filling of the internal urethra then elicits signals that are transmitted through the pudendal nerves to the sacral regions of the cord. In turn, signals from the sacral cord further excite the rhythmic contraction of the internal genital organs and also cause contraction of the ischiocavernosus and bulbocavernosus muscles that compress the bases of the penile erectile tissue. These effects together cause rhythmic, wavelike increases in pressure in the genital ducts and urethra, which ''ejaculate'' the semen from the urethra to the exterior. This process is called *ejaculation*. At the same time, rhythmic contractions of the pelvic muscles and even of some of the muscles of the body trunk cause thrusting movements of the pelvis and penis, which also help propel the semen into the deepest recesses of the vagina and perhaps even through the cervix into the uterus.

This entire period of emission and ejaculation is called the *male orgasm*. At its termination, the male sexual excitement disappears almost entirely within one to two minutes, and erection ceases.

THE FEMALE SEXUAL ACT

Stimulation of the Female Sexual Act. As is true in the male sexual act, successful performance of the female sexual act depends on both psychic stimulation and local sexual stimulation.

As is also true in the male, the thinking of erotic thoughts can lead to female sexual desire, and this aids greatly in the performance of the female sexual act. Such desire is probably based as much on one's background training as on physiological drive, though sexual desire does increase in proportion to the level of secretion of the sex hormones. Desire also changes during the sexual month, reaching a peak near the time of ovulation, probably because

of the high levels of estrogen secretion during the preovulatory period.

Local sexual stimulation in women occurs in more or less the same manner as in men, for massage, irritation, or other types of stimulation of the perineal region, sexual organs, and urinary tract create sexual sensations. The *clitoris* is especially sensitive for initiating sexual sensations. As in the male, the sexual sensory signals are mediated to the sacral segments of the spinal cord through the pudendal nerve and sacral plexus. Once these signals have entered the spinal cord, they are transmitted thence to the cerebrum. Also, local reflexes integrated in the sacral and lumbar spinal cord are at least partly responsible for female sexual reactions.

Female Erection and Lubrication. Located around the introitus and extending into the clitoris is erectile tissue almost identical with the erectile tissue of the penis. This erectile tissue, like that of the penis, is controlled by the parasympathetic nerves that pass through the nervi erigentes from the sacral plexus to the external genitalia. In the early phases of sexual stimulation, parasympathetic signals dilate the arteries of the erectile tissues, and this allows rapid accumulation of blood in the erectile tissue so that the introitus tightens around the penis; this aids the male greatly in his attainment of sufficient sexual stimulation for ejaculation to occur.

Parasympathetic signals also pass to the bilateral Bartholin's glands located beneath the labia minora to cause secretion of mucus immediately inside the introitus. This mucus is responsible for much of the lubrication during sexual intercourse, though much is also provided by mucus secreted by the vaginal epithelium as well and a small amount from the male urethral glands. The lubrication in turn is necessary for establishing during intercourse a satisfactory massaging sensation rather than an irritative sensation, which may be provoked by a dry vagina. A massaging sensation constitutes the optimal type of sensation for evoking the appropriate reflexes that culminate in both the male and female climaxes.

The Female Orgasm. When local sexual stimulation reaches maximum intensity, and especially when the local sensations are supported by appropriate psychic conditioning signals from the cerebrum, reflexes are initiated that cause the female orgasm, also called the *female climax*. The female orgasm is analogous to emission and ejaculation in the male, and it perhaps helps promote fertilization of the ovum. Indeed, the human female is known to be somewhat more fertile when inseminated by normal sexual intercourse rather than by artificial methods, thus indicating an important function of the female orgasm. Possible effects that could result in this are:

First, during the orgasm the perineal muscles of the female contract rhythmically, which results from spinal cord reflexes similar to those that cause ejaculation in the male. It is possible, also, that these same reflexes increase uterine and fallopian tube motility during the orgasm, thus helping transport the sperm toward the ovum, but the information on this subject is scanty. Also, the orgasm seems to cause dilation of the cervical canal for up to half an hour, thus allowing easy transport of the sperm.

Second, in many lower animals, copulation causes the posterior pituitary gland to secrete oxytocin; this effect is probably mediated through the amygdaloid nuclei and then through the hypothalamus to the pituitary. The oxytocin in turn causes increased rhythmical contractions of the uterus, which has been postulated to cause rapid transport of the sperm. Sperm have been shown to traverse the entire length of the fallopian tube in the cow in approximately five minutes, a rate at least ten times as fast as that which the swimming motions of the sperm themselves could achieve. Whether or not this occurs in the human female is unknown.

In addition to the possible effects of the orgasm on fertilization, the intense sexual sensations that develop during the orgasm also pass to the cerebrum and cause intense muscle tension throughout the body. But after culmination of the sexual act, this gives way during the succeeding minutes to a sense of satisfaction characterized by relaxed peacefulness, an effect called *resolution*.

REFERENCES

PITUITARY HORMONES

Brownstein, M. J.: Biosynthesis of vasopressin and oxytocin. *Annu. Rev. Physiol.*, 45:129, 1983.

Conn, P. M., *et al.*: Gonadotropin-releasing hormone: Molecular and cell biology, physiology, and clinical applications. *Fed. Proc.*, 43:2351, 1984.

Doris, P. A.: Vasopressin and central integrative processes. *Neuroendocrinology*, 38:75, 1984.

Gann, D. S., *et al.*: Neural interaction in control of adrenocorticotropin. *Fed. Proc.*, 44:161, 1985.

Keller-Wood, M. E., and Dallman, M. F.: Corticosteroid inhibition of ACTH secretion. *Endocr. Rev.*, 5:1, 1984.

Nissley, S. P., and Rechler, M. M.: Somatomedin/insulin-like growth factor tissue receptors. *Clin. Endocrinol. Metab.*, 13:43, 1984.

Rennels, E. G., and Herbert, D. C.: Functional correlates of anterior pituitary cytology. *In* Greep, R. O. (ed.): International Review of Physiology: Reproductive Physiology III. Vol. 22. Baltimore, University Park Press, 1980, p. 1.

Wass, J. A. H., and Besser, G. M.: The medical management of hormone-secreting tumors of the pituitary. *Annu. Rev. Med.*, 34:283, 1983.

MALE FUNCTIONS

Conn, P. M., *et al.*: Gonadotropin-releasing hormone: Molecular and cell biology, physiology, and clinical applications. *Fed. Proc.*, 43:2351, 1984.

Ewing, L. L., *et al.*: Regulation of testicular function: A spatial and temporal view. *In* Greep, R. O. (ed.): International Review of Physiology: Reproductive Physiology III. Vol. 22. Baltimore, University Park Press, 1980, p. 41.

Habenicht, U. F.: Hormonal Regulation of Testicular Descent. New York, Springer-Verlag, 1983.

Kolodny, R. C., *et al.*: Textbook of Sexual Medicine. Boston, Little, Brown, 1979.

McCann, S. M.: Physiology and pharmacology of LHRH and somatostatin. *Annu. Rev. Pharmacol. Toxicol.*, 22:491, 1982.

Negro, V. A. (ed.): Male Reproduction and Fertility. New York, Raven Press, 1983.

Styne, D. M., and Grumbach, M. M.: Puberty in the male and female: Its physiology and disorders. *In* Yen, S. S. C., and Jaffe, R. B. (eds.): Reproductive Endocrinology, Philadelphia, W. B. Saunders Co., 1978, p. 189.

FEMALE FUNCTIONS

Conn, P. M., *et al.*: Gonadotropin-releasing hormone: Molecular and cell biology, physiology, and clinical applications. *Fed. Proc.*, 43:2351, 1984.

Greenblatt, R. B. (ed.): Induction of Ovulation. Philadelphia, Lea & Febiger, 1979.

Lein, A.: The Cycling Female: Her Menstrual Rhythm. San Francisco, W. H. Freeman, 1979.

Leung, P. C. K., and Armstrong, D. T.: Interactions of steroids and gonadotropins in the control of steroidogenesis in the ovarian follicle. *Annu. Rev. Physiol.*, 42:71, 1980.

McEwen, B. S., and Parsons, B.: Gonadal steroid action on the brain: Neurochemistry and neuropharmacology. *Annu. Rev. Pharmacol. Toxicol.*, 22:555, 1982.

Ochiai, K. (ed.): Endocrine Correlates of Reproduction. New York, Springer-Verlag, 1984.

Pohl, C. R., and Knobil, E.: The role of the central nervous system in the control of ovarian function in higher primates. *Annu. Rev. Physiol.*, 44:583, 1982.

Reiter, E. O., and Grumbach, M. M.: Neuroendocrine control mechanisms and the onset of puberty. *Annu. Rev. Physiol.*, 44:595, 1982.

Index

Page numbers in *italic* type indicate illustrations; page numbers followed by *t* refer to tables.

0246502